Oxford Specialist Handbook of Cardiothoracic Surgery

Second edition

Joanna Chikwe

Associate Professor, Department of Cardiothoracic Surgery, Mount Sinai Medical Center, New York, United States

David Tom Cooke

Assistant Professor, Division of Cardiothoracic Surgery, University of California, Davis Medical Center, Sacramento, United States

Aaron Weiss

Resident, Department of Cardiothoracic Surgery, Mount Sinai Medical Center, New York, United States

T0355164

OXFORD
UNIVERSITY PRESS

OXFORD
UNIVERSITY PRESS

Great Clarendon Street, Oxford, OX2 6DP,
United Kingdom

Oxford University Press is a department of the University of Oxford.
It furthers the University's objective of excellence in research, scholarship,
and education by publishing worldwide. Oxford is a registered trade mark of
Oxford University Press in the UK and in certain other countries

First Edition published in 2006
Second Edition published in 2013

British Library Cataloguing in Publication Data
Data available

Library of Congress Cataloging in Publication Data
Library of Congress Control Number: 2012945092

ISBN 978-0-19-964283-0

Printed in Great Britain by
Ashford Colour Press Ltd, Gosport, Hampshire

OXFORD MEDICAL PUBLICATIONS

Cardiothoracic
Surgery

Oxford Specialist Handbooks

General Oxford Specialist Handbooks
A Resuscitation Room Guide
Addiction Medicine
Day Case Surgery
Perioperative Medicine, 2e
Postoperative Complications, 2e
Renal Transplantation

Oxford Specialist Handbooks in Anaesthesia
Anaesthesia for Medical and Surgical Emergencies
Cardiac Anaesthesia
Neuroanaethesia
Obstetric Anaesthesia
Ophthalmic Anaesthesia
Paediatric Anaesthesia
Regional Anaesthesia, Stimulation and Ultrasound Techniques
Thoracic Anaesthesia

Oxford Specialist Handbooks in Cardiology
Adult Congenital Heart Disease
Cardiac Catheterization and Coronary Intervention
Cardiac Electrophysiology and Catheter Ablation
Cardiovascular Computed Tomography
Cardiovascular Magnetic Resonance
Echocardiography, 2e
Fetal Cardiology
Heart Failure
Hypertension
Inherited Cardiac Disease
Nuclear Cardiology
Pacemakers and ICDs
Pulmonary Hypertension
Valvular Heart Disease

Oxford Specialist Handbooks in Critical Care
Advanced Respiratory Critical Care
Oxford Specialist Handbooks in End of Life Care
End of Life Care in Cardiology
End of Life Care in Dementia
End of Life Care in Nephrology
End of Life Care in Respiratory Disease
End of Life in the Intensive Care Unit

Oxford Specialist Handbooks in Neurology
Epilepsy
Parkinson's Disease and Other Movement Disorders
Stroke Medicine

Oxford Specialist Handbooks in Paediatrics
Paediatric Dermatology
Paediatric Endocrinology and Diabetes
Paediatric Gastroenterology, Hepatology, and Nutrition
Paediatric Haematology and Oncology
Paediatric Intensive Care
Paediatric Nephrology, 2e
Paediatric Neurology, 2e
Paediatric Radiology
Paediatric Respiratory Medicine
Paediatric Rheumatology

Oxford Specialist Handbooks in Pain Medicine
Spinal Interventions in Pain Management

Oxford Specialist Handbooks in Psychiatry
Child and Adolescent Psychiatry
Forensic Psychiatry
Old Age Psychiatry

Oxford Specialist Handbooks in Radiology
Interventional Radiology
Musculoskeletal Imaging
Pulmonary Imaging
Thoracic Imaging

Oxford Specialist Handbooks in Surgery
Cardiothoracic Surgery
Colorectal Surgery
Hand Surgery
Hepatopancreatobiliary Surgery
Neurosurgery
Operative Surgery, 2e
Oral Maxillofacial Surgery
Otolaryngology and Head and Neck Surgery
Paediatric Surgery
Plastic and Reconstructive Surgery
Surgical Oncology
Urological Surgery
Vascular Surgery

Preface to second edition

I wrote the first edition of this book when I was a cardiothoracic surgery resident because I wanted facts, tips, and advice covering the whole spectrum of this brilliant specialty instantly available in my pocket—a compact insurance policy against errors and ignorance in a spill-proof cover. Six years on, the cover has changed, but the aim stays the same—and largely thanks to two simply great new co-authors who totally understood the whole idea. This second edition has been expanded, updated and revised for an international audience.

It is usually much easier to understand stuff if you can see it or simplify it—so the book is full of drawings, lists, and tables. It is nice to have answers for those 'Why do we do that?' moments—this book will give you those, as well as a good framework for further reading and exam revision. But mainly, this handbook is for making sure you have the facts and practical advice you need, in front of you, to provide the best cardiothoracic care you can, in the ICU, at the bedside, and in the operating room.

Now, go save some more lives!

JC
2012

Preface to first edition

This handbook is aimed at doctors embarking on their first job in cardio-thoracic surgery. We hope it will also be useful for junior doctors and allied health professionals working in cardiac anesthesia, cardiothoracic intensive care units, coronary care units, and cardiothoracic theatres.

Cardiothoracic surgery is an exciting, fast-moving, and sometimes daunting speciality. The primary concern of junior doctors is correctly diagnosing and managing the life-threatening problems that can rapidly develop in the postoperative patient. From their first day on a cardiothoracic unit, junior surgeons are also expected to play a part in preoperative decision-making; and they need to rapidly acquire a firm grasp of the principles of operative surgery. This handbook brings together these aspects of this challenging speciality, covering adult and pediatric cardiac and thoracic surgery. It is not intended to be a comprehensive text, or a 'do-it-yourself' guide to cardiothoracics: it is designed to accompany practical training under direct supervision, enabling junior doctors and healthcare professionals to gain the most from their time in the speciality.

The evidence base behind daily practice is outlined in sections that include the basic sciences applied to cardiothoracic surgery, key references from the literature, and a bibliography of text and web-based resources.

JC
EB
BG
2006

Acknowledgements

I would like to record my heartfelt thanks to our many contributors:

Miss N Kahn, Consultant Congenital Surgeon, Birmingham Children's Hospital, completely revised Chapter 12.

Dr A Pawale, Integrated Cardiothoracic Surgery Resident, Mount Sinai Medical Center revised Chapter 11.

Particularly extensive and helpful changes to the first edition were made by Dr P Jones, Consultant Cardiac Anaesthetist and Intensivist, St Bartholomew's Hospital, London, most of which have been retained in chapters 3 and 5.

Prof J Pepper, Professor of Cardiothoracic Surgery, Royal Brompton Hospital, London; Dr K Mandal, Assistant Professor, Cardiac Surgery, Johns Hopkins University School of Medicine, Baltimore; Mr B Sethia, Consultant Cardiac Surgeon, Royal Brompton Hospital, London; and Mr A Cherian, Consultant Cardiothoracic Surgeon, London reviewed initial drafts of the first edition, and their influence carries over into this one.

I am also very grateful to our junior advisers who road-tested early drafts: Dr A Weiss, Dr C Critchley, Dr M Ridgeway, and Dr A Smith.

I thank Mr M Poullis, Consultant Cardiothoracic Surgeon, the Cardiothoracic Centre, Liverpool for allowing us to use images from his library in Chapter 5; the Resuscitation Council UK for permission to reproduce the ALS algorithm from their 2000 guidelines; and the Society of Cardiothoracic Surgeons of Great Britain and Ireland for their permission to reprint the Euroscore table on the inside cover. The table on p361 was adapted from *Kirklin/Barratt-Boyes Cardiac Surgery*, 3rd edition, Volume 1, Nicholas T Kouchoukos, Eugene H Blackstone, Donald B Doty, Frank L Hanley, Robert B Karp, Table 7.7 p391, copyright 2003, with permission from Elsevier.

Illustrations are drawn by me, except where otherwise acknowledged.

Finally I would like to thank the staff at OUP for their help and support, particularly Helen Liepman, Imogen Lowe, Susan Crowhurst, Tessa Eaton, Kate Smith, and Fiona Chippendale.

JC

Acknowledgements

I would like to record my heartfelt thanks to our many contributors.

Contents

Symbols and abbreviations

📖	cross-reference
+ve	positive
−ve	negative
±	with/without
↑	increased
↓	decreased
°	degrees
~	approximately
3D	three-dimensional
2VD	two-vessel disease
3VD	three-vessel disease
5-FU	5-fluorouracil
AA	aortic annulus
AAI	demand atrial pacing
ABG	arterial blood gas
ACAB	atraumatic coronary artery bypass
ACC	American College of Cardiologists
ACE	angiotensin-converting enzyme
AChR	acetyl cholinesterase receptor
ACS	acute coronary syndrome
ADH	antidiuretic hormone
ADP	adenosine diphosphate
AEG	atrial electrogram
AHA	American Heart Association
AI	aortic insufficiency
AJCC	American Joint Committee on Cancer
ALCAPA	anomalous origin of the left coronary artery from the pulmonary artery
AMI	acute myocardial infarction
AP	anteroposterior
APC	antigen presenting cell
APTT	activated partial thromboplastin time
AR	aortic regurgitation
ARDS	acute respiratory distress syndrome
AS	aortic stenosis
ASD	atrial septal defect
ATP	adenosine triphosphate

AV	atrioventricular
AVR	aortic valve replacement
BAL	bronchoalveolar lavage
BARI	balloon angioplasty revascularization investigation
bid	twice a day (*bis in die*)
BIMA	bilateral internal mammary artery
BiPAP	biphasic positive pressure ventilation
BiVAD	biventricular assist device
BMS	bare metal stent
BMV	balloon mitral valvuloplasty
BP	blood pressure
BR	brachioradialis
BSA	bovine serum albumin
BUN	blood urea nitrogen
Ca^{2+}	calcium
CABG	coronary artery bypass graft
CAD	coronary artery disease
CAVH	continuous arteriovenous hemofiltration
CBC	complete blood count
CCF	congestive cardiac failure
CCS	Canadian Cardiovascular Society
ccTGA	congenitally corrected transposition of the great arteries
CDC	Centers for Disease Control and Prevention
CHB	complete heart block
CLL	chronic lymphocytic leukemia
cm	centimeter/s
CMR	cardiac magnetic resonance
CMV	cytomegalovirus *or* controlled mechanical ventilation
CN	cyanide
CNS	central nervous system
CO	cardiac output
CoAo	coarctation of the aorta
COPD	chronic obstructive pulmonary disease
CPAP	continuous positive airway pressure
CPB	cardiopulmonary bypass
CPR	cardiopulmonary resuscitation
CRP	C-reactive protein
CSF	cerebrospinal fluid
CT	computed tomography
CTA	computed tomography angiogram

CVA	cerebrovascular accident
CVP	continuous venous pressure
CVVH	continuous venovenous hemofiltration
Cx	circumflex artery
CXR	chest X-ray
D	diagonal
DA	dopamine
DCM	dilated cardiomyopathy
DES	drug-eluting stent
DHCA	deep hypothermic circulatory arrest
DIC	disseminated intravascular coagulation
DLCO	diffusing capacity of the lung for carbon monoxide
DMSO	dimethyl sulfoxide solution
DO_2	oxygen delivery
DOO	asynchronous dual chamber pacing
DORV	double outlet right ventricle
DSWI	deep sternal wound infection
DVI	dual chamber pacing–asynchronous atrial, ventricular demand
DVT	deep vein thrombosis
EBUS	endobronchial ultrasound
EBV	Epstein–Barr virus
ECF	extracellular fluid
EEG	electroencephalogram
ECMO	extracorporeal membrane oxygenation
EDV	end-diastolic volume
EGD	esophagogastroduodenoscopy
EKG	electrocardiogram
EMG	electromyogram
ENT	ear, nose, and throat
EPO	erythropoietin
ERO	effective regurgitant orifice
ET	endotracheal
EtOH	ethanol (alcohol)
EUS	endoscopic ultrasound
FBC	full blood count
FCU	flexor carpi ulnaris
Fe	iron
FEV_1	forced expiratory volume in 1 second
FFP	fresh frozen plasma
FFR	fractional flow reserve

FiO$_2$	fraction of inspired oxygen
FNR	fine needle aspiration
FVC	forced vital capacity
g	gram/s
GEJ	gastroesophageal junction
GERD	gastroesophageal reflux disease
GFR	glomerular filtration rate
GI	gastrointestinal
HACEK	*Hemophilus*, *Actinobacillus*, *Cardiobacterium*, *Eikenella*, *Kingella*
HAR	hyperacute rejection
HCM	hypertrophic cardiomyopathy
HCV	hepatitis C virus
HGD	high-grade dysplasia
HIT	heparin-induced thrombocytopenia
HITT	heparin-induced thrombocytopenia and thrombosis
HLA	human leukocyte antigen
HLHS	hypoplastic left heart syndrome
HOCM	hypertrophic obstructive cardiomyopathy
HPOA	hypertrophic pulmonary osteoarthropathy
h	hour
HR	heart rate
HTLV	human T-lymphotrophic virus
IABP	intra-aortic balloon pump
ICD	implantable cardioverter-defibrillator *or* International Classification of Diseases
ICU	intensive care unit
IEOA	indexed effective opening area
im	intramuscular
IMA	internal mammary artery
INPV	intermittent negative pressure ventilation
INR	international normalized ratio
Int	intermediate
IPPV	intermittent positive pressure ventilation
ITA	internal thoracic artery
ITU	intensive therapy unit
iv	intravenous
IVC	inferior vena cava
IVUS	intravascular ultrasound
JVP	jugular venous pressure
K	potassium

kg	kilogram/s
L	liter/s
LA	left atrium/atrial
LAD	left anterior descending coronary artery
LAM	left anterior mediastinotomy
LAO	left anterior oblique
LAP	left atrial pressure
LCA	left coronary artery
LFT	liver function test
LGD	low-grade dysplasia
LIMA	left internal mammary artery
LITA	left internal throacic artery
LMS	left main stem
LMWH	low molecular weight heparin
LN	lymph node
LPA	left pulmonary artery
LSV	long saphenous vein
LSVC	left superior vena cava
LUL	left upper lobe
LV	left ventricle
LVAD	left ventricular assist device
LVB	lateral ventricular branch
LVEDP	left ventricle end-diastolic pressure
LVEDV	left ventricle end-diastolic volume
LVOT	left ventricle outflow tract
LVSWI	left ventricular stroke work index
MAC	mitral annular calcification
MAO	monoamine oxidase
MAP	mean arterial pressure
MAPCA	major aortopulmonary collateral artery
MCV	mean corpuscular volume
MDT	multidisciplinary team
MEP	motor evoked potential
mg	milligram/s
MG	myasthenia gravis
MI	myocardial infarction
MIDCAB	minimally invasive direct coronary artery bypass
min	minute/s
mL	milliliter/s
mLAP	mean left atrial pressure
MMF	mycophenolate mofetil

mmol	millimole/s
MMV	mandatory minute ventilation
mPAP	mean pulmonary artery pressure
MR	mitral regurgitation
MRA	magnetic resonance angiography
MRI	magnetic resonance imaging
MRSA	meticillin-resistant *Staphylococcus aureus*
ms	millisecond/s
MS	mitral stenosis
MVO$_2$	mixed venous oxygen saturation
MVR	mitral valve replacement
MVV	maximal voluntary ventilation
Na	sodium
NBM	nil by mouth
NCC	non-coronary cusp
NSCLC	non-small-cell lung cancer
NG	nasogastric
NIBP	non-invasive blood pressure
NIPPV	non-invasive intermittent positive pressure ventilation
NO	nitric oxide
nocte	at night
NPO	withold food and drink by mouth (nil per os)
NSAID	non-steroidal anti-inflammatory drug
NSTEMI	non-ST segment elevation myocardial infarction
NTG	nitroglycerine
NYHA	New York Heart Association
OCP	oral contraceptive pill
od	once a day (*omne in die*)
ODA	operating department assistant
OM	obtuse marginal
OPCAB	off-pump coronary artery bypass
OR	operating room *or* odds ratio
pa	per annum
PA	pulmonary artery *or* posteroanterior *or* physician assistant
PAH	pulmonary arterial hypertension
PAN	polyarteritis nodosa
PAP	pulmonary artery pressure
PAPVC	partial anomalous pulmonary venous connection
PAPVD	partial anomalous pulmonary venous drainage
PAWP	pulmonary artery wedge pressure

PCI	percutaneous coronary intervention
PCR	polymerase chain reaction
PDA	posterior descending artery or patent ductus arteriosus
PDGF	platelet-derived growth factor
PE	pulmonary embolism
PEA	pulseless electrical activity
PEEP	positive end-expiratory pressure
PEG	percutaneous endoscopic gastrostomy
PET	positron emission tomography
PFO	patent foramen ovale
PGE_1	prostaglandin E_1
PICU	pediatric intensive care unit
Plts	platelets
po	by mouth (*per os*)
POBA	plain old balloon angioplasty
PPI	proton pump inhibitor
PPM	permanent pacemaker or patient–prosthesis mismatch
ppo	predicted postoperative
prn	*pro re nata* (as required)
PS	pulmonary stenosis or pressure support
PSV	pressure support ventilation
PT	prothrombin time
PTCA	percutaneous transluminal coronary angioplasty
PTE	pulmonary thromboembolism
PVC	polyvinyl chloride
PVR	peripheral vascular resistance
PVRI	pulmonary vascular resistance index
qid	four times a day (*quater in die*)
RA	right atrium/atrial
RAAS	renin–angiotensin–aldosterone system
RAM	right anterior mediastinotomy
RAO	right anterior oblique
RAP	right atrial pressure
RBB	right bundle branch
RBC	red blood cell
RCA	right coronary artery
RCC	right coronary cusp
RCT	randomized controlled trial
RGEA	right gastroepiploic artery
RIMA	right internal mammary artery
RITA	right internal thoracic artery

RPA	right pulmonary artery
RSPV	right superior pulmonary vein
RSV	respiratory syncytial virus
RUL	right upper lobe
RV	right ventricle
RVAD	right ventricular assist device
RVEDP	right ventricular end-diastolic pressure
RVEDV	right ventricular end-diastolic volume
RVOT	right ventricular outflow tract
RVSWI	right ventricular stroke work index
s	second/s
SA	sinoatrial
SALT	speech and language therapy
SAM	systolic anterior motion
SaO_2	oxygen saturation of arterial blood
SBT	spontaneous breathing trials
sc	subcutaneous
SCBU	special care baby unit
SCLC	small-cell lung cancer
SFJ	sapheno-femoral junction
SIADH	syndrome of inappropriate antidiuretic hormone secretion
SIMV	synchronized intermittent mandatory ventilation
SIRS	systemic inflammatory response syndrome
s/l	sublingual
SLE	systemic lupus erythematosus
SNP	sodium nitroprusside
SPECT	single positron emission computed tomography
SSEP	somatosensory evoked potential
SSV	short saphenous vein
STEMI	ST segment elevation myocardial infarction
STJ	sinotubular junction
SV	single ventricle
SVC	superior vena cava
SVG	saphenous vein graft
SvO_2	mixed venous oxygen saturation
SVR	systemic vascular resistance
SVRI	systemic vascular resistance index
SWI	superficial wound infection
TA	truncus arteriosus
TAPVC	total anomalous pulmonary venous connection
TAPVD	total anomalous pulmonary venous drainage

TAVI	transcatheter aortic valve implantation
TBNA	transbronchial needle aspiration
TEE	transesophageal echocardiography
TEF	tracheoesophageal fistula
TEG	thrombelastography
TGA	transposition of the great arteries
THE	transhiatal esophagectomy
TIA	transient ischemic attack
tid	three times a day (*ter in die*)
TIF	tracheoinnominate fistula
TIMI	thrombolysis in myocardial infarction
TIVA	total intravenous anesthesia
TLC	total lung capacity
ToF	tetralogy of Fallot
TOS	thoracic outlet syndrome
TRAM	transverse rectus abdominis myocutaneous
TR	tricuspid regurgitation
TS	tricuspid stenosis
TTE	transthoracic echocardiography
TTE	transthoracic esophagectomy
U&E	urea and electrolytes
U/S	ultrasound
URTI	upper respiratory tract infection
U	unit/s
VAD	ventricular assist device
VATS	video-assisted thoracic surgery
VAVD	vacuum-assisted venous drainage
VC	vital capacity
VF	ventricular fibrillation
Vit	vitamin
VOO	asynchronous ventricular pacing
VQ	ventilation-perfusion
VSD	ventricular septal defect
VT	ventricular tachycardia
VVI	demand ventricular pacing
WCC	white cell count
WL	window level
WPW	Wolff–Parkinson–White (syndrome)
WW	window width
XM	cross match

Preoperative assessment

Cardiovascular history

There are three main aims of obtaining a cardiovascular history:
- Establish the indications for surgery.
- Identify issues that need management outside standard protocols.
- Define preoperative estimate of risk (mortality, stroke, etc.).

Angina

Angina is frequently not the classic 'central, crushing, chest pain radiating to the jaw and down the left arm'. It may present as heaviness, indigestion, isolated arm, neck or jaw discomfort, nausea, or fatigue. Ask about precipitants such as exertion, stress, emotion, and cold air, as well as relieving factors such as rest and sublingual nitroglycerine (NTG). How many times a day is NTG spray used? Angina is graded (see Box 1.1). *Class III and IV (heart failure) symptoms* are associated with increased risk.

Breathlessness

Ask about exertional dyspnea and classify it (see Box 1.1). *Heart failure is defined as class III or IV symptoms*. Ask about other precipitants: paroxysmal nocturnal dyspnea, orthopnea, palpitations, chest infections, chronic obstructive pulmonary disease (COPD), pulmonary embolism (PE), medication such as β-blockers. Ask about associated symptoms such as peripheral edema, palpitations, wheeze, and sputum. Ask about relieving factors such as NTG, rest, sitting up.

Previous myocardial infarction

Document the number, dates, and anatomy of any previous myocardial infarctions (MIs). Check chart and EKG (Q waves). Risk of surgery is higher after recent ST segment elevation MI (STEMI) than non-ST segment elevation MI (STEMI), and highest early after MI, falling after 1 week (📖 p297).

Previous chest surgery

Ask, check chart, and look carefully at *whole chest and back* for scars. Previous cardiac surgery is associated with incremental operative mortality and requires several changes to standard operative approach (📖 p342). Most patients should undergo CT (computed tomography) chest to evaluate relationship of aorta and right ventricle (RV) to sternum, and location of patient bypass grafts (requires iv contrast). Obtain operative report.

Box 1.1 Functional classifications

Canadian Cardiovascular Society (CCS) applies to angina only
- Class I: no angina with ordinary activity.
- Class II: slight limitation of ordinary activity.
- Class III: marked limitation of ordinary activity.
- Class IV: angina on minimal exertion or at rest.

New York Heart Association (NYHA) dyspnea and/or angina
- Class I: no limitation during ordinary activity (asymptomatic).
- Class II: slight limitation during ordinary activity.
- Class III: marked limitation of ordinary activity.
- Class IV: no physical activity without symptoms.

Previous percutaneous interventions

Note left ventricle (LV) function and coronary anatomy from the angiography report. Document the number, dates, type, and result of previous percutaneous interventions (angioplasty or stenting). Emergency surgery after failed percutaneous coronary intervention (PCI) is high risk. Recent PCI usually mandates at least 1 month of clopidogrel (📖 p18), and can impact conduct of coronary bypass surgery (📖 p651).

Syncope and dizziness

'Black-outs' may be a result of epilepsy, transient ischemic attacks (TIAs), hypoglycemia, vasovagal (standing, emotion, coughing, micturition) syndromes. True *cardiac syncope* from aortic stenosis (AS) is usually exertional. Syncope when the patient is sitting or lying suggests arrhythmias. Dizziness may be associated with syncope (presyncopal episodes), but is fairly non-specific. Common causes are antianginals, antihypertensives, and diuretics causing postural hypotension. Dizziness may reflect low cardiac output states (failure, arrhythmias, ischemia) or cerebrovascular disease. Diabetic autonomic neuropathy is probably an under-recognized cause.

Palpitations and atrial fibrillation

To the patient palpitations may be skipped beats, tachycardia, irregular rhythm, or awareness of their heart particularly at night. Ask about onset: rapid onset and offset suggests paroxysmal arrhythmias, gradual onset and offset suggests sinus tachycardia. Preoperative atrial fibrillation (AF) may require ablation and/ or left atrial (LA) appendage ligation, and warfarin (📖 pp262, 484).

Peripheral edema

This may be associated with changes in diuretic therapy, weight gain, and exacerbations of dyspnea, and helps quantify the heart failure.

Extracardiac arteriopathy

Ask specifically about TIAs, strokes, claudication, and vascular interventions. A history of TIAs warrants a carotid duplex to exclude carotid disease which may be an indication for carotid intervention (📖 p 279). Extracardiac arteriopathy is important for risk scoring (📖 p359), affects the risk of stroke and limb ischemia quoted when consenting the patient, and influences the choice of conduit (📖 p302) and cannulation site (📖 p120).

Coronary risk factors

Reversible risk factors that should be addressed in hospital include: smoking, hypercholesterolemia, obesity, hypertension, and diabetes. Irreversible risk factors include male sex, age, and family history. Be precise: 'non-smoker' is not the same as 'smoked 60 a day, gave up 2 weeks ago.'

Valve patients

Note the type and degree of valve disease, and LV function from the echo. Ask about rheumatic disease and endocarditis. Check that patients have been recently cleared by a dentist (edentulous patients to do not need to be seen by a dentist), check that they have no active sources of infection, they have had an angiogram if they are males >45 years, postmenopausal females, have angina type symptoms or multiple coronary risk factors, and that the *type of valve replacement* (📖 p370) has been discussed.

Systems enquiry

The main aims of the systems enquiry are:
- Identifying problems that alter standard perioperative management.
- Identifying contraindications to elective surgery.
- Identifying problems that could potentially delay discharge.

Previous medical history

Ask about any other medical problems, and repeat the question by asking if the patient has ever been in hospital with any problems other than their heart, and whether they have had any operations, *ever*. Be persistent as patients often forget important chronic illnesses and operations.
- Preoperative management of *diabetic patients* is described on 📖 p31.
- Previous *chest radiotherapy* mandates CT scan: aorta may be calcified.
- *Malignant disease* should be carefully evaluated; in most cases metastatic spread is a relative contraindication to cardiac surgery.
- *Thyroid disease* may dictate the choice of antiarrhythmic (📖 p205).
- Patients with *hip replacements* should be transferred with a pillow between their legs: adducting the hip may result in dislocation.
- Patients with *blood dyscrasias* (thrombocytopenia, factor deficiencies, thrombophilias) should be reviewed by a hematologist.

Medication and allergies

Take full details of all drugs, doses, and regimens as well as allergies to drugs, iodine, contrast, and fish (protamine is made from salmon sperm).
- *Latex allergies* require changes to equipment: warn operating room.
- History of *heparin-induced thrombocytopenia* may require non-heparin (bivalirudin or argatroban) bypass, which mandates careful preplanning.
- Continue *antianginals* until surgery, and stop postoperatively.
- Continue β-*blockers* until surgery, and reintroduce as blood pressure (BP) and rhythm permit postoperatively.
- Stop *ACE inhibitors* 24–48 hours before surgery to avoid profound peripheral dilatation in the immediate postoperative period.
- *Aspirin* and *clopidogrel* are discontinued by many surgeons 5–10 days preoperatively as they predispose to increased postoperative bleeding, but there is a slightly higher risk of acute ischemic events and in high-risk patients (e.g. recent PCI, tight left main stem (LMS)) they may be continued.
- *Warfarin* should be stopped 5 days before surgery (📖 p31). In patients at higher risk of thromboembolic event (e.g. prior TIA, deep vein thrombosis (DVT)) admission 24–48 hours pre-op may be required for iv heparin.
- *Steroids* should be reduced where possible preoperatively: patients taking >5mg of prednisone daily should be prescribed 48 hours 50–100mg hydrocortisone iv 6-hourly, or an equivalent dose continuous infusion, starting with the premedication to avoid Addisonian crisis as a result of adrenal suppression.
- Withhold long-acting *hypoglycemics* on the morning of surgery and commence an insulin sliding scale where appropriate (📖 p31).

Social history

- *Jehovah's witness* patients do not accept blood or blood products, and some may not agree to use of cell salvage: these patients must be identified preoperatively, counselled, preferences clearly documented, and every effort made to ensure preoperative hamatocrit >40%. Several weeks of erythropoietin therapy may be indicated.
- Heavy/binge drinkers are at risk of alchohol withdrawal. Haloperidol lowers the seizure threshold and prolongs the QT-prescribe diazepam 2mg po 8-hourly, thiamine and folate.
- If the patient *lives alone*, plan for rehabilitation. If the patient mobilizes with a walking stick or frame contact physiotherapists early, as sternal union may be compromised even if mobility is not.

Respiratory history

An *active upper respiratory tract infection* (URTI) is sufficient reason to cancel the operation, so ask about cough, colds, and sputum. If you suspect a URTI measure temperature, C-reactive protein (CRP), and white cell count (WCC), and get a chest X-ray (CXR). Assess *COPD* by asking about hospital admissions, inhalers, nebulizers, and home O_2. If dyspnea is the prominent symptom, and the patient has COPD get lung function tests (📖 p652) including blood gases.

Gastrointestinal history

Cardiac surgery patients are at risk of upper gastrointestinal (GI) bleeds from *peptic ulcer disease*, and prolonged ileus, as well as acute deterioration in pre-existing disease, e.g. pancreatitis, and cholecystitis, so ask specifically about GI problems, particularly dyspepsia, ulcers, and pancreatitis. Start all patients on prophylactic proton pump inhibitors (PPIs), and make a note on the drug chart to avoid prescribing non-steroidal anti-inflammatory drug (NSAID) analgesics in at-risk patients. Aspirin should be enteric coated and given with food in these patients.

Renal history

Check the notes for evidence of **renal dysfunction**. If there has been an acute deterioration it may be worth delaying the patient to optimize this by stopping nephrotoxic drugs including angiotensin-converting enzyme (ACE) inhibitors and NSAID analgesia, starting iv fluids with careful fluid balance, and in some cases dialysis. **Dialysis patients** should be dialysed the morning of surgery or the night before. Patients undergoing preoperative cardiac catheterization are at particular risk of temporary impairments in renal function because of the combination of hypovolemia due to preprocedure fasting, and nephrotoxic contrast. Prescribe iv fluid in patients with borderline renal function, and consider iv acetylcysteine prior to contrast studies. Patients with a history suggestive of **prostatic enlargement** should be warned that they may need a suprapubic catheter.

Neurological history

In addition to identifying TIAs, strokes, and residual deficit identify dementia, which in advanced cases is a contraindication to cardiac surgery.

Examination

The main purpose of the examination is:
- To identify disease that needs further investigation and management.
- To help plan surgery.
- To identify problems that may delay recovery.

For the average elective patient a shortened version of the full cardiovascular examination described is sufficient (see Box 1.2).

> **Box 1.2 Short examination**
>
> - Assess pulse rate and rhythm.
> - Document BP.
> - Assess jugular venous pressure with the patient at 45°.
> - Auscultate heart sounds, carotids and breath sounds. Look for scars.
> - Examine the abdomen (tenderness, hernias, organomegaly, scars).
> - Feel peripheral pulses including the abdominal aorta.
> - Asses pedal edema.
> - Assess conduits.

General inspection

From the end of the bed assess whether the patient is comfortable at rest, requiring oxygen, well or moribund, obese or cachexic, or has features suggestive of Down's syndrome (atrial or ventricular septal defect (ASD/VSD), or Marfan syndrome (aortic aneurysms, dissection, and incompetence). Position the patient at 45° in the bed.

Hands and forearms

Look for nicotine staining, stigmata of endocarditis, e.g. splinter hemorrhages, Osler's nodes (tender lumps in the fingertip pulps), Janeway lesions (red macules on the palms or flexor aspects of the wrist), tendon xanthoma. Petechiae may be present in infective endocarditis.

Pulse

Note rate and rhythm at the radial pulse, and character and volume at the brachial or carotid pulse. AS classically has a slow rising, thready pulse. Aortic incompetence has a large volume bounding pulse. Feel the peripheral pulses including the abdominal aorta.

Blood pressure

Note uncontrolled hypertension: systolic >180mmHg should be treated with nifedipine 10mg s/l preoperatively. A wide pulse pressure is suggestive of aortic incompetence. Use a broad cuff for fat arms as BP will otherwise be underestimated. Check BP in both arms if aortic dissection or coarctation is suspected.

Face

Malar flush (cyanosis in a butterfly rash distribution) is characteristic of mitral stenosis. Look at the eyes: jaundice may be caused by hemolysis from prosthetic heart valves; xanthelasma and corneal arcus are common signs of hyperlipidemia, Roth spots may be seen in infective endocarditis, and rarely Argyll Robertson pupils are a feature of syphilitic aortic incompetence. Look at the mouth: check for central cyanosis by examining the tongue and gums, look for the high arched palate of Marfan and check for poor dentition particularly in valve patients.

Neck

Assess the jugular venous pulse with the patient at 45°.

Chest

Inspect the chest for scars (left and right lateral thoracotomy and median sternotomy), implantable cardioverter defibrillator (ICD) and pacemaker insertion, pectus, visible pulsations. Expose the patient adequately or you will miss these.

Palpate the apex beat, which is the point furthest from the manubrium where the heart can be felt, normally 5th intercostal space in the mid-clavicular line. This is shifted laterally in cardiomegaly or mediastinal shift. AS and hypertensive cardiomyopathy results in a sustained, forceful apex beat. A dilated LV (e.g. aortic regurgitation (AR)) normally has a downwards displaced apex beat. In mitral stenosis (MS) the apex beat is described as tapping. Left parasternal heave may be felt in right ventricular hypertrophy. Thrills are palpable murmurs.

Auscultate Timing heart sounds against the radial pulse, use the bell to listen to low-pitched sounds and the diaphragm for high-pitched sounds. Listen over the apex (diaphragm and bell), upper and lower left sternal borders, under the clavicles, over the carotids, and in the axilla (diaphragm ± bell), and then listen again at the apex with the patient in the left lateral position, and at the lower left sternal border with the patient sitting forward in full expiration. Murmurs can be graded on a scale of 1–6: grade 1 is just audible in a quiet room with the patient breath holding, grade 3 is easy to hear without a thrill, grade 6 is audible without a stethoscope. Murmurs and carotid bruits need ultrasound (US) imaging.

Heart murmurs (📖 pp373, 375, 398, 401, 416, 559)

- *Ejection systolic:* AS (loudest in aortic area in expiration, radiates to carotids), aortic sclerosis, pulmonary stenosis, ASD, 'innocent' flow murmur (anemia, hyperthyroid, pregnancy).
- *Pansystolic:* mitral regurgitation (MR) (loudest at apex, radiates to axilla), tricuspid regurgitation (TR), VSD, patent ductus arteriosus (PDA).
- *Early diastolic:* AR, pulmonary regurgitation.
- *Mid diastolic:* MS, tricuspid stenosis (TS), Austin Flint murmur of AR.

Conduit

Stand the patient up so that you can see both legs from ankle to groin. Look for varicosities and decide which distribution they are in (long or short saphenous). To test the suitability of the radial artery perform Allen's test by asking the patient to clench their fist tightly, occluding both radial and ulnar pulses, asking the patient to open their hand and noting how long it takes for the palm of the hand to pink up once the ulnar occlusion is released. Refill time <5s is suitable for harvest.

General examination

Listen to the chest and palpate the abdomen.

Routine laboratory tests

Routine preoperative investigations

- Complete blood count (CBC).
- Coagulation screen (activated partial thromboplastin time (APPT) and prothrombin time (PT)). International normalized ratio (INR) if taking warfarin.
- Biochemistry (Chem 7: Na^+, K^+, Cl^-, HCO_3, blood urea nitrogen (BUN), Cr, glucose).
- Liver function tests (LFTs).
- Cross match blood (XM) 2 units (4 units + fresh frozen plasma (FFP)/platelets (plts) in reoperations or thoracoabdominals).
- Methicillin-resistant *Staphylococcus aureus* (MRSA) screening swab, urinalysis, pregnancy, and sickle cell testing.

Management of common biochemical derangements
See Table 1.1.

Table 1.1 Management of common biochemical derangements

Result	Causes	Management
↑Na >145mmol/L	Commonly diarrhea, vomiting. Less commonly diabetes insipidus.	Oral water or iv 5% dextrose. Discuss with anesthesiologist
↓Na <130mmol/L	Commonly diuretics, diarrhea, vomiting Less commonly nephritic syndromes (congestive cardiac failure (CCF), cirrhosis, renal failure), Addison's, syndrome of inappropriate antidiuretic hormone secretion (SIADH) (common postoperatively)	Assess renal function (📖 p234) and treat accordingly. Fluid restrict if appropriate (📖 p271). Discuss with anasthesiologist
↑K >5mmol/L	Commonly K-sparing diuretics and ACE inhibitors, excess K therapy, artifact (hemolysis in tube) Less commonly renal failure, diabetic acidosis, Addison's disease	See 📖 p271. It should be possible to correct hyperkalemia over 12h
↓K <3.5mmol/L	Commonly diuretics, vomiting, diarrhea Less commonly Conn's, Cushing's syndromes, renal tubular failure	See 📖 p270. It should be possible to correct hypokalemia over 12h

Table 1.1 (*Contd.*)

↑Cr >1.2mg/dL BUN >21mg/dL	Renal impairment. Disproportionately ↑U, suggests dehydration as primary cause. Isolated ↑U occurs with thiazide diuretics, gout, lymphoma, leukemia	See 🕮 p270.
↑LFTs or bilirubin, or gamma GT	Commonly drugs (paracetamol, OCP, co-amoxiclav, chlorpromazine, erythromycin), hemolysis, viral hepatitis, gallstones, Gilbert's syndrome, sepsis, EtOH Less commonly malignancy causing biliary tract obstruction,	Ask about iv drug use, transfusions, travel, EtOH. Examine abdomen for ↑spleen/liver, signs of chronic liver disease, test urine for bilirubin and urobilinogen. Request liver US. Consider serology.

The decision to cancel surgery in order to investigate or treat abnormalities thrown up in preoperative screening is based on judging the risk of delaying surgery against the increased risk of surgery. The symptomatic, unstable patient with a tight LMS lesion is less likely to be cancelled for a mild neutrophilia than the elective valve patient, for example. Discuss any move to cancel with the surgical team.

Management of common hematological derangements
See Table 1.2.

Table 1.2 Management of common hematological derangements

Result	Causes	Management
↓Hb <9.5g/dL	Mean corpuscular volume (MCV) <75: Fe deficiency, thalassemia MCV 75–95: chronic disease, renal failure, bone marrow failure, hemolysis, hypothyroidism, dilutional (acute) MCV >95: ↓B_{12} or folate, EtOH, liver disease, hypothyroidism, myelodysplasias, bone marrow infiltration	Undiagnosed Fe deficiency should be fully investigated as GI malignancy is a common cause in this age group Treat the causes where possible, and avoid transfusion unless Hb ↓↓↓. The perfusionist may want extra blood to prime the pump

(*Continued*)

Table 1.2 (*Contd.*)

↑Hb >14g/dL	Relative (↓plasma volume): dehydration (EtOH and diuretics), Absolute (↑red blood cell (RBC) mass): primary polycythemia rubra vera, secondary to smoking, COPD, altitude, tumours	PCV patients may need formal anticoagulation postoperatively to prevent thromboembolic events
↑WCC >12×10⁹/L	Neutrophilia: bacterial sepsis, trauma, surgery, burns, inflammation, MI, polymyalgia, steroids, hemorrhage	Recheck history and examination for evidence of sepsis, take temperature, look at CXR and urine dipsticks. Elective valve patients: check with team: may cancel. If due to a URTI, start ABCs, and recheck WCC in 2–3 weeks
	Lymphophilia: viral infection (Epstein Barr virus (EBV), cytomegalovirus (CMV)), chronic lymphocytic leukemia (CLL)	
	Eosinophilia: asthma, allergy, parasitic infections, eczema, malignancy	
↓WCC<2 ×10⁹/L	Rarely neutropenic sepsis, steroids, sulfonamides, systemic lupus erythematosus (SLE)	Discuss with hematologist—emergency in sepsis
↑Plts >400×10⁹/L	Essential thrombocythemia, sepsis, inflammatory disease (e.g. rheumatoid arthritis). 50% have malignancy	Discuss with hematologist
↓Plts <120×10⁹/L	Heparin-induced thrombocytopenia (📖 p288), sepsis and DIC (📖 p288), drugs, SLE, lymphoma, bone marrow failure.	Discontinue heparin and request heparin-induced thrombocytopenia (HIT) screen. In septic patients send fibrin degradation products. Request plts
Clotting	↑PT = warfarin, ↓vit K, liver disease	Investigate as for liver disease, measure clotting factors. Talk to hematologist
	↑APTT = heparin, ↓factor VIII, IX	
	↑INR = warfarin, liver disease	
XM	Atypical antibodies may mean more time and further samples are required to obtain blood that gives a satisfactory cross-match.	

Plain chest radiograph

Chest radiograph

PA and AP films

The standard view is posteroanterior (PA). The patient stands facing the film, clasping it in both arms, the X-rays pass through the chest *from posterior to anterior*, and the films are taken in full inspiration to maximize the size of the lung fields. This has advantages over the anteroposterior (AP) view, used for portable X-rays in immobile patients (where the plate is placed under the patient's back and the X-rays pass through the patient from *anterior to posterior*), namely:

- The scapulae are rotated away so they obscure the lung fields less.
- The heart shadow is smaller, so more of the lung fields are visible
- The relative sizes of the lung fields and the cardiac silhouette can be reliably used to comment on cardiomegaly and mediastinal widening.

Lateral chest films

Lateral films are used to further define abnormalities identified in the lung fields on the PA and AP films. A left lateral film is taken to define abnormalities in the left thorax. The patient's left side is placed against the film, which is labelled 'L'. Right lateral views are taken in a similar way (Fig. 1.1).

System for describing chest X-rays

- Confirm the name and age of the patient, and the date of the film.
- Define the film (AP, PA, or lateral, erect or supine, contrast or plain).
- Check that the film is oriented correctly!
- Check that it is correctly aligned (clavicle and ribs should be symmetrically aligned with sternum and spinous processes), shows all of the lung fields from apex to costophrenic angle, and has adequate exposure (you should see the vertebral bodies through the heart).
- Comment on presence and position of endotracheal (ET) or nasogastric (NG) tube, catheters (pulmonary artery (PA) or central line), clips, drains, prosthetic valves, rings, wires.
- Now examine the bony tissues looking for fractures and dislocations, lytic lesions, calcification, erosions, and extra ribs (the ribs are easier to see posteriorly than anteriorly).
- Next assess the soft tissue shadows of the neck, chest wall, breasts, and look at the diaphragms (right normally one rib higher than left).
- Examine the mediastinal shadow (Fig. 1.1: aortic knob 8; pulmonary trunk 9; LA appendage 10, LV 11; inferior vena cava (IVC) 12; right atrium (RA) 13; superior vena cava (SVC) 14).
- Then look at the airways, including the trachea, main bronchi, and lung fields (normal a deep breath in can inflate lungs to 10th rib posteriorly or 6th rib anteriorly), fissures, and vascularity of lung fields.
- Tips:
  - Trachea should be midline, opacities should be symmetrical.
  - It takes 400mL of fluid to blunt the costophrenic angles.
  - In the supine patient fluid level is replaced by diffuse opacity.
  - If one hemithorax is more opaque, either you have a collection on the opaque side, or a pneumothorax on the other side.

(a)

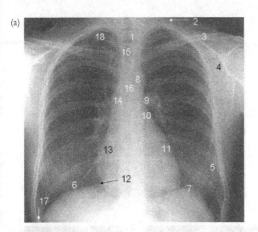

(b)

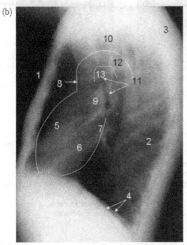

Fig. 1.1 (a) Normal CXR. 1, spinous process of T12; 2, 1st left rib; 3, left clavicle; 4, body of left scapula; 5, left 8th rib; 6, right hemidiaphragm; 7, left hemidiaphragm; 8, aortic knuckle; 9, pulmonary trunk; 10, left atrial appendage; 11, left ventricle; 12, inferior vena cava; 13, right atrium; 14, superior vena cava; 15, trachea; 16, carina; 17, right costophrenic angle; 18, apex right lung. (b) Plain lateral CXR. 1, manubriosternal junction; 2, body of thoracic vertebra; 3, body of scapula; 4, right and left hemidiaphragms; 5, right ventricle; 6, left ventricle; 7, left atrium; 8, ascending aorta; 9, pulmonary trunk; 10, proximal trachea; 11, distal trachea; 12, distal arch of aorta; 13, aortopulmonary window.

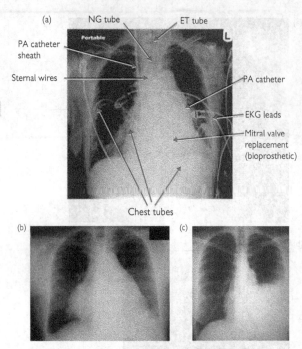

Fig. 1.2 Postoperative films. (a) Early film showing the position of most commonly seen lines and catheters. A portable X-ray is done on immediate arrival in the ICU. Check the position of the ET tube (should be 1 inch (2.5cm) above the carina), NG tube (should be visible in stomach), and PA catheter (usually in right pulmonary artery, check it is not coiled, in too far, or malpositioned, e.g. in IVC). Look for collections (remember these may just be diffuse haze in supine patients), pneumothorax, and lobar collapse. (b) Pericardial effusion—globular heart shadow, CT, and echo are diagnostic, and echo is required for diagnosis of tamponade. (c) Left pleural effusion in erect patient. Note concave upwards meniscus suggestive of fluid. If there is a flat fluid level, this suggests hydropneumothorax.

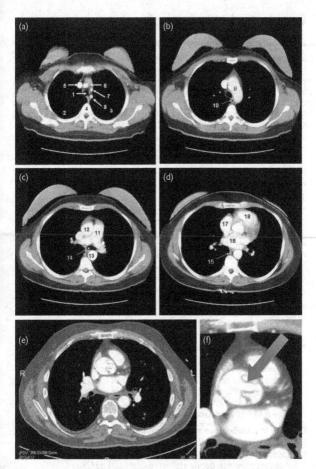

Fig. 1.3 (a–d) Normal contrast CT; 1, trachea; 2, right lung; 3, left lung; 4, body of T3; 5, SVC full of contrast; 6, brachiocephalic artery; 7, left common carotid; 8, left subclavian; 9, aortic arch; 10, esophagus; 11, pulmonary trunk; 12, ascending aorta; 13, descending aorta; 14, carina; 15, hemiazygous vein; 16, left atrium; 17, right atrium; 18, right ventricle. (e) CT with iv contrast showing type A dissection. (f) Detail (arrow indicates obvious dissection flap, which is often less prominent and more concave).

Computed tomography

Principles of computed tomography

CT uses the same radiation as standard X-rays, but moves the X-ray source round the patient. The attenuation of each point is measured on a scale of *Hounsfield units* (HU) which assigns water 0HU, and ranges from +1000 (white) to −1000 (black). Bone is +400 to +1000 (white), contrast is +800 (white), soft tissue is +40 to +80 (gray), lung is −500 (gray to black). As the eye can't distinguish 2000 shades of gray, a limited range of HU or *window width (WW)* is selected for display once images are acquired, around a central *window level (WL)*, depending on the tissue of interest. A *mediastinal or soft tissue window* has a WL of +40 HU (Fig. 1.4a), a **lung window** has a WL of −600 (Fig. 1.4b) showing detailed lung parenchyma, which cannot be seen on soft tissue windows. IV contrast is used to define vascular structures.

Types of CT scanners

* *Conventional CT scanners*: X-ray source and detectors are unable to rotate continuously. The table moves the patient a set distance, stopping between each slice so the next slice can be taken.
* *Spiral CT scanners*: the majority of conventional scanners have been replaced by spiral CT which incorporate 'slip rings' that remove the need for a physical connection between the X-ray tube and the power cables, meaning that the ring can rotate in one direction indefinitely. The table moves the patient continuously while the image is being acquired. Advantages of spiral CT over conventional include:
  * Faster, higher-resolution images allowing angiography—e.g. coronary and pulmonary angiography and standard vascular views.
  * Any plane and 3-dimensional (3D) images can be constructed.
* *Multislice CT scanners*: instead of the single row of detectors used in conventional and spiral scanners, multislice CT scanners have several rows of detectors. Tube rotation is also much faster. Advantages:
  * Image acquisition is several times faster than spiral CT scanners, so they are used in unstable and uncooperative patients, and vascular imaging, as scan time and movement artefact is minimized.
  * Resolution is significantly better allowing video footage, e.g. of valves.

CT scans in perioperative management of cardiac surgery patients

Chest CT is particularly helpful in cardiac surgical patients:
* Reoperations: identifying vascular structures, e.g. patent grafts, aorta, RV at particular risk during sternal re-entry (🕮 p347).
* Valve patients at low risk of coronary disease may elect to have *CT coronary angiography* rather than cardiac catheterization to evaluate coronary disease preoperatively. CT angiography is very specific and sensitive for coronary disease. Any significant abnormality should be evaluated with standard coronary angiography (so little to gain from evaluating higher risk patients with this modality). Contrast load and radiation exposure are very similar for invasive and CT angiography.
* Diagnosis and evaluation of aortic aneurysm and dissection (Fig. 1.3e).
* Evaluation of mediastinitis, sternal dehiscence, PE.

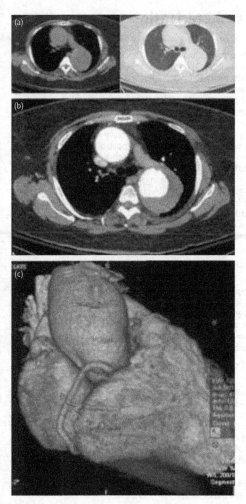

Fig.1.4 (a) Non-contrast CT of chest showing large ascending and descending aortic aneurysm (mediastinal windows on the left and lung windows on the right). Calcification is visible in the wall of the descending aorta but little other information about the vessel lumen can be derived. (b) The same patient and view after administration of iv contrast now clearly showing evidence of a type B dissection, with intraluminal thrombus in the descending aorta. (c) 3D reconstruction of aneurysmal ascending aorta showing right coronary artery (arrowed) in atrioventricular groove.

Cardiac catheterization

Key facts

- Cardiac catheterization may be right and/or left heart, diagnostic or therapeutic and allows:
- *Left heart catheterization* (via the femoral or radial artery):
  - Measurement of LA, LV, and aortic pressures and transmitral and transaortic pressure gradients.
  - Calculation of mitral and aortic valve areas.
  - *Coronary angiography* (the commonest indication) and ventriculography which requires substantially more contrast.
  - PCI, percutaneous balloon mitral valvuloplasty (BMV), transcatheter aortic valve implantation (TAVI), LA appendage occlusion.
- *Right heart catheterization* (via the femoral, internal jugular, or subclavian vein) is essentially the same as floating a Swann–Ganz catheter:
  - Measurement of RA, RV, and PA pressures, pulmonary artery wedge pressure (PAWP) and saturations including SvO_2 (mixed venous oxygen saturation).
  - Calculation of peripheral vascular resistance (PVR), CO, shunts.
  - Pulmonary angiography.
  - Transseptal puncture for LA access.

Contraindications

These are few. The patient may be too unwell (acute type A dissection) to tolerate the procedure. Patients with AS or mobile vegetations should not have ventriculography or pull back gradients performed as crossing the aortic valve carries a risk of stroke, and hemodynamic data can be obtained more safely by echocardiography. Similarly, patients with renal dysfunction should not have ventriculograms as the increased contrast load will exacerbate renal impairment significantly.

Principles of coronary angiography

Technique

The patient is usually awake but sedated and supine. Access is via a sheath using a modified Seldinger technique. Radio-opaque contrast is injected into the coronary ostia in turn via a size 4 Judkins catheter (2–3mm diameter). The X-ray tube and camera are opposite each other on a C-arm, and can be rotated cranially and caudally, and from left to right to achieve a range of views of the coronary anatomy. Biplane imaging uses two cameras to obtain simultaneous images from two different angles, reducing radiation exposure. Moving images are captured on digital CDs which have superseded cine film. Patients may be given 300mg of clopidogrel or 75mg of aspirin pre- and post-PCI.

Complications

- Complications requiring emergency bypass surgery (left anterior descending coronary artery (LAD) dissection, acute LAD occlusion, cardiac tamponade) 1:1000 catheterizations.
- Major adverse events (e.g. stroke) 1%, death 0.01%.
- Failure to occlude the puncture site after removal can result in extensive hematoma, which may be retroperitoneal if femoral puncture high.

Coronary anatomy is described on 📖 pp20–21 and pp46–47. Interpretation of coronary angiograms is described below.

Interpretation of coronary angiography

- Look at each lesion in several views and the whole film.
- Eccentric plaques will look most significant when viewed end on, and may almost disappear when viewed perpendicularly.
- Comment on the vessels systemically.
- Lesions are compared to adjacent 'normal' segments: in diffusely diseased vessels this can lead to underestimating severity.
- A reduction in **vessel diameter** of 50% corresponds to a 75% reduction in **cross-sectional area**, and a 70% reduction in vessel diameter corresponds to a reduction of 90% in cross-sectional area (Fig. 1.5).
- A stenosis is **significant** if it is >50% the lumen diameter as it reduces the normal 3–4 x flow reserve, >70% lumen diameter stenosis eliminates any capacity to increase above resting flow, and >90% stenosis usually means TIMI grade 1 or 2 flow (📖 p22).
- Remember occluded vessels frequently fill late, retrogradely from shots of other vessels: most commonly the PDA and right coronary artery (RCA) from the LAD, and sometimes the LAD from the PDA.
- Beware mistaking a large diagonal for a completely occluded LAD: always look at the left anterior oblique (LAO) view before commenting on the LAD.
  - Start with a summary after viewing **all** views: 'This is a 75-year-old male with 3-vessel disease and moderate LV…'.
  - Describe the LMS, best seen in the right anterior oblique (RAO) view and the LAO caudal.
  - Describe the circumflex system, best seen in the RAO view.
  - Describe the LAD and diagonals, best seen in the LAO cranial.
  - Describe the RCA and PDA, and the dominance.
- Describe the ventricular function, any regional akinesia, MR, and calcification of the coronary vessels or valves.

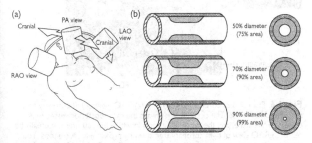

Fig. 1.5 (a) The orientation of the X-ray box and camera for the various views. (b) Relationship between angiographic and actual lumen narrowing.

Interpreting coronary imaging

Key facts

- Recognizing views and vessels rapidly becomes pattern recognition, but following a systematic approach will help avoid common mistakes.
- Identify each view, look at all the views, look at each vessel in multiple views, look at the whole clip for each view (some vessels only fill late).

Which view is it, which vessel is it?

- In a RAO view ribs go down to the right of the image, which is on the right of the spine (catheter in aorta).
- In a LAO view the ribs go down to the left of the image which is on the left of the spine (catheter in aorta).
- In cranial views the diaphragm is superimposed over most of the picture, whereas in caudal views it is hardly seen.
- The circumflex is the vessel closest to the spine (or the catheter in the descending aorta) in every image.
- The LAD is the vessel that travels towards the apex, it is usually the longest vessel, and it has septals coming off it at 90°.

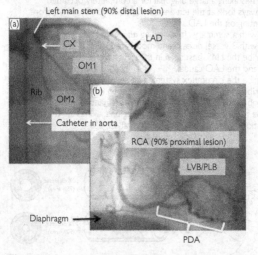

Fig. 1.6 Examples of coronary angiograms. (a) RAO view of left coronary tree showing LMS disease. The circumflex is always the most posterior vessel, i.e., it is closest to the spine, and the descending aorta in which the catheter can usually be seen. (b) RAO view of right coronary tree showing proximal RCA stenosis. You can just about make out the short septals coming off the PDA at 90°. These help distinguish the PDA from the LVB.

Coronary anatomy (see also 📖 pp46–47)

- Branches of the *right coronary artery* in order:
  - 1) Conus branch, 2) SA nodal branch, 3) RV branch, 4) acute marginal, 5) AV nodal artery (60%), 6) in right-dominant patients (85%) the RCA then bifurcates into PDA which gives off inferior septals at 90°, and 7) LVB or posterolateral branches.
  - Proximal RCA is up to the RV branch, mid up to the acute marginal, and distal up to the bifurcation.
- Branches of the *left coronary artery*:
  - 1) LMS which bifurcates (occasionally trifurcates into ramus intermediate branch) into 2) LAD which gives off septals at 90° and diagonals, and 3) Cx which gives off OMs and may give rise to AV nodal artery (40%) and in left-dominant patients PDA (10%) and LVB or posterolateral branches.
  - The proximal LAD is up to the 1st septal, mid LAD until the 2nd diagonal, and distal LAD after the 2nd diagonal.

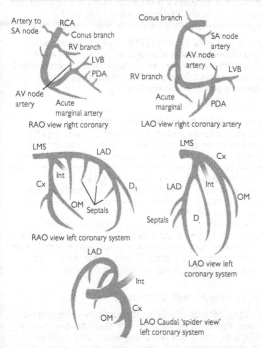

Fig. 1.7 The five common angiographic views. RCA, right coronary artery; RV, right ventricular; SA, sinoatrial; AV, atrioventricular; LVB, lateral ventricular branch; PDA, posterior descending artery; LMS, left main stem; LAD, left anterior descending; D, diagonal; Int, intermediate; Cx, circumflex; OM, obtuse marginal.

Cardiac hemodynamics

Key facts

- Severity of coronary stenosis may be misrepresented by angiography: additional information can be obtained by pressure measurements, e.g., fractional flow reserve (FFR), and intravascular ultrasound (IVUS).
- When echocardiography is equivocal, cardiac catheterization can provide useful additional information on severity of valve lesions, pulmonary hypertension, ventricular function, and intracardiac shunts.

Coronary hemodynamics

Fractional flow reserve

This is essentially the ratio between the BP proximal to and distal to a lesion, when flow is maximal. A FFR <75% (i.e., <75% of maximal flow in a non-diseased coronary) indicates a significant lesion and there is some data to suggest it is safe to watch (rather than intervene) on patients with higher FFRs. The test is performed at maximal blood flow which is induced by giving adenosine or papaverine (and which is 4–5 × resting blood flow in the normal subject), hence it assesses coronary reserve.

TIMI flow

Thrombolysis in myocardial infarction (TIMI) scale grades coronary flow:
- TIMI 0 (no perfusion): absence of antegrade flow beyond a lesion.
- TIMI 1 (penetration no perfusion): incomplete filling distal coronary bed.
- TIMI 2 (partial reperfusion): delayed but complete filling distally.
- TIMI 3 (complete perfusion): normal flow.

Assessment of valve disease

Quantifying valve stenosis by cardiac catheterization

- Transaortic valve pressure gradient is estimated by measuring LV pressure and either simultaneously measuring aortic pressure distal to the valve (mean and peak to peak gradients) or by 'pull-back' where the catheter is then pulled back into the aorta to record pressure. The most physiologic value is the mean gradient (Fig. 1.8).
- Mitral pressure gradients are measured by simultaneous recording of PAWP or LA pressure (LAP) obtained by transseptal puncture, and LV end-diastolic pressure (LVEDP).
- Valve area is estimated using the Gorlin equation (essentially valve area = flow/velocity) or area − cardiac output /√ pressure gradient. Accurate estimation of cardiac output is particularly critical, and particularly open to error in low cardiac output states (□ p492) when dobutamine stress testing can be used as a diagnostic adjunct (□ p25).

Grossman grading of regurgitation

- Grade I: faint opacification of proximal chamber, clears with one beat.
- Grade II: opacification of proximal less than distal chamber.
- Grade III: opacification proximal chamber equals distal chamber.
- Grade IV: complete dense opacification of proximal chamber with a constant density greater than in the distal chamber.

Calculation of cardiac output

There are multiple methods of calculating cardiac output during cardiac catheterization, all with potential errors.

- *Thermodilution* technique (📖 p135) involves injection of a bolus of normal saline into the proximal port, measurement of the pressure gradient between this and a distal port, which is entered into an equation incorporating the specific gravity and temperatures of the fluid and the patient's blood. TR, incorrect injection technique, and low cardiac output are all potential sources of error.
- The *Fick principle* is that the uptake (or release) of a substance (usually VO_2) by a substance is equal to the product of the arteriovenous concentration gradient and the cardiac output. In most labs VO_2 is not measured, and assumed to be $125mL/m^2$. This method is more accurate than thermodilution in low output states, but should not be used in MR or AI, or patients receiving supplemental O_2.
- *Angiographic methods* involve tracing the LV end-diastolic and end-systolic images and converting these to volume using modelling.

Assessment of other pathology

- PVR = (mPAP − mLAP)/CO, where PAWP is substituted for LA pressure in the absence of pulmonary disease. Normal PVR is 3 Woods units. Fixed pulmonary hypertension cannot be reversed with NTG, inhaled NO or Flolan, or exercise (📖 p504).
- Cardiac catheterization is also used to differentiate between restrictive cardiomyopathy and constrictive pericarditis (📖 pp83, 488).
- Shunts can be detected and quantified using sampling of blood oximetry from IVC, SVC, multiple RA locations, PA and coronary sinus and artery: Qp:Qs = (SaO_2 − MVO_2/PVO_2 − PAO_2).

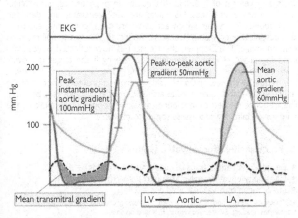

Fig. 1.8 Quantifying valve stenosis by cardiac catheterization.

Echocardiography

Key facts

Echocardiography is ultrasound used to assess cardiac conditions. There are two main approaches: transthoracic (TTE) and transesophageal echocardiography (TEE), and four modalities are used commonly (Box 1.2).

Box 1.2 Terminology in echocardiography

- *B-mode* (brightness mode), also called 2D or real-time, provides a 2D grayscale picture of a single plane across the heart. The intensity of the echo is related to the brightness of signal.
- *M-mode* (motion mode) is more accurate than B-mode, so it is used for measurements, but it only yields a 1D image of structures plotted on the y-axis against time on the x-axis.
- *D-mode* (Doppler) uses Doppler frequency shifts to measure flow velocities and hence calculate gradients and valve areas. Only moving targets are displayed. Duplex US combines Doppler and grayscale images to correlate flow with fixed structures.
- *Colour flow imaging* is a colour-enhanced duplex Doppler echo which combines M-mode and D-mode with blood flow imaging. Most systems code blood flow **a**way from the transducer as **b**lue, and blood flow **t**owards the transducer as **r**ed (BART).
- *3D echo* allows 3D visualization of the cardiac structures. It is particularly useful when viewing the morphology of the mitral valve.

Principles of echocardiography

US is a waveform of 2–5MHz that passes through tissues, with reflection from tissue interfaces. US waves are both generated and detected by piezoelectric crystals which act as transducers, converting electrical to mechanical energy and vice versa. Reflected waves are calibrated to form an image. The Doppler effect describes how reflected waves from a moving target change in frequency, increasing if the target is moving towards the wave source, and decreasing if the target is moving away. The frequency change, or *Doppler shift*, is proportional to the speed of the object, which can be quantified as an audible signal, or color (see Box 1.2). The frequencies used cannot penetrate air or bone, which explains the need for certain views to assess some structures.

Echo quantification of valve stenosis

- Bernouilli equation: transvalvular gradient (mmHg) = $4v_m^2$
- Continuity equation: valve area (cm²) = SV/(ET × 85 × v_m)
- In AS: mean transvalvular gradient = $2.4v_{max}^2$

v_m= mean velocity of blood (m/s), v_{max} = maximum velocity of blood, VF= valve flow, VG = transvalvular gradient, SV = stroke volume, ET= ejection time.

Normal cardiac dimensions

Echocardiography allows precise measurement of cardiac dimensions. Septal and posterior wall thickness in systole and diastole allow calculation of fractional shortening, which is a crude index of LV systolic function (which is expressed as a percentage but should not be confused with ejection fraction), and LV mass. See Table 1.3.

Table 1.3 Normal adult ranges in M-mode echocardiography

Structure	Parameter	Range
Left ventricle	End-systolic diameter	25–41mm
	End-diastolic diameter	35–56mm
	Shortening fraction	30–40%
	Ejection fraction	50–65%
	Mass	60–124g/m^2
Aortic root	Diameter	20–37mm
	Cusp separation	15–26mm
Left atrium		19–40mm
Right ventricle		7–23mm

Assessing LV function

LV function can be assessed quantitatively and qualitatively. Qualitative assessments involve scoring regional wall motion and categorizing LV function as normal, mild, moderate, or severe impairment. Quantitative methods, e.g. fractional shortening and calculations of ejection fraction are still subject to operator variability. The nine-segment model for regional wall motion assessment is shown in Fig. 1.9.

Stress echocardiography

Stress echocardiography stresses the myocardium either chemically or via exercise protocols to gain information about myocardial viability and regional perfusion. Standard treadmill protocols such as the Bruce protocol are used for exercise testing: they give a limited time in which to image the heart and hyperventilation may make imaging difficult. The main drug used in pharmacological stress echocardiography is dobutamine in incremental low- or high-dose protocols.
- Net outward systolic motion and failure of a segment to thicken during systole suggests that the segment is infarcted.
- Reduction of wall motion during stress, in a segment that contracts when the patient is at rest, suggests flow-limiting coronary stenoses.
- During low-dose dobutamine protocols, improvement of function in a segment that is impaired at rest suggests that the segment contains stunned or hibernating myocardium (📖 pp74–75).
- Increase in a moderate gradient across a critically stenosed aortic valve suggests that myocardium will respond well to valve replacement.
- Papillary muscle ischemia may cause MR as a result of an inducible septal or posterior wall motion defect.

Echo interpretation

TEE versus TTE

- TEE has finer resolution than TTE (down to 2–3mm).
- TEE is better than TTE at imaging the posterior heart (e.g., identifying LA appendage thrombus), and the ascending aorta.
- TEE can be carried out under light sedation. Relative contraindications include esophageal strictures (use pediatric probe), pouches and varices, respiratory compromise, and cervical pathology.

Commonly used views

TEE can be distinguished from TTE as: (1) films are usually labelled, (2) in a TEE the left atrium is the chamber closest to the transducer and hence at the apex of the image triangle, and (3) the AV valves are concave downwards in most views. Standard TEE views are shown in Fig. 1.9. Tips for orientating yourself when looking at TEE films.

- The apex of the TEE image is the probe in the esophagus, i.e., posterior and the left atrium is almost always at the apex of the triangle (Fig. 1.9).
- Right ventricle and atrium are the most anterior structures.
- The aortic valve is adjacent to the anterior leaflet of the mitral valve.
- The inter-atrial septum points at the non-coronary cusp of the aortic valve in the short-axis view (see Fig. 1.9).
- In the long-axis view the aortic valve may be on the left or right of the image depending on the probe orientation, but it is always adjacent to the interventricular septum.

Common sources of error

Image quality in TTE is highly dependent on patient build (obese, emphysematous, postoperative patients are difficult to image), patient position, probe position and contact, and machine settings. Other errors include:

- Failure to align the US beam parallel to the flow of blood thus underestimating its velocity and hence transvalvular gradient.
- Aligning the beam obliquely across a chamber and overestimating its size.
- Measuring eccentric jets, or other signals (the jet of MR may be mistaken for AS if views are poor) instead of the main blood flow.

Echocardiographic grading of regurgitation

There are a number of qualitative and quantitative variables each of which can be used to grade regurgitation. This box summarizes some of the more commonly used indices.

Aortic regurgitation
- Mild: central jet width <25% of LVOT, regurgitant fraction <30%.
- Moderate: values intermediate to mild and severe.
- Severe: central jet width >65% of LVOT, regurgitant fraction >50%.

Mitral regurgitation
- Mild: central jet <20% of LA area, regurgitant fraction <30%.
- Moderate: values intermediate between mild and severe.
- Severe; central jet >40% of LA area, regurgitant fraction >50%, jet impinging on wall of LA, systolic flow reversal in pulmonary veins, effective regurgitant orifice (ERO) >40mm.

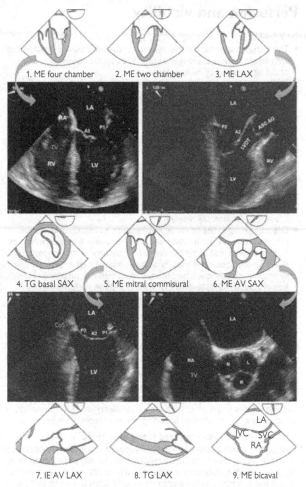

Fig. 1.9 9 of 20 standard TOE views. ME, mid-oesophageal; LAX, long axis; SAX, short axis; TG, transgastric; LV, left ventricle; RV, right ventricle; RA, right atrium; LA, left atrium; CoS, coronary sinus; TV tricuspid valve; N, non-coronary cusp; L, left coronary cusp; R, right coronary cusp; LVOT, left ventricular outflow tract. A1, A2, P1, P3, anterior and posterior mitral leaflets (see 📖 p1 for terminology).

Perfusion and viability

Key facts

- The historic view that chronic ventricular dysfunction was synonymous with infarction was challenged in the 1970s by the observation that it could be reversed by revascularization.
- The term '*hibernating myocardium*' was coined to describe the theory that chronic LV dysfunction was an adaptive response to chronically reduced coronary blood flow at rest.
- More recent studies suggest that hibernation is really due to repetitive *stunning* (📖 pp74–75): myocardium is adequately perfused at rest, but on exercise becomes ischemic because of impaired coronary flow reserve.
- Characteristics of hibernating myocardial include:
  - Reduced contractility (hypokinesis rather than akinesis).
  - Reduced perfusion (usually evident on exercise rather than rest).
  - Viable (i.e., not infarcted) myocardium (evidenced by hypokinesis).
  - Functional improvement with revascularization, which can sometimes be predicted by similar improvement with intropes or exercise (**contractile reserve**).
- Detecting hibernating or viable myocardium is clinically important in patients with poor LV function and predominantly dyspneic symptoms (rather than angina) being considered for coronary artery bypass graft (CABG): the absence of viability suggests much lower prognostic and symptomatic benefit will be obtained from high-risk surgery (📖 p299).
- Key modalities for assessment of viability include nuclear imaging, stress echocardiography, and magnetic resonance imaging (MRI).

Nuclear imaging

Nuclear imaging of the heart allows ventriculography and perfusion studies. Isotopes may either be γ-ray or positron-emitting radionuclides:

Conventional radionuclide imaging

^{99m}Technetium is used to make compounds such as sestamibi and tetrofosmin (Table 1.4), which are replacing cheaper ^{201}thallium-labeled compounds. These radiolabeled compounds are taken up by red blood cells (RBCs). Decay produces γ-rays which hit a sodium iodide crystal causing scintillations detected by a photomultiplier, providing images of regional perfusion.

Single-positron emission computed tomography (SPECT)

Two gamma cameras and computerized reconstruction allow images from technetium or thallium tests to be reconstructed in any plane. Stress imaging (after exercise, dobutamine, dipyridamole, or adenosine) is performed first: if this is normal, subsequent rest imaging does not need to be performed. If it is abnormal, rest images are obtained: fixed perfusion defects represent infarcts, reversible defects suggest hibernation.

Positron emission tomography (PET)

^{18}Fluoro-2-deoxyglucose (^{18}FDG) is most widely used: it is taken up by myocytes, reflecting glucose metabolism during ischemia. PET scans offer much better spatial resolution than the 1cm offered by SPECT but routine use is limited by very high costs.

Table 1.4 Commonly used radiopharmaceuticals

Radionuclide	Compound	Imaging
^{99m}Tc	^{99m}Tc-labeled RBCs	Blood pool studies
	^{99m}Tc MIBI	Ventriculography
	^{99m}Tc pyrophosphate	Myocardial perfusion
^{201}Tl	^{201}TlCl	Hibernation
^{18}FDG		Hibernation
^{13}N		Myocardial perfusion
^{13}O		Oxygen uptake

Interpreting images

Ventriculography

Nuclear imaging can be used to provide an accurate, relatively non-invasive, reproducible ejection fraction and intracardiac shunts.

Myocardial perfusion imaging

Regional blood flow is imaged after stress then at rest. Stressors include adenosine, dopamine, and exercise (see 📖 p25). During stress, territories supplied by a vessel with a flow-limiting stenosis receive relatively less blood than adjoining normal territories. A defect in the post-stress scan which normalizes after rest (reversible defect) usually represents reversible ischemia, which may be improved by revascularization (Fig. 1.10). A photon-deficient area which remains unchanged in both phases of the study is called a fixed defect, and usually represents an area of infarction, which will not be improved by revascularization.

Magnetic resonance imaging

Cardiac magnetic resonance (CMR) imaging can assess myocardial viability through measurement of end-diastolic wall thickness, dobutamine stress (which identifies contractile reserve), and contrast enhancement revealing scar tissue, as well as accurate measurement of LV and RV volumes and ejection fraction. Late enhancement can also be demonstrated on CT along with measurement of wall thickness and volumes.

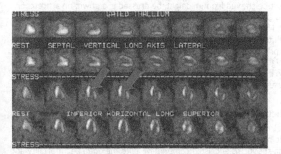

Fig. 1.10 Thallium scan showing apical (A) perfusion defects after stress (arrowed) which reverse on rest images below, suggesting reversible ischaemia.

General pre-op checklist

Box 1.3 contains an overview of planning an elective operating list in cardiac surgery. For emergency surgery, make sure that the following are available: an ICU bed; a surgeon; anesthesiology team; an operating room (OR); two scrub nurses; a perfusionist; blood.

Box 1.3 Elective list checklist

- Always see the patients you are operating on: always take your own history and do your own examination.
- Consent the patient (📖 p257).
- Review the bloods and check that they have been cross-matched.
- Review the CXR and make sure all relevant films are available.
- Review echo/angiography, repeat studies >6 months old.
- Does the patient need any additional investigations?
- Decide on the order of the list with the surgeon:
  - Sick, complex patients who medically will not tolerate cancellation, and who would benefit from admission to ICU early in the day when there is full availability of imaging and support services, are best placed first on the list.
  - Patients with infection risks are placed last on the list.
  - The availability of equipment may dictate the running order.
- Speak to the anesthesiologist, particularly if there are last-minute changes.
- Make sure the nursing staff know the list order: a copy of the list should be on every location with a patient on the list, ICU, and OR.
- When writing the list, in addition to operation, specify radial artery and side, off-pump, redo, femoral bypass, thoracotomy, and side.
- Homografts (📖 p386) may need to be ordered in advance.
- Pacing technicians should be contacted for patients with permanent pacemaker (PPMs).
- Theatres should be notified of patients with latex allergies several days in advance if possible.
- If the patient is an outlier on a ward not used to preparing patients for surgery, make sure that the nursing staff know that the patient must be starved from midnight, be dressed in a gown, on a stretcher, and shaved at least 30 minutes before the send time.
- Let ICU know which patients are appropriate for fast-tracking.
- Tell the perfusionist if the patient is anemic (they may decide to prime the pump with blood and you will need to XM extra), weighs <60kg (they may want to minimize prime volume to avoid hemodilution), and if the patient has a high creatinine (the perfusionist can filter the patient on bypass).

Predicting mortality risk

Several *risk stratification* tools estimate operative risk. Most institutions submit mandatory data to registries which may publish institution and *surgeon-specific risk-adjusted comparative outcome data*, i.e., mortality and complication rates which take into account certain patient comorbidities, demographic factors, and nature of surgery. Data is usually published in the format where raw mortality data for *index operations*, e.g., isolated CABG, is provided for individual institutions or surgeons, highlighting any that fall outside 2 standard deviations above or below the risk-adjusted mean. This may have contributed to lowering mortality rates, possibly through **risk-averse behaviour** leading to bias against high-risk patients. The main risk stratification systems used are:

- *EuroSCORE* (see inside front cover): based on European CABG patients, available as simple additive and as a more accurate logistic version, general tendency to overestimate operative risk.
- *STS* (Society of Thoracic Surgeons): similar model validated in North American patient groups, freely available as online calculator.
- *Parsonnet score*: one of the earliest systems, not widely used now.

Summary of preoperative management

Warfarin: stop 3–5 days preoperatively. In high-risk patients (e.g., mechanical valve) admit early and commence patient on heparin, which should be stopped 6 hours before surgery.

Aspirin and clopidogrel: aspirin should be stopped 5 days pre-op, clopidogrel 10 days pre-op in low-risk patients (see 🔲 p4).

ACE inhibitors: withhold on the day before surgery.

Diabetes: non-insulin-dependent diabetics should have normal medication, but withhold long-acting hypoglycaemics (gliclazide) on the morning of surgery. Insulin-dependent diabetics should be first on the list, and have their morning insulin replaced by a sliding scale and iv fluids.

Carotid bruits: obtain a carotid Doppler if the patient has a history of cerebrovascular accident (CVA), TIA, or severe peripheral vascular disease. Carotid intervention may be indicated for internal carotid stenoses >70% especially if the contralateral side is tightly stenosed, to reduce the risk of CVA (🔲 p279). Discuss with vascular surgeon. Maintain high perfusion pressures.

Murmurs: all patients should have recent pre-op TTE: review it!

Anemia: unexplained anemia requires full outpatient investigation. Surgeon may elect to prime the pump with blood rather than crystalloid. Patients are not normally transfused preoperatively.

Neutrophilia: valve patients should be cancelled and a source of infection found and treated. CABG may go ahead if the WCC <12.0 and the CRP is normal. Always discuss with the surgical team.

Respiratory impairment: admit high-risk patients for physiotherapy, nebulizers, and education.

Renal impairment: acute deterioration should be treated before surgery: stop nephrotoxic drugs including ACE inhibitors. Consider iv fluids.

MRSA: this should be treated preoperatively: consult the infection control team to ensure the appropriate treatment.

Lung lesions: these should be investigated preoperatively with a lateral film and CT. Isolated lung lesions of non-infective origin are not usually a contraindication to coronary artery surgery.

Applied basic science

Anatomy of the chest wall, airways, lungs and pleura, and esophagus are described in more detail on 📖 pp655–661. Embryology is described on 📖 pp528–535.

Surface anatomy

Bony landmarks

- The 1st rib is difficult to palpate as it lies under the clavicle. The 2nd rib articulates with the manubrium, just above the sternal angle. The 1st rib space is palpable just above and lateral to the sternal angle. The costal margin is formed by lower borders of ribs 7–10, and ends of 11 and 12. Important bony landmarks include cricoid cartilage (C6), suprasternal notch (T2), sternal angle (T4/5), xiphisternal joint (T9) anteriorly, and the 1st palpable spinous process (vertebra prominens), C7 (C1–6 are covered by the ligamentum nuchae), and the superior (T2) and inferior angle (T8) and spine (T3) of the scapula posteriorly.

Lines of orientation

The midclavicular line is a vertical line from the midpoint of the clavicle downwards. The anterior and posterior axillary lines are from anterior and posterior axillary folds downwards. The midaxillary line lies midway between the anterior and posterior axillary lines.

Surface markings of thoracic structures

Trachea

This commences at the lower border of the cricoid cartilage (C6), descending in the midline to end slightly to the right, bifurcating at the level of the sternal angle (T4/5) into left and right bronchi.

Lungs and pleurae

The apex of the pleura curves 2.5cm above the medial 1/3 of the clavicle. Lines of pleural reflection pass behind sternoclavicular joints meeting in the midline at the sternal angle. The right pleura passes down behind the 6th costal cartilage whereas the left, displaced by the heart, passes laterally for 2cm at the 4th costal cartilage then descending to the 6th costal cartilage lateral to the left sternal edge. From here both pleura run posteriorly crossing the 8th rib in the midclavicular line, the 10th rib in the midaxillary line and just below the 12th rib at the medial border of the erector spinae muscle posteriorly above the pleural reflections. This varies by 5–8cm in extremes of respiration. Both oblique fissures run from T3 posteriorly to the 6th costal cartilage in the midaxillary line. The horizontal fissure roughly follows the 5th rib.

Heart

The heart is bounded by the 2nd left costal cartilage, the 3rd right costal cartilage, the 6th right costal cartilage, and the 5th left costal cartilage.

Vessels

The internal thoracic arteries descend behind the costal cartilages, 1cm lateral to the sternal edge. The aortic arch arches anteroposteriorly behind the manubrium, the innominate, and left common carotid ascend posterior to the manubrium. The innominate veins are formed by the confluence of the internal jugular and subclavian veins posterior to the sternoclavicular joints. The SVC arises from the left and right innominate veins behind the 2nd and 3rd right costal cartilages.

Diaphragm

The highest part of the right hemidiaphragm reaches the upper border of the 5th rib in the midclavicular line in mid-inspiration. The left dome reaches the lower border of the 5th rib (see Fig. 2.1).

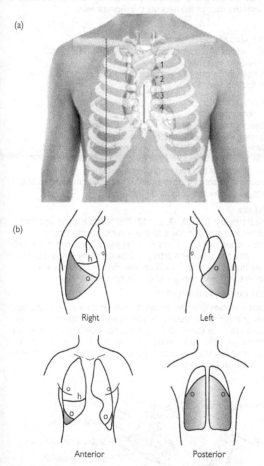

(a)

(b)

Right

Left

Anterior

Posterior

Fig. 2.1 (a) Surface markings of the heart and great vessels. Dotted line represents midaxillary line. Solid line represents standard low midline incision for full sternotomy. Numbers indicate intercostal spaces. (b) Surface markings of the lungs (shaded area represents lower lobe).

Thoracic bony cage

The thoracic cage

This is formed by the sternum and costal cartilages anteriorly, the vertebral column posteriorly, and the ribs and intercostal spaces laterally. It is separated from the abdominal cavity by the diaphragm and communicates superiorly with the root of the neck via the *thoracic inlet*.

Ribs

There are 12 pairs of ribs:
- 7 pairs of true ribs which articulate with the sternum via costal cartilages and the vertebrae.
- The false ribs whose cartilage articulates with that of the rib above.
- The false floating ribs 11 and 12.

Typical ribs

Typical ribs comprise:
- A head bearing two articular facets which articulate with the corresponding vertebrae and the one above.
- A neck which gives attachment to the costotransverse ligaments.
- A tubercle which has a smooth facet for articulation with the transverse process of the corresponding vertebrae.
- A long shaft with a costal groove in which the intercostal vessels and nerve runs, just *below* the body of the rib.

The atypical ribs

- The atypical ribs are 1, 2, 10, 11, and 12. The 1st rib is short and flat. The head has a single facet, the scalenus anterior inserts onto the prominent scalene tubercle. The subclavian vein passes over the 1st rib anterior to this, the subclavian artery and lowest trunk of the brachial plexus pass posteriorly (Fig. 2.2). A *cervical rib* is an extra rib which articulates with C7 posteriorly and the 1st rib anteriorly.

Intercostal nerves and arteries

The intercostal nerves are the anterior primary rami of the thoracic nerves. They give off a collateral muscular branch and lateral and anterior cutaneous branches (see Table 2.1). Posterior intercostal arteries are branches of the thoracic aorta, except for the first two which are arise from the costocervical trunk. The six anterior intercostals are branches of the internal mammary artery (IMA).

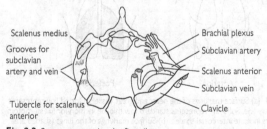

Scalenus medius

Grooves for subclavian artery and vein

Tubercle for scalenus anterior

Brachial plexus

Subclavian artery

Scalenus anterior

Subclavian vein

Clavicle

Fig. 2.2 Structures crossing the first rib.

Table 2.1 The muscles of the thoracic wall, innervation, and attachments

Muscle	Origin/insertion	Nerve (n.)/ artery (a.)	Action
Latissimus dorsi	Vertebral spines T7–sacrum, iliac crest, lower 4 ribs. Intertubercular groove	Thoracodorsal n. and a.	Extends arm, rotates medially
Serratus anterior	Ribs 1–9, medial border of scapula on costal surface	Long thoracic nerve of Bell (C5–7)	Draws scapula forward and rotates
Trapezius	Superior nuchal line, occipital protuberance, spinous processes C7–T12 Lateral 1/3 clavicle, scapular spine	Transverse cervical a. Spinal accessory n.	Elevates, depresses, retracts and rotates scapular superiorly
Diaphragm	Xiphoid, costal margin, lateral and medial arcuate ligaments, vertebral bodies 1–3/central tendon of diaphragm	C3–5 phrenic n. and a.	Descends to produce inspiration
Pectoralis major	Clavicle, manubrium and sternum, costal cartilages 2–6, rectus sheath. Crest of great tubercle of humerus	Pectoral n: C5–T1, pectoral a., thoracoacromial a.	Flexes, adducts, and medially rotates arm
External intercostals	Lower border of rib above/downwards and medially to upper border of rib below	Intercostals n. (T1–11) and a	Elevates ribcage and strengthens wall
Internal intercostals	Upper border of rib below/upwards and laterally to lower border of rib above	Intercostals n. (T1–11) and a.	Elevates and reinforces ribcage
Innermost intercostals	Same as internal intercostals but deep to the intercostal a. and n.	Intercostals n.(T1–11) and artery	Elevates and reinforces ribcage
Levators costarum	Transverse processes C7–11/rib below, medial to angle	Dorsal rami C7–11	Elevates the rib
Levator scapulae	C1–4 transverse processes, medial border scapula	Dorsal scapular n. and a.	Elevates scapula
Rhomboids min and maj	Ligamentum nuchae, spines C7–T1, T2–5 Medial border of scapula	Dorsal scapular n. and a.	Retracts, elevates and rotates the scapula inferiorly
Erector spinae	Iliac crest, sacrum, transverse, and spinous processes, supraspinal ligament, rib angles	Segmental C1–S5	Extends and laterally bends spine

Thoracic incisions

The chest may be entered via anterior, lateral, or posterior approaches.

Anterior incisions

- *Median sternotomy:* vertical midline incision from suprasternal notch
  to lower end of xiphoid. The sternum is divided using a sternal saw.
  - Identify midline: drape symmetrically so you can see landmarks, and
    palpate sternal notch, 2nd intercostal spaces, and xiphisternum
  - 23 blade to divide epidermis barely breaking fat (generally an
    incision from 3 fingerbreadths below sternal notch to the tip of
    xiphisternum is more than adequate for most cardiac surgery).
  - Cautery on 50W (fulgurate). Spread tissue with left hand and
    cauterize down to periosteum.
  - Repalpate midline landmarks and carefully incise midline of
    periosteum with cautery top to bottom: this marks a line for the saw.
  - Sweep pericardiacosternal ligaments from under xiphisternum with
    a finger. Insert sternal saw under xiphisternum, and lifting slightly
    upwards push it forwards to divide sternum. If a low incision you
    will need an assistant to retract skin at top. The saw can be used
    top to bottom, in which case there is no need to sweep under
    xiphisternum—instead, clear sternal notch of tissue.
  - The sternal saw is designed to stop if caught in soft tissue: so do
    not force it as you may end up opening the pericardium or worse.
  - Place pack under bone edges, cauterize periosteum, and use bone
    wax judiciously to stop bleeding marrow.
  - Re-sternotomy is described on 🕮 p345.
- *Transverse cervical or collar incision:* transverse incision midway
  between suprasternal notch and thyroid cartilage, along skin crease.
  This incision is used for thyroidectomy, tracheostomy (smaller and
  more inferior), and upper half tracheal resection and reconstruction.
- *Left anterior to sternocleidomastoid incision:* oblique incision anterior
  to the sternocleidomastoid incision, extending to the sternal notch.
  This incision is used for exposure of the cervical esophagus, or
  anterior cervical spine.
- *Dartevelle:* longitudinal incision along anterior border of
  sternocleidomastoid, continuing transversely across to the medial
  clavicle. The clavicle can be mobilized and distracted from the incision.
- *Anterior mediastinotomy:* transverse incision along 2nd intercostal
  space laterally from parasternal edge. Used for a Chamberlain
  mediastinal biopsy. Often the sternal–rib cartilage junction is removed.
  Care is taken to preserve the internal mammary artery.
- *Anterior thoracotomy:* transverse incision from parasternal edge
  along the inframammary crease to the anterior axillary line in the 4th
  interspace. The pectoralis major muscle can be elevated off the chest.
- *Thoracosternotomy ('clamshell'):* incision from anterior axillary line
  along submammary crease bilaterally elevating in the midline to
  the level of the nipple (🕮 p819). As an anterior thoracotomy, the
  pectoralis major can be elevated and raised a flap. The sternum is
  divided transversely, and reconstructed with wires ± pins.

Lateral and posterior incisions

- *Axillary thoracotomy:* curvilinear incision at the inferior border of axillary hairline between lateral border of pectoralis major and anterior border of latissimus dorsi.
- *Lateral 'muscle-sparing' thoracotomy:* lazy 'S': incision along submammary crease starting below nipple passing upwards towards the axilla.
- *French:* incision along submammary crease from below nipple to 2cm below tip of scapula. The muscle-sparing thoracotomy is characterized by mobilization and preservation of the latissimus dorsi muscle. The serratus anterior muscle is divided in the direction of its fibres.
- *Lateral thoracotomy:* curvilinear incision passing from anterior axillary line to 2cm below tip of scapula.
- *Posterolateral thoracotomy:* curvilinear incision from anterior axillary line passing 3–4cm below tip of scapula and continuing superiorly midway between medial border of scapula and spinous processes of vertebral column. This standard 'workhorse' incision usually involves division of the latissimus dorsi muscle, and distal division (or sparing) of the serratus anterior muscle.
- *Thoracoabdominal incision:* oblique incision as for posterolateral incision but extending anteriorly across the costal margin at the level of the 7th interspace towards the midline.

Operative positions

- *Lateral decubitus position* (side up): most common position used in thoracic surgery. Allows the best surgical access to and control of structures in the hilum. Ventilation of the contralateral dependent lung may be more troublesome than with other positions. The ipsilateral arm is extended, and rested on a cushioned platform or multiple folded blankets. Care must be taken to avoid stretch of the ipsilateral brachial plexus from overextension, as well as crush of the down brachial plexus. This may be avoided by placement of a transverse shoulder roll, just inferior to the down axilla. The bed is flexed to spread the intercostal space, and drop the ipsilateral hip out of the way. All pressure points are padded, and in males the testicles are distracted anteriorly.
- *Prone* (face down): allows access to the posterior structures, specifically the spine and esophagus. Major vessels are furthest away from operator and access to the hilum is limited. Care is taken to avoid ocular pressure.
- *Supine* (face up): sternotomy easier with roll under shoulders.
- *Fowler's:* patient on back, sitting up at about 45–60°, usually with arms extended on boards. Allows video-assisted thoracic surgery (VATS) approach to both pleura, and head-up tilt helps lung fall away from apex to allow apical procedures such as sympathectomy (📖 p804).

Mediastinum

Key facts

- The mediastinum is the space between the pleural sacs.
- It is divided by a line drawn horizontally from the sternal angle to the lower border of T4, into **superior** (bounded by the thoracic inlet above) and *inferior* **mediastinum** (bounded by the diaphragm below).
- The inferior mediastinum is further divided by the pericardial sac into anterior, middle, and posterior (Fig. 2.3a).

Contents of the mediastinum

- *Superior mediastinum:* great vessels, trachea, esophagus, phrenic nerve and vagus nerve, thoracic duct.
- *Anterior mediastinum:* sternopericardial ligaments, thymus, lymph nodes
- *Middle mediastinum:* pericardial cavity, heart, great vessels, phrenic nerve.
- *Posterior mediastinum:* esophagus, descending aorta, azygos veins, thoracic duct, lymph nodes.

Relationships of the heart

- *Anteriorly:* sternum, costal cartilages of ribs 3–5, anterior lungs.
- *Laterally:* lungs and hila.
- *Posteriorly:* esophagus, tracheal bifurcation, main bronchi, descending aorta, and vertebrae T5–T8.
- *Inferiorly:* diaphragm and liver.
- *Superiorly:* great vessels.

Pericardium and its reflections

The pericardium has three layers: one fibrous and two internal serous (parietal and visceral) separated by pericardial fluid. The heart and proximal great vessels are contained within the conical fibrous pericardium. The apex fuses with the adventitia of the vessels and the base fuses with the central tendon of the diaphragm. The fibrous pericardium is lined inside by the parietal serous pericardium which is reflected around the great vessels becoming continuous with the visceral layer of pericardium. The lines of reflection define the oblique sinus (bounded by the IVC and four pulmonary veins) and the transverse sinus (bounded by the SVC, LA, pulmonary trunk, and aorta) posteriorly (Fig. 2.3).

Vagus nerve

The vagus nerve contains visceral afferent fibres from the heart, lower respiratory tract and gut, and efferent pre-ganglionic parasympathetic motor fibres to the pharynx, larynx, heart, and smooth muscles of the bronchi and gut. It passes vertically down from the jugular foramen to the root of the neck lying posteriorly in the carotid sheath between the internal jugular vein and the internal then common carotid. In the neck it gives pharyngeal, superior laryngeal, and superior and inferior cardiac branches.

On the right side the recurrent laryngeal branch arises as the vagus crosses the subclavian artery. The vagus descends through the superior mediastinum passing behind the hilum of the right lung to the pulmonary plexus and then the esophageal plexus. The left vagus crosses the arch of the aorta giving off the recurrent laryngeal nerve, which passes below the ligamentum arteriosum, behind the arch and then ascends in the groove between trachea and esophagus. The vagus passes behind the left lung hilum to form the pulmonary and esophageal plexuses. The vagi leave the thorax via the esophageal diaphragmatic opening. The subclavian loop carries afferents from the stellate ganglion to the eye and head, running adjacent to the subclavian bilaterally.

Phrenic nerve

The phrenic nerve contains visceral afferents from the heart and diaphragm, as well as motor efferents from the dorsal rami of C3–5. It enters the thoracic inlet on the anterior surface of the anterior scalene muscle, lying just posterior to the IMA. On the right side the phrenic travels down the front of the SVC descending anterior to the hilum before reflecting onto the right diaphragm. The left phrenic nerve follows a similar course.

Thoracic sympathetic plexus

This lies lateral to the posterior mediastinum behind the parietal pleurae, crossing the necks of the first ribs, the heads of the 2nd–10th ribs and the bodies of the 11th and 12th vertebrae entering the diaphragm to continue as the lumbar sympathetic trunk. It distributes sympathetic branches to the skin, post-ganglionic fibres to thoracic viscera, and pre-ganglionic fibres to the celiac and renal ganglions below the diaphragm.

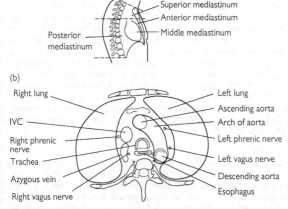

Fig. 2.3 (a) S(ubdivisions of the mediastinum; (b) Cross-section through the mediastinum at T4.

Cardiac chambers

Right atrium

The RA receives venous drainage from four sources:
- The *SVC* superiorly, draining the azygos, jugular, and subclavian veins.
- The *IVC* inferiorly, draining the lower body.
- The *coronary sinus* inferiorly, draining the heart.
- The *anterior cardiac vein* anteriorly, draining the front of the heart.

Running vertically downwards between the IVC and SVC is the *crista terminalis*, a muscular ridge marked externally by the sulcus terminalis. The *sinus node* lies at the superior end of the terminal groove, where the atrial appendage meets the SVC. The crista terminalis separates the smooth-walled posterior RA derived from the *sinus venosus* from the trabeculated appendage, derived from the fetal RA. The IVC and coronary sinus have rudimentary valves (the *Eustachian* and *Thebesian valves* respectively). The Eustachian valve is continuous with the annulus ovalis which surrounds the *fossa ovalis*. It is also continuous with the Thebesian valve via the *tendon of Todaro*.

The triangle of Koch (Fig. 2.4)

The apex of this long narrow triangle identifies the AV node, and proximal portion of the bundle of His. The triangle is formed by:
- *Short base:* coronary sinus and Thebesian valve.
- *Long upper side:* septal leaflet of the tricuspid valve.
- *Long lower side:* tendon of Todaro.

Right ventricle

The RV consists of a large inlet (sinus) and a smaller outlet (conus) portion separated by the *supraventricular crest*. The inlet portion surrounds the tricuspid valve and its subvalvular apparatus. The inflow tract is characterized by *trabeculae carnae*, from some of which *papillary* muscles project, attaching to the inferior border of the tricuspid valve leaflets via *tendinae chordae*. The *moderator band* is a muscular bundle crossing the ventricular cavity from the interventricular septum to the anterior wall, conveying the right branch of the AV bundle to the ventricular muscle. The outlet portion is smooth walled and consists of the *infundibulum* (a muscular structure that supports the *pulmonary valve*), the superior part of the septal band, and a very narrow portion superior to the trabecular septum. The thick, muscular supraventricular crest separates the pulmonary valve from the tricuspid valve.

Left atrium

The LA is smaller than the right with thicker walls. The four pulmonary veins open into the upper part of its posterior wall. On its septal surface there is a 'flap' valve which corresponds to the fossa ovalis. The *left atrial appendage* is characterized by *pectinate muscles*. It is longer and narrower-based than the wide-based right atrial appendage, so in AF blood has a greater tendency to stagnate inside and form thrombi.

Left ventricle

The LV consists of a large trabeculated inlet (sinus) and a smaller smooth-walled outlet portion. In comparison to the well-separated pulmonary and tricuspid valve, the aortic and mitral valve are in **fibrous continuity**. Most of the inlet portion is finely trabeculated with **anterolateral** (anterior) and **posteromedial** (posterior) **papillary muscles** connecting to the mitral valve leaflets via **tendinae chordae**.

Atrial septum

Although at first glance it looks as though the lateral RA wall between the IVC and SVC is the atrial septum, the true septum is virtually confined to the **fossa ovalis**. The superior rim of the fossa is commonly referred to as the **septum secundum**, but it is really an infolding between the right atrium and the pulmonary veins.

Ventricular septum

The ventricular septal surfaces are asymmetrical firstly because of the infundibular portion of the RV, secondly because of the differing long axis of RV (vertical) and LV (oblique), and the pressure differential between RV and LV. It is made up of a **muscular septum, a membranous septum**, and the **atrioventricular septum**. The atrioventricular septum lies between the right atrium and the left ventricle. The **AV node** lies in the atrial septum adjacent to the junction between the membranous and muscular portions of the atrioventricular septum, and the **bundle of His** passes toward the **right fibrous trigone** between these components.

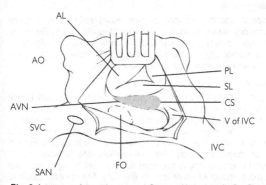

Fig. 2.4 Interior of the right atrium: AO aorta, AL anterior leaflet, PL posterior leaflet and SL septal leaflet of tricuspid valve, AVN atrioventricular node, SVC superior vena cava, FO foramen ovale, IVC inferior vena cava, V of IVC Esutacian valve, CS coronary sinus, T tendon of Todaro, TK triangle of Koch.

Cardiac valves

Key facts

The valves occupy a central position between the mitral and tricuspid valves, with the pulmonary valve slightly superior, anterior, and to the left. The valves are thin folds of endocardium covered by endothelium. All cardiac valves share the same basic histological structure:

- Thin ventricular layer (radially aligned collagen fibers).
- Central spongiosa (loosely arranged collagen and proteoglycans).
- Thick fibrous layer (densely packed fibers arranged parallel to the leaflet edge) which provides structural integrity and stability.
- Thin upper collagenous layer.
- The aortic and pulmonary valve leaflets are nearly avascular: they are thin enough to be perfused from surrounding blood, whereas the mitral and tricuspid valves contain a few capillaries.

Tricuspid valve

This has an anterior, a septal, and a posterior leaflet. The orifice is triangular, larger than the mitral valve, and the annulus is much less well defined. The leaflets and chordae are thinner than the mitral valve. The chordae to the largest anterior leaflet arise from the anterior and medial papillary muscles. The posterior leaflet is the smallest, most inferior, and is usually scalloped. The chordae to the septal leaflet arise from the posterior and septal papillary muscles. The conduction system is closely related to the septal leaflet (Fig. 2.5).

Pulmonary valve

This is made of right, left, and anterior (non-septal) leaflets. The structure of the pulmonary valve is similar to the aortic valve, with three differences. Firstly, the valve leaflets are flimsier than the aortic valve; secondly, coronary arteries do not originate from the sinuses; and thirdly, the valve is not in continuity with the anterior tricuspid valve leaflet.

Mitral valve

This bicuspid valve has a large anterior (aortic or septal) leaflet and a small posterior (mural or ventricular) leaflet. The leaflet area is much greater than the valve area, allowing a large area for coaptation, distinguished as a rough zone. The larger anterior leaflet inserts on only a third of the annulus, through which it is fibrous continuity with the left and half of the non-coronary cusp of the aortic valve. The smaller posterior leaflet inserts into 2/3 of the annulus and is scalloped. Each leaflet is segmented into three for the purposes of nomenclature (Fig. 2.5). The chordae tendinae insert into both leaflets from the anterolateral and posteromedial papillary muscles. There are three orders of chordae: 1st (marginal) insert onto the leaflet free margin, 2nd order insert a few millimeters further back, and 3rd (basal) insert at the base of the posterior leaflet only.

Aortic valve

This tricuspid valve is in fibrous continuity with the anterior leaflet of the mitral valve and the membranous septum. The free edge of each cusp is thickest and at the midpoint of each free edge is a fibrous nodulus arantii,

(a)

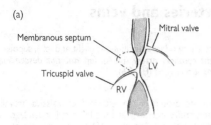

(b)

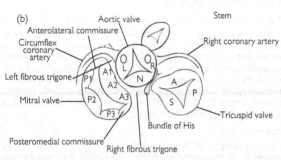

Fig. 2.5 (a) Atrioventricular junction: note the septal atttachment of the tricuspid valve is lower than the septal attachment of the mitral valve. (b) Cardiac valves and their relationships viewed from above, with the atria removed. Note how the commissure of the left (L) and the noncoronary (N) sinuses of the aortic valve points at the midpoint of the anterior leaflet of the mitral valve (A2). The circumflex coronary artery is particularly close to the posterior mitral annulus in the P3, P2 segment. The right coronary artery is close to anterior tricuspid annulus. The bundle of His lies in the membranous septum near the right fibrous trigone located at the junction of the right (R) and the non-coronary cusp (N), extending to the antero-septal commissure of the tricuspid valve.

bordered on either side by crescent-shaped lunula which form the region of coaptation. The aortic sinuses (sinuses of Valsalva) are dilated, relatively thin-walled, pockets of the aortic root, two of which give rise to the coronary arteries. Because of the shape of the cusps the annulus is crown shaped. The cusps are called right, left, and non-coronary, based on the origin of the coronary arteries (Fig. 2.5).

Fibrous trigones

The mitral and tricuspid annuli are in fibrous continuity with each other and the membranous septum, forming the fibrous skeleton of the heart. The central fibrous trigones lie between the mitral and tricuspid valves (Fig. 2.5): the right trigone sits between the mitral and tricuspid annuli, the non-coronary cusp of the aortic valve and the membranous septum. The left fibrous trigone lies between the ventriculoaortic junction and the mitral annulus. The bundle of His pierces the right fibrous trigone.

Coronary arteries and veins

Key facts
The coronary arteries are two main distributions (right and left), supplied by three vessels; *right coronary artery* (RCA), *left anterior descending* (LAD), *and circumflex artery* (Cx) (Fig. 2.6).

Left main stem
The LMS arises from the ostium of the left sinus of Valsalva, travels between the pulmonary trunk anteriorly and the left atrial appendage to the left AV groove, dividing after 1–2cm into LAD, Cx, and occasionally a third artery: the intermediate (Int).

Left anterior descending
The LAD runs down the anterior interventricular groove to the apex of the heart, usually extending round the apex to the posterior interventricular groove and the territory of the PDA. A variable number of *diagonals* are given off over the anterior surface of the LV, small branches supply the anterior surface of the RV, and superior *septals* are given off perpendicularly to supply the anterior 2/3 of the interventricular septum. The first septal is the largest. Some of the RV branches anastomose with infundibular branches of the proximal RCA: *loop of Vieussens*.

Circumflex
The Cx originates at 90° from the LMS and runs medially to the LA appendage for 2–3cm, continuing in the posterior left AV groove to the crux of the heart. In left dominant hearts (5–10%) the Cx turns 90° into the posterior interventricular groove to form the posterior descending artery (PDA). In 85–90% of hearts the PDA arises from the RCA (right dominant). About 5% of hearts are co-dominant. A variable number of *obtuse marginals* (OM) arise from the Cx to supply the posterior LV. They are frequently intramuscular. The first branch of the Cx is the *AV nodal artery* in 45% which courses round the LA near the AV groove.

Right coronary artery
The RCA arises from an ostium in the right sinus of Valsalva, gives off an *infundibular branch* and then a branch to the *SA node* early, and runs immediately into the deep right AV groove where it gives off *RV branches* to the anterior RV wall. The *acute marginal* is a large branch which crosses the acute margin of the heart to travel to the apex. In right dominant hearts the RCA reaches the crux of the hearts where it turns 90° to form the *PDA*, which runs towards the apex in the posterior interventricular groove. *Inferior septals* which supply the inferior 1/3 of the interventricular septum arise at 90° from the PDA. The *AV node artery* is given off by the RCA in 55% at the crux. One or more *right posterolateral branches* (RPLSs) supply the LV.

Venous drainage of the heart
The coronary sinus runs in the posterior AV groove draining into the RA with the great cardiac vein. Thebesian veins empty directly into the heart.

Variations in coronary anatomy

- Right dominant 90%, left dominant 5%, co-dominant 5%.
- Absent LMS with separate ostia for the Cx and the LAD (1%).
- LAD or RCA represented by 2 separate parallel vessels (2%).
- SA node artery arising from the Cx (2–3%).
- SA node artery may travel round the SVC clockwise or anticlockwise, or bifurcate and travel in both directions (Fig. 2.6b).
- AV node artery from RCA (55%) from Cx (45%).

Variations causing ischemia

- *ALCAPA* (anomalous left coronary artery from the pulmonary artery <0.01%) and coronary ostial atresia cause severe ischemia. Untreated, most patients die in infancy. If large collateral network patients may survive to adulthood: treatment for adults is CABG.
- *ACAOS* (anomalous origin of a coronary artery from the opposite sinus), e.g., origin of the LMS from the RCA then passing between RVOT and aorta (or anterior to the PA, or posterior to the aorta) may cause intermittent ischemia and sudden death during or shortly after exercise, due to increased blood flow and pressure in these arteries during exercise, slit-like ostium. CABG traditional approach.

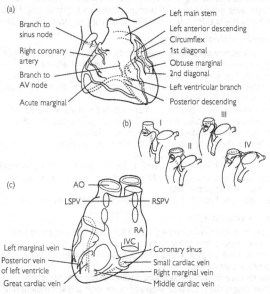

(a)

Branch to sinus node
Right coronary artery
Branch to AV node
Acute marginal

Left main stem
Left anterior descending
Circumflex
1st diagonal
Obtuse marginal
2nd diagonal
Left ventricular branch
Posterior descending

(b) I II III IV

(c)

AO
LSPV — RSPV
RA
IVC
Left marginal vein — Coronary sinus
Posterior vein of left ventricle — Small cardiac vein
Great cardiac vein — Right marginal vein
Middle cardiac vein

Fig. 2.6 (a) Coronary arteries. (b) Variations in the sinus node artery, which may arise from the right coronary artery (60%) and encircle the base of the superior vena cava in a clockwise (I), anticlockwise (II) or both (III) directions, or arise from the left coronary artery (40% of cases) (IV). (c) Coronary veins.

Lung anatomy

Lobes

- The right lung has three lobes: an upper, a middle, and a lower lobe.
- The smaller left lung has two lobes: an upper, and a lower lobe.

The lingular segment of the left upper lobe corresponds to the right middle lobe. An azygos lobe is found in up to 1% of lungs in the right upper lobe. It is formed from varying portions of the apical and/or posterior segments by an aberrant azygos vein and its pleural mesentery. The fissure is visible on the chest radiograph as an inverted comma.

Fissures

- The right lung has two fissures: an oblique and a transverse fissure.
- The left lung has one fissure: the oblique fissure.

The oblique fissure separates the upper lobe (and middle lobe on the right) from the lower lobe on each side. The transverse fissure separates the upper lobe from the middle lobe on the right. It is often incomplete.

Bronchopulmonary segments

- A bronchopulmonary segment is a portion of lung which functions as an individual unit, having its own artery and bronchus. There are 18.
- The right lung is divided into 10 bronchopulmonary segments (Fig. 13.2).
- The left lung is divided into 8 bronchopulmonary segments (Fig. 13.2).

Tracheobronchial anatomy

The trachea commences at the lower border of the cricoid cartilage (C6) and terminates at the carina (T7) dividing into right and left main bronchi.

- Right main bronchus is 1.2cm long.
- After the upper lobe bronchial orifice arises, the bronchus intermedius (BI) is given off. It is ~2cm long.
- The middle lobe bronchus arises from anterior surface of the BI, and the superior segmental bronchus to the lower lobe arises from the posterior wall of the distal BI below the middle lobe.
- The BI then divides to form the basal segmental bronchi.
- The left main bronchus is 4–6cm long.
- After the upper lobe bronchial orifice the left main bronchus continues as the lower lobe bronchus: its first branch is the superior segmental bronchus, arising posteriorly.
- The lower lobe bronchus divides to form the basal segmental bronchi.

Tracheal anatomy

- The average adult male trachea is 10–13cm in length, measured from the lower edge of the cricoid ring to the carina.
- 1/3 of the adult trachea is above the sternal notch, with the balance an intrathoracic structure.
- In the absence of congenital tracheal stenosis, the only complete tracheal ring is the cricoid cartilage; all other rings are incomplete ring of cartilage with a posterior membranous wall.

- There are 18–22 D-shaped partial rings. The cartilaginous rings are softer in the pediatric population, and can become calcified with age.
- The arterial supply of the trachea is segmental, or entering via lateral pedicles. Dissection of the trachea should be limited to anterior and posterior planes. In the absence of tracheal resection, circumferential dissection should be limited to 1–2cm to avoid ischemic necrosis.

Upper half of trachea
- Tracheoesophageal branches of the inferior thyroid artery.
- Rarely, branches from the subclavian arteries.

Middle to lower trachea and carina
- Branches from the supreme intercostal artery, subclavian artery, right internal mammary artery, innominate artery.
- Branches from the bronchial arteries.

Pulmonary vessels

Pulmonary trunk
- This arises intrapericardially from the infundibulum of the RV. It continues superioposteriorly to the left for approximately 5cm as the main pulmonary artery. It bifurcates just below the aortic arch.

Right pulmonary artery
- Passes posterior to aorta and SVC. Initially anterior and inferior to right main bronchus, and superior and posterior to the superior pulmonary vein. It gives off three branches: (1) truncus anterior branch to upper lobe, (2) middle lobe artery arises anteromedially and distal to the truncus anterior, (3) posterolaterally at a similar level the superior segmental branch to the lower lobe arises. The artery distal to this becomes the common basal trunk which divides to form the basal segmental vessels.

Left pulmonary artery
- This passes laterally and posteriorly under the aortic arch before giving off the upper lobe branches, usually four. The most distal branch to the upper lobe is the lingular branch. Posteriorly at the level of the fissure the branch supplying the superior segment of the lower lobe arises. Distal to this the vessel becomes the common basal trunk and subsequently divides into two main vessels supplying the lower lobe segments.

Pulmonary veins
- There are two pulmonary veins on each side, a superior and an inferior. The veins drain into the LA. At the hilum the right superior pulmonary vein is anteroinferior to the artery. It usually drains the upper and middle lobes. Inferoposteriorly lies the inferior vein. It drains the lower lobe and rarely the middle lobe. The middle lobe may have its own vein which enters the right atrium separate to the superior pulmonary vein. At the hilum the left superior vein is anteroinferior to the artery. It drains the upper lobe including the lingular segments. Occasionally the lingular segments drain into the inferior vein.

Bronchial arterial system
- This arises from systemic circulation, from various arterial origins. Drainage is into the pulmonary venous system, azygos, and hemiazygos veins.

Anatomy of the esophagus

The esophagus is a continuation of the pharynx, arising at the level of C6 and the cricoid cartilage, and ending at the stomach at T11. It attaches superiorly to cricoid cartilage and inferiorly to the diaphragm. The average length from cricopharyngeus muscle to gastroesophageal junction is 25cm in males and 23cm in females. The average length from incisor teeth to cricopharyngeus is 15cm in males and 14cm in females (Fig. 13.4). The length from incisor teeth to middle indentation is 24–26cm. These measurements are important landmarks when accurately describing the position of lesions in the esophagus at esophagoscopy. There are three regions of narrowing/indentations along its length:

* At the origin, caused by cricopharyngeus.
* The middle indentation, caused by aortic arch and left main bronchus.
* At the distal end, caused by the lower esophageal sphincter at the diaphragm

Relationships in the thorax

The esophagus enters the thorax through the thoracic inlet. It is intimately related to the prevertebral fascia down to the tracheal bifurcation. It moves slightly to the right just above the bifurcation, then passes posterior to the pericardium in line with the left atrium to reach the esophageal opening in the diaphragm. At the diaphragm the thoracic duct lies behind the esophagus. As it ascends in the thorax it gradually moves to the left of the esophagus. It passes dorsal to the aortic arch and drains into the venous system at the union of the left subclavian and internal jugular veins (see Fig. 2.7).

Musculature of the esophagus

* The upper part consists of striated muscle fibres only. Smooth muscle fibres increase in number on descending the esophagus until they constitute the entire musculature. There is an outer longitudinal and an inner thicker circular layer of muscle, allowing effective peristalsis.

Arterial supply

* Cervical esophagus: inferior thyroid artery.
* Thoracic esophagus: bronchial arteries. Two esophageal branches also typically arise directly from the descending aorta.
* Abdominal esophagus: inferior phrenic and esophageal branches of inferior gastric arteries.
* There is an extensive intramural arterial network allowing mobilization without devascularization.

Venous drainage

* A submucosal venous plexus drains into periesophageal venous plexus which then forms the esophageal veins. In the cervical region the esophagus drains into the inferior thyroid vein, in the thorax into the azygos, hemiazygos, and bronchial veins, in the abdominal region into the coronary vein. There is continuity between esophageal and stomach venous networks, important in portal hypertension.

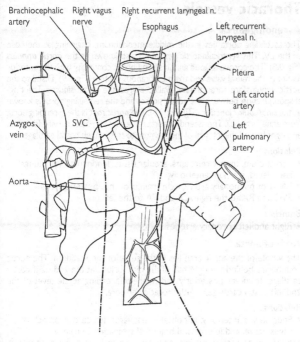

Brachiocephalic artery
Right vagus nerve
Right recurrent laryngeal n.
Esophagus
Left recurrent laryngeal n.
Pleura
Left carotid artery
Azygos vein
SVC
Left pulmonary artery
Aorta

Fig. 2.7 Relationships of trachea, esophagus, and great vessels in the mediastinum.

Nerve supply

Parasympathetic supply
Vagus nerve–recurrent laryngeal nerves superiorly, esophageal plexus inferiorly.

Sympathetic supply
The pharyngeal plexus receives fibres from the superior cervical ganglion. Postganglionic fibres from the cervical and thoracic sympathetic chain then reach the esophagus. The distal esophagus also receives sympathetic fibres from the celiac ganglion.

Thoracic vessels

Ascending aorta

The ascending aorta lies in the middle mediastinum, beginning at the base of the LV. This **ventriculoaortic junction** is also known as the **aortic annulus** (Fig. 2.8). The corona-shaped annulus is in fibrous continuity with the anterior leaflet of the mitral valve and the membranous septum (Fig. 8.9). Distal to the aortic annulus are three thinner-walled bulges: the **aortic sinuses**. The ring-shaped junction between the aortic sinuses and the remaining aorta is known as the **sinotubular junction (STJ)** (Fig. 2.8). The **aortic root** is the ascending aorta from annulus to STJ. The ascending aorta carries on for ~5cm, curving forwards and right behind the left half of the sternum to the 2nd left costal cartilage.

Relations
- Pericardium, thymic remnants, areolar tissue, innominate vein, lungs and pleura, sternum anteriorly.
- LA, right pulmonary artery, right main bronchus posteriorly.
- SVC and RA to the right, LA and PA to the left.

Branches
- Right and left coronary arteries.

Arch of aorta

The whole of the aortic arch lies in the superior mediastinum. The aortic arch begins behind the right half of the manubrium, at the 2nd right costal cartilage. It curves posteriorly and to the left, ending at the level of the 2nd left costal cartilage, or 4th thoracic vertebra.

Relations
- Four nerves anteriorly: left phrenic, left vagus, left cardiac branch of vagus nerve, and left cervical branch of sympathetic chain.
- Four nerves posteriorly: left recurrent laryngeal nerve (given off by left vagus nerve, looping back under the aortic arch), deep cardiac plexus, right vagus nerve and right phrenic nerve (separated from the aortic arch by the trachea and SVC respectively).
- Four structures posteriorly: trachea, esophagus, vertebral bodies, thoracic duct.

Branches
Brachiocephalic artery, left common carotid artery, left subclavian artery, occasionally thyroidea IMA artery, bronchial arteries.

Descending thoracic aorta

The descending aorta lies in the posterior mediastinum. It begins at the level of the 4th thoracic vertebra, ending at the 12th thoracic vertebral border, where it passes through the diaphragm to become the abdominal aorta. It goes from being to the left of the vertebral column superiorly, to being directly anterior to it at the level of the diaphragm.

Relations
- Left pulmonary hilum, LA, esophagus, diaphragm anteriorly.
- Vertebral column and hemiazygos veins posteriorly.
- Azygos vein, thoracic duct, and lower esophagus to the right.
- Pleura and left lung to the left.

Branches
Pericardial branches, right and left bronchial arteries, which run posteriorly on the bronchi, four or five esophageal arteries, mediastinal and phrenic branches, nine paired posterior intercostal arteries (see also 📖 p36), paired subcostal arteries.

Inferior vena cava
Conveys blood to the RA from all structures below diaphragm. Formed by the junction of the common iliac veins, ascends anterior to the vertebral column, to the right of the aorta. It traverses the posterior surface of the liver via a deep groove, piercing the tendinous part of the diaphragm and pericardium to enter the RA. Collateral circulations exist between epigastric, internal thoracic, hemiazygos, azygos, and pelvic veins.

Superior vena cava
Returns blood from upper half of the body. Formed by junction of the brachiocephalic veins, and receives azygos vein before entering the pericardium. It is valveless. Descends behind the 1st to the 3rd right costal cartilage. The right pulmonary hilum is posterior, the right phrenic nerve is right lateral, and the trachea and right vagus nerve lie posteromedial.

Azygos vein
Returns blood from the posterior thoracic wall, esophagus, bronchi, pericardium and mediastinal lymph nodes. Variable origin. Ascends anterior to thoracic vertebrae in the posterior mediastinum to T4, where it arches over the right pulmonary hilum ending in the SVC, which it enters 1–2cm distal to junction with RA posteriorly.

Hemiazygos and accessory hemiazygos veins
The hemiazygos ascends on the left like the azygos vein, crossing the vertebral column posterior to the aorta at a variable level to end in the azygos vein. The accessory hemiazygos vein descends to the left of the upper vertebral column, crossing at T7 to join the azygos vein.

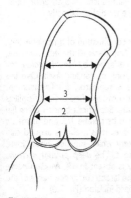

Fig. 2.8 Aortic root dimensions. 1) Annulus, 2) sinuses, 3) sinotubular junction, 4) ascending aorta. Drawn by Marcia Williams.

Vascular anatomy and pathology

Peripheral cannulation sites

Axillary artery and vein

The axillary artery, which is less prone to atherosclerosis or aneurysm than the aorta or femoral artery, is located deep to the deltopectoral groove (Fig. 2.9). Vein lies caudal to artery. The *subclavian artery* becomes the axillary artery at the 1st rib lateral margin. Divided into three parts by *pectoralis minor*. 1st part proximal to pectoralis minor, has one branch: superior thoracic artery. 2nd part posterior to pectoralis minor has two branches: thoracoacromial and lateral thoracic artery. 3rd distal part has three branches: subscapular (largest), anterior and posterior circumflex humeral arteries. Three cords of *brachial plexus* wrap around 2nd part: lateral cord contains C5–C7, medial cord (ulnar nerve) contains C8–T1, posterior cord (axillary and radial nerve) contains C5–T1 contributions.

Femoral artery and vein

Located at midinguinal point: femoral nerve laterally, femoral vein medial. The *profunda femoris* is its largest branch originating from its lateral side in the femoral triangle, and running posteriorly. More vasospastic in young patients, and more atherosclerotic in elderly than aorta or axillary artery.

Conduit

Internal mammary artery

Arises inferiorly from left *subclavian* artery 2cm above the sternal clavicle, opposite the thyrocervical trunk. Descends anteromedially behind the clavicle and *brachiocephalic veins* and 1st costal cartilage, between two venae comitantes. Crossed by *phrenic nerve* from lateral to medial as it enters thorax. Descends vertically over the first six costal cartilages, bifurcating into the *superior epigastric* and *musculophrenic arteries* at the xiphisternal junction. Separated from pleurae after 3rd rib by fascia and transversus thoracis. *Intercostal nerves* cross it anteriorly in each rib space. Pericardiacophrenic artery is proximal branch. Two anterior intercostal branches per rib space. RIMA is more medial proximally.

Radial artery

Smaller than ulnar artery, but a more direct continuation of *brachial artery*, beginning medial to the neck of the radius, 1cm distal to the elbow crease, 1–2cm distal to the bicipital aponeurosis. Overlapped by *brachioradialis* for the proximal 2/3 (Fig. 7.6). Distal 1/3 covered only by skin and fascia. Overlies (from proximal to distal) the tendon of biceps, supinator, distal attachment of pronator teres, radial head of flexor digitorum superficialis, flexor pollicis longus, pronator quadratus, and distal radius. Superficial branch of *radial nerve* is closely related to the radial artery in its middle 1/3, and filaments of *lateral cutaneous nerve* of forearm run over it as it curves around carpus. The 1st branch is *recurrent radial artery* which supplies elbow joint. Muscular branches are distributed throughout. The *deep palmar arch* via which it anastomoses with the ulnar artery is absent in 3%. *Median nerve* lies deep to flexor digitorum superficialis. The lateral cutaneous nerve of the forearm lies lateral and parallel to the standard incision (Fig. 7.6).

Long and short saphenous veins
Continuation of medial marginal vein, 2cm anterior to **medial malleolus**, crossing distal 1/3 of medial surface of tibia ascending just posterior to the tibial border to knee (Fig. 7.1a). Here it lies 2cm posteromedial to medial tibial and femoral condyles. Ascends medial aspect of thigh traversing the saphenous opening to empty into femoral vein. The saphenous opening is located ~3cm inferolateral to pubic tubercle. Receives multiple tributaries, particularly around knee, from superficial and deep veins. The vein may be duplicated in the lower leg, and contains 10–20 valves. The **saphenous nerve** distally and the **median femoral cutaneous nerve** proximally are closely associated, as is the saphenous branch of the genicular artery at the knee. **Short saphenous vein** commences 1cm posterior to lateral malleolus running lateral to Achilles tendon, ascending in midline with **sural nerve**, to join popliteal vein in popliteal fossa (Fig. 7.5a).

Conduit pathophysiology and patency
- Conduit patency (📖 p302) is dictated by three main factors: (1) technical factors (📖 p323), (2) targets, i.e., distal run-off (📖 p323) and severity of stenosis being bypassed (📖 p323), and (3) intrinsic qualities of the conduit
- There are several intrinsic differences between the IMA, radial artery, and SVG that may contribute to the different patency rates observed:
  - IMA has non-fenestrated elastic lamina that may reduce cellular migration and intimal hyperplasia (📖 p323) whereas the radial artery and SVG have fenestrated elastic lamina.
  - IMA thinner and less vasoreactive muscular layer than radial artery (it does not vasoconstrict in response to norepinephrine), and also reduced proliferative response: so less prone to early vasospasm.
  - Unlike SVG and radial, IMA adapts in response to flow over time.
  - SVG has a lower propensity to spasm than arterial conduit, but reduced endothelial resistance to thrombosis and atherosclerosis.

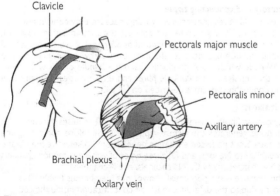

Clavicle

Pectorals major muscle

Pectoralis minor

Axillary artery

Brachial plexus

Axilary vein

Fig. 2.9 The axillary artery.

Myocardium

Specialized cardiac tissues

The heart is composed of three cardiac muscle types: atrial muscle, ventricular muscle, and specialized excitatory and conductive muscle.

Atrial and ventricular muscle

The basic unit of the cardiac contractile apparatus is the *sarcomere*. This is the part of a *myofibril* lying between adjacent Z discs. Cardiac muscle fibres are composed of hundreds of myofibrils containing several thousand *actin* and *myosin filaments*, the protein polymers responsible for muscle contraction. Actin filaments are made of three proteins: actin, *troponin*, and tropomyosin. The ends of the actin filaments connect to a strip of protein filaments called the *Z disk*, which passes from one myofibril to another, connecting to all the myofibrils across the muscle fiber. This arrangement gives cardiac muscle and skeletal muscle its striated appearance. Myofibrils are suspended inside the muscle fiber in a matrix called sarcoplasm, which contains a high concentration of K^+, Mg^{2+}, PO_4, protein enzymes, mitochondria and an extensive sarcolemma. Cardiac muscle differs from skeletal muscle in several ways:

- *Rhythmicity* (see 📖 p58) and resistance to tetany and fatigue.
- Cardiac myofibrils interconnect to form a network or *synctium*.
- Individual muscle cell membranes, called *intercalated disks*, are extremely permeable, allowing the action potential to move unhindered between muscle cells, and across the lattice.
- The action potential does not spread instantly from atria to ventricles because the heart is composed of two separate syncytiums, an atrial and a ventricular one, separated from each other by fibrous tissue which surrounds the valve orifices: the delay between atrial and ventricular contraction is critical for cardiac function.
- Normally the only way that an action potential can be conducted from atria to ventricles is via the specialized conducting pathways.

Excitatory and conducting tissue

These muscle fibres contract very weakly, because they contain few contractile fibrils. They generate and conduct the cardiac action potential. Fig. 2.4 shows the *sinus node (sinoatrial or SA node)* in which the normal rhythmic impulse is generated, the internodal pathways connecting it to the *AV node* which slows conduction, and the *bundle of His* which conducts the impulse to the *Purkinje fibres* and the ventricles. The anatomy of the conducting system is described on 📖 p43.

Excitation

Many cardiac fibres generate automatic rhythmical impulses. Normally the sinus node generates the fastest impulse rate, therefore controlling the heart rate. Sinus node self-excitation depends on: (1) selective membrane permeability to Na ions, and (2) three types of voltage-gated ion channels (fast Na channels, slow Ca/Na channels, and K channels).

- The negative resting potential of myocytes membranes (−80mV) is mostly due to the difference in K^+ ion concentration inside the cell

(140mEq/L) compared to outside (4mEq/L) partially offset by the opposing difference in Na^+ concentrations inside the cell (14mEq/L) compared to outside (142mEq/L).

- The sodium–potassium pump contributes about −4mEq/L to the resting potential by pumping out three Na^+ for every two K^+ pumped in.
- The conductive cells of the heart are normally relatively impermeable to Na^+, which reduces the negative resting potential slightly.
- The sinus node cells are fairly permeable to Na^+, so the negative resting potential is offset to a much greater amount: the resting potential of the sinus node cells is less negative at −55 to −60mV than it is in ventricular fibers at −85 to −90 mV.
- The *action potential* (an electrical nerve or muscle impulse) is generated when the slow leakage of Na^+ into the cell lowers the *resting potential* to −40mV.
- The calcium–sodium channels are activated, causing rapid influx of Ca^{2+} and Na^+: these channels close 100ms later, stopping the influx of positive ions.
- The membrane is now *depolarized*: the potential is no longer negative.
- At this point the voltage-gated K^+ channels open, and large amounts of K^+ leave the cell, terminating the action potential.
- This continues for a longer time than depolarization: the membrane is temporarily much more negative (hyperpolarization): the K^+ channels eventually close, and Na^+ diffuse in slowly, returning the membrane to resting and then threshold potential.

Conduction

An action potential elicited at one point of a conducting tissue, normally excites adjacent portions, resulting in *propagation* of the action potential. This occurs at the same speed in all directions. The specialized conducting tissues of the heart are designed to propagate the impulse in such a way that both atria contract a short time before the ventricles. The impulse is delayed as it passes through the AV node and the bundle of His, firstly because the conducting fibers are much smaller there, secondly because the threshold membrane potentials are much less negative, and thirdly because there a fewer gap junctions connecting fibers together. AV conduction is normally one way, preventing re-entry of cardiac impulses via this route. Purkinje fibers conduct so fast that the cardiac impulse is transmitted throughout each ventricle almost simultaneously. Abnormal pacemakers are described on 📖 p484.

Contraction

The action potential travels along muscle fibers in the same way. The action potential depolarizes the muscle fiber membrane and causes the sarcolemma to release large quantities of calcium into the myofibrils. The calcium ions initiate attractive forces between the actin and myosin filaments, causing them to slide together, resulting in muscle contraction. This process requires energy derived from the conversion of adenosine triphosphate (ATP) to adenosine diphosphate (ADP) in the myosin molecule head. Like any muscle, cardiac muscle generates its maximum force of contraction from its resting length.

The electrocardiogram

Key facts

The action potential, already described on ◻ p56, is shown in Fig. 2.10a for the nodal tissues and non-nodal tissues of the heart. As the cardiac impulses pass through the heart electrical currents spread into surrounding tissues and can be detected by electrodes on the skin surface. The voltages recorded are small: the QRS complex is about 3–4mV compared to the monophasic action potential of 100mV recorded by an electrode inserted into cardiac muscle. Note that no potential at all is recorded in the electrocardiogram (EKG) when the ventricular muscle is completely depolarized or completely polarized. Current only flows during depolarization and repolarization.

The normal EKG

The normal EKG (Fig. 2.10b) is composed of a P wave, a QRS complex, and a T wave. The *P wave* is caused by depolarization of the atria prior to contraction, the *QRS complex* is caused by depolarization of the ventricles prior to contraction (and obscures the atrial T wave caused by atrial repolarization), and the *T wave* is caused by ventricular repolarization. The heart rate is estimated from the *RR interval*. Normal heart rhythm (sinus rhythm) is implied by a normal P wave followed by a QRS complex, with a constant PR interval and a constant RR interval.

- In standard recordings 1 small square of EKG paper = 0.04s.
- The P wave normally lasts for 0.12s (3 small squares).
- The PR interval is normally 0.16s (4 small squares).
- The QRS complex is usually <0.12s (3 small squares).
- The PR segment occupies the *isoelectric point*, and under normal conditions so does the ST segment.
- Inverted waves in certain leads are abnormal. Interpretation of EKGs is outlined on ◻ p212.

Understanding EKG leads

The standard bipolar limb leads (I, II, and III) are not single wires connecting from the body, but a combination of two wires and their electrodes which make a complete circuit through the tissue between them to the electrocardiograph (Fig. 2.10c).

- The augmented (a) limb leads (aVR, aVL, and aVF) are unipolar limb leads where two of the leads are connected to the negative terminal of the EKG and one is connected to the positive.
- The positive terminal may be the right arm (aVR), the left arm (aVL), or the left leg (aVF).
- The six chest leads (V1–V6) consist of one wire connected to the body in the positions shown, and an indifferent wire connected to all three limb leads.
- The chest leads record the potential of the cardiac muscle directly beneath them, and minute changes in particularly the anterior ventricular wall appear in these leads.

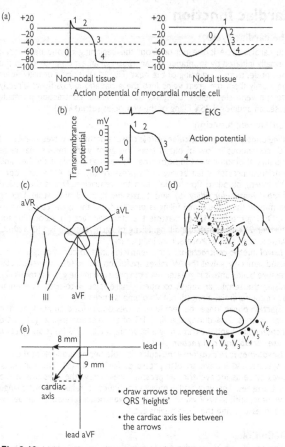

Fig. 2.10 (a) Monophasic action potentials of nodal tissue, and non-nodal tissue, and their relationship to the EKG. (b) ECK superimposed on action potential (c) Axes of the three bipolar and three unipolar limb leads. The axis of a lead is the direction from positive to negative electrode. Lead I is recorded from two electrodes that lie in the horizontal position with respect to the chest: the axis is 0. Lead aVF is 90°. The size of current recorded and the direction (positive or negative) in a lead can be recorded. (d) The chest leads. (e) The mean electrical axis of the QRS complex is normally 60°. The axis of the QRS complex can be calculated by adding the QRS complex in any two leads.

Cardiac function

The cardiac cycle

The cardiac cycle is the period from the beginning of one heart beat, normally initiated by spontaneous generation of an action potential in the sinus node, to the beginning of the next (Fig. 2.11). Blood normally flows continually from the great veins into the atria: about 75% flows directly into the ventricles before the atria contact. Atrial contraction normally causes an additional 25% filling of the ventricles (**atrial kick**).

Ventricular function

Filling phase: during **ventricular systole** closure of the AV valves, combined with continuous inflow of blood from the great veins, means that large amounts of blood collect in both atria. As soon as systole is finished and ventricular pressures fall below atrial pressure (5), the AV valves open (v) allowing blood to flow rapidly into the ventricles. This is the period of **rapid ventricular filling** (6), and it lasts the first 1/3 of diastole. During the middle third additional filling is directly from the great cardiac veins (7). During the final 1/3 of diastole the atria contract (1) accounting for a further 25% of ventricular filling. Filling of each ventricle is 110–120mL. Diastole is an active process, requiring energy.

Isovolumetric contraction: as the ventricles start to contract against the closed semilunar valves the AV valves are forced closed (c). Intraventricular pressure builds until it is greater than the pressure in the great arteries (2), causing the semilunar valves to open. There is apex-to-base shortening and circumferential elongation. LV volume is unchanged.

Ejection phase: once the semilunar valves open blood empties into the great arteries, 70% during the first 1/3 of the ejection period (3) (**rapid ejection phase**) and the remaining 30% during the last 2/3 (4) (**slow ejection phase**) or **isotonic contraction** phase.

Isovolumetric relaxation: ventricular diastole begins suddenly at the end of systole, and intraventricular pressures fall rapidly (5). The semilunar valves close as intraventricular pressure falls below the pressure in the great arteries. The ventricular muscle continues to relax without change in volume, until the AV valves open (v) as ventricular pressures fall below atrial pressure, and the cycle begins again.

Definitions

- **End-diastolic volume** (EDV) = largest ventricular volume (~120mL) immediately prior to the beginning of systole.
- **End-systolic volume** (ESV) = smallest ventricular volume (~40mL) immediately before the beginning of diastole.
- The **stroke volume** = amount ejected per cycle (120 – 40 = 80mL).
- The **ejection fraction** = percentage ejected (80/120mL = 66%).
- The **cardiac output** = stroke volume times the heart rate. The normal heart can increase cardiac output by up to 6x depending on demand, by decreasing ESV, increasing EDV, and increasing heart rate.
- **Compliance** is unit increase in volume/unit increase in pressure. It is a measure of active and passive relaxation and passive stretch.

Pressure–volume loops

Pressure–volume loops (Fig. 8.3) are derived by filling the heart with increasing amounts of blood and then measuring the pressure immediately before systole to obtain the diastolic curve; and by preventing any outflow of blood and measuring the maximum intraventricular pressure to obtain the systolic curve. Normally the heart operates within a much smaller area. The area enclosed within the pressure–volume loop is equal to the net ***external work output*** of the ventricle. The slope of the diastolic curve is inversely proportional to ***compliance*** (the ability of the ventricle to relax). The pressure–volume loops associated with valvular heart disease are shown on 📖 p375.

Preload and afterload

* ***Preload*** is the volume of blood in the ventricle at the end of diastole (the EDV). It is affected by circulating volume, LV compliance, the length of diastole and atrial contraction.
Afterload is the resistance to ventricular ejection. It is affected by the outflow tract area, peripheral resistance and wall stress. Manipulating preload and afterload is described on 📖 pp186–187.

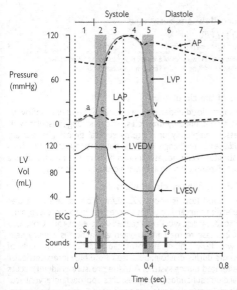

Fig. 2.11 The cardiac cycle. AP, aortic pressure; LVP, left ventricular pressure; LAP, left atrial pressure; LVEDV, left ventricular end–diastolic volume; LVESV, left ventricular end systolic volume. 1, atrial contraction; 2, isovolumetric contraction; 3, rapid ejection; 4, reduced ejection; 5, isovolumetric relaxation; 6, rapid filling; 7, reduced filling.

Circulation

Key facts

Blood flow to body tissues and cardiac output is controlled in relation to oxygen demand. BP control under normal circumstances is regulated so that it is nearly independent of cardiac output and regional blood flow control (□ p64). Flow through a blood vessel is determined entirely by two factors: (1) the **pressure difference** between the two ends of the vessel (ΔP), and (2) the **vascular resistance** to flow (R). The relationship is summarized by **Ohm's law** (see Box 2.1).

- When blood flows through a smooth walled vessel, it flows in concentric streamlines, with the centermost stream moving fastest and streams closest to the vessel wall moving slowest: this is **laminar flow**.
- **Poiseulle's law**, which integrates laminar flow theory, states that flow is proportional to the 4th power of the radius of the vessel: i.e., a slight increase in vessel diameter causes flow to increase by a large amount: any decrease in vessel size causes large reductions in flow.
- Poiseulle's law also states viscosity of blood is inversely proportional to flow. **Viscosity** is mainly determined by hematocrit: the higher the Hb, the higher the viscosity and the slower the flow.

Box 2.1 Pressure, flow, and resistance

- Ohm's law: $Q = \Delta P/R$
- Poiseulle's law: $Q = \pi\Delta Pr^4/8\eta l$

ΔP = pressure difference across two ends of a vessel, R = resistance to blood flow (Q), r= radius of the vessel, l = length of the vessel, η = viscosity of blood.

Functional parts of the circulation

The **arteries** transport blood under high pressure to the tissues. Inflow to the capillary beds is controlled by **arterioles**, whose strong muscular walls can close the vessel completely or dilate by several times. The primary role of the **capillaries** is exchange of fluid, nutrients, electrolytes, hormones, and metabolites. **Veins** act as conduits back to the heart, and as a reservoir: they can expand or contract their volume as necessary.

Physiology of the coronary circulation

Normal coronary blood flow is about 225mL/min, or 5% of the cardiac output. During exertion the cardiac output increases up to six-fold, against an increased afterload: cardiac work is increased up to eight-fold. Coronary blood flow must increase to match as oxygen extraction is already near maximal: this is why flow limiting stenoses cause ischemia. The bulk of coronary flow occurs during diastole, because of the high interventricular wall pressures generated during systole. A tissue pressure gradient occurs across the myocardium: **subendocardial** pressures approach interventricular pressures: **epicardial** muscle pressures are closer to atmospheric pressures. The subendocardial blood supply is most likely to be compromised when coronary blood flow is restricted. A dense subendocardial plexus compensates for this.

Systemic circulation

The overall flow in the circulation (**cardiac output**) is about 5L/min at rest
in an adult. Calculating and manipulating the cardiac output is described on
🕮 p131, p184. Fig. 2.12 shows arterial traces and blood volumes in the various
parts of the circulation. Although the pressure in the veins is shown as near
0mmHg, the weight of a column of blood that exists inside the veins when
a person is standing or sitting still (**hydrostatic pressure**) means that venous
pressure in the lower leg may be as much as 90mmHg. Arterial pressures are
similarly raised. Pressures in the capillaries rise causing interstitial edema: as
much as 15–20% of circulating volume may be lost from the circulation in the
first 15min of standing still. The arrangement of venous valves described on
🕮 p55 means that muscle contraction propels blood proximally, reducing
venous pressure distally behind the valve on muscle relaxation.

Microcirculation

The capillary beds do not obey the same laws of flow and resistance just
described. Once vessels are <1.5mm in diameter red cells tend to **rouleaux**
(line up with each other and move together as a cylinder). The internal
viscous resistance of blood is almost eliminated: this is called the **Fahraeus–
Lindqvist** effect. This compensates for the much slower velocity of blood
(1mm/s) in the low-pressure system. Blood flows intermittently in capillaries as a result of vasomotion, intermittent contraction of **precapillary
sphincters**. This is controlled by local oxygen demand: high oxygen demand
means greater duration of flow periods. **Diffusion** is the most important
method of transfer of solutes between the interstitium and the capillaries.
The rate of diffusion is proportional to the concentration difference: solutes diffuse from areas of high concentration to areas of low concentration.
Four primary forces determine osmotic movement of water and solutes:
the **capillary pressure** and the **interstitial colloid oncotic pressure** which
tend to move fluid out of the capillary, and the **plasma colloid oncotic pressure** and the **interstitial fluid pressure** which tend to move fluid back into
the capillary. Colloid osmotic pressure is caused by negatively charged proteins, which are the only dissolved substances that do not diffuse through
the capillary membrane, and associated Na^+ ions.

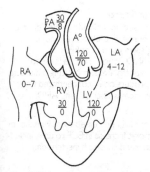

Fig. 2.12 Normal blood pressures (systolic/diastolic (mmHg)) in the cardiac
chambers and great vessels. RA (right atrium), RV (right ventricle), PA (pulmonary
artery), LA (left atrium), LV (left ventricle), Ao (aorta).

Regulation of blood pressure

Overview of factors contributing to blood pressure

Four main physiological mechanisms control normal arterial pressure:
- Autonomic nervous system.
- Capillary shift.
- Hormonal responses.
- Renal regulation of fluid and electrolyte balance.

Autonomic nervous system

This is the most rapid response mechanism. Continuous information is received in the brainstem vasomotor centre from central baroreceptors in the carotid sinus and aortic arch. Decreased arterial pressure activates the sympathetic nervous system resulting in increased cardiac contractility (β-adrenergic receptors), and peripheral arterial and venous vasoconstriction (α adrenergic receptors). Increased heart rate results from inhibition of parasympathetic control.

Capillary shift

Movement of fluid between the vasculature and intersitium is controlled by hydrostatic and oncotic capillary and interstitial pressures (📖 p63). Decreased hydrostatic pressure results in fluid moving from the interstitium across the endothelium into the vasculature increasing blood volume and BP.

Hormonal mechanisms

There are two main hormonal systems, which act on different targets both resulting in rapid response to changes in arterial pressure.
- The adrenal medulla secretes endogenous catecholamines (epinephrine and norepinephrine) in response to sympathetic activation, rapidly increasing cardiac output through increased heart rate and contractility
- Decreased renal blood flow results in increased production of renin and angiotensin which is converted in the lungs to angiotensin II, a potent vasoconstrictor that stimulates production of aldosterone from the adrenal cortex which acts to decrease glomerular permeability and urinary fluid and electrolyte loss.

Renal regulation of fluid and electrolyte balance

- Renal regulation through excretion of sodium chloride (which dictates sodium balance, extracellular fluid volume, and blood volume) is the most important mechanism for long-term control of BP.
- Decreased extracellular fluid (ECF) NaCl concentrations leads to inhibition of ADH secretion by the hypothalamus, producing a diuresis, whereas increased NaCl promotes production of concentrated urine and free water reabsorption through increased circulating AHD.

Long-term sequelae

Chronic increases in the total quantity of NaCl (increased dietary intake, or decreased renal excretion) leads to a chronic increase in ECF volume, including blood volume. This may lead to edema and chronic hypertension.

Response to hypovolemia

Hypovolemia leads to an acute reduction in preload, and hence stroke volume and cardiac output. Reduced cardiac output leads to:

- Reduced carotid and aortic baroreceptor stretch, leading to inhibition of parasympathetic output, and increased sympathetic activity.
- Net result is immediate vasoconstriction, venoconstriction, increased heart rate, contractility, and increased cardiac output.
- Fluid leaves peripheral capacitance vessels and the extravascular space and shifts into the arterial tree, with blood supply to brain, heart, and kidneys maximized by autoregulation.
- Vasoconstriction is augmented by release of angiotensin II through the renin–angiotensin system and ADH. Aldosterone and ADH also lead increased salt and water reabsorption.
- As a result, blood pressure to key organs is maintained through tachycardia, vasoconstriction, venoconstriction, and decreased urine output: this is compensated shock. The patient with decompensated shock shows evidence of end-organ hypoperfusion, e.g., confusion, anuria.

Response to trauma (Fig. 2.13)

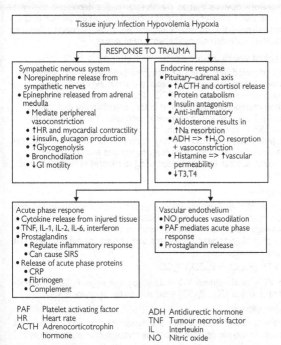

Fig. 2.13 The response to trauma.

Lung and esophageal physiology

Respiratory mechanics

Lung compliance

Lung compliance is change in lung volume per change in pressure. It may be a dynamic or static measurement and measures the distensibility of the lung parenchyma. It is directly related to lung volume, decreasing as lung volume increases. This is in contrast to the chest wall compliance, which increases with increasing lung volume. Diseases which decrease the elastic recoil of the lung increase compliance and those that increase it decrease compliance.

Surfactant

A mixture of phospholipids and protein, it is produced by type II pneumocytes. It is vital for normal lung function. Its reduces the surface tension at the alveolar air interface. Intra alveolar pressure may be measured by:

$$P = 2T/R$$

where P = pressure, T = tension, R = alveolar radius.

It is therefore obvious that as the alveolar radius decreases, the intra-alveolar tension increases. Surfactant reduces the surface tension proportionally to alveolar size, improving lung stability. It also increases pulmonary compliance, hence decreasing the work of breathing.

Control of ventilation

This is performed by a variety of receptors, both central and peripheral.
- **Peripheral chemoreceptors:** situated in the aortic and carotid bodies. They are very sensitive to changes in PCO_2. They also respond to hypoxia.
- **Central chemoreceptors:** situated in the ventrolateral aspect of the medulla. They respond to changes in extracellular or cerebrospinal fluid (CSF) H ion concentration.
- **Intrapulmonary receptors:** Herring–Breuer reflex via stretch receptors, intra-epithelial receptors responding to irritants and J receptors in the pulmonary capillary wall responding to changes in interstitial fluid volume.

Dead space

This is the volume of the respiratory system which is ventilated but does not participate in gas exchange. It includes the anatomical dead space–nasal passages, pharynx, trachea, airways up to the terminal bronchioles, and the physiological dead space—the part of tidal volume not participating in gas exchange.

$$VD/VT = (P_ACO_2 - P_ECO_2)/P_ACO_2$$

where VT = tidal volume, VD = dead space volume, P_ACO_2 = alveolar partial pressure of CO_2, P_ECO_2 = expired partial pressure of CO_2.

Diffusion capacity

This is a measure of the efficiency of diffusion. It is limited by three steps:
- The rate of oxygen passage across the alveolar–capillary membrane.

- The rate of RBC oxygen and hemoglobin combining.
- The difference in PaO_2 between the alveolus and the erythrocyte.

Flow–volume loops (Table 2.2)

Table 2.2 Diagnosis of lung disease (see also Table 13.1)

	Obstructive lung disease	Restrictive lung disease
FEV_1	↓	↓
FVC	Preserved	↓
FEV_1/FVC	↓	↑

Normal esophageal function

Upper esophageal sphincter
Separates the pharynx and the esophagus and prevents regurgitation. Formed from the cricopharyngeus muscle.

Esophageal body
Longitudinal and circular muscle. Circular muscle involved in peristalsis. Commences upon swallowing after which time it is under involuntary control. Peristaltic wave travels at 2–5cm/s along the esophageal body in a cranial to caudal direction, hence propelling esophageal contents towards the lower esophageal sphincter and the stomach.

Lower esophageal sphincter
Has a basal tone to prevent continuous reflux of gastric contents into the esophagus. Relaxes to allow esophageal contents to enter the stomach. Both a physiological and an anatomic sphincter. Relaxation occurs with esophageal distension, swallowing and with distension of the gastric fundus (see 📖 p50, and Fig. 13.4 on 📖 p659 for normal barriers to reflux).

Esophageal pH studies
24h monitoring allows quantitative measurements of acid reflux. It is the standard test when diagnosing gastroesophageal reflux disease (see 📖 p778) and is also useful when investigating patients with recurrent symptoms after surgery for reflux and those with symptoms of reflux following surgery for achalasia. Normal esophageal pH is 4–7. A reading below 4 is registered as an episode of reflux, but cannot identify the cause for the reflux.

- All anti-reflux and antacid medications are stopped prior to the study.
- A probe is placed 5cm above the upper border of the lower esophageal sphincter.
- Patients are advised to be active and to keep accurate diaries documenting meal times, symptoms, and when supine or erect.

Renal homeostasis

Key facts

By controlling solute and water excretion, and hormone production, the kidneys have a key role in control of BP, volume and osmolality, acid–base balance, electrolyte control, and excretion of toxins.

Renal function

GFR is decreased by low renal blood flow, high osmotic plasma pressures, and low hydrostatic capillary pressures, which are determined by afferent and efferent arteriolar resistance. Sympathetic drive reduces renal blood flow and GFR. Creatinine excretion is used to measure GFR.

Clearance and glomerular filtration rate (GFR)

Clearance (Cl) is the volume of plasma completely cleared of solute by the kidney (ml/min) and is the main measure of kidney function.
Cl = (U/P) x V

GFR = clearance, for any substance not metabolized, actively excreted or reabsorbed in the tubules = 125mL/min (in normal adults); U = concentration in urine; P = concentration in plasma of solute; V = urine flow rate.

Body fluid compartments

(See Table 2.3.) In a typical 70kg, 1.80m male:
- Total body water is 42L (60% of body mass).
- Intracellular fluid (ICF) is 27L (40%).
- Extracellular fluid (ECF) is 15L (60%).
- Of the ECF, total blood volume is 5L.
- 2L is contributed by red cell volume.
- Daily intake averages at 2L.
- Insensible loss from the respiratory tract and skin is about 700mL. Daily requirements of solutes are: 160mmol Na^+, 100mmol K^+, 950mmol Ca^{2+}, and 300mmol Mg^{2+}.

Table 2.3 Typical contents of body fluids (mmol/L)

Solute	Plasma	ECF	ICF	Lymph
Na^+	142	145	12	140
K^+	4.3	4.4	150	
Ca^{2+}	2.5	2.4	4.0	
Mg^{2+}	1.1	1.1	34	
Cl^-	104	117	4.0	
PO_4^{2-}	2.0	2.0	40	
$Prot^-$	14	0	54	
HCO_3^-	24	27	12	

Renal tubular function

GFR is autoregulated closely: even a 5% error in matching GFR to body requirements results in rapid accumulation of waste products or excess loss of water and solutes into the urine. Two feedback mechanisms accomplish autoregulation at each glomerulus: (1) an afferent arteriolar vasodilator, (2) an efferent arteriolar vasoconstrictor. These control GFR by controlling blood flow into and out of the individual glomerulus. In this way renal blood flow is kept constant through a wide range of systemic pressures. Urine is formed from the glomerular filtrate by a process of active reabsorbtion, active secretion, changing membrane permeability to water and a countercurrent multiplier (repetitive reabsorption of NaCl by the thick ascending loop of Henle together with continual inflow of new NaCl from the adjacent proximal tubule into the loop of Henle, 'multiplying' the concentration of NaCl).

- Normal pH is 7.35–7.45.
- Normal H^+ concentration is 35–45nmol/L.
- pH is the negative log of H^+ concentration.
- Base excess is the amount of base required to restore 1L of blood to pH 7.0 at a pCO_2 of 5.3kPa.
- Anion gap is the amount of anions other than Cl^- and HCO_3^- (effectively $H_2PO_4^-$ and SO_4^-) needed to neutralize measured Na^+ ions.

Acid–base balance

The kidney controls blood pH by secreting alkaline or acidic urine, by balancing the amount of HCO_3^- reabsorbed and the amount of H^+ secreted. There are three major buffer systems, which act across organ systems: (1) the bicarbonate, (2) the phosphate, and (3) the protein buffer system. The extracellular protein buffers can correct acid–base changes within seconds, the respiratory system can correct changes within minutes, but renal mechanisms (primarily bicarbonate) take hours to days. This longevity makes it more powerful than the other two systems.

Blood

Blood groups

There are 30 commonly occurring and hundreds of rare antigens present on human blood cells. Most do not elicit strong antigen–antibody reactions. The antibodies to two related antigens, *type A* and *type B*, almost always occur in the plasma of people who do not have the antigens on their red cells. These antibodies bind strongly with the red cell antigens to cause agglutination, and form the basis for blood typing. The *rhesus* system is the other important system, but in order for a person to develop rhesus antibodies they must first be exposed to the rhesus antigen, which happens by blood transfusion, or by a Rh −ve mother giving birth to a Rh +ve baby. Of the six rhesus antigens, rhesus D is the most antigenic in the US:

• 37% are blood group O (have neither A nor B antigens on red blood cells, but have anti-A and anti-B antibodies in their plasma).
• 36% are group A (A antigen, anti-B antibodies).
• 9% are group B (B antigen, anti-A antibodies).
• 3% are AB (A and B antigens, no A or B antibodies).
• O Rh −ve patients are *universal donors* (their blood can be given to anyone) because their red cells carry antigens from neither system.
• AB +ve patients are *universal recipients* as their blood contains antibodies to neither system.

Cross-matching blood

• *Type and screen* (or blood grouping) involves adding A and B agglutinins to donated blood to determine blood type.
• *Cross-matching* involves mixing donated blood with the intended recipient blood, to assess compatibility. Cross-matching takes 20min. If no cross-matched blood is available, O −ve blood may be given in an emergency, but rare antigen systems may occasionally cause a transfusion reaction (🕮 p148). Immunocompromised patients may experience a form of *graft-vs-host disease* after transfusion, when donor T cells attack host antigens.

Tissue typing

For lung transplants *major histocompatibility complex (MHC)* antigens, also known as *human leucocyte antigens (HLA)*, must be typed in addition to the *ABO system* if rejection is to be avoided. Chromosome 6 contains the MHC complex that codes for expression of MHC antigens, which originally evolved to enable the body to detect and combat infecting organisms. Most heart transplants do not need an HLA match (🕮 p507).

• MHC class I (A, B, and C) antigens are expressed on the surface of all nucleated cells and platelets.
• MHC class II (DP, DQ, and DR) antigens are expressed on B-lymphocytes, macrophages, monocytes and dendritic cells.
• Each antigen is highly polymorphic: e.g., there are >70 different versions, or alleles, of the DR locus; while there are six ABO phenotypes, there are over 10^{12} MHC phenotypes.
• Tissue typing can be done by using panels of antisera, in a manner similar to blood typing, or by PCR, which allows automation.

Hemostasis and fibrinolysis

There are four phases of hemostasis:

- *A vascular phase:* local BP and flow are reduced by vasospasm in response to direct mechanical and local humoral effects, and local edema and hematoma formation reduces transmural pressure.
- *A platelet phase:* adherence of platelets to damaged endothelium activated by ADP and collagen, and binding von Willebrand factor. Platelet aggregation is mediated by membrane glycoprotein IIb/IIIa and fibrinogen, 5HT, thromboxane A2. Activated platelets release thromboxane A2 and platelet factor.
- *A clotting phase:* the intrinsic and extrinsic pathways happen in parallel *in vivo.*
- *Monocyte activation:* they express tissue factor and factor V.

Fibrinolysis occurs at the same time as clot formation, to limit the process locally (see Fig. 2.14). Fibrinolysis depends on four main molecules. (1) *Plasmin*, a serine protease which is produced by the action of thrombin on plasminogen and attacks unstable bonds between fibrin molecules to generate fibrin degradation products. (2) *Antithrombin III* which binds thrombin, XIIa, IXa, and XI to deactivate them. (3) *Proteins C and S* which prevent thrombin generation by binding factors Va and VIIIa. (4) *Tissue factor pathway inhibitor*, produced by platelets inhibits factors Xa and VIIa.

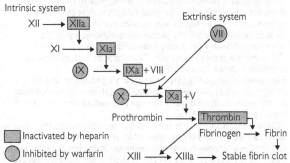

Coagulation casade and the use of heparin

Fig. 2.14 Diagram of the clotting and fibrinolysis cascades.

Ischemic heart disease

Atherosclerosis

Key facts

- Atherosclerosis is a degenerative disease of large and medium-sized arteries characterized by lipid deposition and fibrosis.
- There are **three stages** of atheromatous lesion; **fatty streaks** are linear lesions on the artery lumen, composed of lipid-filled macrophages, and which progress to **fibrolipid plaques** (unstable plaques), and finally **complex lesions** (stable plaques).
- There are multiple lesions throughout the whole vascular tree at all stages of the disease process: the flow-limiting **culprit lesion** responsible for stable angina is usually a stable plaque, whereas the unstable plaques responsible for acute MI are fibrolipid plaques, and are often not due to the flow-limiting lesions visible on coronary angiography.
- Reversible risk factors: smoking, hypercholesterolemia, obesity, hypertension. Irreversible risk factors: diabetes mellitus, male sex, age, family history.

Pathological features

- In sites at risk of atherosclerosis (sites of vessel bifurcation, turbulent flow, post-stenotic areas, areas denuded of endothelial cells) lipid-laden macrophages enter the vessel wall via gaps between endothelial cells.
- A fibrolipid plaque contains a mix of macrophages and smooth muscle cells which migrate into the plaque, capped by fibrous tissue (Fig. 2.15).
- Growth factors, particularly platelet-derived growth factor (PDGF), stimulate the proliferation of intimal smooth muscle cells and the synthesis of collagen, elastin, and mucopolysaccharide.
- Lipid accumulates within the plaque extracellularly, and in the myocytes, ultimately producing **foam cells**.
- Cell death eventually ensues with the release of intracellular lipids, calcification, and a chronic inflammatory reaction.
- High levels of circulating **LDL-cholesterol** are thought to lead to atherosclerosis by damaging endothelium both directly by increasing membrane viscosity, indirectly through **free radical** formation, and by inducing secretion of PDGF.
- In larger vessels such as the aorta, atherosclerotic plaques may release **atheroemboli** and **mural thrombus**, or impinge on the vessel media causing tissue atrophy resulting in **aneurysm** formation or **dissection**.
- **Acute MI** is caused by three processes in coronary vessels: progressive atherosclerosis, disruption of **unstable plaque** with **acute thrombosis**, and acute hemorrhage into the intima around the plaque.

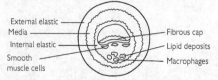

External elastic
Media
Internal elastic
Smooth muscle cells
Fibrous cap
Lipid deposits
Macrophages

Fig. 2.15 Cross-section through an atherosclerotic plaque.

Ischemia and infarction

Key facts

- *Ischemia* is cell damage caused by O_2 supply–demand mismatch.
- *Infarction* is cell death caused by O_2 supply–demand mismatch.
- Normal O_2 supply to the contracting LV is 8mL per 100g muscle per minute. Imbalance in O_2 supply and demand results in ischemia—changes are most acute in the subendocardium as flow mostly occurs in diastole (□ p62). Supply–demand mismatch is caused by:
  - Vascular narrowing (atherosclerosis, thrombus, embolus, spasm).
  - Global hypoperfusion (shock, cardiopulmonary bypass).
  - Hypoxemia (anemia, hypoxia).
  - Vascular compression (increased LVEDP in CHF, distension on bypass).
  - Increased myocardial O_2 demand (exercise, pregnancy, hyperthyroidism, tachycardia, ventricular hypertrophy, ventricular distension).

Pathological features

MIs occur in the right coronary artery territory in 30%, left anterior descending in 50% of cases, and circumflex in 20% of cases.

Changes within seconds of ischemia (reversible)
- Switch to anaerobic glycolysis from oxidative metabolism.
- Decrease in high-energy phosphates (creatinine and ATP)—this can impair recovery after reperfusion, hence need for rapid electromechanical arrest after cross-clamping to avoid depleting myocardial ATP.
- Accumulation of lactic acid and rise in myocardial pH.

Changes within minutes (reversible if oxygen supply restored)
- Decrease in contractility.
- Glycogen stores depleted.
- Cell and mitochondrial swelling.

Changes after 30 minutes of ischemia (irreversible)
- Structural defects appear in the sarcolemma.
- Myocyte death.

Changes after 3 hours
- Coagulation necrosis.
- Changes are only visible macroscopically at 24 hours: muscle appears pale and edematous.

Changes after 3 days
- Inflammatory exudates initially with polymorphonuclear leukocytes.
- Necrotic tissue removed by macrophages.
- Fibroblast infiltration beginning the process of scar formation.
- Macroscopically the infarcted area appears yellow and rubbery with a hemorrhagic border.
- Aneurysm formation and free wall rupture may occur while myocardial wall is weak, before formation of scar tissue.

Changes after 1 week
- Neorevascularization at margins of preserved tissue.
- Scar maturation normally complete by 6 weeks: tough, white area.

Ischemia–reperfusion injury

Key facts

Ischemia–reperfusion injury occurs after angina, spontaneous lysis of coronary thrombi, relief of coronary spasm, thrombolysis, PCI, off-pump coronary artery bypass (OPBCAB), and surgery with electromechanical arrest.

Myocardial stunning

Myocardial stunning

The mechanical dysfunction that persists after reperfusion in the absence of irreversible damage. It is usually a relatively mild and fully reversible injury that is distinct from myocardial infarction, but it contributes to the morbidity and mortality of the ischemic injuries listed in this chapter. The degree of myocardial stunning is proportional to the antecedent ischemia, suggesting that ischemic changes initiate and potentiate reperfusion injury. There are three main mechanisms of injury:

Oxygen free radicals

Generated in the stunned myocardium causing damage during the initial moments of reperfusion. They are produced by several pathways which include increased xanthine oxidase activity, activation of neutrophils, deranged intramitochondrial electron transport systems and auto-oxidative processes. The free radicals react with proteins and fatty acids. Oxygen radical mediated damage of the sarcoplasmic reticulum, sarcolemma, extracellular collagen matrix, and intracellular contractile proteins results in a large rise in intracellular calcium.

Rise in cytosolic free calcium

The rise in cytosolic free calcium activates degradation enzymes such as the phospholipases, further damaging the same intracellular structures and amplifying the damage done by the oxygen free radicals, resulting in reduced myocardial contractility. A prolonged intracellular calcium deficit ensues which is addressed by administration of exogenous calcium.

Excitation-contraction uncoupling

The oxygen radical mediated damage of the sarcoplasmic reticulum, sarcolemma, extracellular collagen matrix and intracellular contractile proteins results in uncoupling of the excitation–contraction mechanism.

The oxygen paradox

This is an irreversible phenomenon. Reoxygenation of ischemic myocardial cells leads to rapid acceleration of the damage described in this chapter. It is characterized by cellular contracture, sudden rupture of increasingly fragile cell membranes, and the release of cell contents as a result of abrupt changes in pH and tissue osmolality, and it seems to occur in the no man's land between reversible and irreversible ischemia. It is an energy-dependent process that does not occur when the cell's ability to generate oxidative energy is abolished, and it only occurs in myocytes. The process is triggered by the re-supply of energy from oxidative phosphorylation to myofibrils, which due to elevated cytosolic calcium are highly activated: hypercontracture and cell death is the result.

Neutrophils and ischemia

Neutrophils accumulate rapidly. In response to acute MI the neutrophil response is apparent at 12–24h, peaking at 3–4 days after permanent coronary artery occlusion. In reperfusion injury neutrophil infiltration begins earlier, is accelerated by reperfusion, and is proportional to the preceding ischemia. Neutrophil depletion or inactivation during reperfusion results in smaller infarct size. Neutrophils probably exacerbate reperfusion injury in three ways:

- Plugging capillaries reducing collateral flow.
- Releasing vasoconstrictors.
- Acting as a source of oxygen free radicals produced by the NADPH-oxidase reaction. 70% of the oxygen used by activated neutrophils is converted to superoxide. This is the basis of their attack on bacteria and damaged cells, but in the myocardium it causes dysfunction.

Quantifying ischemia

- Methods of quantifying ischemia in real-time include:
- Measurement of high-energy phosphates such as ATP, and their breakdown products (purines and pyrimidines) in coronary sinus outflow.
- Measuring levels of lactate in coronary sinus blood.
- Measuring intraoperative myocardial pH with glass electrodes.

Ischemic preconditioning

One or more brief periods of myocardial ischemia followed by reperfusion increases the ability of the myocardium to withstand longer periods of ischemia. Myocardial ATP declines during the first short ischemic periods, but not during subsequent prolonged ischemia. The number of myocytes that die during a period of prolonged ischemia are reduced by up to 75% if the ischemic period is preceded by a shorter period of ischemia. This is because the metabolic changes described in this chapter, when by triggered by a very brief period of ischemia become adaptive rather than maladaptive.

Hibernation

Normally 8mL of oxygen per 100g of muscle per minute is delivered to the contracting left ventricle. Cellular viability is compromised when this falls below 1.5mL oxygen per 100g per minute. With repeated episodes of stunning (such as occurs in stable angina due to coronary artery disease) the metabolic processes of the heart remain intact, but the regional contractility may be reduced. This is *hibernation*: with reperfusion hibernating myocardium may resume normal contraction. Detecting hibernating myocardium is described on 📖 p28.

Pathology of heart failure

Key facts

Heart failure is an inability of the heart to produce an adequate cardiac output despite normal filling pressures. It is characterized by numerous multisystem maladaptive changes. The reduction in cardiac function that underlies these changes may be thought of as *systolic* (a decrease in contractility) and *diastolic* (a decrease in compliance, and hence decreased filling and stroke volume).

Classification

Heart failure may be classified in several different ways:
- Acute and chronic.
- Left, right, and biventricular or congestive.
- High and low output.
- Systolic and diastolic.
- Compensated and decompensated.

40% of patients with heart failure have near normal systolic function: their failure is primarily diastolic.

Etiology

There are many causes of cardiac failure (see Box 2.2), but in the West coronary artery disease and/or hypertension feature in >90% of cases. Severe forms of these disease processes all end in a common pathway of systolic or diastolic dysfunction that results in heart failure.

Box 2.2 Causes of heart failure
- Hypertension.
- Ischemic heart disease.
- Valvular heart disease.
- Toxic: alcohol, cocaine, β-blockers, Ca channel blockers, adriamycin, doxorubicin.
- Viral myocarditis: Coxsackie, HIV.
- The cardiomyopathies: hypertrophic, restrictive, dilated.
- Primary pulmonary hypertension.
- Arrhythmias: AF, sick sinus syndrome.
- Infiltrative: amyloidosis, sarcoidosis.
- Pericardial disease: restrictive pericarditis, pericardial effusion.
- Metabolic: thyrotoxicosis.
- Nutritional: Beri-beri, pellagra.
- High output: anemia, Paget's disease, pregnancy.
- Neuromuscular: Duchenne muscular dystrophy.

Pathogenesis

- The wide ranging changes that occur in heart failure are divided into cardiac and non-cardiac.

Cardiac changes in heart failure

Myocyte
Abnormal excitation–contraction, β-adrenergic downregulation.

Myocardium
Remodelling: regional hypertrophy (eccentric in volume overload, and concentric in pressure overload), thinning and dilatation of infarct zones, increased sphericity, necrosis, fibrosis.

Coronary arteries
Extrinsic compression, inflammation.

Functional changes
MR, ischemia, hibernation, arrhythmias, failure of coordination of right and left ventricular contraction due to heart block.

Non-cardiac changes in heart failure

The fall in cardiac output leads to activation of several neurohumoral systems designed to maintain cardiac output.

- Renin–angiotensin–aldosterone system (RAAS).
- Sympathetic nervous system.
- Brain and atrial natriuretic peptide.

RAAS activation leads to increased circulating renin, plasma angiotensin II, and aldosterone. *Angiotensin II* is a potent vasoconstrictor of renal efferent arterioles and systemic circulation where it stimulates release of *norepinephrine* from sympathetic nerve endings, stimulates release of *aldosterone*, and inhibits vagal tone. The net result is *sodium* and *water retention*, and potassium excretion.

Sympathetic activation occurs early in heart failure via low- and high-pressure baroceptors, providing inotropic support and chronotropic drive to maintain cardiac output. Sustained sympathetic activation activates the RAAS, increasing arterial and venous tone, preload and afterload, and leading to progressive retention of sodium and water. Sympathetic overdrive results in ventricular hypertrophy and focal myocardial necrosis.

Increase in circulating *atrial* and *brain natuiretic peptide* in response to volume expansion leads to *natruiresis* and vasodilation: antagonizing the effects of aldosterone. *ADH* may contribute to hyponatremia. Endothelin, secreted by endothelial cells, acts to conserve sodium and stimulate vasoconstriction.

Valvular heart disease

The pathophysiology of valvular heart disease is described in more detail in 📖 chapter 8. The following section concentrates on the morphology.

Key facts

The content and arrangement of valve fibres (📖 p44) is designed to give maximum strength and flexibility, and minimum obstruction to flow where required. Any pathological process affecting valve structure has a large impact on its function.

Aortic stenosis

Etiology

- Congenital (unicuspid rare, **bicuspid valve** more common around 1–2%). Bicuspid valve morphology varies—may be two equal cusps with central opening, or two unequally sized cusps with raphe in larger cusp indicating where two leaflets have fused. Bicuspid aortic valves usually functionally normal in younger patients, but leaflets may become increasingly sclerotic with age, leading to accelerated stenosis. Around 50% of bicupisd aortic valve are stenotic by age 60 years. Bicuspid valves associated with aortic root dilatation (📖 p428).
- *Rheumatic* (📖 pp372 and 398) due to commissural fusion, leaflet thickening.
- *Calcific degeneration:* commonest cause, occurring in otherwise normal valves. Rheumatic and bicuspid valves eventually calcify.
- Infective endocarditis (rare cause of AS, usually causes AI).
- Hyperlipidaemia (rare).
- Subvalvar (membrane and muscular) and supravalvular.
- Prosthesis failure (pannus, thrombosis, endocarditis, calcification).

Aortic insufficiency

Etiology

- Myxomatous degeneration (common cause, causes leaflet prolapse).
- Rheumatoid (often mixed picture with degree of AS).
- Infective endocarditis (leaflet perforation).
- Root dilatation (quite common—due to rheumatic, atherosclerotic, aneurysmal, Marfan syndrome, syphilis, ankylosing spondylitis).
- Prosthesis failure: paraprosthetic leak, leaflet perforation.

Functional classification

- Disease of the aortic root, e.g., Marfan syndrome.
- Disease of the valve leaflets, e.g., rheumatic, endocarditis.
- Lack of support of the valve commissures, e.g., dissection, trauma.

Mixed aortic valve disease

Mild AI frequently accompanies AS. The commonest causes of mixed aortic valve disease are bicuspid aortic valve, chronic rheumatic valve disease, and infective endocarditis in a stenotic valve.

Mitral stenosis
Etiology
- Chronic *rheumatic* heart disease (commonest cause).
- *Congenital* mitral stenosis (rare).
- *Mitral annular calcification* (MAC) (less usual cause of severe MS).

Mitral regurgitation
Pathophysiologic and functional classifications are described on 🕮 p400.

Aetiology
- Degenerative mitral valve disease. Commonest cause in West. Represents spectrum from fibroelastic deficiency (small valves, single segment prolapse), to Barlow's disease (large valves, multisegment prolapse). Also called floppy valve, prolapse, myxomatous disease.
- Rheumatic heart disease.
- Infective endocarditis
- Connective tissue disorders, e.g. Marfan and Ehlers–Danlos syndromes.
- Ischemic heart disease.
- Congenital cleft valve leaflet (associated with primum ASD).
- Endomyocardial fibrosis (common in sub-Saharan Africa).
- Iatrogenic (balloon valvuloplasty of stenotic valve).
- Prosthesis failure (paraprosthetic leak, leaflet perforation).

Functional classification
Clear understanding of the functional classification (🕮 p400) is required for successful repair. Essentially *Carpentier's functional classification* describes Type I (normal leaflet motion, MR caused by annular dilatation or leaflet perforation), Type II (excess leaflet motion, MR caused by leaflet prolapse due to chordal or papillary muscle elongation or rupture), Type IIIa (decreased diastolic leaflet motion due to leaflet thickening) and Type IIIb (decreased systolic leaflet motion due to chordal tethering or shortening).

Mixed mitral valve disease
- The commonest cause of mixed mitral valve disease is rheumatic. Usually MS predominates.

Tricupid valve disease
TS is rare—usually rheumatoid. TR may be caused by:
- *Functional* secondary to mitral valve disease (commonest).
- *Rheumatic* heart disease.
- *Infective endocarditis*.
- Ebstein's anomaly.
- *Carcinoid* syndrome (usually associated with pulmonary regurgitation).
- Endomyocardial fibrosis.
- Prolapsing cusp.

Pulmonary valve disease
Acquired pulmonary valve disease is unusual. Severe pulmonary hypertension may cause dilatation of the pulmonary valve ring causing pulmonary regurgitation.

Infective endocarditis

Key facts

- Infective endocarditis is a microbial infection of the endocardial surface of the heart.
- Incidence 1.7–6.2 cases per 100 000 person years in the West.
- Men more commonly affected than women.
- In MV prolapse the incidence is 100 per 100 000 person years.
- In iv drug users the incidence is 150–2000 per 100 000 person years.
- Prosthetic valve endocarditis accounts for up to 25% of cases in the West. The cumulative risk is about 1% at 12 months and 3% at 5 years post surgery.

Pathology

Normal cardiac endothelium is resistant to infection. Transient bacteremias occur in everyone but immune mechanisms, particularly platelet thrombocidins, play an effective role in preventing endocarditis. Damage to cardiac endothelium, as a result of trauma, turbulent flow, valvular heart disease, or atherosclerosis results in platelet and fibrin deposition. A sterile thrombotic vegetation is produced. Microbes from peripheral sites can colonize these vegetations to cause infective endocarditis, monocyte adhesion, triggering of the coagulation cascade, and clot formation. Commonest sites of infective endocarditis are:

- Predominantly left-sided (95%).
- Mitral valve (85%), aortic valve (55%), tricuspid valve (20%).
- The pulmonary valve is involved in <1% of cases.
- Jet lesions: atrial surface of the mitral valve in MR, or ventricular surface of the aortic valve in AR.

Microbiology

Staphylococcus

Staphylococci, particularly *Staphylococcus aureus*, are now the commonest cause of infective endocarditis, causing up to 40% of cases of native valve endocarditis, and up to 25% of cases of prosthetic valve endocarditis. Coagulase-negative staph cause up to 30% of cases of prosthetic valve endocarditis but <10% of cases of native valve endocarditis. *Staph. aureus* endocarditis is particularly virulent, and associated with annular and myocardial abscess formation and a higher mortality.

Streptococcus

Viridans streptococci, a group of bacteria usually from dental caries, were until recently the commonest cause of endocarditis. Bacteremias can be caused by tooth brushing and chewing, not just by dental extraction. Streptococci now account for about 60% of native valve endocarditis and up to 10% of prosthetic valve endocarditis. The common isolates are *Strep. sanguis*, *bovis*, *mutans*, and *mitis*. *Strep. bovis* is most common amongst elderly people with bowel pathology.

Enterococci

Enterococci are frequently isolated in hospital-acquired bacteremias and cause about 10% of cases of native valve endocarditis, and a similar proportion of prosthetic valve endocarditis. They are virulent.

HACEK species

HACEK stands for *Haemophilus* species, *Actinobacillus actinomycetem-comitans*, *Cardiobacterium hominis*, *Eikenella corrodens*, and *Kingella kingae*. These organisms are slow-growing oral commensals and their presence in blood cultures is almost pathognomonic of infective endocarditis. HACEK vegetations tend to be large.

Polymicrobial infective endocarditis

This is unusual, and normally associated with iv drug abuse.

Sterile endocarditis

Up to 10% of cases of proven infective endocarditis (proven by operative or postmortem cultures) yield negative blood cultures. Previous antibiotic therapy is the commonest cause. *Coxiella burnetii*, *Bartonella* spp., and *Chlamydia* spp. cannot be grown by conventional blood culture methods.

Clinical features

The clinical presentation is extremely varied. The Duke diagnostic criteria are listed on 📖 p418. Symptoms and signs include:

Bacteremia

Pyrexia, chills, rigors, malaise, anorexia, confusion, arthralgia.

Tissue destruction

Embolic illness, valvular incompetence, root and myocardial abscess and fistula formation, dehiscence of prosthetic valves and false aneurysm formation. Heart block results from erosion of the conducting tissues.

Emboli

Emboli occur in up to 50% of cases of infective endocarditis, commonly resulting in CVA (65% of emboli), acute peripheral limb ischemia, MI, TIA, spleen and kidney infarction, PE, and mycotic aneurysms.

Circulating immune complexes

These are manifested by splinter hemorrhages, Osler nodes, and Janeway lesions (📖 p6), vasculitic rash, Roth spots, splenomegaly, nephritis, and arthralgia.

Mortality

The mortality rate depends on the organism and the valvular pathology:
- Up to 50% for *Staph. aureus* and fungi.
- Up to 15% for viridans streptococci and *Strep. bovis*.
- Up to 25% for enterococci.
- About 10% in right-sided endocarditis in iv drug users.
- The overall mortality for native and prosthetic valve endocarditis is 25%, but late prosthetic endocarditis has a mortality of up to 60%.

The management of infective endocarditis is described on 📖 p418.

Pericardial pathology

Etiology

Pericardial disease can be classified as follows:
- Acute and chronic pericarditis.
- Chronic pericarditis may have constrictive component. Severe constrictive pericarditis may be an indications for surgery (🕮 p488) but should not be confused with restrictive cardmyopathy (Table 2.4) which may present similarly, but requires different management.
- Infective: viral, bacterial, toxoplasmosis, amebiasis, TB, ecchinococcal.
- Inflammatory: Dressler's, post cardiotomy.
- Connective tissue disorders: RA, SLE, PAN, rheumatic fever, sclerosis.
- Systemic disease: uraemia, hypothyroidism.
- Neoplastic: primary or metastatic (🕮 p84).
- Effusion and hemorrhage: trauma, aortic dissection.
- Physical agents: radiotherapy, blunt trauma.

Pathophysiology

Normally the pericardial volume is 10% greater than that of the heart. Slow accumulation of fluid in the pericardial space can be accommodated by changes in the pericardium over time, but acute increases in the amount of fluid by even small amounts, and constrictive pericardial disease processes, produce pericardial compression (cardiac tamponade).

Pulsus paradoxus

This is an exaggeration of a normal physiological phenomenon. In inspiration systemic systolic pressures fall by about 4mmHg. In cardiac tamponade this fall is over 10mmHg. This is because inspiration requires the generation of negative intrathoracic pressures, effectively drawing increased blood volumes into the chest and right heart. The interventricular septum is displaced to the left, reducing left ventricular filling. This translates into reduced stroke volume and reduced systemic pressures. The second impact of reduced intrathoracic pressures is a direct effect on the left ventricle: the force that the left ventricle needs to exert relative to the positive pressure in extrathoracic arteries is greater, and the left ventricle empties incompletely during full inspiration. In cardiac tamponade external compression further reduces ventricular filling (LVEDV decreases by up to 30%) exaggerating the decrease in systolic pressure in inspiration.

Equalization of pressures
- LVEDP and RVEDP are within 5mmHg of each other.

Elevation of mean atrial pressures
- RAP and LAP >10mmHg are diagnostic requirements.

Square root sign

A dip plateau pattern in the ventricular filling pressure curve reflects normal ventricular filling that suddenly reaches the elastic limits of constricted pericardium, as opposed to gradually reaching the limit (Fig. 2.16).

Prominent y descent
- In the jugular venous pressure trace x and y descents are prominent.

Elevated RVEDP
- This is typically more than a third of the RV systolic pressure.

Table 2.4 Differences between restrictive cardiomyopathy and constrictive pericarditis

	Restrictive cardiomyopathy	Constrictive pericarditis
Bedside	Usually no history of surgery	History of previous cardiac surgery common
	Pansystolic murmurs from TR and MR common, with ↑apex beat	Murmurs uncommon.
	Kussmaul sign unusual	Kussmaul sign present
Echo	↑Wall thickness	Normal or reduced wall thickness
	No respiratory variation in transmitral/tricuspid flows	>25% respiratory variation in transmitral/tricuspid flows
	No septal bounce	Septal bounce
Cardiac cath	Square root sign present	
	Elevated RA pressures	
	Pulsus paradoxus	
	LVEDP >RVEDP	Equalization of EDPs and RAP
	Concordance in RV and LV pressure changes with respiration	RV and LV pressure discordance
	Slow early diastolic filling	Rapid early diastolic filling
CT ? MRI	Normal pericardium	Thickened pericardium, sometimes calcified
Endocardial biopsy	Normal pericardium	Inflammatory, calcified (rare to require pericardial biopsy)
	Amyloid on endomyocardial biopsy	

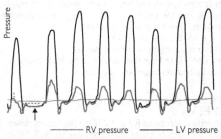

Fig. 2.16 Simultaneous pressure recordings of RV and LV pressures showing equalization of filling pressures (RVEDP and LVEDP), concordance of respiratory variation in RV and LV pressures, and dip and plateau or 'square root' sign (arrowed).

Pressure

——— RV pressure   ——— LV pressure

Cardiac neoplasms

Classification of cardiac neoplasms

Primary
* Benign: myxoma, lipoma, fibroblastoma of valves, rhabdomyoma, mesothelioma of the AV node, hemangioma, teratoma, pheochromocytoma.
* Malignant: angiosarcoma, rhabdomyosarcoma, malignant mesothelioma, fibrosarcoma.

Secondary
* Metastatic: melanoma, sarcoma, bronchiogenic carcinoma, adenocarcinomas of prostate and bowel.
* Direct spread: from lung, breast, esophagus, thymus, hepatic, adrenal, uterine, and renal cell carcinomas.

Myxoma

Definition
Myxoma is a neoplasm of endocardial origin, derived from either subendocardial pluripotential mesenchymal cells or endocardial nerve cells.

Etiology
* Incidence 1:100,000, Commoner in women.
* Comprises 50% of benign cardiac tumors in adults (15% in children).
* Peak incidence 3rd–6th decades.
* 5% show a familiar pattern of autosomal dominant inheritance.
* Myxomas have developed after cardiac trauma.

Pathological features
Myxomas are usually smooth, ovoid, polypoid, and mobile. Less common forms are sessile, villous, and papillary. Most are firm, but some may be gelatinous and friable. Most contain areas of hemorrhage, cyst formation or necrosis. The average size is about 5cm, but many are larger. Histology reveals polygonal cells and capillaries within a mucopolysaccharide matrix. Myxomas tend to grow into the overlying cardiac cavity rather than the surrounding myocardium. They occur in all chambers:
* 75% are LA, 20% are RA, 8% are ventricular.
* Multicentric tumors are commoner in familial disease.
* Atrial tumors commonly arise from the borders of the fossa ovalis.
* RA tumors tend to be broader based and calcified.

Clinical features
* **Embolism:** 30–40% of patients, mostly systemic but also cerebral (including retinal). PE is rare.
* **Intracardiac obstruction:** decreased RV or LV filling (lie patient down to dislodge tumor from outflow tract), pulmonary edema, RVF, syncope, sudden death, MR 'wrecking ball', patent foramen ovale (PFO) and shunting cyanosis. Removal described on p473.

- *Constitutional:* fatigue, fever, rash, pyrexia, arthralgia, myalgia, decreased weight, decreased Hb, increased CRP and ESR.
- *Infective:* infected myxoma and septic emboli.

Other primary benign tumors

Myxomas account for 40% of benign tumors, lipomas, papillary fibroelastomas, and rhabdomyomas account for another 40% of benign tumors, and a number of rarer tumors account for the remaining 20%.

Lipomas

Lipomas are encapsulated tumors of fat cells occurring predominantly in the pericardium, subendocardium and interatrial septum. RA and LV are the sites most commonly affected. The tumors are slow growing and usually asymptomatic. Subendocardial tumors may produce chamber obstruction, most commonly of the RA and LV. Non-encapsulated lipomatous hypertrophy of the interatrial septum is more common than cardiac lipoma. It is encountered in elderly, obese, and female patients. It is not an indication for surgery.

Papillary fibroelastomas

These tumors arise from the cardiac valves or endocardium. All four valves are affected equally frequently, and the villous tumors may occasionally produce flow obstruction and more commonly emboli. These tumors should be resected to prevent embolic complications.

Rhabdomyomas

Rhabdomyomas are probably myocardial hamartomas. They classically occur in children. 90% are multiple, and most are ventricular. They tend to present with flow obstruction, and early operation is recommended.

Primary malignant tumors

These tumors are rare, and largely incurable. They usually arise in adults over the age of 40. Angiosarcomas are 2–3 times commoner in men and 80% arise from the RA. They are bulky tumors which aggressively invade local tissues and metastasize to lung, liver, and brain. Resection is rarely justified and 90% of patients are dead 12 months after diagnosis. Rhabdomyosarcomas are multicentric in 60% of patients, and are also bulky tumors with a strong tendency to invade local tissue and metastasize.

Secondary tumors

Secondary tumors are over 30 times more common than primary cardiac tumors. Approximately 1 in 10 malignant tumors eventually spread to heart or pericardium. The commonest malignancies that metastasize to heart or pericardium are leukemias, lymphomas, breast, lung, melanoma, and various sarcomas via blood and lymphatics. Direct spread from adjacent lung, breast, esophageal, and thymic tumors is common. Subdiaphragmatic tumors including uterine, renal, hepatic, and adrenal may invade the RA via the SVC. 10% of renal cell carcinomas invade the IVC and 40% of these reach the RA.

Cardiac anesthesia

Monitoring, and respiratory and cardiovascular support are
discussed in Chapter 5—Cardiac ICU (📖 pp157–252)

Basic principles of anesthesia

Anesthesia may be general, regional, or local. The vast majority of cardiac surgery is performed under general anesthesia.

General anesthesia

A general anesthetic has three components: *hypnosis* (reversible state of unconsciousness), *analgesia*, and *muscle relaxation*

Hypnosis

* Hypnosis has three phases: *induction*, *maintenance*, and *emergence*.
* Induction and maintenance can be by iv or inhaled drugs.
* Intravenous induction is faster than inhalational induction.
* Some of the iv drugs used for hypnosis are the same as those used for analgesia—just in higher doses.
* As the hypnotic effect of iv anesthetic drugs is short, iv maintenance is by continuous infusion.
* Most induction agents are associated with a degree of *cardiorespiratory depression*, and usually cause *vasodilation*: particular care must be taken when inducing patients with acute tamponade, or critical AS to avoid acute decompensation requiring emergency intervention.

Analgesia

* Analgesia reduces both somatic and autonomic response to pain.
* Analgesics used in general anesthesia are usually opiates.
* Opiate analgesics are associated with respiratory depression.

Muscle relaxation

* Muscle relaxants are classified as depolarizing or non-depolarizing.
* Non-depolarizing muscle relaxants competitively bind with acetylcholine receptors at the neuromuscular junction and last up to 60min.
* They are reversed by *neostigmine*, an anticholinesterase.
* Depolarizing muscle relaxants non-competitively depolarize the muscle end plate causing *fasciculation* and rapid onset paralysis.
* They are effective for 5–15min.
* Choice is dictated by duration and cardiovascular effects (vecuronium and rocuronium have no cardiovascular side effects).

Examples of anesthesia for cardiac surgery

Regime A
* Premed: temazepam 10–20mg po 1h preoperatively.
* Induction: fentanyl 5–10 micrograms/kg and etomidate 10–20mg.
* Maintenance: isoflurane 1–2%, or further boluses of fentanyl.
* Muscle relaxant: pancuronium 0.1mg/kg.

Regime B Total intravenous anesthesia (TIVA)
* Premed: hyoscine 0.3mg im and 5mg morphine im 1h preoperatively.
* Induction: propofol 4–10 micrograms/kg/h.
* Maintenance: propofol 4–10 micrograms/kg/h + remifentanyl 0.3 micrograms/kg/min.
* Muscle relaxant: rocuronium 0.6–1mg/kg.

Fasting

- Elective patients should be fasted for 6–8h preoperatively to allow gastric emptying (NG feeds should be stopped 6h pre-op), reducing the chances of regurgitation and aspiration, although it is ok to take oral medication.
- Pain and opiates slow gastric emptying.
- Rapid sequence induction is used in an emergency to minimize the risk of gastric aspiration.
- Be explicit about fasting to nursing staff otherwise your outliers may get breakfast on the morning of surgery.

Preoperative assessment

- In addition to assessment that covers much of the ground described in Chapter 1 the anesthesiologist assesses the patient with particular regard to adverse reaction to general anesthesia, family history of malignant hyperpyrexia, dentition, and airway.
- The anesthesiologist explains the anesthetic plan, monitoring, induction and intubation, the possibility of awareness during surgery, and emergence while intubated on ITU, and potential complications.

Airway assessment

Ease of intubation has been graded according to the best possible view obtained on laryngoscopy. Grades 3 and 4 are difficult intubations. Difficult intubations can usually be predicted in advance by the presence of a combination of signs. In the *Mallampati scoring system* (📖 p644) the patient sits with mouth open and tongue protruded opposite the anesthesiologist, who assesses the structures visible at the back of the mouth. In Class 1 patients the faucial pillars, soft palate, and uvula are visible. In Class 4 patients none of these soft tissues are visible: these patients are extremely likely to be difficult intubations. In addition to the Mallampati scoring system the following predict difficult intubation:

- Thyromental distance <3 finger breadths with the neck extended.
- More than 2 Wilson risk factors; obesity, restricted head and neck movement, restricted jaw movement, receding mandible, buck teeth.
- Inability to flex the chin onto the chest.
- Reduced jaw opening (<2 finger breadths).
- Radiological features including mandibular depth.

Scoring preoperative condition

Although risk scoring for cardiac surgery has its own dedicated systems (Euroscore and STS Score, 📖 Inside cover) all surgical patients are also allocated an ASA grade (Box 3.1) preoperatively.

Box 3.1 American Society of Anesthesiologists (ASA) score

Grade I: healthy patient.
Grade II: mild systemic disease, no functional limitation.
Grade III: moderate systemic disease, significant functional limitation.
Grade IV: severe systemic disease that is a constant threat to life.
Grade V: moribund patient unlikely to survive 24h.

Conduct of anesthesia

Premedication

There is wide variation in choice of premedication, which is normally given an hour before the patient is transferred to the surgery area. Options include:
- A benzodiazepine, e.g. temazepam 10mg po, or lorazepam 2–4mg po: lorazepam has a half-life of 10–20h, temazepam is shorter acting.
- Intramuscular morphine 0.1mg/kg and scopolamine 4–8 micrograms/kg.
- Intramuscular morphine 0.1mg/kg and hyoscine 0.3 mg.

Transfer

Prior to transfer to the surgical area the following are verified:
- The patient's identification in the form of a wristband with name, date of birth, and a hospital number.
- The patient's name, date of birth, hospital number, operation details, signature, and date of signing, on the consent form.
- Availability of and patient details on cross-matched blood.
- Presence of responsible surgeon.

Prior to induction

The anesthesia area is prepared well in advance of the patient's arrival to ensure that all necessary equipment is present and working, and that the specific drugs required for induction are drawn up and labelled. Practice varies, but most anesthesiologists establish all monitoring, with the exception of the central venous catheter, prior to induction, as this ensures that any hemodynamic or respiratory compromise occurring as a result of induction will be rapidly detected and treated.
- The patient is sat at 45°.
- Oxygen is given by face mask.
- A pulse oximeter is attached and oxygen adjusted appropriately.
- EKG leads attached, checked and II and V5 used for display.
- A 14-gauge venous cannula is placed at the left wrist under local anesthesia, unless the left radial artery is to be harvested.
- A radial arterial catheter is placed under local anesthesia, transduced and a baseline blood gas is measured.

Patients at high risk of hemodynamic instability

Patients with the following lesions are at high risk of hemodynamic decompensation during the induction sequence, and a surgeon should be immediately available, and in the case of acute tamponade the patient prepped and draped ready for incision prior to induction:
- Tight LMS stenosis.
- Severe aortic and mitral stenosis.
- Acute cardiac tamponade or mediastinal bleeding.
- Severe pulmonary hypertension.
- Very poor LV function or cardiogenic shock.
- Pregnancy.

Induction

There is a wide choice of induction agents, and techniques. Use of fentanyl is described here: fentanyl has all the advantages of morphine (overdose is rare, it is not a myocardial depressant, it is non-explosive compared to inhalational agents, it facilitates postoperative management) as well as being a short-acting agent that is safe in the management of critically ill patients. The disadvantage is a risk of awareness.

- The patient is placed flat on a single pillow.
- Preoxygenation with 100% O_2 by face mask helps to avoid pulmonary hypertension in at-risk patients, as well as giving a safety margin by filling the functional residual capacity with O_2 if there are any problems establishing a secure airway later.
- 1mg of pancuronium may help avoid narcotic-induced rigidity.
- Induction: fentanyl 5–10 micrograms/kg and etomidate 10–20mg iv.
- As soon as the patient is unresponsive an appropriate dose of muscle relaxant up to a maximum of 0.1mg/kg of pancuronium is given.
- It may be necessary to give volume or a vasopressor such as metaraminol to treat hypotension at this stage.
- The trachea is intubated, and the ET tube secured.
- The table is placed in Trendelenburg position so that the central venous catheter, and pulmonary artery catheter if indicated, can be inserted.
- The urinary catheter is inserted, and the patient shaved.
- The table is levelled, and the pressure transducers adjusted.
- Prophylactic antibiotics are given: vancomycin is run an hour before incision to maximise serum concentrations.
- The EKG leads for the defibrillator and any TEE probe are placed, and an electrocautery pad is placed.
- The patient's arms are carefully secured to avoid compression injury.

Problems during induction

Respiratory
- Failure to secure an airway.
- Difficult intubation.
- Aspiration.
- Bronchospasm.
- Pulmonary hypertensive crisis.

Cardiovascular
- Cardiac arrest (critical AS and/or LMS, acute tamponade).
- Hypotension or hypertension.
- Ischemia.
- Arrhythmias.

Other
- Anaphylaxis
- Complications of with invasive monitoring (📖 p173, 175, 177).
- Dental and oropharyngeal trauma.
- Brachial plexus, ulnar and radial nerve injury, occipital alopecia, heel and sacral tissue necrosis may result from improper positioning.

Pre-bypass anesthesia

Key facts

Anesthesia management is aimed at optimizing several parameters over a period of time when surgical activity results in variable levels of sympathetic stimulation, as well as manipulation that impact cardiac function, namely:

- The ratio of myocardial oxygen supply: demand to prevent ischemia.
- Preload and afterload, particularly in patients with valvular defects.
- Heart rate, rhythm, and ventricular contractility
- Systemic and pulmonary vascular resistance, particularly in patients with pulmonary hypertension or congenital heart disease.

Median sternotomy

Skin incision, sternal division, sternal retraction, and dissection of the adventitia over the aorta result in high levels of sympathetic stimulation. An adequate depth of anesthesia is necessary to avoid tachyarrhythmias and hypertension. The surgeon should check that the anesthesiologist is happy with the level of anesthesia before starting. Sternotomy occasionally results in significant blood loss. Some surgeons ask for the lungs to be deflated prior to sternal division to reduce the minimal risk of damage to the lung parenchyma. A baseline ACT may be measured at this point.

Redo-sternotomy

This is discussed on 📖 pp344–347. The main differences in redos are:

- The patient must have **external defibrillator pads** on.
- Check cannulation and conduit plan with the surgeon as this dictates possible sites for siting arterial lines (e.g., patient will need left radial line if right axillary artery cannulation or radial harvest planned).
- There is a risk of injuring grafts, ventricle, or great vessels on sternal division: in high-risk cases the patient will be cannulated and even placed on bypass prior to resternotomy to reduce the risk.
- The dissection that must take place before the heart can be cannulated is longer, and involves more mechanical disturbance and bleeding.

Conduit harvest

- This is a period where sympathetic stimulation is minimal, and the anesthesiologist may need to treat bradycardia and hypotension.
- Compression of the left subclavian artery by sternal retractors may mean left radial lines do not accurately reflect systemic pressures.
- Major **occult blood loss** may occur into the pleurae or the leg wound.
- Brachial plexus injury can result from overabduction of the arm when positioning it for radial artery harvest.
- For harvesting the IMA the table needs to be raised, sometimes tilted away from the surgeon, and sometimes the lungs deflated temporarily.
- Heparin (300 units/kg iv) is given before the IMA is divided otherwise it could thrombose: the surgeon will ask for heparin to be given and the anesthesiologist should acknowledge the request.
- Check the ACT 3min after heparin is given (📖 p93).
- If the surgeon injects papaverine directly into the IMA it may be necessary to give phenylephrine to counteract vasodilation and hypotension.

> **Heparin and protamine: avoiding catastrophic drug errors**
> Principles of bypass are discussed in detail on 📖 pp102–124.
> * Acknowledge all communication, and repeat back key instructions e.g., 'give protamine' verbatim.
> * The ACT must be >400 before bypass.
> * Protamine must *never* be given while the patient is on bypass.

Preparing to cannulate

* Hitching the pericardium to the sternal edges frequently leads to transient hypotension as a result of vagal stimulation, and mechanical constriction of the SVC and IVC: if this does not respond to adequate volume resuscitation the surgeon should 'drop' the pericardium. TEE is helpful to reassess valve and ventricular function, guide coronary sinus catheter (Fig. 3.1) and assess aorta.
* Handling the RA while placing purse-strings may result in AF: *synchronized DC cardioversion* 10–50J with internal paddles is safest when patient is heparinized and cannulated as VF is occasionally induced.
* Blood pressure should ideally be <100mmHg systolic at aortic cannulation to reduce the risk of aortic dissection and bleeding.
* Once the aorta is cannulated and pipe connected, volume can be given rapidly by the perfusionist if necessary. Blood loss can be drained by pump suckers directly back to the pump if the ACT is >400.
* Once the venous cannula is in and connected the patient can be put on bypass if needed, but in order to minimize bypass time the surgeon will usually check condut and site additional vents first.

Management of conditions which affect bypass

Antithrombin III deficiency
If ACT remains <400 despite large heparin dose, give FFP to treat antithrombin III deficiency and recheck ACT.

Pregnancy
Although maternal mortality is the same as for a non-pregnant patient, fetal mortality approaches 50%. Placental ischemia occurs as a result of microemboli, elevated IVC pressure which reduces venous drainage, and pump flows inadequate for the hyperdynamic circulation associated with pregnancy. Uterine blood flow is not autoregulated. Dilution of progesterone may result in induction of labour. Management is targeted at establishing adequate pump flows, and avoiding hypoxia and hypothermia.

Heparin-induced thrombocytopenia
Heparin substitutes such as danaparoid may be used (📖 p288).

Sickle cell
Cardiopulmonary bypass exacerbates the tendency of erythrocytes to sickle because of vasoconstriction due to hypothermia, stasis, hypoxia, and acidosis. Even patients with sickle cell trait are at risk of a bypass-induced sickle cell crisis. This condition is managed with preoperative partial exchange transfusion to reduce Hb-S from 100% to less than 33%. Hypoxemia, acidosis and dehydration must be avoided preoperatively.

Anesthesia on bypass

Maintenance of bypass

Blood concentrations of drugs are diluted by the prime in the bypass circuit, and additional muscle relaxant and anesthetic agent may be required on bypass. Once full flow is achieved the patient is disconnected from the ventilator (just switching off the ventilator can result in air trapping, leaving the lungs inflated, interfering with the operative field).

Routine checks during bypass

- *Anticoagulation:* the ACT is checked after initiating bypass and every 30min thereafter, with additional heparin given in 5000-unit increments if necessary to maintain the ACT >500.
- *Blood gas and acid base status:* this is checked after initiating bypass and every 20min thereafter, with the PaO$_2$ maintained at >14kPa (105mmHg) by adjusting FiO$_2$ to the oxygenator, and pH adjusted according to whether management is pH stat or alpha stat (📖 p124).
- *EKG:* checked for inappropriate electrical activity during arrest and ischemic changes and arrhythmias pre-and post-arrest.
- *CVP and MAP:* these are recorded at 5–10min intervals, and should be 1–10mmHg and 50–70mmHg respectively (arterial pressures are maintained 70–80mmHg in elderly/arteriopathic patients).
- *Urine output:* the bag is usually emptied before bypass so that total urine output during bypass can be measured.
- *Face:* periodically check that there is no facial edema, or asymmetry in colour or temperature, and no pupil asymmetry, due to misplacement of the venous or aortic cannulas (📖 p110). Sweating, lacrimation, mydriasis may indicate inadequate depth of anesthesia.
- *Core and peripheral temperature:* nasopharyngeal or tympanic temperature probes measure core temperature which the perfusionist maintains at the temperature requested by the surgeon.

Common abnormalities on bypass

Problems of high line pressures, poor venous drainage and poor electromechanical arrest are discussed on 📖 pp113, 123. Management of catastrophic bypass problems is described on 📖 pp116–119.

Hypotension

- Flow rate deliberately decreased by perfusionist, e.g., when surgeon clamping aorta or dealing with bleeding.
- Inadequate flow as a result of inadequate arterial cannula size for patient's BSA, kinked or clamped arterial line, poor roller head occlusion.
- Low SVR due to vasodilation (give phenylephrine) or hemodilution.
- Cytokines in sudden return of pooled blood via pump suckers.
- Transducer error, calibration error, tubing disconnection, kinking or compression of subclavian, brachial or radial artery.
- Arterial cannulation problems including selective cannulation of carotid arteries, aortic dissection, or rarely reversed cannulation.

Hypertension

- High SVR due to vasoconstriction mediated by endogenous catechol-amines, hypothermia, awareness, and hyperoxia: treat the likely cause.
- Pump flows deliberately increased by perfusionist, e.g., to speed rewarming.
- Selective cannulation of subclavian proximal to radial artery catheter.
- Transducer too low.

High CVP

Poor venous drainage (📖 p113), inadvertently snaring SVC (📖 p111) proximal to cannula, obstructing venous return.
- Catheter abutting SVC wall, venous pipe or snared by surgeon.

Slow nasopharyngeal cooling or rewarming

- Excessive vasoconstriction.
- Low pump flows.
- Temperature probe misplaced or malfunctioning.
- High CVP impeding cerebral perfusion pressure gradient.
- Carotid artery malperfusion (e.g., inadvertent selective cannulation).
- Rarely increased intracranial pressure.

Hypoxemia

- Inadequate FiO_2 to the pump oxygenator.
- Low pump flows.
- Pump oxygenator malfunction (📖 p117).
- Causes of low SvO_2 are as given earlier, and $\uparrow O_2$ consumption secondary to hyperthermia, shivering, and rarely malignant hyperpyrexia.

Oliguria

- Post-renal problems such as kinked catheter tubing, misplacement, clamping, and catheter occlusion by gel or clot.
- Decreased glomerular filtration rate as a result of decreased renal perfusion due to inadequate pump flows, hypotension, renal vasoconstriction by drugs and hypothermia, increased IVC pressures, non-pulsatile perfusion, clamping of descending aorta and circulatory arrest.
- Pre-existing renal impairment.

Hemoglobinuria

- Hemolysis due to pump and pump sucker trauma.
- Trauma to urinary tract in setting of heparinization.
- Blood transfusion reaction.
- Rarely contamination of pump circuit with water from heat exchanger.

Electrolyte imbalance

- $\uparrow K^+$ due to administration of cardioplegia, impaired renal function.
- $\downarrow K^+$ due to dextrose and insulin administration, polyuria.

Awareness

About 1% of patients have recall of intraoperative events. This is due to a combination of dilution of anesthetic agents by the pump prime and absorption of fentanyl into the prime circuit: some patients are too unwell to tolerate higher doses of anesthetic agent. It is commonest when the patient is warm, as hypothermia induces unconsciousness. Variation between individuals means there is no dose of drug that guarantees unconsciousness. Careful titration of anesthetic agents is critical.

Anesthesia post-bypass

Criteria for discontinuing bypass

- No conditions that require CPB, e.g., residual valve leak, bleeding.
- Satisfactory rhythm, ventricular rate >60, paced if necessary, with adequate cardiac function, and minimal intracardiac air.
- Nasopharyngeal temperature 36.5–37.5°C.
- K^+ 4.0–5.0.
- pH 7.30–7.50.
- pO_2 >16kPa (120 mmHg).
- Anesthesiologist has resumed ventilating the lungs.

Weaning from bypass

Weaning from bypass is discussed in more detail on 📖 pp114–115. The anesthesiologist and perfusionist ensure that all parameters are suitable for discontinuing bypass without delay once surgery is completed.

The usual sequence of events for the anesthesiologist is:
- The perfusionist begins rewarming during the last surgical anastomosis. Core temperature should be 36.5–37.5°C as the patient loses heat once off bypass; overshooting may be bad for neurocognitive function.
- Place the table in Trendelenburg position for de-airing.
- Hand ventilate carefully ensuring the IMA graft is not placed under tension by lung inflation, and checking that the lungs expand fully.
- Place the patient on the ventilator. Surgeon de-airs heart (📖 p114).
- The perfusionist gradually allows the heart to fill and eject by progressively occluding the venous line at the same time as reducing pump flows, until pump flow ceases and the patient is 'off bypass'.
- Bypass can be terminated immediately at any point during this procedure, and it is usually better to come off relatively underfilled as excessive preload and afterload increase myocardial oxygen demand at the time when the heart is least able to deal with this.
- Rapid, controlled transfusion is given by perfusionist in aliquots of 50–100mL from the pump via the arterial line on request, and pump suckers can still be used to return blood to the pump, so there is no need to give volume intravenously.
- Inotropes, chronotropes, vasodilators, or vasoconstrictors are titrated.
- If hemodynamic instability or evidence of ischemia it may be necessary to return go back on bypass for a period to reduce the demand on the heart, and allow it to recover from stunning.
- Failure to wean from bypass is discussed on 📖 p117.
- Protamine slow push (3mg/kg/iv or dose calculated by Hepcon®) is given to reverse heparin **after** bypass is finally terminated.
- The surgeon will spend a period of time checking hemostasis while protamine is given, allowing time for full reversal of heparin.
- The surgeon decannulates the aorta once the pump is empty or the heart is full: systemic pressure should be <110mmHg systolic to reduce the risk of hemorrhage or dissection at this point.

Giving protamine

Management of **protamine reactions** is described on p116. Once the surgeon is sure that bypass will not be required again they will ask the anesthesiologist to give the protamine. It is good practice not to draw up protamine until this request is made as bypass has been inadvertently and catastrophically terminated by giving protamine by mistake instead of a drug in a nearby syringe. Although bypass is terminated blood can still be transfused to the patient from the pump via the arterial line if required, but use of pump suckers should be discontinued once protamine starts.

Avoiding catastrophic pump failure
- Do not draw up protamine until asked to give it.
- Never give protamine while the heart is on bypass.
- State clearly when you start to give the protamine: pump suction *should* be discontinued immediately by perfusionist or surgeon.

Variations in sequence

Decannulating before protamine is given
- If the surgeon expects that attempting to decannulate the aorta may cause sufficient hemodynamic compromise that bypass must be reinstituted, they may elect to decannulate before protamine is given. Some surgeons routinely decannulate the aorta before protamine is given to eliminate any risk of thrombus formation at the tip of the cannula.

Placing the aortic cannula into the right atrium after decannulation
If the surgeon anticipates substantial bleeding from the aortic cannulation site, they may elect to place the arterial cannula into the RA via the purse-string previously used for the venous cannula, so that blood transfusion from the pump may be continued if required.

Surgical maneuvers that cause hypotension
Always look at the operative field before treating hypotension: the cause is usually surgical and temporary.
- Aortic decannulation: (1) surgeon may compress heart or occlude venous inflow to deliberately lower arterial pressure in order to decannulate safely, (2) if significant bleeding occurs.
- Oversewing the atrial purse-string if arrhythmias or bleeding result.
- Lifting the heart to inspect anastomoses.
- Packing the pericardium.
- Hitching the pericardium: most surgeons unhitch at this stage.
- Approximating the sternal edges if there are packs around the heart.
- Deliberate occlusion of the IVC by the surgeon to reduce BP rapidly (see aortic decannulation).
- Pacing problems: use of electrocautery while on demand pacing if slow (or no) underlying rhythm, deliberate or inadvertent disconnection.
- Use of electrocautery interfering with IABP in EKG mode.

Anesthesia for off-pump surgery

Key facts

While off-pump surgery confers the benefits listed on 📖 p305, it presents surgeon and anesthesiologist with two major challenges, which anesthetic and surgical technique must overcome:
- Reduction in cardiac output when positioning the heart.
- Interruption to coronary blood flow during each distal anastomosis.

Anesthetic technique

One important reason for choosing off-pump surgery is that patients can sometimes be extubated earlier, but this can only be accomplished with appropriate choice of anesthetic agents and analgesia.
- Smaller doses of short-acting benzodiazepines are given as premedication, which may be supplemented by midazolam if necessary.
- Fentanyl and remifentanil are shorter-acting anesthetic agents that may be used in preference to propofol and opioids.
- Lines inserted by the anesthesiologist are the only means of giving rapid transfusion in the absence of an aortic cannula: there *must* be adequate wide-bore venous access.
- To help maintain cardiac output when the heart is positioned, patients are actively hydrated.
- Heparin is frequently given at a lower dose but check with the surgeon: doses vary between 100–300 units/kg iv.
- Most units routinely use TEE to assess LV function intraoperatively, and routinely place PA catheters to help detect ischemic changes (e.g., ischemic MR, elevated PA pressures).
- Continual measurement of ST segment changes is a very useful adjunct.
- Make sure that a sterile warming blanket is placed on the patient, as there will be no other way of securing normothermia intraoperatively.

Hemodynamic management during anastomoses

Hemodynamic changes occur rapidly, but can be anticipated by knowing the sequence of surgery, as well as by adjuncts to standard monitoring: ST segment analysis, TEE, and cardiac output measurements. Pressor support may be required during the distal anastomosis, during which preload must be optimized. The systemic pressure needs to be relatively high prior to the distal anastomoses, as positioning the heart inevitably results in a decrease in cardiac output. For the proximal anastomoses the systemic pressures need to be lower, to minimize the risk of aortic tears and dissection. It is possible to perform the proximal anastomoses first: this may be indicated to minimize the period of relative ischemia, and exploit low systemic pressures. The use of intracoronary shunts helps to reduce myocardial ischemia while performing distal anastomoses. The use of TEE may allow the anesthesiologist to assess whether the heart is likely to tolerate particular positions, by identifying valvular regurgitation, and ventricular impairment before the heart decompensates. Tachycardia makes distal anastomoses more difficult. It is easier to maintain hemodynamic stability when the pH is physiological. BP and cardiac output should return to baseline between each anastomosis.

Respiratory management

Sometimes it is necessary to stop ventilating for short periods to optimize surgical exposure. This is usually during anastomoses to the obtuse marginal vessels. The table will also be placed in steep Trendelenburg position for the right-sided anastomoses, which results in a reduction in pulmonary compliance and functional residual capacity. This may result in hypoxia, hypercarbia and atelectasis, which should be addressed by careful hyperventilation.

Postoperative management and extubation

Not all surgeons choose to reverse heparinization with protamine. If the patient is normothermic, not acidotic, and adequately ventilating, hemodynamically stable and not bleeding once the sternum is closed, they are candidates for waking and extubation in theatre, or shortly within intensive care. Adequate analgesia is imperative. Although intrathecal morphine has been used in some centres, most units use patient- and nurse-controlled analgesic iv morphine infusions. High O_2 flows, bronchodilator therapy, and chest physiotherapy are important adjuncts. Patients with good ventricular function and a full revascularization are usually hypertensive and tachycardic. They do not produce a diuresis as they are often relatively underfilled. A significant metabolic acidosis frequently develops during the first 6h postoperatively, resolving within 12h. The cause of the acidosis is unclear but may reflect an intraoperative low cardiac output state. As bypass cannot be used to warm these patients they may be hypothermic.
• Ensure these patients are adequately filled.
• Use warming blankets and infusion warmers to achieve normothermia.

These patients sometimes receive a reduced dose of intraoperative heparin depending on surgical preference, and should therefore receive early aspirin (75mg po) and low-molecular-weight heparin (5000 units sc) to ensure graft patency and avoid thromboembolic complications.

Epidural anesthesia in cardiac surgery

This technique is also used in cardiac surgery requiring cardiopulmonary bypass. An epidural is sited at either T1/2, T2/3, or T3/4. This may be done as early as the night before surgery. 8mL 0.5% ropivacaine with 20 micrograms of fentanyl is infused before induction of anesthesia so that sensory spread can be assessed. After induction the infusion is continues at 5–15mL/h. A sensory blockade of T1–T10 can be achieved. The epidural is discontinued on postoperative day 3. The most important complication is *paraplegia* from a spinal cord haematoma (risk approximately 1:3000). The benefits of this technique include:
• Large improvement in pain relief.
• Reduced opioid and NSAID requirement.
• Improved physiotherapy compliance.
• Improved respiratory function.
• Reduced length of ITU and hospital stay have been claimed.
• Reduced incidence of depression.

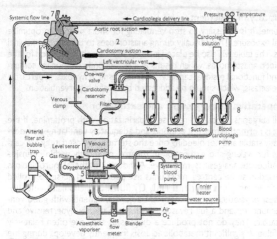

Fig. 3.1 Standard cardiopulmonary bypass circuit. Venous cannulae (1), vents and pump suckers (2) drain blood from the patient into the venous reservoir (3) which is then pumped (4) through an oxygenator (5) and then filtered (6) and returned at arterial pressure into the arterial cannula (7) (aorta, femoral or axillary).

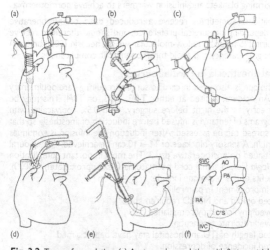

Fig. 3.2 Types of cannulation. (a) Aortocaval cannulation with 2-stage atrial cannula (note 2 levels of perforations, one at IVC and one within RA). (b) Bicaval cannulation. (c) Direct bicaval cannulation with right angled venous cannula. (d) Antegrade cardioplegia cannulae with root vent. (e) Retrograde cardioplegia cannula with syringe of saline to inflate balloon and manometry line. (f) Labelled heart: superio vena cava (SVC), pulmonary artery (PA), aorta (AO), right atrium (RA), inferior vena cava (IVC).

Cardiopulmonary bypass

Complications of bypass are discussed together with
off-pump surgery on 📖 p305. ECMO is described on 📖 p500.
Ventricular assist devices are discussed on 📖 p496. Myocardial
ischemia-reperfusion injury, stunning, and hibernation are
discussed on 📖 pp74–75. Spinal cord protection is discussed in
more detail on 📖 p436.

Cardiopulmonary bypass circuit 1

Key facts

Cardiopulmonary bypass (CPB) provides a still, bloodless heart while circulation to the rest of the body is maintained. Alternatives to standard cardiopulmonary bypass, including circulatory arrest and off-pump surgery, are discussed on p121. There are three essential functions of CPB:

- Oxygenation.
- Ventilation.
- Circulation.

The other important function of CPB is temperature control.

The CPB circuit

Desaturated blood drains from the RA or vena cava via venous cannulas and the venous line (1) to a reservoir (3). A pump (4) propels blood from the venous reservoir through a membrane oxygenator (5), followed by an arterial filter (6), into the patient's aorta via the arterial line and the aortic cannula (7). Adjuncts to the basic circuit include:

- Venous occlusion (an adjustable clamp on the venous line).
- Ports for drug and fluid infusions to the venous reservoir.
- Cardioplegia delivery system using a separate roller pump.
- Source of oxygen, air, CO_2 and anesthetic gases.
- Sampling ports, and in-line blood gas and temperature monitors.
- Bypass line around the arterial filter in case the filter obstructs.
- Low-level reservoir alarm.
- Ultrafiltration.
- Suction tubing leading to cardiotomy reservoir via a pump for removing blood from heart (vents) or the surgical field (pump suckers).

The standard components of the CPB circuit

- Atrial cannula (right atrial, caval, femoral and/or axillary).
- Venous line (PVC ½ inch diameter 12mm).
- Venous reservoir (integrated with oxygenator).
- Venous outlet (PVC ⅜ inch 8mm).
- Pump (peristaltic roller pump or centrifugal).
- Oxygenator (membrane oxygenator, defoamer and heat exchanger).
- Arterial filters macro and micro (300 micrometer) and bubble detector.
- Arterial line (PVC ⅜ inch).
- Arterial cannula (aortic, femoral, or axillary).

Venous cannulas

The technique of venous cannulation is described on p110. There are four main types of venous cannulas: Ross basket, two-stage, bicaval (single stage), and peripheral venous cannulas. The Ross basket is a large thimble-shaped metal tip, perforated with several large holes, designed to sit in the RA, so that the rim of metal is flush with the atrial purse-string. The two-stage venous cannula is tapered and reinforced with wire to prevent kinking. It is placed in the RA (usually so that an external marker is flush with the atrial purse-string) ensuring its perforated tip in the IVC, and the proximal perforation sits close to the SVC. Bicaval cannulas can be placed in each cava either directly (metal tipped) or via the right atrium (PVC). **Total CPB** completely eliminates venous return to the RA by placing snares around the caval cannulas. Two-stage cannulation is quick, and provides good venous drainage of the heart in a range of positions.

- Total CPB (bicaval cannulation with IVC and SVC snared) provides better myocardial cooling, but can result in poor SVC or IVC drainage if either cannula malpositioned or blocked, causing venous congestion.
- Total CPB prevents myocardial rewarming as a result of systemic venous return more effectively than other venous cannulation.
- Total CPB prevents airlocks (📖 p118) when opening the right side of the heart, although if using vacuum-assisted venous drainage (VAVD) airlocks occur only very rarely so snares are not necessary.
- Direct bicaval cannulation allows best exposure of the mitral valve.
- Ross basket avoids the risk of damaging the IVC during cannulation.
- For most surgery (coronary, aortic root, ascending, and arch work) a two-stage cannula provides good drainage and access.
- Various combinations of open or percutaneous femoral, internal jugular, and axillary venous cannulas are useful in minimally invasive (📖 p346) and reoperative (📖 p344).

Venous drainage

Venous drainage is by: (1) gravity siphonage: *the venous reservoir must be below the level of the patient, and the line must be full of fluid*, or (2) vacuum assist (VAVD). Inadequate venous drainage leads to the heart distending with blood, increasing myocardial oxygen demand which can lead to ischemia (📖 p113). Venous drainage is increased by ensuring the cannulas are in the correct position, and by increasing:

- The amount of vacuum assist (maximum of −60mmHg).
- CVP which is dependent on intravascular volume and compliance.
- Difference in height between the patient and the venous reservoir.
- Lumen of venous cannulas (36F for two-stage, up to 34F for bicaval).

Problems with venous drainage

- Inadequate venous drainage is caused by:
  - Malposition of the venous cannula: the CVP should be <2–6mmHg. If it is higher always check venous cannula for problems (📖 p113) as cerebral edema can result from inadequate SVC drainage.
  - Positioning the heart, kinking, or clamping the lines
  - Hypovolemia and vasodilation.
  - Airlock interrupting siphon drainage, loss of vacuum assist (📖 p118)
  - Tearing the IVC during insertion of a two-stage cannula (📖 p118).
- 'Chatter': venous drainage may be faster than blood return, leading to intermittent collapsing of the cava and atrium against the cannula, stopping drainage, rapidly alternating with atria filling with blood, causing juddering. To correct this, the perfusionist reduces venous drainage by increasing the amount of clamp or occlusion of the venous line.
- Hemolysis results from excessive VAVD and air admixture.

Cardiopulmonary bypass circuit 2

Arterial cannulas

The key is that the narrowest section of the bypass circuit is the part of the arterial cannula that enters the aorta; this limits flows and it should therefore be as short as possible. High flows through narrow cannulas generate high-pressure jets which may dislodge atheroma, and pressure gradient >100mmHg causing hemolysis, turbulence, and cavitation. Most standard 24F adult arterial cannulas provide adequate flows at gradients <100mmHg in patients of any size. A variety of options is available:

- Diffusion tips (several side perforations rather than one central one) are designed to reduce high-pressure jets. The Sarns Soft-Flow® is an example (vs. the Sarns bevelled tip).
- Vents to allow additional de-airing once connected.
- Flanges that may or may not be removable to improve hemostasis.
- Flexible lumen so cannula can be positioned out of the field.
- Seldinger technique for very small incisions (Edwards Fem-Flex®).
- Removable intra-aortic filter to capture debris (Edwards EMBOL-X®).

Tubing and connectors

Tubing and connectors are biocompatible, i.e., non-toxic, non-immunogenic, non-allergenic, and non-mutagenic. They should be waterproof, transparent, flexible but strong, inert, smooth, and easy to manufacture in bulk. Tubing is usually PVC and may be heparin bonded (which reduces complement activation). Traditionally *venous tubing diameter is ½ inch (12mm), and arterial tubing is ³/₈ inch (9mm)*: the large tubing size reduces resistance to blood flow, and the difference also minimizes the risk of incorrect connections.

Pumps

Pumps are either peristaltic or centrifugal. *Peristaltic or roller pumps* consist of a section of tubing inside a metal housing. Two rollers mounted at 180° to each other rotate so that one roller is compressing the tubing at all times. Blood flow is achieved by pushing the blood ahead of the moving roller. Excessive compression causes hemolysis. Inadequate compression also induces hemolysis and reduces forward blood flow which depends on the size of the tubing, the length undergoing compression, and the rpm. Roller pumps are used to provide arterial flow to the patient, for administering cardioplegia and for providing suction (by reversing the direction of tubing in the metal housing). If the line becomes occluded the roller pumps continue to exert pressure (positive or negative). Tubing and connector rupture is avoided by using pressure regulators. High negative pressures are avoided by the perfusionist either asking the surgeon to reposition occluded lines or by reducing the rpm.

Centrifugal pumps consist of a nest of smooth plastic cones located inside plastic housing, which is rotated at 2000–3000rpm generating a pressure differential. Centrifugal pumps are totally non-occlusive and afterload dependent: increase in downstream resistance decreases the rate of the pump and arterial return to the patient. When the pump is connected to the patient's arterial system, but is not rotating, the arterial line must be clamped as blood and potentially air will flow back into the pump from the patient. These pumps also become deprimed and stop working if >50mL of air is entrained.

Oxygenators

There are two main types of oxygenator: *membrane oxygenators* which are widely used, and *bubble oxygenators* which are no longer widely used. Most oxygenators come as part of an integral unit housing a heat exchanger, venous reservoir, arterial filter, gas inlet, infusion and sampling ports. Membrane oxygenators can either be true membrane oxygenators that completely separate blood and gas phases, with gas exchange occurring by diffusion, as in the lungs; or the membrane can be full of micropores which increase diffusion. Because the surface area required for adequate gas exchange is so much larger in true membranes, microporous membranes are used in clinical practice. There are two designs of microporous membrane oxygenator: the hollow fibre design with blood flow either inside or outside the fibres, and the folded envelope design.

Bubble oxygenators consist of two chambers. Venous blood flows into the first mixing chamber, and gas is pumped into it through a screen causing thousands of tiny bubbles to form: it is these across which gaseous exchange takes place. The mixture then flows into a defoaming chamber where it comes into contact with defoaming agents silicone Antifoam A and particulate silica. The main practical differences between membrane and bubble oxygenators are:

- Most of the damaging complement activation and inflammatory response occurs in the first few minutes of use of a membrane oxygenator, reducing as blood proteins coat the membrane (compared to bubble oxygenators where the blood–gas interface changes with every new bubble): membrane oxygenators are therefore preferred for long bypass procedures.
- There is a big pressure drop over the membrane oxygenator and the arterial pump is therefore placed after it in the circuit, as opposed to before the bubble oxygenator where the pressure drop is small.
- Ventilation and oxygenation are relatively independent in membrane oxygenators, and it is easier for the perfusionist and anesthesiologist to achieve set parameters by adjusting FiO_2.

Heat exchangers

Heat exchangers can cool or warm blood, controlling the temperature of the patient and of cardioplegia if required. Heat exchangers are an integral part of most oxygenators. They are located proximal to the oxygenator to avoid releasing gas bubbles into the blood, which can occur when the saturated blood is warmed. Water circulates within the heat exchanger between 2–42°C: temperatures outside these ranges risk denaturing proteins. As a result blood can be cooled (at 0.5–1.7°C per minute) more quickly than it can be rewarmed (0.2–0.5°C per minute) as greater temperature differentials can be maintained while cooling. Cooling is slower at lower temperatures for the same reason. The temperature of the patient lags behind the temperature of the perfusate, and the difference between the two is maintained at <15°C.

Pathophysiology of bypass

The pathophysiological changes associated with bypass are due to more than activation of the whole-body inflammatory response as a result of the passage of blood through the non-endothelial circuitry. Changes in temperature, acid–base balance, hemodilution, non-pulsatile flow, drugs, circulating volume, and the mechanics of bypass all contribute to dysfunction of blood constituent cascades and whole organ systems.

Activation of blood constituents

Plasma protein systems

CPB activates five plasma protein systems: the contact system, the intrinsic and extrinsic coagulation pathways, and the complement and fibrinolytic cascades. When blood encounters the non-endothelialized surfaces of the CPB circuit and the operative field, plasma proteins are instantly adsorbed onto the surface to produce a protein layer that varies with the material and the duration of exposure. A dynamic between circulating and adsorbed proteins is established. Heparin-coated circuits change the reactivity of adsorbed proteins but do not reduce thrombogenicity.

- *The contact system* (factors XII, XI, prekallikrein, and kininogen) is activated by non-endothelial surfaces, which in turn activates the intrinsic coagulation pathway, the complement pathway and neutrophils.
- Activated factor XI initiates the *intrinsic coagulation pathway* (📖 p71) which eventually converts prothrombin to thrombin, and fibrinogen to fibrin, providing a major stimulus to coagulation during bypass.
- Tissue factor produced by the damaged tissue surfaces of the wound triggers the *extrinsic coagulation pathway* by activating factor VII.
- Factor XIIa produced by the contact pathway activates C1 of the classic *complement pathway*, augmented by the alternative complement pathway which predominates during CPB, to produce anaphylotoxins that increase capillary permeability; alter vasomotor tone; impair cardiac function; activate neutrophils, mast cells, and platelets; and mediate cell and platelet lysis.
- Thrombin produced by activation of the coagulation cascade stimulates endothelial cells to produce tissue plasminogen activator, which cleaves plasminogen to plasmin resulting in progressive *fibrinolysis*.

Cellular systems

CPB activates five cellular systems which mediate systemic inflammation.

- *Platelet activation* via the glycoprotein IIb/IIIa receptor complex by heparin, thrombin, complement, plasmin, platelet activating factor, and hypothermia results in a decrease in platelet numbers and function, and is a major cause of postoperative bleeding.
- Although dilution decreases neutrophil counts during CPB, activation by complement, kallikrein, factor XIIa, and interleukin 1B results in *neutrophils* accumulating in the lungs where they mediate increased capillary permeability and interstitial edema.
- *Monocytes* are activated more slowly than other cellular elements by complement, endotoxins and contact with the CPB circuitry, producing tissue factor and cytokines, and conjugating with platelets.

- *Lymphocytes* including B-lymphocytes, natural killer cells, and T-helper cells are collectively reduced by CPB, reducing γ-interferon production, phagocytosis, and the response to infection for days.
- *Endothelial cells* produce tPA in response to circulating thrombin, activating the fibrinolytic pathway.

Systems dysfunction

Hemostatic

Bleeding and thrombotic complications associated with CPB are related to activation of platelets and plasma proteins, protamine and heparin. Bleeding times after CPB and full reversal of heparinization do not return to normal for 4–12h after bypass. Disseminated intravascular coagulation (DIC) and heparin-induced thrombocytopenia (HIT) and thrombosis (HITT) are discussed on 📖 pp288–289.

Fluid balance

Massive fluid shifts, largely into the interstitium, result from increases in systemic venous pressure, volume loading, reduction in plasma protein concentration as a result of dilution and adsorption onto the CPB circuit, and the inflammatory increase in capillary permeability described.

Endocrine

The combined stressors of surgery, hypothermia, CPB, and non-pulsatile flow trigger a hormonal stress response. Levels of cortisol, epinephrine and norepinephrine rise during bypass and remain raised for at least 24h afterwards, as does blood glucose. Circulating T3 falls below normal range. Release of numerous vasoactive substances, in addition to those described, that act throughout organ systems mean that CPB turns homeostasis into 'physiologic and biochemical chaos'.

Heart

This is described on 📖 p136.

Lung

Pulmonary edema is caused by activation of complement and sequestration of neutrophils in the pulmonary vasculature where they mediate increase in capillary permeability which is compounded by the fluid shifts described. CPB reduces the effect of natural surfactant, compounding the effects of general anesthetic and median sternotomy that predispose to pulmonary dysfunction (📖 p136). CPB increases shunts, reduces compliance and functional residual volume, and can cause ARDS (📖 p163).

Central nervous system

Stroke is mostly due to emboli from cannulating and clamping the aorta.

Kidney

Hemodilution, microemboli, catecholamines, low perfusion pressure, diuretics, hypothermia, and hemolysis impair renal function.

Gastrointestinal

Peptic ulceration is a response to stress, not to CPB per se. Pancreatitis and mild jaundice are not uncommon. Greater permeability of gut mucosa leads to endotoxin translocation, adding to the inflammatory response.

Technique of aortic cannulation

- There are many techniques of cannulation. The one described is a commonly used, safe way of cannulating the heart without an assistant.

Basic cannulation sequence

- Give heparin before dividing the LIMA, or after completing the median sternotomy if no IMA, and secure the CPB lines on the field.
- Hitch the pericardium and place side-towels.
- Palpate aorta and use epiaortic US to assess aortic atheroma.
- Place the aortic purse-strings.
- Check with perfusionist, clamp and divide the CPB lines (📖 p112).
- Check that the systolic pressure is <100mmHg.
- Place a pump sucker to the left of the PA if the ACT is >300.
- Warn the anesthesiologist that you are cannulating.
- Cannulate the aorta and connect the arterial line.
- Check that there is a good swing, and that the line pressure is okay.
- Place the right atrial purse string and cannulate the atria.
- Connect the venous line.
- If the ACT >400 you are now ready to go on bypass (📖 p112).

Aortic cannulation

- Palpate the aorta and use epiaortic ultrasound to identify atheromatous plaques. Pick a soft, clean spot, on the inner curve of the intrapericardial aorta, which is thought to be more resistant than the greater curve and the extrapericardial aorta to dissection and tears.
- Make two diamond-shaped purse-strings with a greater transverse diameter, about 1cm², using double-ended 4/0 Ethibond. The easiest way of doing this is two forehand partial-thickness stitches followed by two backhand partial thickness stitches, then the second purse-string, just outside the first, is four forehands. The trick to ensuring that the needle does not go full thickness is to mount it so that it is effectively flat and drive it parallel to the surface of the aorta.
- Place a snare on the sutures and place a clamp on the sutures.
- Now clamp and divide the lines (📖 p112), and check the arterial line for air.
- Take a Debakey's in your left hand and grasp the adventitia caudal to the planned arteriotomy. With an 15-blade in your right hand, and after clearing the adventitia from the cannulation site, scratch the aorta transversely until there is a 5mm incision down to the intima. Insert the blade full thickness. Pull the adventia over the aortotomy to maintain control while you pick up the aortic cannula.
- Hold the cannula so that the bevel is pointing towards the arch, and slide it firmly into the aortotomy up to the flange. Keep hold of the cannula with your right hand and tighten the snare with your left (you can't do this one-handed if you put the mosquito on the snare).
- Now still holding the snare tight with your left hand put a tubing clamp on the aortic cannula with your right hand positioning the clamp against the horizontal bar of the sternal retractor, propping the aortic

cannula in place so that you can tie it firmly to the snare with a heavy silk tie. Remove the plastic cap occluding the cannula.
- Partially release the tubing clamp to fill a gallipot with blood, completely de-airing the cannula. Replace the clamp on the aortic cannula.
- Remove the tubing clamp from the arterial line, and ask the perfusionist to wind up the level of fluid so that you can join the aortic cannula to the arterial line without any air. You can get rid of the air in the arterial line without the perfusionist winding up by cutting the line flush with the clamp and squeezing hard as you connect it to the cannula, but seeing the arterial fluid 'come up' confirms you have the right line flowing in the right direction.
- The perfusionist should confirm that there is a swing and, after infusing a small amount of prime, that the line pressures are satisfactory.

Problems with aortic cannulation

Poor exposure of aorta (short, high aorta or small, low incision)
Clamping aortic adventia, or passing a tape around the aorta, and retracting towards the feet improves exposure for cannulation. Use a McIndoe scissors to develop the plane between the PA and the ascending aorta, extend it by encircling the aorta with your finger and thumb, and pass a Sem clamp carefully from right to left under the aorta, opening it gently so that you can place a wet tape in the jaws.

Can't get the aortic cannula into the aortotomy
If your aortotomy is big enough, difficulty inserting the cannula is usually due to a flap of adventitia. If the systolic BP is low, the aorta will tend to slide away as you cannulate it. Control bleeding using a forceps or a finger, place a pump sucker to the left of the PA, and slide a closed McIndoe scissors into the aortotomy to confirm free passage. If the McIndoe scissors passes easily up to a 1cm, a 24 gauge cannula will.

Cut the purse-string
Should have used two purse strings. Either your purse sting was too small, or visibility was compromised by hematoma. Take a second suture, then ask the scrub nurse or assistant to hold the cannula in place, pushing down gently so that the flange helps control bleeding from the aortotomy. Sew a second purse-string around the aortic cannula, and snare as usual.

Adventitial hematoma
Caused by bleeding from full thickness purse-strings. Divide adventitia with McIndoe scissors. If bleeding is profuse place an extra purse-string.

Aortic root cardioplegia
Siting the cardioplegia cannula depends on whether it will be used as a root vent, proximal anastomosis site, or incorporated into an aortotomy. As a rule of thumb it needs to be far away enough from the sinotubular junction so that the aortic leaflets are not inadvertently damaged, at the highest point of the aorta if is going to be used as a vent, but far enough away from the aortic cannula that the cross clamp can be applied without difficulty. Stockert cannulas require a partial thickness purse-string with 4/0 proline. Flush the plegia so that there is no air in the circuit before connecting.

Technique of venous cannulation

The main advantage of having the aorta cannulated before you put in your atrial purse-strings is the ability to give rapid and controlled transfusion from the pump if handling the right atrium destabilizes the patient.

Atrial cannulation

Place a full thickness purse-string about 2×2cm (2×4cm if a Ross basket is being used) in the face of the atrial appendage, avoiding the right coronary artery in the AV groove, so that the free ends are at 12 o'clock. Snare these and hang them away from you so that their weight pulls the purse-string taut if you grasp the purse-string at 6 o'clock with a Debakey's. Open the purse-string vertically with an 11-blade, widen the incision using a McIndoe scissors, insert the cannula (or Ross basket attached to the end of the venous line) up to the appropriate mark. If you are using a two-stage venous cannula remove the obturator and quickly check that it is in the IVC by palpation. If it does not pass easily into the IVC do not force it. Snare the purse-string and tie it firmly to the venous cannula with a silk tie. Finally connect the venous line to the atrial cannula. There will be some air in the venous line: this does not matter unless you have enough (several feet) to cause an airlock.

Bicaval cannulation

Indirect

Site the first purse-string in the manner described. Site the other one 1–2cm away from the IVC (higher if you plan to 'cross' the caval cannulas). You need to gently retract the right atrium with your left hand, while placing a 2cm² triangle sized purse-string where the RA wall seems thick enough to hold it. The heart will decompensate as filling is impaired, so be prepared to release the right atrium in between stitches so that the heart can recover. Pass one cannula into the SVC and the other into the IVC—this can be done through either purse-string. 'Crossing' the cannulas is where the cannulas are placed via the purse-strings furthest away from the respective cavae, which can help exposure if a mitral retractor is not used. Ensure that the cannula in the SVC is rotated so that the bevel faces left, otherwise drainage of the left jugular and subclavian vein will be inadequate. Palpate the SVC and IVC to check that the cannulas are no further than 1cm into the cavae, snare and tie.

Direct

Dissect the pericardium off the SVC, being careful not to injure the phrenic nerve lying on the pleural side, and place a long narrow diamond purse-string on the SVC, well away from the sinoatrial junction. If exposure is poor ask the anesthesiologist to hold ventilation, retract the aorta using the tape or a nerve root retractor in your assistant's right hand, and have your assistant hold the SVC adventia with a forceps in their left hand. Place a pump sucker to the right of the SVC. Hold the SVC opposite your assistant with a forceps and make a 1cm longitudinal incision with an 11-blade. You control bleeding by pushing your forceps against the assistant's, while taking the cannula (which you should bend into an 'L' shape) and inserting the tip into the SVC. Tie it in place with two heavy silks to stop it spinning out of position. The IVC cannula is placed in the same way as for indirect cannulation. Connect the caval cannulas with a 'Y' connector. Some surgeons clamp the SVC cannula initially while going on bypass via the IVC to avoid a risk of entraining air, but it is just as easy to exclude air from the circuit using venous pressure before you connect it.

Taping the cavae

It is usually quite easy to pass a Sem round the IVC and SVC in order to tape them. Make it even easier by partially dissecting away the pericardial reflection superiorly from both vessels. This will also improve exposure of the mitral valve as the atria can be lifted further away by the retractor.

Retrograde cardioplegia

Site a $1cm^2$ triangular purse-string a few cm to the right of the atrial append-age. Bend the cannula 120°, point it away from you, and drop it through the purse-string. It should find its way naturally into the coronary sinus, and you will feel the cannula through the posterior surface of the heart. A man-ometry line is attached: coronary sinus pressure should be 30–50mmHg while plegia is being given. A drop in pressure implies that the balloon tip has deflated, the catheter is no longer in position or the sinus is perforated. The coronary sinus catheter also can be easily placed under direct vision by opening the RA once on bypass if you are bicavally cannulated.

Problems with venous cannulation

Can't get the venous cannula into the right atrium
If the purse-string and incision are not too small, trabeculae may prevent smooth passage. Put your little finger (middle finger if using a Ross basket) into the atriotomy, then try inserting the cannula again.

Can't get the venous cannula into the IVC or SVC
Either a prominent valve blocks passage of the cannula, or the cavo-atrial junction is distorted by putting the pericardium under too much tension. Try gently probing the IVC with the cannula using your right hand to pal-pate it and guide it from outside the RA.

Can't get the retrograde cannula into the coronary sinus
Orient the cannula so that it is not twisting around and pointing towards you and away from the coronary sinus once it enters the right atrium: use an external marker such as the position of the plastic handle as a guide. Place your hand under the hearts so you can feel the catheter. If you place a two-stage cannula first it may obstruct easy passage. TEE guidance can be helpful. *Never force it: placing it under direct vision is easier than repairing a perforated coronary sinus.*

Right atrium tears easily
Avoid placing purse-strings too close to the SVC and IVC unless you plan to cannulate them directly. Pick the white, thicker patches of atrial wall. Trying to primarily close tears in dilated, thin-walled atria can rapidly make them significantly worse. Use pledgets. If you make a significant tear, place a second purse-string to prevent entraining air during bypass.

Conduct of bypass

Heparinization

- The ACT should be >300 in order to cannulate.
- The ACT must be >400 in order to commence CPB.
- The ACT must be >480 for hypothermic CPB.
- 3mg/kg (300 units/ kg) is given iv by the anesthesiologist.
- 1mg of protamine is given for every 100U heparin for reversal.
- The ACT is checked after 3min.
- The pump contains 3 units/mL of pump prime (about 5000U).

Prime

Before institution of bypass the tubing is filled with crystalloid (or occasionally blood) to exclude air from the system. This is called priming, and takes ~2L of fluid (usually crystalloid based ± colloid ± 5000U heparin, which causes initial hemodilution, but blood can be used if needed). Large-bore tubing minimizes the gradients needed to achieve adequate flow rates. Minimizing tubing length reduces the amount of prime required. *Retrograde autologous prime* is where the patient's blood is allowed to flow back through the arterial cannula into the tubing, oxygenator, and reservoir displacing up to 1L of prime, with vaso-constrictors to maintain BP if needed. The aim is to reduce hemodilution and transfusion requirements: supporting evidence that this is achieved is mixed.

Dividing the lines

The arterial and venous lines are in continuity when they are handed out by the perfusionist, so that prime can be circulated continuously round the pump. The lines should have been completely de-aired by the perfusionist. Check that there is no residual air, tap connectors to dislodge any bubbles, and check that the perfusionist is ready for you to 'clamp and divide' the lines. Divide them so that tubing length is minimized and they sit flat on the drapes without kinking.

- If you clamp while prime is still being circulated by a roller pump you will cause the pressure behind the clamp to increase until either the perfusionist spots your error or the circuit ruptures.
- If you divide the lines before the perfusionist has clamped their end of the venous line, all the prime in the venous line will be siphoned into the reservoir leaving an empty venous line: refill from the table.

Commencing bypass

Connecting the lines to the cannulas is described on 🕮 p109. Try to ensure that that the venous line is uppermost (as this is often mobilized during surgery), that the arterial line is lowest (as this reduces the risk of it being dislodged) and that the cardioplegia and vents are between the two. It is customary not to give heparin until a satisfactory length of conduit is exposed, and not to go on bypass until all conduit has been checked in coronary artery surgery. The ACT >400 cut-off is based on early observational data that no thrombosis occurred in the reservoir at this ACT.

- Check the ACT >400 and that any line clamps are removed.
- Tell the perfusionist to 'Go on bypass.'

- The perfusionist gradually removes venous occlusion at the same time as gradually increasing the perfusion flow up to about 2.2L/min, taking care to balance venous return with arterial inflow.
- At full flow the anesthesiologist should stop lung ventilation.

High line pressures

This is when pressures >300mmHg are generated when the perfusionist attempts to transfuse volume from the pump into the aorta before bypass, or on commencing bypass. The aortic cannula may be abutting plaque, up against the opposite wall, not in the aorta, or have caused an aortic dissection (📖 p118). Stop transfusing immediately, check the line is not clamped or kinked, and evaluate the cannulation and aorta site directly, as well as with TEE.

Poor venous drainage

The perfusionist is receiving inadequate venous return, usually because the venous cannula is malpositioned (📖 p103, or because of low venous pressure. Adjust the venous cannula: the RA and RV should collapse. If they are already flat, then poor venous return is due to low CVP (📖 p103).

Sources of blood returning to the heart on bypass

Blood returns to the RA past the caval cannulas if they are not snared, and via the coronary sinus, great cardiac vein, and Thebesian veins. Blood returns to the RV via the RA and the Thebesian veins which drain the myocardium. Blood returns to the LA via the bronchial veins which empty into the pulmonary veins. This flow may be up to 200mL/min, and even greater in patients with COPD. Blood returns to the LV from the aortic root if there is AI (no clamp) or the aortic clamp is not fully on, from the left atrium and the Thebesian veins. Abnormal sources include persistent LSVC (📖 p121), patent ductus arteriosus, systemic to pulmonary artery (Blalog–Taussig) shunt, ASDs, VSDs, and anomalous systemic venous drainage. This blood is warmer and may cause myocardial rewarming.

Venting

Effective venting prevents left heart distension and reduces myocardial rewarming, both reducing the risk of myocardial ischemia; it also improves visibility and exposure, and helps in de-airing. Vent sites are:
- Aortic root (often as a sidearm on the cardioplegia cannula).
- Right superior pulmonary vein (placed into across mitral valve into LV).
- LV apex.
- Pulmonary trunk (left heart venting less satisfactory, via collaterals).

Cardiopulmonary bypass during operation

Flows are maintained at 2.2–2.4L/min/m², and the patient is cooled (or the temperature allowed to drift) down to 32°C for most CABG and valve operations. Lower flows are possible at temperatures below 28°C, as oxygen demand (VO_2) decreases. The peripheral vascular resistance is manipulated with vasodilators (NTG) and vasoconstrictors (metaraminol) so that systemic pressure is 60–80mmHg. Choice of temperature and hypothermia is discussed on 📖 pp124–125.

Weaning from bypass

Criteria for discontinuing bypass

• No condition (e.g., bleeding, residual regurgitation, ischemia) that requires bypass to correct.
• Heart largely free of air.
• Ventilating.
• Satisfactory rhythm, ventricular rate >60, paced if necessary.
• Nasopharyngeal temperature 36.5–37.5°C.
• K^+ 4.0–5.5mmol/L.
• pH 7.30–7.50.
• pO_2 >16kPa (120mmHg).

Standard rewarming

Rewarming occurs more slowly than cooling at 0.2 0.5°C/c ([] p105). Most surgeons ask the perfusionist to rewarm when they are on their last distal anastomosis (CABG), closing the aortotomy (AVR) or the atriotomy (mitral). As the perfusionist increases flows to speed up rewarming and supply increasing oxygen demand, there is an increase in coronary flow which may impair visibility slightly. Once bypass is discontinued the only means of warming the patient is using a sterile warming blanket. With the chest open there is net heat loss, but overwarming to 38°C is associated with adverse neurological outcomes. Hemostasis and chest closure should be carried out efficiently to reduce further heat loss.

De-airing the heart

This is a critical process, particularly important after valve surgery. De-airing in CABG normally consists of needling the grafts proximal to bulldog clamps, and releasing the clamps once air and no longer be seen in the conduit. There are a variety of ways of de-airing after valve surgery. A sensible way is to de-air the heart chambers sequentially is:

• Use CO_2 insufflation into the field for valve surgery.
• As the aortotomy or atriotomy is closed, stop venting the LA and LV.
• Close the suture line as blood completely fills the chamber.
• Vent the aortic root (venting earlier will just suck air into the heart).
• Release any caval snares and ask the perfusionist to 'fill the heart' (the perfusionist partially clamps the venous line, so that the right side of the heart fills with blood, displacing any air present on the right).
• Ask the anesthesiologist to 'inflate the lungs', which dispels air from the pulmonary veins into the LA, which can be aspirated from the dome of the LA or by loosening the LA suture line temporarily.
• Some surgeons shake the patient to dislodge air from underneath valve leaflets and trabeculae, bringing to it to the surface of the chambers: agitating the heart has a similar purpose.
• If a mechanical mitral valve is being frustrated with a Foley catheter, deflate the balloon, remove the catheter and close the atriotomy.
• Lift the heart gently so that the LV apex can be aspirated.
• If an LV vent has been used, agitate the heart until micro air bubbles stop leaving the ventriculotomy, which should then be oversewn.

- 'Empty out' the heart, stop ventilating, put the patient head-down.
- Reduce flows temporarily as the aortic clamp is released.
- Continue venting the aortic root.
- Defibrillate the heart if it is not beating and pace if necessary.
- Agitate the ventricles again, and ask the perfusionist to gently fill the heart so that it is ejecting, and reassess air using TEE.

Sudden arrhythmias and ST segment changes during this period usually reflect coronary air embolism. Resume full bypass and increase MAP to >80mmHg. Re-ops need more aggressive de-airing as adhesions distort tissue, creating pockets of air particularly in the pulmonary veins which take longer to shift.

Discontinuing bypass

The perfusionist, anesthesiologist, and surgeon should work together to monitor the effect of gradually reducing CPB flow on the heart. The perfusionist gradually increases occlusion on the venous line at the same time as reducing arterial flow. Increasing occlusion fills the heart. Ventricular function can be assessed by the surgeon (the RV should still wrinkle, the heart should not rise much above the pericardial reflection and the PA should feel reasonably soft to palpation), and by the CVP which should be 10–12mmHg. It is possible to come completely off bypass at any time during weaning. If is usually safest to come off with the heart underfilled rather than overfilled, as the increased afterload and preload increases myocardial oxygen demand at a time when myocardial stunning may mean that the heart is poorly equipped to deal with this. Once you are off bypass, if the heart appears to be contracting well you can ask the perfusionist to transfuse some of the remaining volume in the venous reservoir. Some teams give vasodilators so that all of the volume remaining in the venous reservoir can be transfused back to the patient. Poor LV is managed by a period of partial bypass while preload, afterload and contractility is carefully adjusted using inotropes, pressors, and filling. The goal is MAP 75–80 and CVP 6–12mmHg.

- Once bypass is discontinued the venous cannula can be removed.
- The blood in the venous line is siphoned by the perfusionist.
- The venous cannulation site is snared.
- Protamine is given slowly, and hemostasis secured.
- Volume is transfused as appropriate into the aorta.
- The aortic cannula is removed and both cannulation sites oversewn.

Protamine

Giving protamine on bypass leads to catastrophic thrombus formation in the circuit causing systemic emboli and failure of the oxygenator. Protamine is given once bypass has been permanently discontinued, in a slow iv push. 1mg of protamine is given for every 100U of heparin given. Pump suckers should be removed as soon as protamine is started. The ACT is checked after 5min and further protamine given if required. Protamine is usually associated by a transient drop in systemic pressures, and occasionally with one of four types of adverse reaction (📖 p116).

Emergency bypass scenarios 1

Protamine reaction

Protamine is a polycationic protein derived from salmon sperm, which binds ionically with anionic heparin in a 1:1 ratio, to produce a stable precipitate. Protamine contains two active sites, one that neutralizes heparin and one that has a mild anticoagulant effect. There is therefore a theoretical risk that excess protamine is anticoagulant: it is probably only clinically relevant at 3× the appropriate dose. Protamine has a mild direct antiplatelet effect. Bleeding may occur 2–3h after protamine administration due to heparin rebound (heparin is resorbed from plasma proteins after protamine has been cleared from the circulation) which is treated by additional protamine administration. The **Horrow classification** lists three main types of protamine reaction.

Horrow classification of protamine reactions

- I: hypotension from rapid administration.
- II: anaphylactic reactions.
- III: catastrophic pulmonary vasoconstriction.

Type II reactions are subdivided into IIa true anaphylaxis, IIb immediate anaphylactoid, and IIc delayed anaphylactoid reactions.

Type I reaction

Protamine induces hypotension independently of the heparin–protamine complex, mediated by histamine release. This is dependent on the rate of administration. The fact that some patients become much more hypotensive than others probably reflects reduced myocardial reserve. Give heparin slowly (over 5min). Treat hypotension with careful volume transfusion from the pump. Inotropic support may be necessary.

Type II reactions

True anaphylaxis to protamine (Horrow type IIa) is mediated by a specific antiprotamine IgE antibody, and does not require the heparin–protamine complex. It requires previous exposure to protamine and is commoner in diabetics taking protamine-zinc insulin, patients with prior protamine exposure, and possibly patients with fish allergies. Vasectomized men are theoretically at higher risk because of cross-reactivity between antibodies to human sperm protamine and fish sperm protamine. Massive release of histamine and other inflammatory mediators (leukotrienes, kinins, prostaglandins) leads to acute bronchospasm, hypotension as a result of coronary vasospasm and systemic vasodilation, and angioedema. Respiratory and circulatory collapse can ensue. Anaphylactoid reactions are similar but less dramatic, and probably mediated by the complement pathway. Management for anaphylactic collapse is:

- Discontinue protamine immediately.
- 10mL of 1:100,000 adrenaline iv.
- 100mg hydrocortisone iv.
- 10mg chlorphenamine (Piriton®) iv.
- 100% O_2 if necessary, with nebulized bronchodilators.

Type III reaction

Acute pulmonary vasoconstriction leading to RV failure, circulatory collapse, and sometimes bronchospasm is caused by activation of the complement pathway and massive release of thomboxane A2 (a potent vasoconstrictor) in the lungs, after even minute doses of protamine, in <1% of patients. Acute RV failure due to poor myocardial protection causes a similar picture, with similar timing, and is managed the same way:

• Discontinue protamine infusion and give full dose of heparin.
• Give 10mL of 1:100,000 epinephrine.
• Start NTG and consider milrinone to reduce pulmonary hypertension.
• The initial episode usually may resolve, but if the heart is too compromised to weather this period recannulate (with internal massage if needed) and go back on bypass as soon as safe to do so.
• Slow administration of protamine is usually well tolerated a second time.

RV or LV failure

Failure of the heart to wean from bypass is manifested by low systemic pressures, high filling pressures, PA that feels very firm to touch, and a distended and dyskinetic ventricle. Myocardial stunning ($\square$ p74) accounts for an acute deterioration in LV function. Repair of severe mitral regurgitation may unmask poor LV function by removing the low-resistance regurgitant pathway ($\square$ p401). Incomplete revascularization or inadequate myocardial protection results in reduced LV and/or RV function.

• If you have already started protamine, stop and give full-dose heparin.
• Go back on bypass, ensure the heart is fully decompressed (vent PA).
• Some surgeons recommend a period on bypass equal to 1/3 of the ischaemic (cross-clamp) time to allow stunned myocardium to recover.
• Escalate inotropic support ($\square$ p198).
• If necessary, pressure in the aortic root, pulmonary artery and LA can be measured directly using a manometry line handed out to the anesthesiologist and a 23G (blue) needle, to help assess preload and afterload, and confirm invasive monitoring.
• If the heart fails to wean with appropriate support, insert an IABP.

Pump failure

Pump failure is unusual. Causes include electrical failure (rare because most operating rooms have back-up generators, and many CPB consoles have their own battery packs), and oxygenator failure (0.25 per 1000 pump runs), which is associated with the inadvertent administration of protamine during CPB that causes massive clot throughout the bypass circuit and oxygenator. In the event of total electrical failure the bypass circuit can be hand cranked. Oxygenator failure (characterized by inadequate oxygenation despite increasing FiO_2, and high transmembrane pressures) requires circulatory arrest (maximum of 5min safe at 36°C, longer at lower temperatures $\square$ p125) to replace the oxygenator and recirculate: a drill that all perfusionists are taught and rehearse regularly. *Inadvertent administration of protamine requires a new pump circuit as well as administration of heparin. To avoid this potentially lethal error protamine is never drawn up until the instruction to give it is made.*

Emergency bypass scenarios 2

Aortic dissection

Aortic dissection from aortic cannulation has an incidence of about 0.05%. It can occur at the clamp or antegrade cardioplegia, but more commonly at aortic cannulation where it is recognized by:
- Purple hematoma with bleeding at a distance from the cannula site.
- Blood does not rise up the aortic cannula on cannulation.
- On removing the tubing clamp, blood does not flow normally.
- The patient becomes profoundly hypotensive with low RAP.
- Ischemic changes develop on the EKG.
- 'No swing' on connecting up the arterial line with the aortic cannula.
- Low systemic pressure confirmed by the Teicos and palpation.
- High line pressures on infusing prime via the aortic cannula.
- Poor venous return.
- *TEE or epiaortic ultrasound shows dissection flap.*

▶ If bypass has to be discontinued for any reason always clamp the venous line, or the patient will exsanguinate into the venous reservoir.

The patient needs emergency repair of the dissection, usually with an interposition graft, in addition to the planned surgery. Stop bypass immediately. Clamp the aortic cannula. Place the aortic cannula into the RA so volume can be given rapidly as required, and proceed to femoral-caval bypass immediately, or occasionally cannulation of distal arch. Survival of aortic dissection recognized intraoperatively is about 85%.

IVC laceration

The IVC may be lacerated by passage of venous cannula, attempts at snaring the cavae, or dissection during redo surgery. Intrapericardial tears are obvious from venous hemorrhage into the pericardial sling, classically after termination of bypass. Intra-abdominal tears result in:
- Poor venous return.
- Low systemic and filling pressures.
- Loss of volume from the bypass circuit requiring volume replacement.

Perform a patch repair with autologous pericardium or saphenous vein graft as the tissue is usually too friable to close primarily, and to avoid stenosis. Endovascular stents have been used for intra-abdominal tears.

Airlock

If substantial amounts of air enter the venous lines (from perforation of the RA or cavae, dislodged venous cannula, or communication between an open LA and a cannula in the RA) the siphon may be interrupted, resulting in cessation of venous return, emptying of the venous reservoir and interruption of bypass if not addressed quickly. Reposition the cannula if grossly displaced. Chase the air down to the venous reservoir by elevating each section of the venous line from heart to pump in turn. It may be necessary to refill the venous line from the table. Vacuum-assisted venous drainage almost eliminates this problem: airlocks only occur with substantial air during periods of low flow.

Air embolism

In contrast to venous air, arterial air can be catastrophic. Air can enter the heart from the operative field, the pump, or anesthetic lines. Fatal air embolism can occur from amounts as small as 0.25mL/kg entering the left side of the heart and the coronary and cerebral circulation. Although right-sided air embolism is better tolerated in the absence of PFO, it can lead to severe pulmonary hypertension. Surgical sources of air include aortic cannulation, cardiotomy for valve surgery, entraining air with aggressive RSPV venting, entraining air from opened LAD when venting the aortic root. Air tends to collect in the LA, in the right superior pulmonary vein, and within the trabeculae of the LV, which explains the rationale for standard de-airing techniques (📕 p114). Air embolism from the CPB circuit can occur if the CPB reservoir empties: maintaining volume of the reservoir by interrupting bypass if necessary is a fundamental safety principle. Accidental disconnects, punctures, taps open to air, oxygenator or vacuum-assist malfunction can all potentially result in air embolism. The treatment of air embolism depends on the severity and timing:

- Coronary air embolism is best managed by continuing CPB, if appropriate pinching the aorta distal to the aortic cannula to increase coronary perfusion pressures for a few minutes.
- Hypothermia, retrograde coronary and cerebral perfusion (see Box 4.1) and de-airing procedures (📕 p114) are useful adjuncts.
- Ventilating the patient with 100% oxygen and decreasing cerebral oxygen demand by packing the patient's head in ice may help.
- If air embolism occurs before or after CPB with cardiac arrest, place the patient head down in the left lateral position and institute CPR.
- Drug therapy is first aimed at increasing BP to 'flush' air through to the venous circulation, and then limit tissue damage with steroids, diuretics, antiplatelet agents, anticonvulsants, and barbiturates.
- The surgical procedure should be completed regardless of the timing.
- Compression in a hyperbaric chamber and ventilation with 100% oxygen is the definitive management, but logistics make this difficult.

Box 4.1 Treatment of massive air embolism on bypass
- Stop bypass immediately
- Clamp venous and arterial lines, aspirate air, start cardiac massage.
- Put patient head down, occlude carotids and place ice around head.
- Remove aortic cannula from ascending aorta.
- Connect venous and arterial lines together so that air can be purged from the bypass circuit by the perfusionist, or fill from table.
- If large quantities of air have entered the cerebral circulation insert the aortic cannula into the SVC and snare it.
- Begin retrograde cerebral perfusion at 20°C at 1–2L/min for 1–3min, until no more froth is seen entering the aorta.
- Otherwise reconnect the lines to the appropriate cannula and resume bypass with active aortic root venting.
- Give 2–4g methylprednisolone and 25g mannitol.

Alternative approaches

Alternatives to ascending aortic cannulation

There are several alternative arterial cannulation sites if the ascending aorta is unsuitable for any of the following reasons:

- Porcelain aorta (a completely calcified aorta).
- Severe atherosclerosis with or without liquid intramural disease.
- Surgery involving the distal ascending aorta or aortic arch.
- High-risk re-do surgery (p344).
- Small incision surgery (p458).

Elsewhere on the aorta or innominate artery

- Underside of the distal aortic arch is most likely to be disease free.

Femoral artery: left or right.

- Useful in emergency, re-ops, and minimally invasive approaches.
- Vasculopathy relative contraindication.
- Disadvantages: increased risk of stroke with retrograde arterial perfusion in patients with atherosclerotic aortic disease. Risk of peripheral limb ischemia almost eliminated by cannulating via an 8mm Dacron side graft sewn end-to-side onto the artery with 5/0 Prolene.
- *Technique*: 3–4cm incision in skin crease over femoral pulse, blunt dissection down onto femoral artery (may be very adhesed if prior arterial punctures), give 5000U of heparin. Either modified Seldinger insertion of 22F FemFlex cannula or sidegraft (see axillary). Arteriotomy should be repaired at end of case.

Axillary artery: usually right

- Particularly useful for selective perfusion in arch surgery (pp125, 449), but also good for same indications as femoral cannulation.
- Less likely to be involved in vasculopathy, and antegrade arterial perfusion means stroke risk greatly reduced compared to femoral.
- Disadvantage is proximity to brachial plexus and obvious incision.
- Lower risk of peripheral ischemia as more collaterals than femoral.
- *Technique*: 4–5cm oblique incision 1cm below lateral 1/3 of clavicle, divide pectoralis major with cautery down to pectoralis minor, divide pec minor for easiest exposure, axillary artery lies immediately beneath pec minor. Give 5000U of heparin. Silastics to control 2–3cm of artery avoiding brachial plexus fibres, and ligate all arterial branches (if you use silastic ties these can be removed at end of case). Apply vascular clamps proximally and distally, longitudinal arteriotomy, sew 8mm Dacron sidegraft with continuous 6.0 Prolene, and cannulate with 24F Sarns (remove cuff). Multiple silk ties around graft and cannula. Clamp cannula, remove vascular clamps from axillary artery, de-air and connect in usual fashion. Use distal axillary sling to prevent hyperperfusion of arm. Staple or oversew graft at end of case.

Alternatives to caval cannulation

If it is not ideal to cannulate centrally (minimally invasive, or re-operative surgery), the femoral or axillary vein can be cannulated after heparinization, percutaneously or under direct vision, passing a long perforated venous cannula carefully up into the RA under TEE guidance using Seldinger technique. If done open, place a 5/0 purse-string for easy closure at the end of the case.

- Fem-fem bypass is bypass via femoral artery and vein.
- Fem-caval bypass is via the femoral artery and RA.
- Aorto-femoral bypass is via the aorta and femoral vein.
- Axillo-caval bypass is via the axillary artery and RA.

Alternatives to cross-clamping the ascending aorta

- If the aorta cannot be clamped (porcelain aorta, severe atherosclerosis, imminent rupture) there are several options:
- **Beating heart on bypass**, where the aorta is not clamped and the coronaries are perfused with blood from the aortic cannula for the duration of surgery can be used to perform coronary mitral, tricuspid, or pulmonary valve surgery. If there is more than minimal aortic insufficiency it can be quite difficult to get decent visualization of the mitral valve because of blood flooding the field.
- **Fibrillating heart on bypass** can be used in conjunction with beating heart or on its own. If the aortic valve is incompetent the LV must be adequately vented as soon as the heart stops beating to prevent distension. Fibrillating the unclamped heart on bypass may occur as part of a deliberate hypothermic protection strategy (usually < 32°C), or can be done using a fibrillator at normothermia, in order to minimize the risk of air being ejected from the LV during mitral surgery performed without a cross-clamp.
- Neither of these are options for aortic valve or aneurysm surgery. In this case **deep hypothermic circulatory arrest** (DHCA) (📖 pp124–125) must be instituted if it is impossible to clamp the aorta, via any of the cannulation strategies outlined opposite. It is possible to resume cardiopulmonary bypass once a graft has been sewn onto the transected distal aorta, de-aired and clamped. (📖 p125, 📖 p449).
- **Off-pump coronary surgery** (📖 pp304–305, 335).

Persistent left superior venal cava

A left SVC is present in 0.3–0.5% of the general population, and in 2–10% of patients with congenital heart disease. It drains the left subclavian vein and jugular veins into the RA via the right coronary sinus in 90% of cases, and into the LA in 10% of cases. Suspect the presence of a LSVC if the innominate vein is small or absent; TEE may show an enormous coronary sinus.

- If the right heart is not opened and a two-stage cannula is used, a LSVC poses no problems. Retrograde cardioplegia will not work.
- If bicaval cannulation is used, the problem of blood flow into the RA causing right heart distension, or occluding the operative field can be solved by snaring the LSVC, unless there is absence of the RCVC or innominate vein in which case cerebral edema would result.
- If the LSVC cannot be snared, it can be cannulated via the coronary sinus, vented or cannulated distally with a caval cannula.
- Induction of deep hypothermic circulatory arrest with a single venous cannula is used in infants.

Myocardial protection

Key facts

- Myocardial protection should minimize myocardial ischemia and damage during bypass, primarily by reducing myocardial O_2 consumption.
- This is usually achieved by rapid diastolic arrest, mild or moderate hypothermia, buffering, avoiding substrate depletion, and intracellular edema using cardioplegia, but there are alternative options (Box 4.2).

Cardioplegia

Rapid diastolic arrest reduces MVO_2 by 90% and minimizes depletion of high-energy phosphates. Reducing the arrested heart from 37°C to 32°C drops MVO_2 by 90%: lower achieves little extra benefit. Most strategies rely on concentrated K^+: St. Thomas' and Bretschneider are crystalloid solutions. Blood cardioplegia, e.g., Buckberg, is used for its intrinsic O_2 carrying and buffering capacity: it may better protect in poor LV or long ischemic times. Crystalloid plegia is given from a pressurized bag. Blood plegia is given from the pump enabling accurate control and monitoring of volume, pressure, flow and temperature, and is made up from the patient's blood once CPB is commenced.

Antegrade cardioplegia

Root cardioplegia

Plegia is given into the aortic root via a simple trocar, e.g., Medicut, or via a cannula with a side arm root vent, e.g., Stockert, which needs a partial-thickness 4/0 Prolene purse-string 2cm from the sinotubular junction.

- Flush the cardioplegia line so that it is completely free of air.
- Insert the cannula taking care not to damage the back wall of the aorta.

Box 4.2 Types of myocardial protection

- Myocardial protection may or may not involve cardioplegia.
- Non-cardioplegic methods include 'cross-clamp fib' (🔲 p325), fibrillating (🔲 p121) or beating heart (🔲 p325) on bypass, and DHCA (🔲 pp124–125).
- Cardioplegia may be given intermittently or continuously, given antegradely or retrogradely, be crystalloid (which can be intracellular, e.g., Bretschneider or extracellular, e.g., St. Thomas'), or blood (warm or cold) and high (20mmol/L) or low (10mmol/L) K^+.

Protection in high-risk cases

In cases with long ischemic times or severe RV and LV dysfunction protect the heart by maintaining a uniform cold temperature using systemic cooling, topical hypothermia, insulating pads (to stop liver warming base of heart), venting to prevent collateral flow warming heart, total CPB (🔲 p103), myocardial temperature monitoring, frequent (15min) doses of cardioplegia, running cold blood the rest of the time. Retrograde cardioplegia facilitates this. A hot shot is given (🔲 p123).

- Snare to the purse-string, remove the trocar, and clamp the cannula.
- Ask the perfusionist to trickle the plegia and connect the cannula.
- Ask the perfusionist to reduce flows while you cross-clamp the aorta between the aortic cannula and the antegrade cardioplegia cannula.
- Ask the perfusionist to give cardioplegia—either until complete electromechanical arrest is achieved, or a standard volume (800mL–1L).
- Check the LV and RV intermittently to ensure they are not distending and are cooling uniformly, and that the aortic root is pressurized.
- Once all cardioplegia is given and the heart is arrested, clamp or remove the cardioplegia cannula and empty the LV by venting the aortic root and/or gently squeezing the ventricles.

Ostial cardioplegia

This technique requires an aortotomy. The aorta is opened after clamping, and pump sucker placed in the LV, and the ostia visualized. A balloon-tipped cannula is attached to the cardioplegia line: size 6–7 for the left main, size 5–6 for the smaller RCA. If plegia does not run well, adjust the angle, or try a smaller cannula. Beware of inadvertently selectively cannulating the circumflex or LAD in the patient with a short LMS.

Retrograde cardioplegia

Insertion is described on 🕮 p111. Retrograde cardioplegia does not protect the RV if the cannula is inserted too far, bypassing the great cardiac vein. It is a useful adjunct when high-grade coronary stenoses make antegrade delivery inefficient, or there is a need to give continual cardioplegia during long surgery (e.g., root replacement, complex mitral repair) without adjusting the heart or stopping the flow of surgery. Venovenous channels mean up to 60% drains back into the heart via the Thebesian veins. Satisfactory administration can be confirmed by: (1) decrease in myocardial temperature; (2) sustained increase in coronary sinus pressure from 0–10mmHg to 50mmHg while giving 100mL/min; (3) filling the cardiac veins over the RV; (4) dark blood issuing from both coronary ostia.

Terminal warm blood or 'hot shot'

Before unclamping (and usually while performing proximal anastomoses or closing heart, warm blood (no extra K^+) is usually or retrograde which may restore energy stores and may improve ventricular recovery (although data is very mixed), as well as help with de-airing.

Failure of the heart to arrest

- High-grade proximal RCA lesion (no plegia reaching sinus node).
- Blood cardioplegia is slower to arrest than crystalloid, and retrograde arrest is slower than antegrade.
- Cross-clamp not properly applied (plegia diluted with aortic blood— stop giving, reduce bypass flows, and reapply clamp more carefully).
- L/RV distension (vent, improve drainage, check clamp, caval snares).
- AI (plegia filling LV—pinch root, give ostial plegia or give retrograde).
- Cardioplegia incorrectly made up, or not cold (check temperature).

Cerebral and spinal protection

Key facts

- *Cerebral protection* is necessary when bypass cannot supply the head vessels, e.g., during surgery of the distal ascending aorta and arch.
- There are two modalities: hypothermia, which is by far the most important, and retrograde or antegrade selective cerebral perfusion.
- *Spinal cord protection* includes hypothermia and CSF drainage aimed at reducing risk of paraplegia in thoracoabdominal surgery (📖 p436).

Hypothermia

During coronary and valve surgery most surgeons cool actively or passively (drift) to about 32°C. At 37°C irreversible cerebral damage occurs after 2–3min of ischemia. Cerebral O_2 consumption is reduced by approximately 5% per 1°C drop between 37°C and 22°C. At 20°C cerebral O_2 consumption is 20% of normothermia. Although this suggests a safe circulatory arrest time of 15–20min, clinical evidence suggests that 30min is tolerated, rising to 45min at 18°C as other factors including pH and suppression of neuronal function may pay a role.

Acid–base changes with hypothermia

Normal pH is 7.40 and normal $PaCO_2$ is 5kPa in blood at 37°C. A sample of arterial blood in an airtight syringe has a PCO_2 that varies directly with temperature: decreasing the temperature of a solution increases the solubility of a given gas, decreasing its partial pressure. pH, on the other hand, varies inversely with temperature: the greater the CO_2 content in solution, the more H^+ in solution. CPB is not an airtight system: CO_2 can be added or taken away. So as hypothermia is induced the perfusionist has the choice of leaving total blood CO_2 constant, and letting pH and $PaCO_2$ find their own levels dictated by the temperature, or adding CO_2 to maintain $PaCO_2$ at 5kPa and maintain pH at 7.40. The former is known as *alpha-stat* CPB, and the latter is known as *pH-stat* CPB (Box 4.3). pH-stat management seems logical as most enzymes depend on optimal pH for their function, but the depression of metabolism that occurs with increasing acidosis characterized by alpha-stat management may be beneficial in terms of cerebral and myocardial protection. Recent evidence suggests that alpha-stat management gives better results in moderate hypothermic CPB. During deep hypothermic CPB best results may be achieved with a mixed strategy: pH stat during cooling, alpha-stat during rewarming, reperfusion and termination of bypass.

Deep hypothermic circulatory arrest

After institution of bypass the patient is cooled to a point where bypass can be discontinued. This technique is used in distal ascending aorta and

---

Box 4.3 Alpha-stat and pH-stat

- *PH-stat* tries to keep the pH stable by adding CO_2 as temperatures fall and removing it as they rise.
- *Alpha-stat* does not add anything. $PaCO_2$ rises and pH falls with falling temperature.

arch repair (p448), and sometimes during pulmonary embolectomy and stage II elephant trunk. Due to decreased tissue metabolism and O_2 demand, even a small degree of systemic hypothermia allows lower pump flows, less blood trauma, better myocardial protection, and better organ protection than normothermic perfusion. Hypothermia decreases blood flow to vascular beds in proportion with reduced metabolic demands, most pronounced in skeletal muscle and the extremities.

Left heart bypass

This is a useful adjunct in surgery on the descending aorta, where the heart does not need to be arrested, but the distal descending aorta and lower limbs need perfusion during the period of descending aorta cross-clamp. The LA is cannulated and oxygenated blood is siphoned into a reservoir, and pumped into a femoral line. An oxygenator is not required as blood is oxygenated by the lungs. A heat exchanger is optional as the patient is allowed to cool passively. Without these components there is less need for heparinization: 100U/kg heparin is normally given, and the ACT is maintained at <200s. Flows are maintained at 75% of full flow and MAPs distal to the clamp at 55–70mmHg.

Safe duration of circulatory arrest
- 36°C < 2–3min.
- 32°C 3–5min.
- 28°C 10min (moderate hypothermia).
- 20°C 30min (DHCA).
- 15°C 45min (DHCA).

Cerebral perfusion

Retrograde cerebral perfusion

Bicaval cannulas and a venous to arterial bridge are required: when retrograde perfusion is required bypass is discontinued, the IVC cannula is clamped, the SVC cannula is snared, and the perfusionist uses the bridge to pump oxygenated blood up the venous line. Deoxygenated blood is drained from the head and neck vessels. Low, near-continuous flow is used by some surgeons during hypothermic circulatory arrest. The common observation of dark, deoxygenated blood flowing out of the neck vessels suggests that cerebral oxygen utilization occurs.

Antegrade (selective) cerebral perfusion

This is used in arch surgery to reduce DHCA time. The brachiocephalic artery and left common carotid artery can be directly cannulated with a retrograde cardioplegia cannula. Or, if the axillary artery has been cannulated and the head and neck vessels anastomosed to a trifurcation graft the head can be selectively perfused from the axillary artery (p449). This reduces the risk of embolization from instrumenting the vessels, and keeps the field clearer. Flows are maintained at 10mL/kg, MAPs 40–50mmHg, and temperature around 20°C.

Cardiac ICU

Managing the five commonest calls to ICU

Atrial fibrillation

(📖 pp218–219)
- Give 10–20mmol K^+ via central line to get serum K^+ 4.5–5mmol/L
- Give empirical 20mmol Mg^{2+} via central line if none given post-op.
- Give 300mg amiodarone iv over 1h in patients with good LV, followed by 900mg amiodarone iv over 23h.
- In patient with poor LV function give digoxin in 125-microgram increments iv every 20min until rate control is obtained, up to a maximum of 1500 micrograms in 24h.
- Synchronized DC cardioversion for unstable patients (📖 pp224–225).

Bleeding

(📖 pp144–145)
- Get immediate help if bleeding is >400mL in 30min.
- Give colloid to get CVP 10–14 and systolic BP 80–100mmHg.
- Order 4 units of blood, 2 units FFP, and 2 pools platelets.
- Send coags and CBC, request a CXR stat.
- Transfuse to achieve Hb >8.0g/dL, platelets >100 × 10^9/L, APTT<40.
- Give empirical protamine 25mg iv, consider desmopression (DDAVP®).
- Emergency re-exploration is indicated for excessive bleeding.

Profound hypotension

(📖 pp142–143)
- Get immediate help. Check that reading is correct (📖 p173)
- Quickly assess pulse, rhythm, rate, CVP, O_2 sats and bleeding.
- Defibrillate VF or pulseless VT, treat AF as described.
- Treat bradycardia with atropine 0.3mg iv or pace (📖 p28).
- Give colloid to raise CVP to 12–16mmHg, place bed head-down.
- If you suspect cardiac tamponade (📖 p144) prepare for re-sternotomy.
- If patient warm and vasodilated draw up 10 micrograms of metaraminol into 10mL of saline and give *1mL* through a central line, and flush.
- If patient still very hypotensive repeat, or give 1mL 1:10,000 epinephrine iv and start infusion of presssor e.g., norepinephrine 0.1mcg/kg/min.

Poor gases

(📖 pp160–163)
- If sats <85% and falling get immediate help.
- Increase the FiO_2 to 100% temporarily, check the pulse oximeter.
- Look at expansion, auscultate the chest, check PaO_2.
- If you suspect a tension pneumothorax treat immediately (📖 p162).
- Suction the ET tube, check that the patient is not biting on it.
- Check that the drain tubing is patent, and drains are on suction.
- Treat bronchospasm with albuterol 2.5mg nebulizer.
- Disconnect from the ventilator and hand-ventilate the patient.
- Get a CXR: look for pneumothorax, hemothorax, atelectasis, ET tube position, and lobar collapse, and treat appropriately (📖 p162).

Poor urine output
(📖 pp234–235)
- Check that the Foley catheter is patent.
- If the patient is hypotensive treat this first (📖 pp142–143).
- Give a fluid challenge of colloid to raise the CVP to 14mmHg.
- If you are confident that the patient is not in a low cardiac output state (📖 pp142–143, p183), and is adequately filled, it is not unreasonable to treat profound oligura with 20mg furosemide iv (📖 pp208–209), and repeat if indicated.

Assessing cardiac output
- Cardiac output is defined on 📖 pp130–131, and is essentially a measure of cardiac function.
- When you're reviewing a patient it's always good to step back and ask yourself 'Is the cardiac output normal, high or low?' and treat any problems in that context. For example, if you are called to treat hypotension: the warm patient with bounding pulses and a high cardiac output, is going to need very different management to the patient that is cold, mottled, and oliguric, with a low cardiac output.
- There are many useful indicators of cardiac output (Table 5.1)—some may not fit (most are not isolated measures of cardiac output and can be affected by other issues including operator error), but you will usually get it right if you look at the whole picture, don't just treat one number, and go back and reassess the patient frequently (📖 p143).

Table 5.1 Assessment of cardiac output

Normal/high output state	Low cardiac output state
Peripheries warm	Peripheries cold
Brisk capillary refill	Extremities pale, mottled
Palpable/bounding distal pulses	Unable to feel distal pulses
If awake – patient appropriate	Patient obtunded
Wide pulse pressure, low CVP	Narrow pulse pressure, high CVP
Urine output >1ml/kg/hour	Urine output<1/2ml/kg/hour (📖 p234)
EKG normal	Dysrhythmias, ischemia on EKG (📖 p220)
CO>4l/min, CI>2.2l/min/m²	CO<3l/min, CI<2.0l/min/m²
SVO2>75% (📖 p178)	SVO2<65% (📖 p178)
Lactate <2.0	Lactate >2.5
Not acidotic	Metabolic acidosis (📖 pp168–171)
Creatinine, LFTs normal	Elevated creatinine, LFTs
Normal LV and RV on TEE/TTE	Poor LV or RV function on echo.
No effusion	Pericardial effusion (📖 p265)
No valve dysfunction	Valve dysfunction e.g. SAM (📖 p190)

Definitions of common terms

Basic concepts

- Instead of referring to systolic and diastolic BP, arterial pressure is frequently described as a single figure: the *mean arterial pressure* (MAP) which is calculated by adding 1/3 of the difference between diastolic and systolic pressures to the diastolic pressure.
- The MAP on its own does not adequately describe cardiac function: a number of other parameters are frequently used.
- *Cardiac output*: the volume of blood ejected by the heart per minute.
- *Stroke volume*: the volume of blood ejected by the heart per beat.
- Cardiac output equals heart rate × stroke volume.
- *Cardiac index* is the cardiac output adjusted to take into account the size of the patient, and is a more accurate reflection of cardiac function.

Preload

- Stroke volume depends on *preload, afterload,* and *contractility*.
- *Preload* is a measure of the wall tension in the LV at the end of diastole, but it is difficult to quantify directly.
- *Central venous pressure* (CVP), *pulmonary artery wedge pressure* (PAWP) and *left atrial pressure* (LAP) are indirect measures of preload: they are sometimes referred to as 'filling pressures'.
- *Left ventricular end-diastolic volume* (LVEDV), and *left ventricular end-diastolic pressure* (LVEDP) are better measures of preload, but they are rarely measured in clinical practise.

Afterload

- *Afterload* is a measure of the wall tension of the LV during systole.
- It is determined by preload, which determines the maximum 'stretch,' and by the resistance against which the heart must eject, which is a function of *systemic vascular resistance* (SVR), *vascular compliance, mean arterial pressure*, and any LVOT pressure gradient.
- SVR, which usually reflects the amount of peripheral vasoconstriction, is a commonly used indirect measurement of afterload.

Contractility and compliance

- *Contractility* is a measure of the strength of myocardial contraction at a given preload and afterload.
- MAP and cardiac output are commonly used indirect measures of contractility.
- *Compliance* is a measure of the distensibility of the LV in diastole: stiff, hypertrophied ventricles have low compliance.
- Compliance is difficult to quantify in the clinical setting.
- LVEDP, which may be measured at preoperative cardiac catheterization or estimated by preoperative echo, is an indirect measure of compliance.

Important hemodynamic formulas

Cardiac output = SV × HR
Cardiac index = CO/BSA
Mean arterial pressure = DP + (SP − DP)/3
Systemic vascular resistance = ((MAP − CVP)/CO) × 80
Systemic vascular resistance index = SVR/BSA
Pulmonary vascular resistance = ((PAP − PAWP)/CO) × 80
Pulmonary vascular resistance index = PVR/BSA
Mixed venous = SaO_2 − (VO_2/(Hb ×1.39 × CO)) × 10

CO = cardiac output	4.5–8L/min
SV = stroke volume	60–100mL
BSA = body surface area	2–2.2 m²
CI = cardiac index	2.0–4.0L/min/m²
SVI = stroke volume index	33–47 mL/beat/m²
MAP = mean arterial pressure	70–100mmHg
DP = diastolic pressure	60–80mmHg
SP = systolic pressure	110–150mmHg
SVR = systemic vascular resistance	800–1200 dyne/s/cm⁵
CVP = central venous pressure	0–12mmHg
SVRI = systemic vascular resistance index	400–600 dynes/s/cm⁵/m²
PVR = pulmonary vascular resistance	50–250 dynes/s/cm⁵
PAP = pulmonary artery pressure	20–30mmHg
PAWP = pulmonary artery wedge pressure	8–14mmHg
PVRI = pulmonary vascular resistance index	20–125 dynes/s/cm⁵/m²
SaO_2 = arterial saturation	95–100%
VO_2 = oxygen consumption	200–250mL/min

Oxygenation and ventilation

- *Oxygenation*, the amount of oxygen in arterial blood, is described in terms of the *partial pressure of* oxygen in arterial blood (PaO_2), and the *percentage saturation of arterial hemoglobin with oxygen* (SaO_2).
- *Ventilation*, the movement of air in and out of the lungs, is described in terms of minute volume, and assessed by measuring the partial pressure of carbon dioxide in arterial blood ($PaCO_2$).
- Oxygenation is independent of minute volumes until they are very low.
- In postoperative patients the primary cause of hypoxia is atelectasis and this must be reversed before the patient can benefit from increasing the fraction of oxygen in inspired air (FiO_2).
- *Positive end expiratory pressure* (PEEP) and *continuous positive airway pressure* (CPAP) (📖 pp158–159) treat and prevent atelectasis.
- The balance between oxygen consumption and delivery is assessed by measuring the *percentage saturation of mixed venous hemoglobin with oxygen* (SvO_2) or 'mixed venous', which is dependent on cardiac output, hematocrit, oxygenation, and oxygen consumption.
- Loss of functional residual capacity through atelectasis, supine position, lobar consolidation and collapse, effusions and obesity, results in hypoxia: CPAP, PEEP, and physiotherapy are aimed at limiting this loss.

Transfer and admission to ICU

It is easy for the surgeon to take this process for granted. Don't.

Patient requirements during transport to ICU

- Monitoring: EKG, MAP, and pulse oximetry.
- Respiratory support: E tank (most common portable size) of O_2 (check it is at least half full) connection tubing, 3L self-inflating reservoir bag, PEEP valve.
- Pharmacological support: all drugs infusing prior to transport: sedatives or anesthetics, inotropes, antihypertensives.
- Other support: IABP, other assist devices.
- Portable defibrillator.

Transfer

The postoperative patient can decompensate suddenly and catastrophically at any time during this process. The surgeon is responsible for the patient's safe arrival in ICU: surgery does not end with skin closure.

In the operating room

- Before unscrubbing, glance at the monitors to check that the patient remains in a stable rhythm, with isoelectric ST segments, satisfactory MAPs and oxygen saturations, and check the mediastinal drains: there should be no more than 100mL of blood.
- It will take several minutes for the anesthesiologist to disconnect, re-zero, and re-calibrate the monitors, and transfer the infusion pumps and ventilation to portable systems. At no stage should the patient be without electrocardiographic and hemodynamic monitoring. A surgeon should be present at all times.
- Lifting the patient can cause arrhythmias and hypotension in the volume-depleted patient, and hypertension in the waking patient.
- Make a note of what infusions are running.
- Ensure that the mediastinal drains do not become disconnected, and are placed below the level of the patient so that they continue to drain by gravity during transfer.
- Mediastinal drains should not be clamped during transfer, and if there is a significant air leak an underwater seal must be used in preference to cell salvage as tension pneumothorax is a risk.
- The patient must have an adequate rhythm, systemic pressure, and level of oxygenation before leaving the operating room.

Transport

- The anesthesiologist should have a clear view of the monitor at all times.
- During transport, manual ventilation of patients with a self-inflating bag and 100% O_2 is the anesthesiologist's responsibility: oxygenation is monitored with continuous pulse oximetry.
- All drug infusions should have been topped up and switched to battery-operated infusion pumps: running out of infusions with short half-lives such as norepinephrine during transfer can be catastrophic.

Admission to ICU

The key here is meticulous transfer of information to ensure continuity of care. The anesthesiologist, surgeon, and ICU staff ensure that the patient monitoring is transferred, re-zeroed, and re-calibrated, and transfer the portable infusion pumps and ventilation to ICU set-up. Check that hemodynamic and ventilatory parameters are acceptable, ensure that the mediastinal drains are placed on 10cmH$_2$O wall suction, and then outline preoperative status, operation, and the plan to the admitting team.

Typical postoperative handover

'Mr A is a 56-year-old man with good LV, three-vessel disease, smoker but no comorbidity, who has had an elective aortic valve replacement for tight aortic stenosis with a 23mm carbomedic mechanical valve and coronary artery bypass grafting times three under Dr A. Off bypass in sinus rhythm on dobutamine at 4 micrograms/kg/min. He has two atrial and two ventricular pacing wires, a mediastinal and right and left pleural drains, crossed. Aim for filling pressures of 14–16mmHg and MAPS 70–80mmHg. Wake, wean, and extubate as per protocol.'

Respiratory and cardiovascular monitoring

This is described in detail on 📖 pp156–157, and 📖 pp172–181 respectively.

Renal function

All cardiac surgical patients are catheterized. Suprapubic catheters should be used if strictures make insertion of urethral catheters difficult. Urine output is measured and recorded hourly, as are total crystalloid and colloid infusion volumes, surgical drainage, NGT aspirates, and infusions. Total fluid balance is calculated hourly. Serum electrolytes are checked on arrival in ICU and at 6–12h. Serum potassium is checked hourly.

Neurological function

Pupil size, afferent and efferent reflexes are usually checked after admission to the ICU and at 3-hourly intervals.

Temperature

Core temperature

This represents the temperature of the vital organs. The best estimate is obtained from the PA catheter thermistor. Nasopharyngeal temperature and tympanic temperature provide an accurate measure of brain temperature. Bladder temperature can be used but is inaccurate in oliguria.

Peripheral temperature

This lags behind core temperature during warming and cooling, and is affected by local factors, e.g., warmers and peripheral vasoconstriction.

Mediastinal drainage

Mediastinal and pleural drainage is recorded hourly until the drains are removed (📖 p254).

Fast-track patients

Patients undergoing CABG surgery with low preoperative risk scoring, no major comorbidity, and a straightforward operative course should be eligible for 'fast-tracking' (see Box 5.1).

Box 5.1 Exclusion criteria for 'fast-tracking'

Many units have minimal exclusion criteria, fast-tracking all but the most complex patients. Exclusion criteria used by other units include:
- Age >75 years.
- Poor LV.
- Previous history of CABG or valve surgery.
- Left bundle branch block.
- Previous problematic general anesthesia.
- Inotropic support preoperatively
- MI within 3 weeks.
- Active congestive cardiac failure.
- IABP.
- Severe COPD.
- Pulmonary hypertension.
- Severe hepatic or renal insufficiency.
- Peripheral vascular disease or stroke.
- Ongoing bleeding.

Although patient selection and care varies widely between centers, the goal is rapid progress through hospital from operation to discharge. At the perioperative stage this mandates:
- Selection of short-acting anesthetic agents.
- Sustained normothermia.
- Effective control of postoperative pain, nausea, and vomiting.
- Early waking and extubating.
- Rapid weaning of any inotropic support.
- Early independence from invasive monitoring.
- Early mobilization.

These patients are frequently awake and extubated within 6h of arriving in ICU. Bleeding is minimal so mediastinal drains can be rapidly removed following extubation. They are hemodynamically stable with no need for inotropic support, with satisfactory respiratory, renal, and neurological function. They may be transferred to a high-dependency unit within 12h, to the floor within 24h, and discharged home within 4 or 5 days. There is often additional provision for early follow-up.

Postoperative pathophysiology

Key facts

- The majority of patients exhibit a broadly similar pattern of pathophysiological derangements in the hours following cardiac surgery. Intensive care protocols are designed to enable medical and nursing staff to avoid, recognize, and treat these changes.
- This section summarizes this process system by system. This should enable you to recognize and manage patients that fall outside these predictable response patterns.

Hemodynamic

The cardiovascular system is the system that undergoes the greatest physiological stresses during both bypass and beating heart surgery, even uncomplicated cardiac surgery.

- Myocardial compliance falls because of myocardial edema. Higher filling pressures are required to generate the same stroke volume.
- Contractility is impaired as a result of myocardial edema, metabolic derangements, myocardial stunning, and ischemia (which may be caused by coronary artery and arterial conduit spasm, air and particulate emboli, manipulation of the heart post bypass, periods of hypoperfusion during transfer, and factors affecting gas exchange).
- Myocardial function continues to decline for 6–8h postoperatively as a result of ischemia-reperfusion injury, before returning to baseline.
- Hypothermia is common as it is difficult to keep up with heat loss from an open chest in theatre, and it is detrimental as it predisposes to ventricular arrhythmias, coagulopathy, and metabolic acidosis, and raises afterload increasing myocardial oxygen demand.
- The high SVR helps, however, to maintain MAPs until the patient is rewarmed: it is vital to ensure that adequate volume replacement and if necessary pharmacologic support are given, to avoid hypotension during rewarming.
- Patients may 'overshoot' to temperatures above 37.5°C because of abnormalities in central thermoregulation or systemic inflammatory response syndrome (SIRS) resulting in peripheral vasodilatation and hypotension, and associated with a poorer neurological outcome.
- Vasodilatation and capillary leak mean that there is a progressive requirement for volume resuscitation to achieve satisfactory filling pressures that must be balanced against volume overloading the patient, which has a particularly deleterious effect on respiratory function.

Respiratory

Patients have a high preoperative incidence of obstructive airway disease: smoking is a common risk factor. Pulmonary function may be further compromised by pre-existing pulmonary edema, post-perfusion lung syndrome, administration of protamine, anaphylaxis, intrapulmonary shunts, mechanical factors such as pneumothorax, hemothorax, and obstruction of the tracheobronchial tree by blood or mucus plugs (p163). Functional residual capacity is further reduced by supine position.

- Most patients arrive in the ICU heavily sedated, anesthetized, and paralysed. They require mechanical ventilation for a variable time.
- The anesthesiologist will frequently pre-oxygenate the patient prior to transfer with an FiO_2 of 100%. The FiO_2 is gradually weaned to 40% as long as the PaO_2 remains above 10kPa, and the rate of ventilation is reduced as the patient wakes.
- Fluid shift into the interstitial space, exacerbated by fluid overloading the vasodilated patient during rewarming, impairs oxygenation.
- Hypercapnia occurs in patients who are waking, shivering, or warming: increasing the tidal volume and/or the respiratory rate of ventilation is normally sufficient to treat this.
- The awake, neurologically appropriate patient who is stable hemodynamically and not bleeding is extubated if gases and respiratory rate are satisfactory after a period of pressure support ventilation.

Bleeding

Multiple perioperative factors predispose the patient to bleeding: preoperative antiplatelet therapy, residual heparin effect, platelet depletion and dysfunction post bypass, hypothermia, hypertension, clotting factor depletion, and surgical technique (🕮 p144).
- Bleeding should taper quickly after a few hours.
- Prevention, recognition, and treatment of abnormal bleeding patterns and their sequelae is a key part of the recovery process (🕮 p145).

Renal

Cardiopulmonary bypass results in major changes in fluid distribution and renal function, moderated by pharmacological agents employed primarily for hemodynamic support. The importance of correct fluid management cannot be overstated: it is the difference between a satisfactory postoperative course and one complicated by multisystem dysfunction.
- Most patients arrive in ICU in a state of total body sodium and water overload, which becomes more pronounced with the additional volume given as the patient warms and vasodilates, even though the patient may have a relatively depleted intravascular volume.
- The aim of fluid management is to ensure adequate intravascular volume to maintain perfusion. Volume resuscitation in isolation may not be enough to achieve this, and in excess will have a deleterious effect on both cardiac and respiratory function: low-dose vasoconstrictors are useful in this setting.
- Glomerular filtration rate and hence urine output is a sensitive measure of cardiac function.
- Patients with normal preoperative renal function should maintain a diuresis of at least 1ml/kg/h: renal dysfunction is uncommon in these patients in the absence of prolonged perioperative hypotension.

Neurological

Patients should be alert and oriented prior to extubation: grossly abnormal cognitive function at this stage requires resedation and continued ventilation so that the cause can be identified and treated. Agitated, confused patients commonly consume more oxygen than they will accept from a ventilator, and may remove critical lines and tubes.

Common ICU scenarios: CABG

Key facts

- In the immediate postoperative period most patients tend to follow one or more of several common clinical patterns. These are determined by the preoperative disease process, the nature of the surgery, and the body's response to the complex pathophysiological processes outlined earlier in this chapter. Common cardiac surgical intensive care scenarios are outlined in the following pages.
- Older patients, and those with more comorbidity or undergoing more complex surgery, often do not fit a single clinical pattern.

On-pump coronary artery bypass

Patients with good ventricular function and a full revascularization have an initial tendency to hypertension and tachycardia, and may also produce a large initial diuresis. Usually hypertension resolves quite quickly as the patient warms, vasodilates, and diureses.

- Early hypertension can be managed with:
  - Sedation: give 25–100 micrograms iv fentanyl bolus if the patient is agitated or in pain, and not otherwise ready to wean from the ventilator.
  - Nitrates: a continuous infusion of nitroglycerine (5–200 mcg/min iv) reduces coronary artery vasospasm, increases coronary flow to ischemic regions increasing contractility and the threshold for ventricular fibrillation, and decreases systemic vascular resistance and myocardial oxygen consumption ($\square$ p202). Especially useful in patients with borderline EKG changes.
  - Diltiazem: start infusion at 5mg/h to a maximum of 15mg/h (250mg in 250mL 5% dextrose) to provide similar effect on coronary blood flow, often reducing atrial tachycardias.
  - Hydralazine and β-blockers are useful later in the postoperative period in stable patients. They are not routinely used early on as they are difficult to titrate in patients with labile hemodynamics.
- The disadvantage of starting nitroglycerine routinely is that hypotension secondary to vasodilation may then be treated by giving volume to a patient who is already volume overloaded.
- Tachycardia is common, and heart rates of 90–100bpm achieve maximal cardiac output, but rates above this reduce cardiac output as diastolic filling times decrease.
  - Except in patients with LV hypertrophy ($\square$ p140) or SAM ($\square$ p190) who may be compromised by tachycardia there is no need to treat
  - Look for and address underlying causes—commonly hypovolemia, pain, anxiety, acidosis, hypercapnia, chronotropic agents (epinephrine, dobutamine), occasionally tamponade.
- 1/3 of patients go into AF, but not usually within the first postoperative day if K^+ is maintained at 4.5–5.0mmol/L ($\square$ p218).
- Many patients become hypotensive as a result of vasodilation in response to warming, or the long half-life of preoperative ACE inhibitors: if the patient is peripherally warm, with CI >2.2L/min/m^2

and SVO_2 >70, and CVP<14mmHg a small amount of norepinephrine 0.03–0.05 micrograms/kg/min) is usually sufficient to treat this.

• Patients with poor ventricular function or incomplete revascularization may also become increasingly hypotensive with poor urine outputs, as stunned myocardium is transiently further depressed in the first 6–12h post surgery. Look for:
  • Worsening lactic acidosis.
  • Rising filling pressures.
  • EKG changes, e.g., ST segment elevation.

• In this case dobutamine (250mg in 50mL 5% dextrose at 3–5 micrograms/kg/min) is the first-line choice, alternatively epinephrine (250mg in 250mL 5% dextrose at 0.03–0/05 micrograms/kg/min) will improve contractility.

• Ischemic EKG changes (ST segment elevation or depression, T-wave inversion, new bundle branch block) suggest poor myocardial protection, vasospasm of arterial grafts, incomplete revascularization, or acute graft occlusion: management is discussed on 🕮 p185.

• Failure to respond to appropriate inotropic support mandates accurate assessment of cardiac indices with a pulmonary artery catheter if not already *in situ*, and echocardiography (🕮 p185): an IABP or re-exploration may be indicated.

Early warning signs in CABG patients

Correct metabolic abnormalities, talk to the surgeon—do you need echo to evaluate regional wall motion abnormalities (ischemia) or collection (tamponade)?
• Frequent extrasystoles, ST segment changes.
• Hypotension, rising filling pressures, rising PAPs.
• Low cardiac output, low mixed venous, rising lactate, acidosis.
• Oliguria (do not empirically treat with diuretics).

Coronary artery bypass—off-pump

Patients with good ventricular function and a full revascularization are usually hypertensive and tachycardic. They do not produce a diuresis as they are often relatively underfilled. A significant metabolic acidosis frequently develops during the first 6h postoperatively, resolving within 12h. The cause of the acidosis is unclear but may reflect an intraoperative low cardiac output state. As bypass cannot be used to warm these patients they are often hypothermic.

• Ensure these patients are adequately filled.
• Use warming blankets and infusion warmers to achieve normothermia.
• These patients sometimes receive a reduced dose of intraoperative heparin depending on surgical preference, and should therefore receive early aspirin (81mg po) and low-molecular-weight heparin (5000U sc) to ensure graft patency and avoid thromboembolic complications.

Common ICU scenarios: valves

Aortic stenosis

These patients have a stiff, hypertrophied ventricle that is dependent on synchronized atrial contraction to provide 30% of stroke volume and therefore cardiac output. Shortened filling times reduce cardiac output.

- AF and tachyarrhythmias cause these patients to decompensate rapidly: have a low threshold for synchronized DC cardioversion if antiarrhythmic drugs do not achieve cardioversion quickly. It may be worth prophylactically loading these patients with 300mg iv amiodarone followed by 900mg over 24h.
- Sequential AV pacing achieves a much better cardiac output than ventricular pacing alone, and both atrial and ventricular epicardial pacing leads should be placed during surgery as debridement of heavily calcified valves frequently results in complete heart block, which may eventually require permanent pacing in 2–3% of all aortic valve replacements.
- Ensure adequate preload by filling to CVP 14–16mmHg: as the ventricle is small and non-compliant, very little volume may be required to achieve this.
- Hypertension usually develops after 6–8h as the heart recovers from bypass, and responds to the removal of the outflow gradient.
- In order to reduce myocardial oxygen demand, preserve suture lines and reduce the risk of hemorrhagic stroke, mean systemic pressures should be maintained at 70–80mmHg using diltiazem or nitroglycerine (5–200 mcg/min iv).
- Anticoagulate mechanical valves if chest tube output minimal, starting the second evening after surgery by commencing warfarin: the risk from thrombosis is negligible in the first 2–3 days post-op so there is no reason to start iv heparin at this stage.

Aortic regurgitation

These patients have dilated, compliant ventricles, and also rely on AV conduction.

- Compliant, dilated ventricles mean that large volumes are often required to raise filling pressures.
- Removal of the regurgitant fraction means LV performance improves compared to RV function: filling pressures are therefore lower postoperatively than they are in AS.
- Anticoagulate as described above.

Mitral stenosis and mitral regurgitation

Both types of patient are commonly in chronic AF and have a variable degree of pulmonary hypertension, which may be associated with RV dysfunction postoperatively. Patients with MS usually have small LVs and well-preserved function. Correcting MR, on the other hand, may unmask severe LV dysfunction as the low-resistance regurgitant pathway is removed: the preoperative ejection fraction usually overestimates LV function.

- Treatment is directed at reducing pulmonary hypertension and RV dysfunction, which may be exacerbated intraoperatively by poor myocardial protection, and postoperatively by factors which raise pulmonary resistance: positive pressure ventilation, bronchospasm, pulmonary edema, reduction in functional residual capacity and vasoconstrictors such as norepinephrine.

- Higher filling pressures are required to ensure adequate cardiac output, but right-sided filling pressures may not correlate with left-sided pressure because of RV dysfunction and pulmonary hypertension.
- Large fluid volumes may be needed because of increased atrial or ventricular compliance, but giving volume may exacerbates RV dysfunction without achieving optimal LV filling pressures: inotropic support is commonly required.
- Systolic anterior motion may complicate mitral repair (📖 p190): the mainstay of medical management is avoiding tachycardia and hypovolemia, giving volume and β-blockade. SAM in the setting of significant RV dysfunction is a difficult problem, as the management of the two problems is completely opposed (📖 pp190–191).
- TEE or a PA catheter should be used to assess RV dysfunction.
- Respiratory dysfunction is common as a result of pulmonary hypertension and volume overload, and it must be managed aggressively with a diuresis and particularly careful ventilatory weaning.
- Dobutamine and milrinone result in pulmonary vasodilation and reduce pulmonary hypertension in addition to their inotropic effect: inhaled nitric oxide decreases PVR and helps in severe RV dysfunction.
- Some patients with chronic AF come off bypass in sinus or junctional rhythms, particularly if ablation has been performed: amiodarone should normally be started to maintain freedom from AF.
- Patients with mechanical valves do not normally need therapeutic anticoagulation in the first 48h.

Aortic surgery

Aortic dissection and aneurysm repair involves suturing Dacron graft to friable tissues. The proximal false lumen is obliterated, but distal extension of the dissection can occur with end-organ ischemia. Surgery often involves a period of hypothermic circulatory arrest. Postoperatively paraplegia can result from hypoperfusion of spinal cord (📖 pp436–437).

- Avoid extremes of BP: aim for MAPs 90–100mmHg using either antihypertensives that reduce the rate and force of contraction e.g. labetolol in hypertensive patients or vasoconstrictors and fluid in hypotensive patients.
- Bleeding may be a significant problem: long bypass times and hypothermia contribute to a significant coagulopathy. Fragile suture lines result in increased bleeding rates during periods of hypertension, and are often not improved by further surgery: there will be a higher threshold for re-sternotomy. Correct coagulopathy (📖 p145).
- Poor renal function, or worsening metabolic acidosis refractory to adequate perfusion pressures should be investigated by imaging the descending aorta; percutaneous fenestration of the dissection flap may salvage ischemic end-organs. Deteriorating lower extremity neurology may respond to increase perfusion pressure or spinal drainage (📖 pp436–437).

Common hemodynamic scenarios

Normotensive but low cardiac output

Peripheries are cold to touch. (If the patient is warm, with good peripheral pulses and normotensive, it is almost impossible for their cardiac output to be low.) Mean arterial and filling pressures are initially adequate. One of the conditions for terminating bypass is a core temperature of 36.6–37.5°C. After bypass the chest remains open while the surgeon establishes satisfactory hemostasis: although the anesthesiologist may make vigorous efforts to maintain core temperature using warming blankets and warming iv fluids, patients usually reach ICU hypothermic and vasoconstricted. Shivering increases filling pressures, and can double oxygen consumption, causing SVO_2 to fall in the hypovolemic patient.

- These patients should be managed with aggressive volume replacement to maintain preload which tends to fall as warming causes vasodilatation: as much as 3L of fluid are often required in the first few hours on ICU in response to capillary leak, diuresis, rewarming, and the fact the perfusionist may have hemoconcentrated the patient by filtering several litres of fluid off during bypass.
- Warming blankets correct core temperature slowly, mainly by minimizing peripheral heat loss. Avoid infusion of cold fluid.
- Nitroglycerine infusion reduces coronary artery vasospasm, increases coronary flow to ischemic regions increasing contractility and the threshold for ventricular fibrillation, and decreases systemic vascular resistance and myocardial oxygen consumption (📖 p202).
- The vasodilated patient equilibrates with external temperatures faster than the vasoconstricted patient.
- Stop shivering, which increases oxygen demand and compromises ventilation, by warming the patient and giving a muscle relaxant (vecuronium 0.1mg/kg iv) in the sedated, intubated patient.
- In the awake patient shivering can be treated with pethidine (25mg iv) which has an antispasmodic effect as well as its analgesic effect.

Hypotensive with low CVP despite giving volume

Warm patient with good cardiac output

If peripheries are warm to touch with good pulses, CVP is <10mmHg despite being >1–2L positive, cardiac index is >2.2L/min, although mixed venous saturation may be low, this suggests primary issue is vasodilation. As patients warm to 37°C they vasodilate. Falling filling pressures require volume to maintain systemic pressures.

- In a young patient, if urine >1mL/kg/h, mixed venous and pH are ok, and patient warm and well perfused, MAPs 55–60mmHg may be adequate for organ perfusion: less likely in elderly.
- Colloid is the first choice: blood to maintain the hemoglobin levels >8.0g/dL: Gelofusine®, Hespan®, or albumin where the hemoglobin is satisfactory, blood products in the bleeding patient.
- Fill to achieve RAPs of 12–14mmHg: MAPs should improve significantly and quickly.
- If the patient is mounting a large diuresis, "replace crystalloid with crystalloid": use normal saline in older patients who may have impaired

ability to conserve sodium, and are therefore at risk of hyponatremia, but look out for hyperchloremic acidosis in these patients (📖 p169).

• If the patient has low MAPs, low filling pressures, and poor urine output despite being over 2–3L positive, *and is not bleeding*, this reflects abnormally high cardiac compliance and capillary permeability rather than a need for continued fluid challenges, which will adversely effect pulmonary function: start a small dose of a vasoconstrictor such as norepinephrine (4mg in 50mL 5% dextrose at 0.03–0.3 micrograms/kg/min)which should reduce the volume requirement.

Poor cardiac output, cool peripheries

• Recheck fluid balance—look for bleeding, which may be in the **chest, groin, leg drains, gut, abdomen, or the bed, not just the chest tubes.** Is the hematocrit falling rapidly? Is the patient polyuric?

• Look for causes of low cardiac output while starting a low-dose epinephrine (4mg in 250mL 5% dextrose at 0.03–0.05 micrograms/kg/min) and continuing fluid resuscitation.

Hypotensive with high filling pressures

The causes of this scenario range from benign to acutely life-threatening.

• Fluids being run through CVP transducer port (most common).
• Cardiac tamponade (📖 p144).
• Other causes of pump failure (📖 pp184–185, 188–191).
• Patient waking: shivering and 'fighting' the ventilator (📖 p165).
• Massive PE (rare in patients without pre-op risk factors) (📖 p476).

Useful rules of thumb

Always look at the whole picture, and examine the patient—treating one number in isolation is almost always a mistake.

• Remember that the picture is dynamic—go back and reassess.
• If you are not sure what is going on, change one thing at a time, wait and reassess—making multiple changes at once can confuse the clinical picture. It's rare you have time to do this safely.
• If the numbers don't make sense, recheck them: check the arterial line pressure against a cuff pressure, check the CVP off a different port, check the cardiac output against clinical findings.
• If the patient is warm, with good peripheral pulses, and normotensive it is virtually impossible for their cardiac output to be low.
• If the patient is cold, with barely palpable peripheral pulses, their cardiac output is not adequate, whatever the number recorded.
• Remember that mixed venous saturation, is dependent on oxygen consumption (is the patient shivering, or agitated?), hematocrit and oxygenation—not just cardiac output. Treat the underlying causes, and do not just escalate inotropes without confirming cardiac output is inadequate.
• Low filling pressures mean hypovolemia: this is usually due to capillary leak, diuresis, rewarming, and vasodilatation, but don't forget to look for bleeding, which is not always evident in the chest tubes.
• High filling pressures are cause for concern: they may be due to a patient shivering or waking up, but can indicate RV or LV dysfunction, MR or TR, ischemia, tension pneumothorax or tamponade.

Bleeding

Key facts

• Excessive bleeding is bleeding that falls outside the 'normal' pattern of bleeding post cardiotomy (see Box 5.2), and except in rare cases should not be acutely life threatening if correctly managed.

• Every effort must be made to prevent excessive bleeding with good surgical technique, and careful correction of coagulopathy pre- and postoperatively, as bleeding and transfusion are associated with potentially major morbidity and mortality.

Cardiac tamponade

Cardiac tamponade is a surgical emergency. It is an indication for urgent re-sternotomy (🕮 p150). It is not always an easy diagnosis to make, as severe LV or RV dysfunction may result in similar picture. Tamponade is suggested by.

• Hypotension *and* high filling pressures.

• Additional features may include:
  • Worsening urine output and acidosis despite diuretic therapy.
  • Equilibration of cardiac filling pressures.
  • Sudden cessation of bleeding.
  • Excessive widening of the mediastinum on CXR.
  • Decreased EKG voltage; pulseless electrical activity (PEA) is a very late sign.
  • TEE may show clot in pericardium, collapse of RV in diastole, and underfilled hyperdynamic LV, but is operator dependent and not 100% accurate: a negative echo does not rule out tamponade.

Box 5.2 'Normal' bleeding

Mediastinal bleeding should be greatest in the hours immediately after surgery, tailing off to near zero over the course of the following 6–12h. Acceptable rates of bleeding are: up to 2mL/kg/h for the first 2–3h, up to 1mL/kg/h for the next 3h, and <0.5mL/kg/h by 12h post closure. The trend should be downward.

Etiology

• *Preoperative:* medication, e.g., aspirin, clopidogrel, warfarin, thrombolytics, coagulopathy (ITP), age, previous sternotomy, infective endocarditis. Preoperative pleural effusions mimic bleeding if not drained in surgery.

• *Operative:* surgical technique, bypass causing platelet dysfunction, thrombocytopenia and fibrinolysis (🕮 p106), residual heparin, open chest.

• *Postoperative:* dilutional, massive transfusion with red cells, hypothermia, hypertension, sepsis, DIC, ECMO, old collection.

Management

Prevent perioperative blood loss by identifying and correcting pre-existing coagulopathies (🕮 p145). Some surgeons give prophylactic aminocaproic acid (Amicar®) or tranexamic acid (🕮 p147). Meticulous operative technique is usually the most important factor.

Investigation

- If the chest looks wet on closing ask for TEG, heparin level, repeat ACT and platelet works in OR and treat. Check Hb, platelets, APTT, PT, and fibrinogen levels on arrival in ICU, and after each batch of blood products when treating bleeding.
- *Look* at the patient; are they hemodynamically unstable, is blood rising very rapidly up the drains, does drainage look arterial, are the conduit harvest sites bleeding, are line sites bleeding?
- Bleeding frequently needs treating empirically, before the results of clotting studies are known: replace blood loss with blood products.
- If bleeding does not decrease despite corrected APTT, PT, and platelets, consider re-exploration (📖 p150).
- A CXR will show pleural collections and may show excessive mediastinal widening (📖 p14, Fig. 1.2b).
- If you suspect that the drainage is bloodstained fluid (if the patient had pleural effusions preoperatively, or the chest was washed out at the end of the procedure) measure the hematocrit of the drain fluid (<10 suggests effusion rather than frank bleeding).

Treatment

- If bleeding approaches 500mL in 30min, or the patient is hemodynamically unstable, prepare for emergency resternotomy (📖 p150).
- Order 4–6 units of blood, FFP, platelets, and cryoprecipitate.
- Give blood, or colloid if no blood available, to maintain MAPs.
- Put the bed flat or head-down if patient very hypotensive.
- Control hypertension with adequate sedation and vasodilation (📖 p202), and control shivering with sedation and paralysis (📖 p142).
- Increasing PEEP can reduce bleeding, but also reduces cardiac filling causing hypotension.
- Check coagulation and treat the bleeding patient with platelets, FFP, blood, protamine, or cryoprecipitate as indicated (📖 p146): if there is no coagulopathy the bleeding patient needs to be re-explored
  - Give desmopressin(DDAVP®).
  - Give 2 units of platelets for functional platelet count <90 × 10^9 /L.
  - Give 2–4 units of blood to maintain Hb >8.0g/dL.
  - Give 1 pool of cryoprecipitate to maintain fibrinogen >400.
  - Give 2 units FFP to maintain APTT 25–35s.
  - Give 25mg iv protamine to reduce residual heparin level to 0.
- Withhold postoperative aspirin and any anticoagulants.
- Ensure patency of chest drains by milking them regularly.
- Avoid giving large volumes of cold fluid: use infusion warmers.
- Warm the patient to 36°C: hypothermia suppresses coagulation mechanism and platelet function.
- If a drain appears blocked, clamp and disconnect it and quickly remove any clot with forceps: using a sterile fine-bore aspiration tube under wall suction may help but exposes patient to risk of sepsis and should be reserved for emergencies.

Blood products, antifibrinolytics

Blood

- 1 unit of blood increases Hb by about 1g/dL in a 70kg adult.
- Blood is normally provided as packed red cells (1 unit = ~350mL).
- Cross-matched blood can normally be provided within 20min: it contains blood from a single donor.
- In dire emergencies O −ve blood (universal donor) can be given to recipients of any ABO Rh group without incompatibility reaction.
- Some centers use autologous blood transfusion to avoid the complications described on 🕮 p148: up to 2 units of blood are withdrawn from patients preoperatively, which may be stored for up to 5 weeks.
- Additionally *cell salvage* reduces the need for allogeneic blood. Shed blood is collected intraoperatively and postoperatively, 5000U of heparin are added to collected blood which is spun with normal saline to remove all material, including residual heparin, platelets, and clotting product, to produce RBCs suspended in saline.

Platelets

- 1 unit of platelets increases platelet count by 10^9/L in a 70kg adult.
- Platelets are provided as units (1 unit = ~50mL).
- Platelets do not need to be cross-matched but they should be ABO compatible (and rhesus matched in females of childbearing age).
- 1 unit contains platelets from a single donor.
- They are stored at 22°C, and have a shelf life of 5 days.

Fresh frozen plasma

- 1 unit of FFP contains all the coagulation factors except platelets.
- 1mL of FFP per kg will raise most clotting factors by 1% in a 70kg adult.
- 1 unit of FFP = 150–250mL, and 5–10mL/kg is normally given.
- 1 unit of FFP usually contains product from a single donor but is sometimes pooled, in which case it may be from several donors.
- FFP does not need to be cross-matched but should be ABO compatible (and Rhesus matched in females of childbearing age).
- FFP must be stored at <−18°C; it must be thawed, usually over 20min, before giving, and discarded if not used within 2h.
- FFP treats heparin resistance due to antithrombin III deficiency (🕮 p93).

Cryoprecipitate

- I bag of cryoprecipitate contains 150–250mg fibrinogen, and factors VII and VIII, and von Willebrand factor.
- 10 bags of cryoprecipitate raises fibrinogen 0.6–0.7 mg/L in a 70kg adult.
- I bag of cryoprecipitate = 20mL: 5–10 pooled bags are normally given.
- ABO and rhesus compatibility is not relevant.

Recombinant activated factor VII

- Potent agent acting at site of tissue injury, binds to exposed tissue factor, activating platelets and leading to fibrin and clot formation.
- Few small studies showing significant reduction in blood loss, need for transfusion. Risk of adverse thrombotic sequelae and cost mean this

agent generally reserved for bleeding without a surgical solution that is refractory to two or more rounds of blood products.
- *Dose*: 50–90mcg/kg after discontinuation of bypass (discuss with hematologist).

Antifibrinolytics

There are two types of antifibrinolytic:
- Synthetic lysine analogues, e.g., tranexamic acid and aminocaproic acid (Amicar®).
- The non-specific serine protease inhibitor aprotinin (Trasylol®) which was withdrawn from world markets in May 2008 after several non-randomized studies raised safety concerns.

Aminocaproic acid (Amicar®)
- *Action*: inhibits fibrinolysis by blocking lysine binding sites on plasminogen, inhibiting formation of plasmin
- *Pharmacodynamics*: renal elimination.
- *Dose*: loading dose ranges from 75–150mg/kg and maintenance dose range is 12.5mg/kg/h to 30mg/kg/h over varying timeframe.
- *Indication*: prophylactic prevention of bleeding.
- Randomized controlled trials and meta-analyses show blood loss reduced on average by 200mL per patient, and blood transfused by 1.3 units per patient, but no impact on reoperation for bleeding.
- No apparent increase in death, stroke, myocardial infarction, renal failure, or pulmonary embolism

Tranexamic acid (Cyklokapron®)
- *Action*: binds to plasminogen and plasmin to inhibit fibrinolysis. It promotes clot stability
- *Pharmacodynamics*: renal elimination.
- *Indication*: prophylactic prevention of bleeding.
- *Dose*: normally given as an iv infusion 1–2g on induction, or up to 1g an hour during operation. Can be given postoperatively as a single dose of 1–2g iv.
- RCTs and meta-analyses show blood loss reduced on average by 300mL per patient, and blood transfused by just under 1 unit per patient, but no impact on reoperation for bleeding.
- No apparent increase in death, stroke, myocardial infarction, renal failure, or PE.

Desmopressin (DDAVP)
- *Action*: releases von Willebrand factor from endothelial cells, increasing vWF and factor VIII: main indication in hemophilia A and von Willebrand disease, but also used after cardiac surgery.
- *Dose*: slow infusion 0.3g/kg.
- *Indication*: prophylactic prevention of bleeding.
- One early study showed 30% reduction in blood loss and transfusion requirements, subsequent studies show blood loss reduced on average by 115mL per patient, but no impact on transfusion requirements, or reoperation for bleeding.
- No significant increase in death, stroke, myocardial infarction, renal failure, or PE.

Transfusion reactions

Acute hemolytic reaction

ABO incompatibility as a result of clerical, bedside, sampling or laboratory error is the most common cause. May also be caused by incompatibility within other antigen systems (Duffy/Kidd). **Donor erythrocyte A or B antigens** bind to the recipient's anti-A or anti-B antibodies, resulting in complement formation, membrane attack complex, and immediate hemolysis. Cytokine and chemokine release mediates sympathetic inflammatory response characterized by sudden onset of hypotension, tachycardia, pyrexia, breathlessness, tachypnea and back pain. Bilirubinemia, anemia, and hemoglobinuria as a result of hemolysis ensue.

- Stop the transfusion immediately and give basic life support if required.
- Keep the bag and giving set for analysis, inform haematology.
- Give crystalloid and furosemide to encourage a diuresis.
- Dialysis may be required.

Anaphylaxis and allergic reactions

Normally *IgE-mediated* histamine release reactions to plasma, platelets and red blood cells. Mild allergic reactions are relatively common, and are characterized by erythematous papular rashes, wheals, pruritus and pyrexia. These are treated by stopping the transfusion and administering chlorphenamine (piriton) (10mg iv). Anaphylaxis characterized by hypotension, bronchospasm and angioedema occasionally occurs.

- Stop the transfusion immediately and disconnect connection tubing.
- Basic life support may be required.
- Treat bronchospasm and angioedema with epinephrine (1mL of 1:10,000 iv), chlorpheniramine (10mg iv), and hydrocortisone (100mg iv).

Non-hemolytic febrile reaction

These common and normally mild reactions are caused by recipient antibodies directed against **donor HLA and leukocyte specific antigen on leukocytes and platelets.** Cytokine release mediates a mild pyrexia, typically over an hour after transfusion is started. Antipyrogens such as acetaminophen 500mg–1g po/pr limit pyrexia, but antihistamines are not helpful. Severe reactions feature high grade fever, rigors, nausea, and vomiting. The severity of symptoms is proportional to the number of leukocytes in the transfused blood and the rate of transfusion. Leukocyte-depleted blood helps prevent these reactions.

Delayed extravascular hemolytic reaction

Although pretransfusion antibody testing is negative (a satisfactory XM) these patients experience accelerated destruction of transfused red blood cells 7–10 days following transfusion. This is an antibody-mediated reaction, usually by a patient antibody (commonly rhesus E, Kell, Duffy, and Kidd), present in levels too low to be detected clinically until produced in larger amounts on exposure to **circulating donor antigen**. As hemolysis is extravascular, hemoglobinaemia and hemoglobinuria are uncommon: it is characterized by an unexpected fall in haematocrit a few days post transfusion, hyperbilirubinemia and positive Coombs test.

Transfusion-related acute lung injury (TRALI)

Non-cardiogenic pulmonary edema typically within 6h of transfusion is mediated by recipient antibodies against **donor HLA**. Activated recipient leukocytes migrate to the lung, releasing proteolytic enzymes that cause a localized capillary leak syndrome and pulmonary edema (📖 p163).

Infection

Bacterial

Serious bacterial contamination of stored blood may occur, although platelets, which are usually stored at room temperature, are at greater risk. Common organisms are *Staphylococcus* spp., *Enterobacter*, *Yersinia*, and *Pseudomonas* spp. Contamination is difficult to detect. The recipient is pyrexial >40°C, and hypotensive. This may occur during or hours after transfusion, and unlike febrile transfusion reactions is not self-limiting.

- Volume resuscitation.
- Culture the patient and send bag and giving sets to microbiology.
- Start empirical broad-spectrum antibiotics.

Non-bacterial

- Pretransfusion testing includes screening for Hep B (HbsAg, anti HBc), hepatitis C (anti HCV), HIV (anti HIV-1/2, HIV-1 p24 antigen), HTLV (anti TLC-1/2) and syphilis. HIV can be transmitted by an infective but seronegative donor for about 15 days after infection. The HCV window is 20 days. CMV is common in the donor population (40–60%) and immunocompromised recipients must receive leukocyte-depleted or CMV negative blood. Malaria may be transmitted by blood transfusion as may nvCJD.

Fluid overload

Characterized by hypotension, high filling pressures, and poor gases.

- Stop the transfusion.
- Give high-flow O_2 and loop diuretics (40mg furosemide iv).

Massive transfusion

Massive transfusion is replacement of the patient's circulating volume within 24h. Blood is stored at 4°C for up to 5 weeks, but this is associated with a variety of abnormalities including depletion of ATP, 2,3 DPG and leakage of potassium from RBCs. ↓Ca^{2+} (citrate used to store blood binds Ca^{2+}): ↑K^+, hypothermia (if blood is not warmed), and dilutional coagulopathy are complications of massive transfusion.

- Use infusion warmers and a warming blanket.
- Monitor central circulation and respiratory function closely.
- Give CaCl iv slowly (10mL of 10%) after 8–10 units of blood: calcium gluconate provides 1/3 less ionized calcium.
- Check platelets, APTT and fibrinogen: replace empirically if needed.
- Check K^+ regularly.

Re-exploration for bleeding

Key facts

- The re-sternotomy rate for bleeding or tamponade following first pericardiotomy is ~1–2%.
- Resternotomy is best performed in OR (sterility, light, equipment), but if patient too unstable to transfer can be performed at bedside on ICU.

Indications for emergency re-exploration

1. *Incipient or actual cardiac arrest* due to cardiac tamponade, or torrential hemorrhage.
2. *Excessive bleeding*: re-exploration is indicated for grossly excessive bleeding. The following rates are given for guidance only. The decision is a subjective one as the factors listed below must also be taken into account. Consider emergency resternotomy for bleeding rates of:
- >500 mL in <30min.
- >7 mL/kg for 1h.
- >5 mL/kg for 2 consecutive hours.
- >3 mL/kg for 3 consecutive hours.
- >2 mL/kg for 5 consecutive hours.

Re-exploration versus medical management

Higher bleeding rates are accepted where there is a correctable coagulopathy, where there are known risk factors for bleeding (□ p144), where the surgeon is particularly sure that there is no surgical source for bleeding (e.g., where prolonged efforts were made to secure hemostasis in theatre), or where the surgeon feels that the source of bleeding is not surgically correctable (raw surface, needle holes). If bleeding is excessive but the trend is reducing, it may be acceptable to delay the decision to reopen. The following factors indicate that re-exploration is needed:

- Torrential hemorrhage or increasing rate of bleeding, tamponade.
- Hemodynamic instability (e.g., escalating pressor requirement).
- Large hemothorax.
- Minimal coagulopathy.

Technique of re-exploration

Be familiar with the location and contents of the emergency re-exploration set. If you can stabilize the patient and transfer to the OR, do so. It is much more difficult operating over an ICU bed, with poor light and poor sterility, and no scrub nurse, and results reflect this.

Items that are often NOT on the re-exploration set in ICU:
- Prep: pour over patient before putting on gown and gloves.
- Scalpel blades: open up a disposable pre-mounted one first.
- Suction: pass out the tubing so it can be connected to wall suction.
- Light: send someone to get a portable overhead light.
- Defibrillator: don't forget to connect the internal paddles.

Think! Do you need a perfusionist? Ask someone to phone the senior surgeon responsible for the patient.

- Patient must be intubated and sedated (📖 p90) as you prep and drape.
- Open the wound down to the sternum with a knife. Suction ready.
- Cut the sternal wires with a wire cutter: if there is no wire cutter use a heavy needle holder to grab and twist the wires until they fracture.
- Pull *all* the wires out: leaving fragments of wire risks lacerating the right ventricle and makes it more difficult to get good exposure.
- Lever the sternum open with your fingers, and check edges well clear of any grafts, pacing wires, etc.
- Place the sternal retractor (use the Finochietto if you are on your own as this needs least assembling) and carefully expose the heart.
- You should see an immediate improvement in perfusion pressures.
- The commonest finding is a mass of clot with a liquid component: suction this, and remove the clots carefully: filling pressures should fall.
- If there is a source of major bleeding, put a finger over it if you cannot rapidly gain control, and get more senior help.
- If no source of bleeding is immediately apparent, wash the chest out several times with saline (this physically reduces the bacterial load, and helps highlight continued bleeding points) and pack, systematically looking for bleeding at the surgical sites listed (see Box 5.3), taking great care not to avulse grafts while manipulating the heart: inspection of the inferior aspect of the heart is difficult, and it must be swift as it causes significant hemodynamic instability.
- The suprasternal veins sometimes only bleed as the retractor is closed, releasing tension from the surrounding tissues.
- Remove the packs, noting whether they come out 'red, pink or white'.
- Go back and concentrate the search where swabs are 'red': if bleeding is from needle holes or you cannot see an obvious source of bleeding, pack again with dry swabs. Wait. Pack again.
- If 'non-surgical' bleeding persists despite appropriate clotting factors try a topical procoagulant such as Surgicel®, or a tissue glue such as Floseal®.
- Before closing flush the chest drains through with a 60mL 'bladder' syringe filled with saline to remove clot, and replace them in the chest.
- On the rare occasion that significant 'non-surgical' bleeding persists one option is to pack the chest and close the wound with a 'Bogota' bag (the sterile inside bag of iv fluid, or Goretex® membrane), cut to shape and stitched over the open wound using running 3/0 Prolene. The sternum can be splinted open using a 10mL syringe, with the ends cut off and shaped to fit using eye-cautery.

Box 5.3 Sites of bleeding

- *Venous:* atrial cannulation sites, innominate vein, thymic vein, suprasternal veins, cardiac veins, mammary bed, bone marrow, left pulmonary artery if aorta 'taped', pacing wire sites, 'raw' surface of myocardium, right ventricle, right atriotomy.
- *Arterial:* aortic cannulation site, aortotomy, top-ends, left atriotomy, vent sites (aortic, right superior pulmonary vein, LV apex), vein/IMA side-branch, IMA stump, coronary anastomosis, periosteal arteries.

Respiratory physiology

Normal values

- PaO_2 >10.5kPa (75mmHg)
- $Pa\,CO_2$ 4.7–6.0kPa (35–54mmHg)
- SaO_2 >97%
- SvO_2 65–80%
- O_2 delivery = CO × [(Hb × SaO_2 × 1.39 × 10) + (PaO_2 × 0.0225 × 10)]

(Hb is in g/dL, and PaO_2 is in kPa.)

Basic concepts of oxygen carriage

Definitions of common terms are listed on 🕮 pp130–131.

- Oxygen consumption is about 250mL/min O_2 in the adult at rest, rising to over 4L/min during exercise.
- Oxygen diffuses from alveolus to pulmonary capillary until arterial PO_2 (PaO_2) = alveolar PO_2 (P_AO_2).
- The solubility of oxygen in blood is low (0.000225mL O_2 per mL of blood per kPa): at a normal PaO_2 of 13kPa, there is only 0.3mL O_2 dissolved in 100mL of blood.
- Each gram of hemoglobin combines with 1.34mL O_2: at a normal Hb 13g/dL there is 20mL O_2 bound to hemoglobin in 100mL of blood.
- Hence the percentage of arterial hemoglobin binding sites bound to oxygen (SaO_2) or 'oxygen sats' is the main determinant of the O_2 content of arterial blood.
- A fall in pH, a rise in $PaCO_2$ or increased temperature cause a right shift in the oxygen dissociation curve, encouraging oxygen release in metabolically active tissues (the Bohr effect).

The relationship between PaO_2 and SaO_2 is non-linear. As each O_2 molecule binds to 1 of the 4 heme groups on the hemoglobin molecule, the affinity of the remaining heme molecules for oxygen increases, increasing the steepness of the *oxygen-hemoglobin dissociation curve* (Fig. 5.1). The curve flattens out at partial pressures above 8kPa because there are few remaining sites. Above 8kPa (60mmHg) rises and falls in PaO_2 make very little difference to O_2 saturation. Below 8kPa small drops in PaO_2 result in dramatic drops in SaO_2. PaO_2 is an effective measure of changes in oxygenation where SaO_2 plateaus, which is why it is used as a measure of oxygenation. Below this falling PaO_2 heralds profound desaturation, reflecting a dangerous drop in O_2 content of arterial blood.

Other points about oxygen carriage

- Increasing hemoglobin has a major impact on oxygen content.
- Maintaining the PaO_2 well above 10kPa (75mmHg) maintains a slight safety margin for oxygenation in the event of a drop in cardiac output, acute respiratory compromise, or bleeding.
- In non-cardiac patients, a rise in cardiac output can compensate for SaO_2 >80%, so SvO_2 remains at normal levels. In cardiac patients this does not happen to the same extent. Using inotropes to increase cardiac output to compensate for hypoxemia risks myocardial ischemia.

Basic concepts of carbon dioxide transport

Ventilation has two goals: (1) achieving satisfactory PaO_2 and (2) regulation of $PaCO_2$. It has a major bearing on acid–base balance (📖 pp168–169). CO_2 is transported in the blood as bicarbonate ions (HCO_3^-), and car-bamino compounds combined with proteins and dissolved in plasma. As can be seen from the CO_2 dissociation curve (Fig. 5.1) the amount of CO_2 that can be carried in blood is much more than the amount of O_2, and it does not plateau. This is because CO_2 is highly soluble. 60% of CO_2 is transported in the form of bicarbonate:

$$CO_2 + H_2O \Leftrightarrow H_2CO_3 \Leftrightarrow H^+ + HCO_3^-$$

The left-hand side of the equation proceeds slowly in plasma. Carbonic anhydrase, an enzyme present in red cells, accelerates the reaction. The right-hand side of the equation is rapid in any phase. HCO_3^- diffuses out into plasma, but the red cell membrane is impermeable to H^+. To maintain electrical neutrality Cl^- ions diffuse into the cell: the *chloride shift*. H^+ binds avidly to deoxygenated hemoglobin, which acts as a buffer. Oxygenated hemoglobin does not bind H^+ so well.

- The *Haldane effect* means that for any given $PaCO_2$ the CO_2 content of deoxygenated blood is greater than that of oxygenated blood: CO_2 is appropriately taken up in respiring deoxygenated tissues, and released in the oxygenated blood of the lungs.
- Treating metabolic acidosis by administering *sodium bicarbonate* drives the equation to the right: it is important not to give excessive sodium bicarbonate, and to ensure that the patient is adequately ventilating otherwise a paradoxical intracellular acidosis results as CO_2 accumulates.

Other points about carbon dioxide carriage

- CO_2 is 20 times more soluble than O_2.
- At any given metabolic rate doubling the alveolar ventilation halves alveolar and arterial PCO_2, and vice versa, whereas the relationship between ventilation and PaO_2 is more complicated: hypo- and hyper-ventilation are therefore defined in terms of $PaCO_2$.

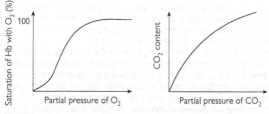

Fig. 5.1 The oxygen and carbon dioxide dissociation curves.

Lung function after heart surgery

Key facts

- Pulmonary dysfunction is maximal for 24h postoperatively, and normally improves over the week following surgery.
- Factors causing changes in pulmonary function can be classified as preoperative, intraoperative, and postoperative, resulting in ventilation-perfusion mismatch and intrapulmonary shunting.

Preoperative factors and respiratory function

- The vast majority of coronary patients have a history of **smoking**.
- Chronic smokers almost invariably have evidence of chronic obstructive airway disease: exertional dyspnea, sputum production, or wheeze is associated with over 5× the rate of pulmonary complication, and 1/3 of these patients will have pulmonary complications requiring additional therapy.
- Stopping smoking 8 weeks or more before surgery has been shown to reduce some of the chronic changes in the bronchopulmonary tree and decrease the rate of pulmonary complications to <15%, but pulmonary complications are probably *increased* in patients who stop smoking <8 weeks before surgery.
- A *recent respiratory infection* is an indication for cancelling non-emergency cardiac surgery, as increased or purulent secretions can lead to atelectasis, pneumonia, bronchial plugging, and eventual occlusion of smaller endotracheal tubes requiring reintubation.
- Resting PaO_2 decreases linearly with age: *older patients* >75 years of age are at greater risk of pulmonary problems.
- *Obesity* increases the risk of postoperative atelectasis: in the morbidly obese sleep apnea and chronic atelectasis may lead to pulmonary hypertension.
- *Pulmonary hypertension* contributes to respiratory insufficiency post-op.

Intraoperative factors and respiratory function

- Both median sternotomy and thoracotomy are associated with *decreased lung capacities* postoperatively: *left lower lobe collapse* occurs in over 50% of on-pump coronary bypass patients.
- *Selective lung ventilation* on bypass for thoracotomy approaches appears to be associated with increased lung injury in the deflated lung.
- The increased *pain* associated with a thoracotomy further predisposes patients to *atelectasis*: an epidural is a key part of improving respiratory function in the postoperative period.
- Either pleura may be opened during surgery: the evidence is mixed as to whether this increases the risk of postoperative atelectasis and *effusions*, but increased handling of the lung is probably detrimental.
- Cardiopulmonary bypass results in increased intra and extravascular fluid and *pulmonary edema*: pulmonary vascular resistance is increased, *lung compliance is decreased*, atelectasis is increased, and *intrapulmonary shunting* is frequently increased as a result.
- *Transfusion-related acute lung injury* (TRALI) 📖 p149: blood and FFP post a higher risk than platelets and cryoprecipitate.
- Damage to either phrenic nerve when opening the chest, harvesting the internal mammary artery, creating a window in the pleura, or

using topical cooling results in **phrenic nerve paresis** which may be temporary or permanent (📖 p269).

Postoperative factors

72h postoperatively **vital capacity may be less than 50%** of preoperative values: it takes 2 weeks to return to normal. **Total lung compliance** falls by 25%, and **dead space is increased**. Atelectasis is present in >50% of patients and is associated with increased intrapulmonary shunts, and raised PVR. Over 50% of patients consequently have a PaO_2 on room air of <7.5kPa (55mmHg).

- **Narcotics, opioid analgesics and sedatives** depress ventilation.
- **Anticholinergics** dilate the airways, increasing dead space.
- **Inotropes and catecholamines** with alpha activity increase PVR.
- **Beta-blockers** can cause bronchoconstriction.

Hemodynamic effects of ventilation

Reduced cardiac output

Increased intrathoracic pressure increases RAP, decreasing venous return and therefore preload. Right ventricular and therefore LV stroke volume and cardiac output are decreased. Induction and sedative agents (fentanyl, propofol) cause vasodilatation which reduces preload and cardiac output. The interventricular septum is displaced leftwards, decreasing LV compliance, LVEDV, and stroke volume.

Increased peripheral vascular resistance (PVR)

Air space dilatation and blood vessel compression caused by PEEP increases PVR by approximately 10%, most of which is at end-inspiration.

Decreased O_2 requirement

Although the work of breathing in normal circumstances utilizes <5% of the body's total O_2 requirements, in respiratory failure this may increase to 50%. Ventilation reduces the total O_2 requirement.

Negative inotropic effect

Hyperinflation occasionally causes reflex vasodilatation, bradycardia and negative inotropic effect.

Intubating hemodynamically unstable patients

As a result of the hemodynamic effects of induction and sedative agents, and ventilation described, intubating patients who are already hemodynamically compromised can precipitate cardiac arrest. This sometimes occurs postoperatively, but must also be anticipated in certain patients being anesthetized for surgery:

- Cardiac tamponade.
- Critical AS.
- Critical left main stenosis, emergency CABG.
- Pulmonary edema.
- Hypotension (hemorrhage, sepsis).

Initial ventilator settings for post-op patients

- FiO_2: 70–100%, mode: SIMV or pressure control.
- Tidal volume: 8–10mL/kg, respiratory rate: 8–14 breaths/min.
- Minute volume: 100–120mL/kg/min.
- PEEP: 5–7.5cmH$_2$O, pressure support: 8–10 cmH$_2$O.
- Inspiratory–expiratory ratio: 1:2, inspiratory flow rate: 30–60L/min.

Respiratory management

Key facts

- Pulmonary dysfunction is maximal for 24h postoperatively, and normally improves over the week following surgery.
- Most patients need mechanical ventilation for at least 4–6h.

Standard ventilator settings

Ventilation should improve the efficiency of gas exchange and reduce the work of breathing in the sedated, paralysed patient who is pre-oxygenated prior to leaving the OR with a FiO_2 of 100% to ensure oxygenation is adequate during any problems in transfer. The FiO_2 is slowly weaned to 30–40% as long as the PaO_2 stays >10.0kPa (75mmHg).

- Any patient can be ventilated safely using SIMV, but pressure control may be used initially: modes of ventilation are described on 📖 p158.
- A tidal volume of 0–10mL/kg helps prevent atelectasis, but excessive tidal volumes risk barotrauma, and can place a borderline LIMA graft under tension as it crosses the upper lobe of the left lung to the LAD.
- A respiratory rate of 8–14 breaths per minute is adequate for most patients, but patients with higher metabolic demands (shivering, sepsis) may benefit from higher rates which help prevent respiratory acidosis.
- 5 cmH$_2$O of PEEP is added to prevent atelectasis, dramatically reducing FiO_2 requirements.
- Patients with COPD benefit from lower respiratory rates and higher tidal volumes, allowing time for the longer expiratory phase, avoiding air trapping ('autoPEEP') which can cause high intrathoracic pressures, barotrauma, and reduced venous return causing hypotension.
- Increasing PEEP to 10cmH$_2$O helps to reverse atelectasis improving oxygenation, but can reduce venous return and MAPs in patients.
- Higher levels of PEEP are sometimes used in the hemodynamically stable, bleeding patient to tamponade chest wall bleeding: this probably works primarily by reducing MAPs.
- The inspiratory–expiratory (I:E) ratio is 1:2., allowing optimal peak inspiratory pressures and reducing the risk of air trapping: in selected patients that are difficult to oxygenate the intensivist or anesthesiologist will change or even reverse these ratios.
- Peak inflation pressures in the adult are usually <30 cmH$_2$O, and the usual inspiratory flow rate is 30L/min, higher peak inflation pressures occur in obesity, active resistance from the patient, or a mechanical obstruction to airflow such as bronchospasm, endobronchial intubation or mucus plugging with lobar collapse.

Pulse oximetry

Pulse oximetry allows non-invasive continuous measurement of SaO_2. Only available since 1990, it is now mandatory in every ventilated patient.

Principles

- Oxygenated (HbO$_2$) and deoxygenated hemoglobin (Hb) have different absorption spectra. HbO$_2$ absorbs less red light (wavelength 660nm), and more infrared light (wavelength 980nm) than Hb.

- The pulse oximeter probe consists of two light-emitting diodes (LEDs) emitting red and infrared light pulses and a photocell detector.
- The probe is placed on a well-perfused extremity, e.g., digit or pinna.
- It detects maximal (systole) and minimum absorption (diastole), and subtracts the constant, non-arterial component from the pulsatile (arterial) component: the ratio of the two wavelengths passing through the tissue is compared to an algorithm derived from experimental data to give a measure of the relative amounts of HbO and Hb (SaO_2).
- A pulse waveform is displayed with the SaO_2.

Sources of error

- Inaccurate at SaO_2 <70% as not calibrated in volunteers at these levels.
- Loss of the pulsatile component in hypoperfusion, peripheral vasoconstriction, narrow pulse pressure, non-pulsatile cardiopulmonary bypass and venous congestion leads to loss of readings.
- Carboxyhemoglobin (in heavy smokers and carbon monoxide poisoning) gives falsely high readings. Jaundiced patients, and patients with systemic methylene blue, give falsely low readings.
- Movement and electrical artifact, interference from direct, bright ambient light, and absorption by substances such as nail varnish and nicotine staining can distort measurements.

Capnography

Capnography is also mandatory in ventilated patients.

Principles

- Similar principles to pulse oximetry: different gases absorb different amounts of infrared light. Systems can be in-line (in the ET tube) or sampling (withdraw gas from the ventilator circuit and sample it at a remote site), and consist of an infrared LED and a photocell detector.
- The fraction of infrared light absorbed is compared against reference values before the trace is displayed: regular calibration against known CO_2 concentrations is essential.

Interpreting the trace

- Adequate ventilation is indicated by normal end-tidal CO_2. *No CO_2 trace* suggests ET tube displacement, tubing disconnection, CO_2 sampling tubing occlusion, esophageal intubation, or circulatory arrest.
- Low or falling end-tidal CO_2 indicates hyperventilation, PE or low cardiac output; high or rising end-tidal CO_2 indicates inadequate ventilation, and hypermetabolic states in which CO_2 production increases (sepsis, shivering) and rarely malignant hyperpyrexia.
- A slow upstroke and slowly rising plateau is seen in COPD.
- Inspiratory dips indicate that the patient is initiating breaths.

Respiratory support modes

Invasive methods

Intermittent positive pressure ventilation (IPPV); controlled mechanical ventilation (CMV); pressure control ventilation

IPPV or CMV is the mode commonly used during routine surgery. Raising airway pressure forces air into the lungs via an endotracheal or tracheostomy tube. Expiration occurs when airway pressures are allowed to fall to zero. This mode is poorly tolerated by the awake patient.

Positive end-expiratory pressure (PEEP)

Instead of allowing airway pressures to fall to zero, a small positive airway pressure is maintained throughout expiration (PEEP), preventing collapse of small airways and alveoli that occurs at the end of expiration. Functional residual capacity, shunts, lung compliance and PaO_2 are improved, and the work of breathing is reduced. High levels of PEEP (>10cmH₂O) may be necessary to reverse established atelectasis, but increase intrathoracic pressure, reducing venous return and cardiac output, which may reduce PaO_2. Barotrauma is a complication of high PEEP. PEEP as low as 5cmH₂O may cause hemodynamic compromise in the patient with poor LV. Physiological PEEP is normally provided by an intact glottis: patients with COPD sometimes purse their lips during expiration to increase physiological PEEP.

Synchronized intermittent mandatory ventilation (SIMV)

One variation of IPPV is SIMV, where positive airway pressure may be synchronized with patient-initiated breaths. Mandatory (machine initiated) breaths are given if no spontaneous breaths occur in a preset time, but do not occur at the same time as patient-initiated breaths. This mode is used in patients that are awake, but any patient may safely be ventilated on SIMV.

Mandatory minute ventilation (MMV)

Another variation of IPPV is MMV where the ventilator initiates breaths only if patient-initiated ventilation falls below a preset minute volume.

Pressure support (PS); assisted spontaneous breathing (ASB)

Patient-initiated breaths can be supported with a preset positive airway pressure of 6–20cmH₂O. The ventilator detects the drop in airway pressures as the patient generates negative intrathoracic pressures at the beginning of inspiration and assists air inflow with a positive airway pressure. This is lower than the preset inflationary pressures in IPPV, as the patient is making some inspiratory effort. At high levels of pressure support (>20cmH₂O) the patient, although controlling the timing and frequency of respiration, is effectively on IPPV. Pressure support of 8cmH₂O is usually the last stage of weaning prior to extubation.

Continuous positive airway pressure (CPAP)

In CPAP a standing airway pressure, continuous throughout all phases of respiration is applied via the ET tube. It is more commonly used in the extubated patient via a tight-fitting face mask (see 📖 p159).

Non-invasive methods

Intermittent negative pressure ventilation (INPV)

Virtually never used today, INPV involves placing the patient inside a tank ventilator sealed at the neck. Tank pressure is intermittently lowered, expanding the chest and lowering intrapleural pressure.

Non-invasive intermittent positive pressure ventilation (NIPPV)

This is IPPV delivered by face mask, or more commonly, nasal mask. The patient must be cooperative in order to understand how to synchronize their breathing with the ventilator. It is sometimes used in the tiring COPD patient where the primary concern is not recruitment of alveoli, but reducing the work of breathing, without resorting to intubation.

Continuous positive airway pressure (CPAP)

In CPAP a standing airway pressure, continuous throughout all phases of respiration, is applied via an endotracheal tube, tracheostomy, nasal mask or, more commonly, face mask to a spontaneously breathing patient. This results in a kind of non-invasive PEEP, where additional alveoli are recruited with the benefits described on 🕮 p158. CPAP is a useful adjunct in the extubated patient with COPD, atelectasis, pulmonary edema or ARDS. It cannot produce ventilation by itself.

Biphasic positive pressure ventilation (BiPAP)

BiPAP is a solution to the problem of air trapping that can occur in patients, particularly those with COPD, on CPAP. Airway pressure is cycled at preset rates between high and low levels.

High-flow (Venturi) face mask (fixed performance)

The key part of the Venturi facemask is the Venturi valve which draws in an amount of air through calibrated inlets, which is mixed with oxygen flowing into the valve, before entering the mask. More mixed air (up to 30L/min) is delivered to the mask than the patient can use: the excess escapes though holes in the mask. The FiO_2 is set by the choice of valve, not by the patient's breathing pattern (hence the term fixed performance). The maximum FiO_2 that can be delivered by a Venturi mask is about 60%. There is a minimum flow rate of O_2 for each Venturi.

Low flow (Hudson) face mask (variable performance)

Oxygen flows at a set rate (e.g., 2L/min) into the mask. It is diluted by air drawn into the mask, which depends on the patient's minute volumes which can range from 5–30L/min. The FiO_2 achieved thus depends primarily on the patient, and the delivery system should therefore not be used when accurate control of FiO_2 is required. The maximum FiO_2 that can reliably be delivered in this fashion is about 30%. Use of a non-rebreathing mask and reservoir bag, into which 100% O_2 is drawn during expiration and inhaled during inspiration, increases FiO_2 to up to 60%. The reservoir bag must be filled with O_2 before the patient uses it.

Nasal prongs

Nasal prongs deliver a FiO_2 that is determined primarily by the patient, as in a low-flow mask, but they are less obtrusive, allowing the patient to expectorate and eat. They increase tracheal FiO_2 to barely more than room air levels, particularly if the patient breathes through their mouth.

Poor gases in ventilated patients

Key facts

- Most patients recover respiratory function and are weaned from ventilatory support within 24h.
- 5% require additional and prolonged support, often due to multiple risk factors for postoperative respiratory dysfunction (📖 p155).
- Common causes of respiratory insufficiency in ventilated patients are listed on 📖 pp162–163 together with management.

'Poor gases' or respiratory insufficiency

These depend on the context: on FiO_2 of 100% O_2 a 'normal' patient should be able to achieve PaO_2 >400mmHg. Generally the following definitions apply:

- *Hypoxia*: PaO_2 <10.5kPa (80mmHg), SaO_2 >90%.
- *Hypercapnia*: $PaCO_2$ >6.5kPa (50mmHg).
- *Hypocapnia*: $PaCO_2$ <3.5kPa (25mmHg).

Basic assessment and management

- *Look at the patient*: is the ET tube obviously displaced, is the patient biting the ET tube or fighting the ventilator, is chest expansion asymmetrical, can you see or feel subcutaneous emphysema? What is the hemodynamic status of the patient? Poor pulse oximeter readings may reflect low cardiac output and peripheral vasoconstriction.
- *Auscultate the chest* for bilateral breath sounds, and the stomach: is the ET tube advanced too far past the carina resulting in single lung ventilation, or misplaced in the esophagus?
- *Compare SaO_2* from pulse oximeter with SaO_2 from new blood gas, and PaO_2: pulse oximetry may give falsely low reading (📖 p157).
- *Increase the FiO_2* to 100% O_2 which can be given for short periods without causing oxygen toxicity, and usually reverses hypoxia.
- If the O_2 sats do not start quickly rising to >95%, *disconnect the patient from the ventilator and manually ventilate* with 100% O_2. This allows you to:
  - Identify if the ventilator is the source of the problem.
  - Perform recruitment maneuvers to treat atelectasis.
  - Reassess whether both sides of chest moving symmetrically.
  - Assess the patient's airway compliance directly: reasons a patient may be 'difficult to bag' include kinked or blocked tubing, including biting on ET tube, ET tube up against carina or in one main bronchus, bronchospasm, pulmonary edema, tension pneumothorax.
  - Suction the patient to look for and treat mucus plugs or bleeding: suctioning can cause rapid desaturation in patient dependent on PEEP, as well as coughing and agitation.
- Is the patient biting on the ET tube? If they are uncooperative they are not ready for weaning and should be resedated: *sedation or paralysis* improves gas exchange by improving efficiency of ventilation and reducing the energy demands of spontaneous ventilation.

- *Treat bronchospasm with* nebulized albuterol 5mg.
- *Get a CXR.* Assess the position of the ET tube. It should be at least 2cm above the carina—pull it back 2cm if this is not the case.
- Look for *pneumothoraces* or *pleural collections* which should be treated with a formal chest drain, and *atelectasis* or *mucus plug* (complete whiteout lobe or hemithorax—can look similar to hemothorax 📖 p14, Fig. 1.2c) which should be managed with intermittent ET tube suction and increased PEEP.
- Change the *ventilator settings* (see Box 5.4).
- If you suspect mucus plugging (copious secretions, CXR showing lobar collapse or complete whiteout hemithorax) perform fiberoptic bronchoscopy at bedside (📖 pp654–655).

Box 5.4 Impact of ventilator settings on PaO$_2$ and PaCO$_2$
- FiO$_2$: 0.7–1.0 (↑ to increase PaO$_2$).
- Tidal volume: 8–12mL/kg (↑ to reduce PaCO$_2$).
- Respiratory rate: 8–14 breaths/min (↑ to reduce PaCO$_2$).
- Minute volume: 100–120mL/kg/min (↑ to reduce PaCO$_2$).
- PEEP: 5–10cmH$_2$O (↑ to increase PaO$_2$).
- Pressure support: 8–10cmH$_2$O (↑ to increase PaO$_2$).
- Inspiratory–expiratory ratio: 1:2.
- Inspiratory flow rate: 30–60L/min (↑ to increase PaO$_2$).

Respiratory failure on ventilator

Management

Basic assessment and management of acute respiratory insufficiency is described on 📖 pp160–161. Treatments of the various causes of respiratory failure listed in Box 5.5 are outlined here.

> **Box 5.5 Etiology of respiratory failure**
> - *Inadequate O_2 delivery to patient:* ventilator malfunction, incorrect ventilator settings, endotracheal tube problems.
> - *Pulmonary dysfunction:* pneumothorax, hemothorax, pulmonary edema, atelectasis, consolidation, bronchospasm, COPD, ARDS.
> - *Inadequate O_2 delivery to tissues:* low cardiac output, anemia.
> - ↑ O_2 demand: Shivering, sepsis, pyrexia, hyperalimentation, drugs.

Ventilator malfunction: manually ventilate with 100% O_2, which should improve oxygenation immediately and also give an indication of pulmonary compliance. If oxygenation does not improve seek other causes.

Incorrect ventilator settings: inadequate FiO_2, PEEP or pressure support will result in low PaO_2. High $PaCO_2$ may be caused by too low a tidal volume and/or respiratory rate. Check inspiratory flow rate, and increase in COPD. Standard ventilator settings are described on 📖 p155.

ET tube problem: is the tube occluded by sputum plugs, kinking or patient biting, or misplaced in the esophagus, larynx or main bronchus; is there a cuff leak? Listening to both lungs and the epigastrium should confirm placement. A CXR should show the end of the ET tube 2cm above the carina. Suction the pharynx, deflate the cuff, withdraw the tube as appropriate, re-inflate, and look for symmetrical chest expansion. Suction the tube. Be aware in long-term intubated patients that the lumen of the tube can be reduced to little more than the diameter of the fine-bore suction tube by solidified secretions. A Guedel airway stops the patient biting the ET tube.

Low cardiac output: optimize cardiac output (📖 pp184–185).

Anaemia: an Hb >8.0g/dl is adequate for most patients post cardiac surgery. Reduced blood viscosity improves perfusion of microvasculature and leads to reduced risk of graft occlusion. In patients with borderline SaO_2 such as those with COPD, increasing Hb has a large impact in oxygen delivery, seen in increased mixed venous O_2 saturations.

Pneumothorax: increasing $PaCO_2$ and decreasing compliance suggest a pneumothorax, which occurs in approximately 1% of ventilated patients post cardiac surgery. Causes include trauma during central line insertion, median sternotomy, or barotrauma. Breath sounds are audible on the side of the pneumothorax until it is >50%. Get a CXR. If you suspect tension pneumothorax, place an immediate intercostal drain (📖 p248). A pneumothorax is unlikely if there is a patent pleural drain.

Hemothorax: increasing $PaCO_2$, falling Hb, falling CVP and pleural drainage suggests hemothorax which can be confirmed by CXR. Even if the pleura was not opened during surgery, trauma to neck vessels during central venous catheterization or to internal mammary vessels at chest closure may cause a hemothorax. Insert a chest drain (🕮 p248).

Pulmonary edema: cardiogenic or non-cardiogenic. Treat the cause. Loop diuretics are an important temporizing measure (🕮 p209). Failure of mitral valve repair, paraprosthetic leaks, conduit occlusion, cardiac tamponade and endocarditis are causes of acute postoperative pulmonary edema. Non-cardiogenic causes include fluid overload and renal failure.

Atelectasis: prevent with PEEP or CPAP, and treat with physiotherapy.

Consolidation: prevent with early mobilization, prophylactic antibiotics. Do not deflate the cuff on a tracheostomy tube until speech and language assessment is satisfactory. Treat with organism-specific antibiotics. Aspiration pneumonia, suggested by a history of aspiration of vomitus or NG feed while the ET cuff deflated, and bibasal shadowing on CXR, should be treated with cefuroxime 750mg and metronidazole 500mg iv 8-hourly. Prevent mucus plugging by giving humidified oxygen or saline nebulizers. Treat mucus plugs with physiotherapy, suctioning and if necessary bronchial toilet via bronchoscopy.

Bronchospasm and COPD: the ET tube touching the carina, and suctioning can precipitate bronchospasm, as can β-blockers. It is characterized by wheeze, high inflationary pressures, low PaO_2 and high $PaCO_2$. Treat with nebulized albuterol 5mg prn (🕮 p161). Aminophylline infusions are used in refractory cases. Withdraw the ET tube if indicated.

ARDS: diagnostic criteria: (1) progressive hypoxemia (PaO_2 (mmHg): FiO_2 (fraction not percentage) ratio <200). (2) Predisposing cause (cardiopulmonary bypass, pancreatitis, SIRS, aspiration of gastric contents, pulmonary trauma, fat embolism, smoke inhalation), without pre-existing lung disease. (3) Bilateral infiltrates on CXR. (4) Reduced pulmonary compliance. (5) Normal LVEDP—excluding cardiogenic pulmonary edema. Treatment: There is no specific therapy for ARDS. Management is supportive. PEEP maintains lung volumes, decreases shunt and reduces V/Q mismatch. Lowest FiO_2 consistent with O_2 delivery. Nitric oxide and ventilation prone are occasionally used.

Shivering: increases O_2 demand and CO_2 production. Warm patient with warming blanket and use a warmer for iv infusions. Paralyze, and consider improving peripheral perfusion with vasoconstrictors (🕮 p143). Pethidine 25mg iv has an effective antispasmodic effect.

Sepsis: increases O_2 demand and CO_2 production. Culture everything: blood, sputum, urine, wounds, stools, line tips. Treat the cause. Consider hemofiltration to remove cytokines in hyperpyrexia.

Drugs: drugs which exacerbate pulmonary shunting by preventing hypoxic pulmonary vasoconstriction (NTG, SNP) reduce PaO_2. Excessive or rapid administration of sodium bicarbonate leads to ↑CO_2 production (🕮 p153).

Weaning from ventilation

Key facts

- Weaning is normally completed within 6–12h of surgery.
- Patients with poor ventricular function or pulmonary hypertension may take longer as will patients with surgical problems, e.g., bleeding.
- Waking causes vasoconstriction, increased afterload, and tachycardia, thus increasing myocardial oxygen demand.

The weaning process

Short-term ventilated patients

Withhold or minimize narcotics. Reduce the ventilator rate by 2 breaths per hour. At a ventilator rate of 4 with FiO_2 <0.6, check ABGs. If these remain satisfactory the patient can be weaned onto CPAP of $5cmH_2O$, or onto pressure support ventilation of $8cmH_2O$ which is gradually reduced, and then onto a T-piece. ABGs are checked after 45min. Proceed to extubation if the patient meets the extubation criteria.

Long-term ventilated patients

The same process described for short-term ventilated patients occurs over days to weeks (📖 p281). CPAP may be delivered via the tracheostomy, for several hours in between shortening periods of SIMV.

Extubation

All the equipment necessary for emergency re-intubation should be to hand and checked. Have post-extubation oxygen mask and connection tubing to hand, checked and ready. Grade III or IV intubation patients (check the anesthetic record) should be extubated with an anesthesiologist present. The patient should satisfy the criteria in Box 5.6.

- Position the patient upright at 45°.
- Suction the ET tube, mouth, and pharynx. Treat any resultant hypoxia.
- Deflate the ET tube cuff, remove the tube and suction mouth again.
- Apply face mask with $8L/min$ O_2 and $4L/min$ via nasal cannulas.
- Patient should be carefully observed for 20min following extubation with continuous pulse oximetry, and ABGs after 10–15min.
- If the post-extubation gas is good, begin to titrate FiO_2 downwards.
- Keep patient nil by mouth for 4h to allow any vocal cord irritation to settle, then start oral hydration with sips of water, and monitor.

Postextubation management

Oxygen delivery may be compromised by respiratory dysfunction, fluid overload and hemodynamic compromise (📖 p162). *Give 4–6L humidified O_2 by face mask for several hours.* Most patients rapidly progress to lower FiO_2, O_2 delivery via nasal cannulas and then room air. Breathing is compromised by pain and decreased chest wall compliance. Shallow breathing, splinting, and poor cough predispose to atelectasis. *Ensure adequate analgesia, and mobilization, and educate the patient.* A cough cushion held against the chest when coughing helps reduce pain and sternal movement (the abstraction force of pectoralis major is reduced).

Box 5.6 Criteria for weaning and extubation

Respiratory criteria

Ventilation and gas exchange

- *Criteria for weaning*: PaO_2 >10kPa on FiO_2 30%, $PaCO_2$ <7kPa; arterial pH >7.35 unless cause of acidosis known and improving; PEEP <5cmH$_2$O; awake and initiating breaths.
- *Criteria for extubation*: Negative inspiratory pressure >−20cmH$_2$O, vital capacity >10mL/kg, tidal volumes >5mL/kg, resting minute volume >8L, respiratory rate 10–25, PEEP < 5cmH$_2$O.

Safe airway: adequate cough for sputum and secretion clearance.

Lung compliance: compliance should be > 25ml/cmH$_2$O.

Rapid shallow breathing index (frequency/tidal volume (L) <100: patients who fail tend to breathe rapidly and shallowly, so RSBI >100.

Hemodynamic criteria

The EKG should be satisfactory. Cardiac failure with pulmonary edema will impair gas exchange, and may worsen with extubation. High or escalating inotropic requirements mean that myocardial function may be compromised by weaning too soon.

Neurological criteria

Patient should be awake, cooperative, with an adequate gag reflex.

Surgical criteria

Adequate hemostasis: mediastinal drainage <1mL/kg/h. Adequate pain relief. No further surgical procedures planned.

Additional factors

Multiorgan failure, renal failure with fluid overload, ARDS are relative contraindications to weaning. Patients should be normothermic. A base deficit is not a contraindication if cause known and treatable.

Common weaning problems

Drowsiness

Patients may show good respiratory parameters when awake but become apneic, bradycardic, and hypotensive when they sleep. Titrate opioids carefully. Naloxone 0.2–0.4mg iv prn provides emergency reversal.

'Fighting the ventilator'

These patients are unable to breath in synchrony with delivered breaths. Awake patients may bite the ET tube, causing hypoxia. Coughing, gagging, and fighting the ventilator result in raised intrathoracic pressures, which lead to sudden rises in CVP and falls in MAPs which mimic cardiac tamponade. If the patient is confused, with very poor cardiopulmonary parameters, resedate, ventilate, and paralyze if no improvement. In uncooperative but otherwise stable patients early extubation may be beneficial.

Failure to wean from ventilation

In addition to the causes of respiratory failure listed on p162, late failure to wean from ventilation is caused by myocardial ischemia, valvular heart disease, sternal non-union, stroke, and critical illness neuropathy.

Tracheostomy

Key facts

- A tracheostomy is normally performed electively, if the patient proves difficult to wean from ventilation after 7–10 days.
- It can be done as a formal surgical procedure (📖 p664), as a percutaneous ICU procedure (see 📖 p166), or on the HDU as a minitracheostomy (📖 p249) for tracheal toilet (not used for ventilation).

Indications

- Airway protection.
- Prolonged ventilatory support likely—facilitates gradual weaning.
- Tracheobronchial toilet (particularly in pneumonectomy patients).

Contraindications

- Local sepsis and hemodynamic instability are relative contraindications.

Technique of percutaneous tracheostomy

Percutaneous tracheostomy is based on a modified Seldinger technique. It is usually performed in selected patients (thin patients with long necks and good extension) by an intensivist. In about 50% of units a second intensivist routinely monitors the procedure via a fiberoptic bronchoscope as it is easy to perforate the posterior wall of the trachea.

- The patient is preoxygenated.
- With the patient positioned with the neck straight and extended, and the cuff on the ET tube deflated, the midline is carefully identified: this is critical to prevent malpositioning of the tracheostomy tube in the soft tissues adjacent to the trachea.
- The isthmus of the thyroid overlies the 2nd–4th tracheal rings: an approach higher than this avoids the isthmus but is associated with greater incidence of tracheal stenosis.
- Most practitioners elect to enter the trachea below the 2nd or 3rd ring.
- After infiltrating carefully with 10mL 1% lidocaine a skin incision is made over the 2nd ring in the midline.
- A hollow needle is inserted into the trachea, and the guidewire passed through it.
- Progressively larger dilators enlarge the diameter of the hole until it will accept a definitive tracheostomy tube; alternatively, a specially designed dilating forceps can be passed over the guidewire.
- At this point the indwelling ET tube is withdrawn slowly until the tracheostomy tube can be fed over the guidewire into position.
- Secure the tube by suturing it to the skin as well as tying it in place.
- The cuff is inflated, the tube is connected to a bag reservoir and the chest checked for symmetrical inflation while the patient is manually ventilated and suctioned if necessary.

Complications

Percutaneous tracheostomy has a complication rate of 5–7%, lower than that for surgical tracheostomy. Use of fiber optic bronchoscopy does not affect the rate of complications, but appears to protect against the more serious complications. Complications are immediate, early and late.

Hemodynamic instability: this is common due to wide variation in the level of autonomic stimulation during the procedure.

Bleeding: bleeding during or immediately after insertion of the tracheostomy tube is usually due to bleeding from thyroid veins. Correct any coagulopathy. If bleeding does not settle with pressure, surgical exploration is indicated. Late bleeding from around the tube suggests erosion of the tube into the thyroid gland or neck vessels.

Failure to intubate the trachea: creation of a false passage can be avoided by careful positioning of the patient and constant reference to the surface landmarks of the midline. Difficulty ventilating the patient, absence of an end-tidal CO_2 trace, and surgical emphysema all suggest failure to intubate the trachea. Loss of an airway can be avoided by withdrawing the ET tube only as far as necessary to allow insertion of the tracheostomy tube, and leaving the ET tube in place until the tracheostomy tube has been checked and secured.

Esophageal perforation: simultaneous fibreoptic bronchoscopy is designed to avoid this by preventing laceration of the posterior wall of the trachea. Leaving the indwelling ET tube in situ while performing tracheostomy also helps protect against inadvertent damage.

Barotrauma: pneumothorax, pneumomediastinum, and surgical emphysema result from direct injury to the apex of the lung, excessive negative intrathoracic pressures in awake distressed patients, or excessive positive pressure manual ventilation. Management of pneumothorax is described on 📖 p162, pneumomediastinum on 📖 pp731, 790.

Tracheoinnominate fistula (TIF): Catastrophic late bleeding suggests formation of a tracheoinnominate fistula. It is often preceded by a small herald bleed, and may be associated with a pulsating tracheostomy. To gain emergency control compress the innominate artery against the sternum by removing the tracheostomy and placing a finger inside the stoma. ET intubation must be carried out with a cuffed tube to achieve airway control. Repair is via median sternotomy (📖 p665).

Tracheoesophageal fistula (TEF): erosion of the tube cuff through the membranous trachea is less common now that low-pressure cuffs and lighter weight connection tubing are in wide use. Repair is usually delayed until the patient no longer requires ventilatory support. Placing the tracheostomy tube so that the cuff rests below the fistula provides airway protection from gastric contents.

Infection: positive cultures from a tracheostomy tube represent clinical infection and should be treated. Treat cellulitis with antibiotics.

Inadvertent extubation and loss of airway control: in tracheostomies over 7 days old a tract makes re-insertion of the tracheostomy tube relatively easy. Where there is no tract get anesthetic help to attempt oral intubation. If this fails, cricothyroidotomy should be performed.

Tracheal stenosis and granulomas: these can occur at the site of the stoma or the site of the cuff. Management is described on 📖 p751.

Acid–base balance

Key facts

- The pH of arterial blood is maintained at 7.35–7.45. Normal functioning of the body's complex enzyme systems depends on this stability.
- Derangements are due to *respiratory and/or metabolic* dysfunction. Compensatory mechanisms are also divided into metabolic and respiratory. The true clinical picture is usually mixed.

Diagnosing acid–base abnormalities

pH <7.35 is an acidosis: pH>7.45 is an alkalosis

- Look at the pH—is there an acidosis or an alkalosis?
- Look at the $PaCO_2$—is there a change *in keeping with* the pH derangement? If so, the derangement is a respiratory one.
- Look at the base deficit (or anion gap). This will tell you if there is a metabolic derangement: if pH is normal it is fully compensated.
- The *Flenley nomogram* (Fig. 5.2, ☐ p171) is a useful diagnostic aid where mixed metabolic and respiratory derangements are present.

Acid–base physiology

Acids

An *acid* is a substance that can donate a hydrogen ion or proton (H^+) to another substance. Some molecules are stronger donors than others. Acids produced by the body are conventionally divided into *metabolic or fixed acids*, e.g., lactic acid, and *respiratory or volatile acids*, i.e., CO_2 which forms carbonic acid in solution(☐ p153). The production of respiratory acids is many times greater than the production of metabolic acid. Excretion of respiratory acid occurs rapidly through the lungs, whereas excretion of metabolic acid occurs more slowly through the kidneys.

Bases

A *base* can be loosely defined as a substance that accepts a hydrogen ion. Some molecules have higher affinity for H^+ and are stronger bases than others. The most important base is sodium bicarbonate ($NaHCO_3$).

Buffers

Buffers are usually made up of a weak acid, the salt of that acid, and a strong base, and can bind or release H^+ according to the pH, helping to maintain pH stability. The body has an enormous and immediate buffering capacity, which conceals huge changes in H^+ production. This is vital because small changes in pH lead to big changes in the amounts of ionized substances in solution, and speed of enzyme-catalysed reactions. The most important buffers in blood are hemoglobin (Hb) and bicarbonate (HCO_3^-), which is produced and excreted by the kidneys. CO_2 carriage in blood and its removal in the lungs is the most significant factor in acid–base homeostasis. The strength of a buffer or pKa (in this case for HCO_3^-) is described by the *Henderson–Hasselbach equation*:

$$pH = pK_A + \log ([HCO_3^-]/[H_2CO_3])$$

Base excess, base deficit, and anion gap

These are derived numbers, calculated by blood-gas analysers, quantifying changes in metabolic or fixed acids but, because they depend on several assumptions, they do not always reflect the true acid–base balance.

- **Base excess** is defined as the millimoles per litre of *acid* required to titrate the blood pH back to pH 7.4, if the pCO_2 were normal.
- **Base deficit (negative base excess)** is defined as the millimoles per litre of *base* to titrate the blood pH back to pH 7.4, if the pCO_2 were normal.
- A base deficit is negative and a base excess is positive by convention. Normal values are −2mmol/L to 2mmol/L. A base deficit greater than this (e.g., −6mmol) indicates a metabolic acidosis.
- The **anion gap** is the difference between measured cations and measured anions (= $[K^+ + Na^+] - [Cl^- + HCO_3^-]$). This is made up of metabolic acids: ketones, lactate and phosphates. The anion gap is normally 8–16mmol/L: an increase in anion gap indicates a metabolic acidosis.

Metabolic acidosis

Uncompensated: ↓pH, ↔pCO_2, ↓HCO_3^-.
Compensated: ↓ ↔pH, ↓pCO_2, ↓HCO_3^-.

Metabolic acidosis due to increased metabolic acids (increased anion gap)

- Lactic acid (global and/or regional hypoperfusion, hypoxia, sepsis, hepatic failure as the liver normally metabolizes lactate).
- Uric acid (renal failure).
- Ketones (diabetic ketoacidosis, alcoholic and starvation ketoacidosis).
- Drugs/toxins (salicylates, SNP overdose).

Due to loss of bicarbonate or hyperchloremia (normal anion gap)

- Renal tubular acidosis (loss of bicarbonate).
- Diarrhea, high-output ileostomy (loss of bicarbonate).
- Pancreatic fistulae (loss of bicarbonate).
- Hyperchloremic acidosis (excessive saline administration).

Metabolic alkalosis

- Uncompensated: ↑ pH, ↔pCO_2, ↑HCO_3^-.
- Compensated: ↑ ↔pH, ↑pCO_2, ↑HCO_3^-.
- Loss of H^+ from gut (vomiting, NG tube suction).
- Renal loss of H^+ (diuretics), ↑reabsorption of HCO_3 (hypochloremia).
- Administration of base (NaHCO_3, citrate in blood transfusions).

Respiratory acidosis

- Uncompensated: ↓pH, ↑pCO_2, ↔HCO_3^-.
- Compensated: ↓ ↔pH, ↑pCO_2, ↑HCO_3^-.
- Any cause of respiratory failure, or hypoventilation (📖 pp162–163).
- Increased production of CO_2, e.g., sepsis, malignant hyperpyrexia.
- Rebreathing CO_2 (circuit misconnections, soda lime exhaustion).

Respiratory alkalosis

- Uncompensated: ↑pH, ↓pCO_2, ↔HCO_3^-.
- Compensated: ↔↑pH, ↓pCO_2, ↓HCO_3^-.
- Hyperventilation: deliberate, inadvertent, or in non-ventilated patients caused by stroke, anxiety, PE, pneumonia, asthma, pulmonary edema.

The acidotic patient

Key facts

- Acid–base disturbances not only indicate profound hemodynamic, respiratory, and metabolic dysfunction, but also exacerbate myocardial and pulmonary dysfunction.
- It is usually easy and important to distinguish between a metabolic and a respiratory acidosis (📖 pp168–169).

Common causes of acidosis after cardiac surgery

See 📖 p169. Low cardiac output states predispose to poor peripheral perfusion, which may result in lactic acidosis. This is exacerbated by vasoconstriction caused by hypothermia, reflex response to hypotension, or vasoconstrictors such as norepinephrine. Respiratory acidosis is common in obtunded patients without ventilatory support (📖 p281). Other important causes of metabolic acidosis after surgery include diabetic ketoacidosis, regional ischemia including mesenteric and peripheral limb ischemia, sepsis, renal failure, and hyperchloremic acidosis.

Basic investigation and management

Review the diagnostic criteria outlined on 📖 pp168–169.

- In addition to pH, you need to know the pCO_2.
- Base excess or anion gap (📖 p169), and blood glucose and lactate will help you diagnose and treat the causes more accurately.
- Treat respiratory acidosis by increasing respiratory rate and tidal volumes of the ventilator settings: aim for a minute volume of 100mL/kg/min.
- The weaning process should be reversed in the patient that develops a respiratory acidosis while being weaned from ventilation.
- It is sometimes reasonable to support hypoxic extubated patients with CPAP to reduce the work of breathing, but careful attention should be paid to ruling out other reversible causes of hypoxia in addition to atelectasis, and deciding whether in fact they would benefit more from elective rather than emergency reintubation.
- Check the *blood sugar*, and dipstick urine: start an iv insulin sliding scale if serum glucose >140g/dL (8.0mmol/L), or if there are ketones in the urine: many units routinely run patients on sliding scales to achieve tight glycemic control (blood glucose between 80–110mg/dL).
- *Treat peripheral hypoperfusion* by using a warming blanket if necessary to achieve core temperatures 36.5–37.5°C.
- Optimize preload by filling to maintain CVP 14–16mmHg.
- Optimize cardiac output: dopamine 250mcg in 250mL 5% dextrose at 3–6.0 micrograms/kg/min is a good first choice.
- Dopexamine and dobutamine cause peripheral and splanchnic vasodilatation which helps prevent end organ hypoperfusion.
- If the patient is still vasoconstricted with cold peripheries start a NTG infusion (5–200mcg/min).
- *Optimize urine output* by giving loop diuretics in the adequately filled patient to maintain a diuresis >1mL/kg/h, and inotropes if indicated.

- *Give sodium bicarbonate* 25–50mL 8.4% iv (📖 p163). There are situations where the underlying cause of acidosis cannot immediately be treated (off-pump patients who develop a metabolic acidosis possibly as a result of hypoperfusion in theatre, patients requiring high doses of epinephrine or norepinephrine, and patients with sepsis, renal failure and end organ ischemia. Sodium bicarbonate helps to normalize pH temporarily but will increase $PaCO_2$: ventilation must be adequate.
- A deteriorating base deficit, refractory to medical management, in the patient with renal failure is an indication for urgent *hemodialysis*.
- Look for and investigate signs of regional ischemia (📖 p185).

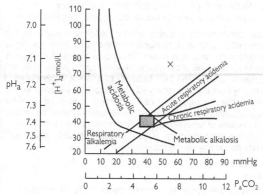

Fig. 5.2 The Flenley nomogram.

Arterial cannulas

Key facts

- All cardiac surgical patients should have an arterial catheter intraoperatively and for the first 12–24h postoperatively.
- Anesthesiologists insert a radial or axillary artery cannula in the non-dominant arm prior to induction.
- Intra-arterial pressure monitoring allows continuous and more precise measurement and control of BP than non-invasive cuff measurement in an environment where rapid changes are commonplace. It also facilitates frequent sampling of ABGs.

Contraindications

Absolute: infection at the site of insertion, distal limb ischemia.
Relative: coagulopathy, proximal obstruction, surgical considerations.

Allen's test demonstrates a patent palmar collateral circulation: the patient clenches a fist to exclude blood from the palm, while you firmly compress both ulnar and radial pulses. The patient then opens his palm, which should be blanched. You release the ulnar compression while still occluding the radial pulse: the palm becomes pink in <5s if there is good collateral supply from the ulnar artery (📖 p7). About 3% of people do not have a collateral palmar supply, and hand ischemia is a potential risk if the radial artery is cannulated. Although the radial artery is most commonly cannulated because of accessibility, pressure readings are more accurate from axillary and femoral artery, especially after long cases when radial line becomes damped by peripheral vasoconstriction.

The arterial waveform

(See Fig. 5.3.)
- The MAP is the average pressure over 1 cardiac cycle. As you can see from the waveform, systole is shorter than diastole, hence the equation MAP = DP + (SP − DP)/3.
- The slope of the upstroke reflects contractility (dP/dt).
- The slope of the diastolic decay reflects resistance to outflow: a long gentle slope is seen in vasoconstriction.
- The stroke volume and CO can be calculated by measuring the area from the beginning of the upstroke to the dicrotic notch.

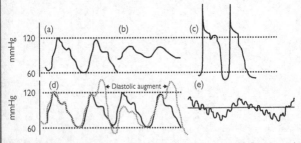

Fig. 5.3 The arterial waveform. (a) Normal. (b) Underdamped. (c) Overdamped. (d) IABP 1:2. (e) Respiratory variation.

Complications

Ischemia, thrombosis, distal embolism, bleeding, damage to radial and median nerve. Inadvertent intra-arterial injection of drugs.

Interpretation and common problems

Low-amplitude trace

This may be due to *poor cardiac output*: palpate a major pulse and ensure a non-invasive cuff measurement is obtained at 30s intervals from the opposite arm. If cardiac output is satisfactory exclude *occlusion* by flushing with 5mL heparinized saline and check that it is easy to aspirate. Ensure the wrist is extended (altering the position of the wrist may help get a good trace if the cannula is *against the vessel wall*). Check cannula and connecting tubing are not *kinked* and that all three-way taps between the patient and transducer are open. *Damping* is caused by cannulas that are too small, excessive lengths of compliant connection tubing, excessive use of three-way taps, air bubbles, and blood clots.

Exaggerated respiratory variation ('respiratory swing')

This suggests that the patient is hypovolemic, in respiratory distress, or cardiac tamponade (📖 p144).

Problems related to other sites

Brachial artery thrombosis has particularly severe consequences. Femoral artery cannulas are more prone to *infection*. Thrombosis has potentially very severe sequelae. A longer catheter is required which may result in *damping*. It is *less accessible* intraoperatively. Dorsalis pedis artery cannula pressure is 10–20mmHg higher than in the central circulation.

Intra-arterial injection

This is a serious mishap. The awake patient will complain of pain in the affected hand. Early signs include pallor, mottling, and cyanosis due to arterial spasm. Late signs included trophic skin changes, ulceration, and edema. Gangrene or contractures are a late feature of severe cases.

The management depends on the injectate:
- Leave the cannula in place.
- Inject 1000U heparin down cannula to reduce risk of thrombosis.
- Inject warm normal saline down cannula to dilute substance.
- Dexamethasone 8mg iv may reduce arterial edema.
- Maintenance anticoagulation for 7–14 days.
- Discuss with plastic surgeons early.
- Antispasmodics such as papaverine may have a role: theatres will have papaverine as it is used topically on harvested arterial conduit intraoperatively to prevent vasospasm. Topical NTG patches may help.

Insertion

Techniques of arterial cannulation are described on 📖 p244.

Removal

Arterial cannulas are routinely removed 24–48h after surgery if the patient is hemodynamically stable, off inotropic support, and has satisfactory ABGs. Firm pressure should be applied to the insertion site for 5min after removal to prevent hematoma formation.

Central venous catheters

Key facts

- All cardiac surgical patients should have central venous pressure monitoring intraoperatively and for the first 12–24h postoperatively.
- Anesthesiologists insert a central line into the right internal jugular vein immediately after intubation.
- Central venous pressure cannulas not only allow continual RAP measurements which are used to guide filling status and assess RV function but also act as an:
  - Infusion port for some drugs which cannot be given peripherally.
  - Insertion port for pulmonary artery catheter.
  - Insertion port for transvenous pacing wires.
  - Infusion port for TPN.
  - Large-bore side arm for rapid infusion volume if required.

Cannulas can be single or multilumen, sheaths (for insertion of PA catheters and pacing wires), tunnelled, or long lines.

Contraindications

- *Absolute*: SVC syndrome, infection at the site of insertion.
- *Relative*: coagulopathy. Undrained contralateral pneumothorax. Uncooperative patient. DVT of the head and neck vessels may make insertion difficult. Patients with ASDs and VSDs are at risk of CVA from air emboli caused by poor technique.

The central venous waveform

(See Fig. 5.4.)

- The waveform is composed of three upstrokes (the 'a', 'c', and 'v' waves) and two descents (the 'x' and 'y' descent).
- The 'a' wave is due to atrial systole.
- The 'v' wave is due to venous return filling the RA before the tricuspid valve opens.
- The 'c' wave is due to bulging of the closed tricuspid valve into the RA at the start of isovolumetric ventricular contraction.
- The 'x' descent occurs in atrial diastole.
- The 'y' descent occurs in ventricular diastole as the tricuspid valve opens.

See 📖 p175 for conditions that cause changes to the normal waveform.

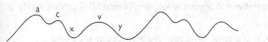

Fig. 5.4 The normal pressure waveform.

Complications

Immediate

Damage to nearby structures (carotid artery puncture, pneumothorax, hemothorax, chylothorax, brachial plexus injury, arrhythmias) air embolism, loss of guidewire into right side of heart.

Late

Sepsis, thromboembolism, AV fistula formation.

Common problems

Poor trace

This may be caused by arrhythmias. Check the EKG. A damped waveform can be caused by excessive lengths of compliant connection tubing, three-way taps, air bubbles, and blood clots. Check that all the three-way taps between patient and transducer are open, that the tubing is not *kinked*, and that no infusions are running into the central line. Check that the central line is still secured in its original place and that you can freely aspirate and flush all ports. Try the pressure transducer on a different port. If there is any suspicion that the central line is *misplaced* (central lines can migrate rostrally, and into the axillary vein) a CXR will confirm placement.

CVP too low

Hypovolemia, peripheral vasodilation, transducer too high.

CVP too high

LV and/or RV failure, cardiac tamponade, fluid overload, TR, AV dyssynchrony, tension pneumothorax, rarely pulmonary embolus. Commonly patient Valsalva-ing or fighting the ventilator, transducer too low, or fluids running through the central line.

Bleeding Apply direct pressure. Correct coagulopathy.

Sepsis Avoid by using good insertion technique. Remove catheter as described.

Insertion

Technique of insertion of internal jugular catheters is described on 📖 p244.

Removal

Central venous catheters are routinely removed 24–48h following surgery if the patient is not requiring inotropic support, and has no rhythm disturbances requiring central infusions or transvenous pacing wires. The patient is placed flat on the bed, and the catheter removed with pressure applied locally for 1min to prevent hematoma formation. Routine change of central venous catheters for patients requiring them longer avoids infection. Most units do this at 7 days unless indicated before. Change by railroading a new catheter over a guidewire placed down the old catheter may be sufficient in the patient with a neutrophilia or pyrexia, with a clean site.

Pulmonary artery catheter

Key facts

- In many units most cardiac surgery patients have PA catheters.
- A right heart catheterization is a one-off set of measurements from a PA catheter.
- This is indicated in patients with hypoperfusion states refractory to 1st- and 2nd-line inotropic support, and should be placed after induction in patients likely to present problems in terms of inotrope and fluid management: patients with pulmonary hypertension, poor ventricular function, transplant and VAD patients, multivalve surgery, and in off-pump CABG to guide intraoperative management.
- Uses include:
  - Pressure monitoring: RAP, RVP, PAP, PAWP.
  - Flow monitoring: cardiac output.
  - Mixed venous oxygen saturations.
  - Derived parameters: SVR, SVRI, PVR, PVRI, LVSV, VO_2, DO_2.
  - RV ejection fraction and RVEDP.
  - Temporary atrial and ventricular pacing.
  - LVSWI and RVSWI less commonly used to guide management.

Contraindications

As for central venous catheters (📖 p174). Those specific to PA include:
- *Absolute*: tricuspid or pulmonic valve stenosis/mechanical prosthesis, RA and RV masses which may embolize, tetralogy of Fallot (the RVOT is hypersensitive: hypercyanotic episode may be induced by the catheter).
- *Relative*: severe arrhythmias, coagulopathy, new intracardiac pacemaker wires which may become dislodged before they have become embedded.

Waveform

(See Fig. 5.5.)
- There is a sudden increase in systolic pressure as the catheter enters the RV.
- As the catheter enters the PA the diastolic pressure increases.
- There is a decrease in mean pressure as the catheter enters the wedge position.
- The PA waveform should reappear if the balloon is deflated at this point.

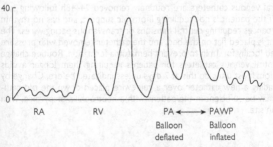

Fig. 5.5 Waveform progression during correct insertion of the PA catheter.

Catheter

Measurements may be continuous or based on intermittent bolus methods, depending on the calibration system. The catheter has four lumens:

• A proximal lumen 25cm from the tip which sits in the RA.
• A distal lumen connected to a pressure transducer sitting in the PA.
• A balloon lumen allowing balloon inflation.
• A thermistor lumen connecting to the gauge 4cm from the tip.

Complications

Complications are those of central venous cannulation (📖 p175) and those specific to PA catheters including: arrhythmias (complete heart block and VF), pulmonary artery rupture, and endobronchial hemorrhage, pulmonary infarction, knotting of catheter, valve damage, infection, thrombocytopenia, thrombus formation, balloon rupture, malplacement.

Common problems

Unable to get good trace

Check that the connection tubing to pressure transducer is free of air, kinks, clots, and closed taps. Flush and aspirate. Deflate balloon, withdraw the catheter and start again: no more than 15–25cm should pass before the waveform changes. If not, deflate balloon, withdraw and try again. Note the natural curve of the catheter, so that you know where the tip is pointing once it is inside the heart. If the catheter is failing to advance to the next chamber: (1) rotate the catheter slightly within the sheath, (2) retry with the patient in the left lateral position, (3) advance catheter slowly with balloon deflated.

Unable to wedge

The catheter is in an incorrect position. Deflate, withdraw, and try again.

Coiling and knotting

This can be avoided by not inserting excessive length: if the trace has not changed after 20cm of catheter deflate, withdraw and try again. If a loose knot is detected on CXR, insertion of a guidewire under fluoroscopy may unravel it. Alternatively, tighten the knot and withdraw the catheter with the balloon deflated, along with the introducer sheath.

Arrhythmias

Placing the patient slightly head up with right lateral tilt may help. Withdraw the catheter 1–2cm when arrhythmias occur, to terminate them.

Difficulty calibrating continual measurement systems

Common pitfalls include failure to enter the correct height and weight data, failure to provide a SvO_2 sample to calibrate, and LED not working. If basic measures don't help, change the box, leads, and catheter.

Insertion

Technique of insertion is described on 📖 p174.

Removal

PA catheters are removed as soon as practicable. The sheath may be left. The balloon **must** be deflated to avoid trauma to the tricuspid valve.

Mixed venous oxygen saturation

Key facts

- The *percentage saturation of mixed venous hemoglobin with* O_2 (SvO_2) or 'mixed venous', is sampled from blood in the pulmonary artery and reflects the balance between O_2 consumption and delivery.
- SvO_2 is dependent on cardiac output, hematocrit, oxygenation, and oxygen consumption.
- In normal physiologic states cardiac output can increase up to 6–10× to compensate for changes in the other three parameters, maintaining SvO_2 within a normal range: this is not true following cardiac surgery.

Measurement of SvO_2

- It can be measured continuously using an oximetric pulmonary artery catheter fitted with an instrument that operates on similar principles to a pulse oximeter (□ p156), or intermittently by withdrawing blood from the distal PA port and passing it through a standard blood gas analyzer.
- It is not adequate to sample SVC or RA blood, because the maximally deoxygenated blood from the coronary sinus will not be fully admixed, and SvO_2 will normally be overestimated. Peripheral venous blood sampling reflects the perfusion and oxygenation of peripheral tissue, and is not a good indicator of cardiac output.

Interpretation of SvO_2

From the equation (see Box 5.7) it is clear how an increased cardiac output can compensate for a low SaO_2, and how increased oxygen extraction can compensate for a low cardiac output.

- A low SvO_2 (<60%) indicates inadequate oxygen delivery. The lower the SvO_2, the more severe the deficit: SvO_2 <40% suggests a pre-terminal state.
- Cardiac output can increase by up to 6 times to compensate for low blood oxygen content, and oxygen extraction can increase by a similar amount to compensate for poor cardiac output: a low SvO_2 suggests that the limits of cardiac compensation have been reached.
- A normal SvO_2 (65–80%) does not always equate with adequate oxygen delivery: an overwedged PA catheter, regional hypoperfusion, left-to-right cardiac shunts, and carbon monoxide poisoning may all give falsely reassuring readings.
- A high SvO_2 (>90%) is most commonly caused by readings being taken from an overwedged PA catheter, but could also be caused by left-to-right shunt
- SvO_2 is a very dynamic measure of cardiac output, tissue perfusion and oxygenation: Fig. 5.6 shows the effects of simple clinical maneuvers on SvO_2.
- Oxygen consumption can easily increase 10-fold in shivering, septic or agitated patients, or in patients with seizures. In normal patients cardiac output can increase up to 10-fold to compensate. This is neither possible nor desirable in post-cardiac surgery patients: so oxygen extraction increases and SvO_2 falls.

- Always look at the SvO_2 in context—a low SvO_2 may indicate poor contractility, or respiratory compromise, hypovolemia, profound anemia, status epilepticus, or sepsis, etc. Similarly a normal SvO_2 does not always equate with a normal cardiac output.

High SvO_2
- Artifact:
  - Overwedged PA catheter.
  - Sampling from SVC, left-to-right shunt.
- Increased systemic O_2 delivery:
  - High FiO_2.
- Decreased systemic O_2 extraction:
  - Hypothermia.
  - Sepsis.
  - Pharmacological paralysis.

Low SvO_2
- Decreased systemic O_2 delivery:
  - Hypoxia, e.g. after suctioning.
  - Anemia.
  - Low cardiac output (hypovolemia, arrhythmias, poor contractility).
- Increased systemic O_2 extraction:
  - Hyperthermia.
  - Sepsis.
  - Shivering, seizures, agitation.

Examples	VO_2 (mL/min)	Hb (g/dL)	CO (L/min)	SaO_2 (%)	SvO_2 (%)
Shivering	1000	13	10	95	45
Anemia	250	6	5	95	36
Low CO	250	8	3	95	26
Hypoxia	250	7.5	5	90	43

Box 5.7 Calculation of SvO_2

$$SvO_2 = SaO_2 - [VO_2/(CO \times Hb \times 13.9)]$$

SvO_2 = mixed venous saturation	65–80%
SaO_2 = arterial saturation	95–100%
VO_2 = oxygen consumption	200–250mL/min
Hb = hemoglobin concentration	10–13g/dL
CO = cardiac output	4–6L/min

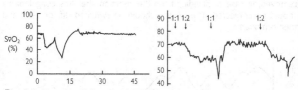

Fig. 5.6 Changes in SvO2 with (a) ET tube suctioning, (b) weaning an IABP.

Other forms of monitoring

Left atrial pressure

Key facts
- LA catheters are indicated where reduced LV compliances or pulmonary vascular disease, congestion, and edema mean that PAWP measurements are no longer a good approximation of LA pressures and LV preload.
- They are also indicated in corrective surgery for congenital lesions where PA placement is impossible.

Contraindications
Sepsis and coagulopathy are relative contraindications.

Insertion
Insertion is done intraoperatively via the right superior pulmonary vein, the root of the LA posterior to the SVC and aorta, or in infants via the LA appendage. The fine-bore catheter is usually passed anterior to the heart and out to the skin at the base of the median sternotomy incision in the same way as a temporary pacing wire.

Waveform
(See Fig. 5.7.)
- Normal LAP is 10–14mmHg.
- PAWP normally exceeds LAP by 2–3mmHg, and the difference increases in the first 12h post bypass, possibly due to pulmonary edema and the effects of ventilation.
- LA pressure does not reflect LVEDP in the presence of mitral disease.
- MR can be detected on the trace as increased 'v' waves, and an increase in the mean LAP. This may be a sign of ischemia, arrhythmias, or overfilling.

Problems
- These are similar to those described for central lines: transducer setting, damping. Particular care must be taken to keep air and clots excluded from the system, as even small amounts of systemic emboli could cause myocardial ischemia and stroke.

Removal
Normally the LA catheter should be removed within 48h, preferably before the patient is extubated and the mediastinal drains have been removed, in case of bleeding from the insertion site. Any coagulopathy should be corrected. The LA line should be switched off for 2–3h and then removed.

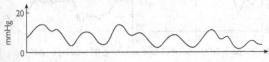

Fig. 5.7 Left atrial pressure waveform.

Doppler hemodynamic monitoring

Key facts

- Blood velocity can be measured by using the change in frequency of an ultrasonic beam as it reflects off a moving object, i.e., erythrocytes. This can be done using a small transesophageal US probe.
- To achieve accurate measurements of cardiac output, three conditions must be met:
  - The cross-sectional area of the aorta must be known.
  - The ultrasound beam must be parallel to the flow of blood.
  - The beam should be stable between measurements.
- Newer probes contain two transducers, one of which is an M-mode transducer which continuously measures the aortic diameter, while a second pulsed Doppler measures beat-to-beat flow. A continuous measure of cardiac output and derived parameters are displayed. The instruments indicate if positioning is poor.

Indications

Where a PA catheter cannot be floated, and cardiac output measurements and derived parameters are needed to guide inotropic therapy.

Contraindications

Esophageal rupture, esophageal varices, recent esophageal surgery.

Insertion

- Sedate the patient.
- Measure approximate insertion depth on the patient (the 3rd intercostals space anteriorly corresponds to T5/6).
- Insert probe facing the patient so that the probe is just beyond T6.
- Withdraw to obtain best signals.
- Rotate to gain Doppler signal of flow in the aorta, and image proximal and distal aortic walls.
- Validate the combined M-mode and Doppler signals.

Interpretation

Aortic diameter (which may be measured or calculated from patient nomograms) continual measurement of cardiac output, stroke volume, and systemic vascular resistance can be displayed. Aortic stroke volume is about 70% of total stroke volume. Maximal acceleration, normally $8–12m/s^2$, is the initial acceleration in blood flow before the effect of systemic vascular resistance comes into play. It is a sensitive indicator of left ventricular contractility. Maximal acceleration $<5m/s^2$ indicates very poor contractility.

Problems

The main problem with transesophageal Doppler is that measurements are positional, and in inexperienced hands they can be highly user dependent.

Cardiac function after surgery

Key facts

Pathophysiological changes postoperatively were summarized on ▢ p186. Changes in the cardiovascular system are reiterated here.

- **Myocardial compliance falls** because of myocardial edema: higher filling pressures are required to generate the same stroke volume.
- **Contractility is impaired** as a result of myocardial edema, metabolic derangements, myocardial stunning, and ischemia.
- **Myocardial function continues to decline for 6–8h** postoperatively as a result of ischemia-reperfusion injury, before returning to baseline.
- **Hypothermia** is common, predisposing to ventricular arrhythmias (VF is common at temperatures below 32°C), coagulopathy and metabolic acidosis, and also raising afterload increasing myocardial O_2 demand. Hypothermia does, however, provide neuroprotection.
- The high SVR helps, however, to maintain MAPs until the patient is rewarmed: it is vital to ensure that adequate volume replacement and if necessary inotropic support are given, to avoid **hypotension during rewarming**.
- Patients may **overshoot** to temperatures above 37.5°C because of abnormalities in central thermoregulation, resulting in pronounced peripheral vasodilatation and hypotension, and associated with a poorer neurological outcome.
- Vasodilatation and capillary leak mean that there is a **progressive requirement for volume** resuscitation to achieve satisfactory filling pressures which must be balanced against volume overloading the patient which has a particularly deleterious effect on respiratory function.
- Electrolyte and acid–base disturbances and myocardial irritability mean that **arrhythmias** are common: a third of patients will have AF postoperatively.

Low cardiac output

The aim of cardiovascular management postoperatively is to achieve a satisfactory cardiac output. If cardiac output measurements are available (PA catheter or transesophageal Doppler) a cardiac index of >2.5L/min/m² is satisfactory. In the absence of cardiac output measurements a MAP of 70–80mmHg, with a urine output of 1mL/kg/h, base deficit of <2, skin temperature of 36.5–37.5°C, and palpable pedal pulses (if these were present preoperatively) mean that cardiac index is most likely > 2.5L/min/m².

Causes of low cardiac output

The causes of low cardiac output and hypoperfusion states are summarized in Box 5.8. The etiology can be divided into:

- Preoperative.
- Operative.
- Postoperative causes, which can be further divided into pump failure (contractility, arrhythmias, mechanical), decreased preload, and increased afterload.

Box 5.8 Causes of low cardiac output

Preoperative
- *Previous MI* resulting in localized or global hypokinesia.
- Recent myocardial infarction resulting in global hypokinesia.
- Right or left ventricular systolic or diastolic dysfunction secondary to valvular heart disease or cardiomyopathy (📖 pp76–77).

Intraoperative
(Ask the surgeon and the anesthesiologist.)
- *Poor myocardial protection.*
- Incomplete revascularization.
- Kinking or occlusion of coronary artery (e.g. Cx during mitral).
- Air embolus down coronaries (usually resolves before transfer).
- Incomplete repair of valvular lesions.
- Hypotension before or after bypass.

Postoperative
(1) Pump failure
Decreased contractility:
- *Myocardial stunning,* poor myocardial protection.
- *Myocardial ischemia* due to coronary artery or conduit spasm.
- Hypoxia, hypercarbia, *acidosis,* hyperkalaemia.
- Drugs including propofol, amiodarone, β-blockers.

Arrhythmias:
- *Tachycardias* reducing filling time (sinus tachycardias, AF, VT).
- *Bradycardias.*
- *Loss of atrial 'kick'* (AF, flutter, junctional rhythms, CHB, VVI pacing).
- Ventricular arrhythmias (VT, VF).

Mechanical:
- Incomplete repair of valvular lesions, *SAM* (📖 p190).
- Ventricular rupture, atrioventricular dehiscence, aortic dissection.

(2) Decreased LV preload
- *Hypovolemia (hemorrhage, polyuria, inadequate fluid replacement)*
- *Vasodilatation (warming, sepsis, vasodilating drugs, e.g. NTG, milrinone, SNP, sedatives, narcotics, protamine, blood products).*
- *RV dysfunction, pulmonary hypertension.*
- *Cardiac tamponade,* tension pneumothorax.
- Sepsis, anaphylaxis, adrenal insufficiency, protamine reaction.

(3) Increased afterload
- Excessive vasoconstriction (hypothermia, vasoconstrictors).
- Fluid overload.
- Poor IABP timing.
- Valve obstruction, e.g., mechanical leaflet blockage.

More frequently seen problems in *italics.*

Managing low cardiac output

Management of common postoperative scenarios is described on 📖 pp128–129. Causes of low cardiac output are described on 📖 p183. The general management of low cardiac output is described here.

Key concept

Don't treat one number: look at the whole patient, and look at trends.

Signs of low cardiac output

Low cardiac output is a cardiac index <2.0L/min/m², but any of the following problems may be a sign of a low cardiac output state:

- Hypotension (MAPs <60mmHg).
- Tachycardia (heart rate >90bpm).
- Oliguria (urine output <1mL/kg/h).
- Metabolic acidosis (pH <7.4, lactate >3.0mL/L, base deficit >−2).
- Low mixed venous O₂ saturations (<65%).
- Pale or mottled, cold extremities.
- Pulmonary congestion and hypoxia.

Assessment of low cardiac output

Make sure you know the perioperative history: look for poor or hypertrophied LV, operation, difficulty weaning from bypass, coagulopathy risks

- Examine the patient: chest tube drainage, SaO₂, breath sounds, murmurs, peripheral perfusion, skin temperature, occult bleeding. agitation.
- Reassess hemodynamics: MAPs, CVP, PAWP, cardiac index, SVRI.
- Look at concentration of inotropes, pressors, sedation.
- Look at fluid balance: amount in vs. urine output, blood loss, etc.
- Look at EKG: heart rate and rhythm, ST segment changes.
- Look at blood gases: pH, PaCO₂, PaO₂, SVO₂, lactate, base deficit, blood glucose, hematocrit, potassium.
- CXR: pneumothorax, hemithorax.
- Echo: tamponade, LV and RV dysfunction, SAM (📖 p141).

Management of low cardiac output

Low cardiac output with low CVP (<14–16mmHg)

- Cardiac contractility is usually *not* the problem.
- Look for and treat the commonest causes which are *hypovolemia* (bleeding or polyuria) and *vasodilatation*.
- (1) Stop or reduce vasodilating infusions, e.g. NTG, milrinone, diltiazem.
- (2) Give 500mL of NS or colloid—one of three things will happen:
  - CVP and MAPs rise and cardiac index normalizes.
  - CVP rises dramatically with little improvement in MAPs or cardiac index: stop giving fluid and look for other problems (see 📖 p143).
  - CVP and MAPs rise transiently: watch CVP and repeat fluid bolus until hemodynamics are better, or you have given >2L fluid with low CVP in which case start a low dose of vasoconstrictor (e.g. norepinephrine 0.03 micrograms/kg/min), or you have high CVP (see 📖 p142).

Low cardiac output with high CVP (>18mmHg)

- This is more worrying as cardiac contractility is usually the problem.
- Look for and treat the commonest causes:
  - LV and/or RV dysfunction.
  - Arrhythmias.
  - Tamponade.
- (1) Correct respiratory or metabolic acidosis, electrolyte abnormalities, anemia and hypoxia (📖 p189). Inotropes are relatively ineffective at low pH, and the myocardium is much more prone to arrhythmias.
- (2) Check EKG for ischemia and treat aggressively (see 📖 p185).
- (3) Treat arrhythmias: if bradycardic pace at 80–90bpm: beware loss of atrial kick in hypertrophied LV (📖 p140) which may result in lower cardiac output, if AF aim to convert to sinus (📖 p218).
- (4) Treat poor contractility with inotrope (see 📖 p198 for choice), e.g., 0.03–0.05 micrograms/kg/min epinephrine, or 3–5 micrograms/kg/min dobutamine, or if high SVR consider milrinone 0.3–0.5 micrograms/kg/min.
- (5) *Escalating inotrope requirements mandate an echo to look for:*
  - Tamponade requiring re-exploration (📖 p144).
  - Severe LV or RV dysfunction requiring IABP (📖 p194) or NO (📖 p191).
  - Ongoing ischemia requiring intervention (📖 p185).
  - SAM requiring more volume and contraindicating inotropes (📖 p190).

Postoperative myocardial ischemia

Etiology

- Kinking of conduits that are too long or follow a tortuous path.
- Vasopasm of coronary arteries, or arterial conduits: increased α-adrenergic tone, adrenergic agents such as norepinephrine, air emboli.
- Thrombosis of grafts: hypercoagulable and low-flow states (such as peri-arrest) predispose to graft thrombosis.
- Endarterectomized vessels are prone to thrombosis.

Diagnosis

ST segment elevation, ventricular arrhythmias, heart block, and deteriorating cardiac output. The differential diagnosis includes the causes of low cardiac output states described on 📖 p183. TEE may demonstrate regional wall motion abnormalities.

Prevention

Good operative technique (everted anastomoses, exclusion of air from the coronary circulation, minimal handling of the conduits and coronary endothelium). Some units give all CABG patients NTG infusion (📖 p138).

Management

- Optimize oxygenation (📖 p189), preload, contractility and afterload (📖 p186).
- Start NTG infusion (200mg in 250mL 5% dextrose at 5mcg/min).
- Persistent ischemia with hemodynamic compromise is an indication for an IABP (📖 p194) if there is no surgical option (e.g., very poor or inaccessible targets) and the patient has no contraindications (📖 p194).
- Otherwise ischemia with hemodynamic instability mandates re-exploration in the first 12h if a surgical cause is suspected or cardiac catheterization if cause is unclear (>12h irreversible infarct).

Optimizing preload and afterload

Key facts

- The aim is to augment cardiac output while minimizing the work of the heart and hence myocardial oxygen demand.
- The most important determinant of myocardial oxygen demand is LV wall tension. The more pressure the LV is required to generate, the greater the myocardial oxygen demand. Wall tension is determined by preload and afterload. Optimizing these parameters, so that LV contraction occurs at smaller LV end-diastolic volume and against less resistance, reduces myocardial oxygen demand most effectively.

Preload

Optimizing preload so that the heart functions in the upper part of the Frank–Starling curve, before the plateau, increases contractility.

Definition of preload

- Preload is a measure of left ventricular end-diastolic fiber length, which is proportional to left ventricular end-diastolic volume (LVEDV) and pressure (LVEDP). It is determined by filling pressure, filling time, and ventricular compliance.
- In the clinical setting this is assessed indirectly by measuring *LAP*, *PAWP*, and *RAP* (LAP is closest and RAP least close to LVEDP).

- Optimize preload by giving *colloid* to increase it or *loop diuretics* to decrease it, aiming for an RAP of 12–16mmHg, a PAWP of 10–14mmHg.
- Patients with chronic MR, or LV hypertrophy (AS, MS, HOCM), require higher filling pressures, sometimes over 20mmHg.
- Trends are more important than absolute values.
- If filling pressures do not noticeably increase with filling, or increase and quickly fall back, then it is likely that the patient is still relatively hypovolemic, even if the absolute pressures are quite high.
- If filling pressures rapidly increase with volume and remain raised, with systemic pressures remaining the same or even decreasing, then the patient is overfilled, even if absolute filling pressures are relatively low.
- In patients with *poor ventricles* there may be very little margin between euvolemia and overfilling. Use small fluid challenges (<250mL colloid) and monitor filling and arterial BP closely.
- *Excessive preload* is deleterious for a number of reasons: it increases ventricular wall tension which exacerbates ischemia as MVO_2 is increased and myocardial perfusion is decreased, and it leads to pulmonary edema, splanchnic congestion, and potentially cerebral edema.
- Failure of filling pressures to rise with adequate volume may be due to *vasodilatation or capillary leak*: it is sometimes necessary to vasoconstrict a patient with a small amount of norepinephrine (4mg in 250mL 5% dextrose at a rate of 0.03–0.06 micrograms/kg/min) to achieve satisfactory preload (📖 pp200–201).

Afterload

The aim here is to optimize afterload. Reducing afterload reduces the work of the heart: the pressure work of the LV (wall tension) is the major determinant of myocardial oxygen demand.

- Care is required in *low cardiac output* states when using vasodilators to reduce afterload: a high SVR is sometimes the only mechanism by which BP, and hence coronary perfusion, is maintained when cardiac output is marginal.

Definition of afterload

- Afterload is a measure of LV wall tension during systole: it is determined by preload (see 📖 p130) and systemic vascular resistance (SVR).
- In the clinical setting SVR can be calculated from measurements of *cardiac output* and *BP* (📖 p131), or estimated from palpation of peripheral pulses and skin temperature.

- *Coronary perfusion pressure* is the difference between aortic diastolic pressure and coronary sinus or right atrial pressure: excessive reduction in afterload will contribute to myocardial ischemia by reducing aortic BP and hence coronary perfusion pressure.
- Afterload is raised in the *hypovolemic* patient because of reflex vasoconstriction. It may be possible to correct this with careful volume infusion often combined with inodilators, e.g., milrinone.
- *Hypothermia* is a common cause of raised SVR postoperatively. Warm the patient using warming blankets, and consider infusion warmers, particularly if large-volume transfusions are needed.
- A variety of *vasodilators can be used to lower SVR* (📖 p202): NTG (200mg in 250mL at a rate of 5mcg/min) is commonly used in most units as it has a beneficial effect on myocardial perfusion, in addition to its effect on the peripheral vasculature; SNP is a particularly potent vasodilator that has a less beneficial effect on myocardial perfusion than NTG and as such is reserved as a second-line adjunct in the control of hypertension (📖 p202).
- There are a number of *inotropes with vasodilatory properties* that reduce afterload: these are milrinone, dopexamine, and dobutamine in decreasing order of ability to reduce afterload and they should be considered in the context of low cardiac output.
- An increase in SVR (and hence afterload) may be the aim: patients with good cardiac outputs (CI >2.5) and poor systemic pressures as a result of *peripheral vasodilatation* are treated with vasoconstrictors such as norepinephrine (4mg in 50mL at a rate of 0.03–0.3 micrograms/kg/min).
- Beware of reducing afterload in patients with a *residual LVOT obstruction*, such as those with septal hypertrophy, or small aortic valve prostheses, as reducing SVR will lead to reduced diastolic pressures resulting in reduced coronary blood flow and myocardial ischemia.

Contractility

Key facts

- The ability to change contractility is unique to cardiac muscle: skeletal muscle cannot change intrinsic contractility.
- Several factors increase myocardial contractility (positive inotropes, e.g., endogenous catecholamines, β_1-adrenergic agents, Ca^{2+}) or decrease it (negative inotropes, e.g., β-blockers, acidosis, hypoxia).
- Although the official definition implies 'fixed preload and afterload', in the clinical setting contractility equates with force of contraction, and optimizing preload and afterload will help increase this.
- Force of contraction is maximal at the midpoint on the Frank–Starling curve which corresponds to a small but not empty LVEDV.

Definition of contractility

- Contractility is formally defined as a measure of the strength of myocardial contraction, at a given preload and afterload.
- It is assessed in the clinical setting by measuring ejection fraction, cardiac index, and LVSWI.
- MAPs and SVO_2 are very indirect measures of contractility.

Positive inotropic effect

Contractility can be increased through two mechanisms. There is a fast acting mechanism important in clinical practice, which involves an increase in Ca^{2+} uptake by myocytes. This can occur through increased stimulation of α_1- and β_1-adrenergic receptors, or via direct effects on electrolyte concentrations. The second process, less important in immediate postoperative care as it takes place over several weeks, results in upregulation of ATPase receptors, which has a similar effect on myocyte electrolyte concentration gradients. Positive inotropes include:

- Sympathetic nerve stimulation (both mechanisms).
- Epinephrine (α_1- and β_1-adrenergic agonist).
- Norepinephrine (very strong α_1 and weaker β_1-adrenergic agonist).
- Dopamine (weaker α_1- and β_1-adrenergic agonist, DA agonist).
- Dobutamine (very weak α_1- and stronger β_1-adrenergic agonist).
- Ephedrine (weak α_1- and β_1-adrenergic agonist).
- Metaraminol (strong α_1- and weak β_1-adrenergic agonist).
- Milrinone (increases Ca^{2+} influx by inhibiting inactivation cAMP).
- Calcium (increases Ca^{2+} influx).
- Digoxin (inhibits Na^+/K^+ ATPase to raise intracellular Ca^{2+}.

Negative inotropic effect

These work through mechanisms, including α_1- and β_1-adrenergic receptor blockade, reduction in uptake of Ca^{2+}, reduction in the speed of spread of the myocardial action potential, and reduction in energy dependent processes governing contraction. Negative inotropes include:

- Parasympathetic nerve stimulation.
- β-blockers and calcium channel blockers.

- Amiodarone.
- Acidosis.
- Hypoxia.
- Inflammatory cytokines.
- Electrolyte abnormalities including $\uparrow\uparrow K^+$, $\downarrow\downarrow K^+$, $\downarrow Mg^+$, $\downarrow Ca^{2+}$.

Optimizing contractility

- Treat hypoxia and hypercapnia (📖 pp160–161).
- Optimize myocardial perfusion (📖 p185).
- Tread acidosis and metabolic abnormalities (📖 pp170–171).
- Treat sepsis (📖 p284).
- Optimize preload and afterload (📖 pp186–187).
- Select inotropic support (📖 pp198–199).
- Mechanical support (📖 pp194, 496, 500) may be required.

Optimizing myocardial oxygen supply: demand

Optimizing preload, contractility and afterload (📖 p186, 📖 p188)
The more pressure the LV has to generate, the greater the MVO_2. Optimizing preload and afterload, so that LV contraction occurs at smaller LVEDV and against less resistance, reduces MVO_2 most effectively.

Peripheral vascular resistance
- Intense peripheral vasoconstriction due to hypothermia, hypovolemia, or α_1- agonists can maintain adequate MAPs despite low cardiac output. End-organ perfusion is compromised leading to mesenteric ischemia, ATN, and hepatic ischemia, which has a poor prognosis. Excessive afterload increases work for the heart, increasing MVO_2 and risk of ischemia.

Arrhythmias
- Poor myocardial function may be disguised by reflex tachycardia that compensates for small stroke volumes to maintain cardiac output. Tachycardia may be a sign of failing LV and exacerbates myocardial ischemia. Management of arrhythmias that cause low CO is described on 📖 pp216–221.

Intra-aortic balloon pump (📖 pp192–195)
An IABP (📖 p192) improves the ratio between myocardial oxygen supply and demand by reducing afterload and improving coronary perfusion.

Improving myocardial perfusion
Coronary perfusion pressure is equal to aortic diastolic pressure minus coronary sinus or right atrial pressure. Myocardial perfusion is also dependent on diastolic filling time.
- If diastolic pressures are low because the patient is profoundly vasodilated, rather than because of a low cardiac output state, start a norepinephrine infusion to raise diastolic pressure >55mmHg.
- If diastolic pressures are low because of low CO state, despite optimizing preload, afterload, and contractility, an IABP may eventually be necessary to treat myocardial ischemia.
- In both cases treat tachycardia aggressively to optimize diastolic filling time: the optimum heart rate postoperatively is 80–100bpm (📖 p222).

Vasoplegia, SAM, and RV failure

Vasoplegia

- Vasoplegia is profound vasodilatation causing hypotension refractory to high dose vasoconstrictors despite normal or high cardiac output.
- It complicates 10% of patients post cardiopulmonary bypass: risk factors include preoperative ACE inhibitors, β-blockers, critical preoperative states, sepsis, low EF, and inodilators such as milrinone.
- High-dose norepinephrine and Pitressin® may not adequately restore arterial pressure and can cause splanchnic, mesenteric, and peripheral malperfusion and ischemia, despite low overall SVR.
- *Methylene blue* (bolus 2mg/kg, infusion 0.6mg/kg/h) blocks cGMP-mediated vasodilatation leading to rapid restoration of vascular tone.

Systolic anterior motion

- SAM is abnormal motion of the anterior leaflet of the mitral valve into the LVOT during systole (Fig. 5.8) resulting in:
  - Anterior displacement of leaflet coaptation.
  - LVOT obstruction (gradients can reach 80mmHg).
  - Mitral regurgitation (posteriorly directed jet).
- It is usually due to excess mitral leaflet tissue compared to the size of the mitral annulus, and the LVOT—*inotropes, tachycardia, and hypovolemia make this problem worse!*

Risk factors

- SAM occurs in hypertrophic obstructive cardiomyopathy.
- It is encountered on ICU as a complication of about 5–10% of mitral valve repairs where it is usually confined to patients with degenerative disease and excessive redundancy of the anterior and/or posterior leaflets, usually with an undersized rigid ring. It is not a feature of:
  - Ischemic mitral repair (where leaflet tissue is deficient and tethered).
  - Mitral valve replacement (where the anterior leaflet is resected).
- SAM may occur more commonly with a rigid annuloplasty ring, possibly as a result of reduction of the anteroposterior annulus diameter, but it does also occur with flexible rings, and in repairs without rings.

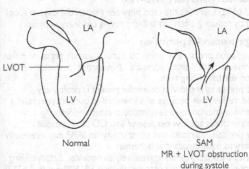

Normal   SAM
                          MR + LVOT obstruction
                          during systole

Fig. 5.8 Longitudinal section across the mitral and aortic valve and left ventricle, showing abnormal systolic anterior motion of the mitral valve.

- Small (underfilled), hyperdynamic (inotropes), hypertrophic, tachycardic left ventricle exacerbate the problem.

Assessment and management

- Hemodynamic compromise (high CVP, high PAWP, low cardiac output, poor MAPs) and a pansystolic murmur after degenerative mitral repair should raise the suspicion of SAM, particularly if a tendency towards SAM was noted on the post-CPB TEE.
- Assess the LVOT gradient, and degree of MR by TEE.
- Treatment consists of careful volume loading, reducing inotropic agents, and increasing afterload, under TEE guidance
- Mild to moderate SAM is treated conservatively: it normally resolves.
- In severe LVOT obstruction, removal of the annuloplasty ring and/or placing neochordae to move coaptation posteriorly improves SAM.
- Aggressive quadrangular resection and sliding leaflet plasty removes redundant posterior leaflet tissue so that the line of coaptation is well away from the LVOT: these are used in conjunction with accurately sized rings (📖 p411) to avoid SAM in high-risk cases.

Right ventricular failure

Risk factors

- Preoperative severe RV dysfunction (look for preoperative markers such as RV dilation, severe TR, congestive liver dysfunction).
- Poor myocardial protection, very long cross-clamp time, injury to right coronary button during root surgery even in non-dominant RCA, air.

Assessment and management

- Hemodynamic compromise (high CVP, RVEDP equalizing with CVP suggesting no RV pressure augment) with low to normal PAWPs and low cardiac output because of inadequate LV filling, often arrhythmias.
- *This picture is similar to tamponade: get an echo to make diagnosis.*
- This will usually respond to a similar approach to poor LV function but with some important differences, that reflect the fact that systemic perfusion pressure has a greater role in RV perfusion, the RV is much more sensitive to over-filling, and pulmonary vascular resistance:
  1 Correct respiratory or metabolic acidosis, electrolyte abnormalities, anemia and hypoxia (📖 p189). Inotropes are ineffective at low pH, and the myocardium is much more prone to arrhythmias.
  2 Check EKG for ischemia and treat aggressively (see 📖 p185).
  3 Treat arrhythmias: if bradycardic pace at 80–90bpm: if AF aim to convert to sinus (📖 p218).
  4 Start inotrope, e.g. 0.05–0.1mcg/kg/min epinephrine, ± norepinephrine or Pitressin® aiming for MAPs >80–90mmHg.
  5 Do not fluid overload: if CVP >25mmHg consider diuresing patient, or placing bed in reverse Trendelenburg position.
  6 Minimize PVR: inhaled NO or epoprostenol for intubated patients run less risk of dropping MAPs than inodilators, e.g., milrinone
  7 IABP will improve coronary perfusion and help failing RV, although in extreme circumstances a temporary RVAD may be needed (📖 p496).
- The occasional patient with SAM and RV dysfunction is a challenge as the treatments are completely opposite: a definitive surgical solution, and inhaled NO (📖 p203) are the mainstays of treatment.

IABP insertion

Key facts

- The IABP is a long polyethylene balloon filled with helium, 2–50mL in size, that sits in the descending aorta just distal to the left subclavian artery (see Fig. 5.9a, p194).
- The balloon inflates in early diastole improving coronary perfusion, and deflates just before systole reducing afterload.
- The MVO_2 supply:demand ratio, and cardiac output are improved.

Indications

- Preoperatively: cardiogenic shock, myocardial ischemia or for high-risk coronary angiography, e.g., pinhole left main stem with angina.
- Intraoperatively to assist weaning from bypass if very poor LV or RV.
- Postoperative poor cardiac output refractory to inotropic support, or myocardial ischemia without surgical or interventional solution.

Contraindications

- ≥2+ AI (balloon inflation during diastole will worsen AI).
- Aortic dissection (may worsen dissection or cause free rupture).
- Severe peripheral vascular and aortic atherosclerosis.

Insertion

The IABP is usually inserted percutaneously with a Seldinger technique. In addition to the IABP pack and the balloon pump console, you will require four large sterile drapes, prep, sterile gown and gloves, hand-held suture, 11 blade, and 10mL of 1% lidocaine if the patient is awake.

- Locate the femoral artery pulse (mid-inguinal ligament).
- Prep and drape. Check that the wire runs smoothly through the wire holder. Draw back firmly on the 60mL syringe connected to the IABP to ensure that the balloon is collapsed, remove the IABP firmly from its packaging, and withdraw the wire from the sidearm.
- Advance the large pink needle from the IABP set on a 10mL syringe, at 45° into the femoral artery until you can easily aspirate arterial blood.
- Remove the syringe, insert and advance the guidewire which should advance without resistance. Withdraw 2cm if ectopics appear.
- Nick the skin over the wire with the 11 blade and advance the smallest of the three dilators provided with the set over the wire and into the femoral artery: you only need the largest dilator if using IABP sheath.
- Leave the dilator *in situ*, and measure IABP so that the tip is at the 3rd rib space, advancing the proximal end of the plastic guard to the groin.
- There is usually a wire inside the IABP that needs to be completely removed first before the IABP will pass over the femoral guidewire.
- Withdraw the dilator, press firmly over the guidewire to prevent bleeding and insert the IABP over the wire and into femoral artery, up to the proximal guard, keeping tension on the end of the guidewire.
- Remove the guidewire.
- Now quickly take the manometry line, flush it and connect with a three-way tap to the IABP, aspirate blood and when the system is free of air, open it to the IABP console: an arterial trace should be visible.

- If this is not done rapidly the manometry lumen may clot off (the manometry lumen is very small to minimize impact on the flow of helium) and a new IABP will need to be inserted.
  - Newer models transduce pressures without a manometry line.
- Next remove the yellow internal marker and attach the port in the pack to the side arm and hand out to the balloon console.
- In an emergency the IABP can be operated at once, using the augmentation trace to decide if positioning is adequate; a TEE is helpful to check positioning; otherwise a CXR should show the proximal tip of the IABP just distal to the left subclavian.

Alternative methods of insertion

- If the femoral artery is difficult to palpate, a cut-down is necessary (📖 p120). Using 5/0 Prolene place a small purse-string in the femoral artery, and insert needle through skin into artery under direct vision.
- Rarely peripheral vascular disease is so severe that femoral insertion is impossible. The IABP can be inserted retrogradely via the ascending aorta. Either a purse-string is created as for aortic cannulation, with short snares left *in situ*, for later removal, or the IABP inserted through a Dacron graft is anastomosed to the ascending aorta. If the graft is brought to the skin, the IABP can be removed without resternotomy.

Complications

Vascular: distal limb ischemia is the commonest complication, causing IABP removal in >10% of patients. Risk is reduced by not using a sheath for insertion as this occupies a large proportion of the femoral artery lumen. Vascular complications also result from aortic dissection, iliac artery rupture, hematoma, and embolization of atherosclerotic plaques, thrombus, and cholesterol microemboli. Renal ischemia may result if the balloon is too low. Regular assessment of distal pulses by palpation or Doppler is mandatory, as is heparinization. If the balloon is left on a 1:3 ratio for over an hour, or deflated, thrombus is likely to form on the balloon leading to embolic complications. If distal limb ischemia develops either remove or place the IABP in the contralateral artery without a sheath (or very rarely directly into the aorta).

Thrombocytopenia: the mechanical action of the IABP destroys circulating platelets, which may be further depleted by HIT. Check platelet counts daily and consider alternative anticoagulation and/or IABP removal if platelet counts fall below 60.

Sepsis: sepsis is rare but associated with a high mortality. Positive blood cultures require removal of the IABP.

Balloon rupture: if blood appears in the balloon tubing it is likely that the balloon has ruptured. In view of the risk of releasing helium into the systemic circulation, inflation should be discontinued immediately and the balloon removed. Place the patient in Trendelenburg to minimize cerebral air emboli. Helium is an inert gas that is quickly absorbed.

- *Other complications*: AV fistula, false aneurysm, and hematoma formation following removal may require surgical exploration and repair. If the patient flexes hip or sits up the IABP tip can migrate and perforate the aortic arch or occlude the left subclavian or left common carotid.

IABP management

IABP basics

- The IABP end-diastolic pressure (A) is lower than the patient's aortic end-diastolic pressure without the balloon pump (a) showing that balloon deflation is well timed: deflation offloads the LV (Fig. 5.9b).
- IABP diastolic augmentation (C) occurs at the dicrotic notch (c): it should be higher than the patient's diastolic pressure (c), is ideally higher than systolic pressure (b): it is the coronary perfusion pressure.
- Assisted systolic pressure (B) is lower than the patient's unassisted systolic pressure (b) because augmented end-diastolic pressure and afterload are reduced by the IABP (Fig. 5.9b, bottom panel).
- The improvement in cardiac output and myocardial oxygen supply: demand ratio is the key: systolic pressures are often higher with the IABP switched off but cardiac function may be worse.

Which pressure to go by? Use systolic not mean pressures. The patient monitor is usually used, but it does not distinguish between diastolic augmentation and systole (denoting the higher as systolic pressure). The IABP console can ('Aug' on the IABP console is the diastolic augmented pressure (C), console 'systolic' is unassisted systole (b)): but *always* check that the IABP transducer is correctly levelled if you are using that.

IABP timing

- IABP should inflate at beginning of diastole and deflate at the end of diastole: there are several triggering modes that can be used.
- *EKG:* EKG leads attached either to the patient or the bedside monitor are plugged into the IABP console. Inflation occurs at the peak of the T wave and deflation on or just before the R wave. Use bipolar cautery.
- *Pressure:* inflation occurs at the dicrotic notch and deflation just before the beginning of the aortic upstroke. Use this mode if interference from monopolar electrocautery, or a poor EKG, makes EKG timing ineffective.

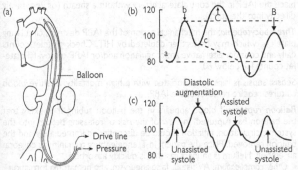

Fig. 5.9 (a) Correct IABP position just distal to left subclavian, and above renal arteries. (b) Top: 1:2 IABP augmentation trace, bottom: 1:3 IABP trace.

- *Pacing*: inflation occurs at the peak of the T wave, deflation occurs on the R wave as for EKG timing, but pacing spikes are filtered out so that that they are not misinterpreted as QRS complexes.

Common problems

Ineffective augmentation: (Fig. 5.10). Too short an augmentation time reduces coronary perfusion pressure. Too early inflation increases LV afterload, too late and coronary perfusion is suboptimal. Arrhythmias, rapid heart rates, and pacing spikes may cause ineffective augmentation or prevent balloon functioning altogether. Move the sliders on the console to obtain the optimal augmentation trace (Fig. 5.10). In older models rapid heart rates require augmentation to be dropped to 1:2.

Volume loss: this will be indicated by the console alarms and is caused by a gas leak in the system, or by incomplete unwrapping of the balloon. Check the connectors are secure. If the alarm persists there may be a gas leak from the balloon, in which case it should be replaced.

Weaning

Wean when pharmacological support has been reduced to moderate levels, and patient can tolerate lying flat. Inflation is reduced to 1:2 for 6h. *If no angina, ST segment changes, fall in urine output, increase in heart rate or PVCs, cardiac index maintained >2.0, SVO_2 >65, minimal rise in PAWP,* the ratio is decreased to 1:3. Heparin is stopped and coagulation checked. If platelets >90 and the APTT <50 the IABP may be removed. 1:3 mode should not last >1h because of the risk of thrombus.

Removal

Balloons inserted surgically should be removed surgically. Balloons inserted percutaneously may be removed with aseptic technique, by cutting the sutures fixing them to the skin. *Ensure IABP is deflated*.

- Press the assist-standby button on the console, and *check the trace again to ensure the balloon is not inflating*.
- With plenty of sterile gauze swabs available swiftly pull the IABP out in the direction of insertion and press firmly over the arteriotomy which is 1–2cm *proximal* to the skin insertion for 15–30min.
- Monitor the patient for the next 24h for hematoma formation and distal limb ischemia.

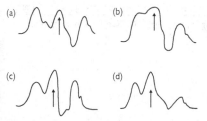

Fig. 5.10 Poor arterial IABP 1:2 augment traces: (a) Late inflation, (b) early inflation, (c) early deflation, (d) late deflation.

Pharmacological support

Calculating drug doses

Conversion to milligrams (mg) or micrograms (µg or mcg) per millilitre
- A drug labelled x% contains xg/dL. Multiply **x** by 10 to get the number of grams per litre, or the number of milligrams per millilitre.
- Concentrations stated as a ratio are converted to milligrams or micrograms per millilitre: 1:1000 = 1g/thousand mL = 1 milligram/mL; 1:1,000,000 = 1g/million mL = 1 microgram /mL.

Examples
- Lidocaine 2% contains 2g/dL, or 20g/L, or 20mg/mL.
- Epinephrine 1:10,000 = 1g/10,000mL = 0.1 mg/mL, or 100mcg/mL.

Calculating infusion rates
- First calculate the *desired dose* to be infused per minute by multiplying the patient's weight in kilograms by the dose in micrograms per kilogram per minute.
- Next calculate the *concentration* (micrograms/mL) of the drug in the syringe driver or infusion bag by multiplying the amount of the drug (micrograms) in the infusion unit by 1000 divided by the amount of diluent (mL).
- Finally calculate the *infusion rate* (mL/min) by dividing the desired dose rate (micrograms/min) by the concentration (micrograms/mL). Multiply this by 60 to get the infusion rate per hour (mL/h) (see Box 5.9 for an example). Common infusions are listed in Tables 5.1 and 5.2.

Box 5.9 Example infusion calculation
- A 70kg patient requires a norepinephrine infusion at 0.03 micrograms/kg/min. The syringe driver is prescribed at 4mg in 50 mL 5% Dextrose.
1) The *desired dose* is 70 × 0.03 = 2.1 micrograms/min
2) The *concentration* is 4 × (1000/50) = 4 x 20 = 80 micrograms/mL
3) The infusion rate = 2.1/80 = 0.026mL/min
or 0.026 x 60 = 1.5mL/h

Infusion rate = Wt (kg) **x** prescribed dose (micrograms/kg/min) **x** 60 (mL/h)

Drug in pump(mg) × (1000/diluent in pump (mL))

Table 5.1 Concentrations, rates, and starting doses for vasoactive drug infusions

Drug	Mg in 250 mL	Dilution (micrograms/mL)	Range (micrograms/kg/min)	Patient wt (kg)		
				50	70	100
Epinephrine	4	16	0.03–0.5	9.5	13	19
Dopamine	250	1000	3.0–10.0	9.0	12.6	18
Dobutamine	250	1000	3.0–10.0	9.0	12.6	18
Dopexamine	250	1000	3.0–10.0	9.0	12.6	18
Norepinephrine	4	16	0.03–0.3	9.5	13	19
Milrinone	40	160	0.3–0.9	9.0	13	18
Isoprenaline	25	100	0.01–0.3	0.5	0.7	1.0
Nitroglycerine	25	100	5–200 micrograms/min	1.5	1.5	1.5
SNP	50	200	0.1–10.0	8	11	16
Diltiazem	250	1000	5–10	5	5	5
Labetalol	250	1000	1–4mg/min	2	2	2
Pitressin® (vasopressin)	250 units	1 unit/mL	2.4–8 units/h	2.4	2.4	2.4

The numbers in Table 5.1 under patient weight heading show the drug infusion rate in mL/h required to achieve the stated starting dose. Not all drips are adjusted by patient weight.

Table 5.2 As regimes used at various institutions vary, this table is blank so that alternative infusion regimes can be entered

Drug	Concentration	Range

Inotropes

Inotropes increase inotropy (contractility)

- α-adrenergic receptor stimulation leads to ↑SVR and PVR.
- β$_1$-stimulation leads to increased contractility, heart rate, and conduction.
- β$_2$-stimulation causes peripheral dilatation and bronchodilation.
- DA stimulation causes coronary, renal, and mesenteric vasodilatation.

Epinephrine (adrenaline) 0.03–0.2 mcg/kg/min

Catecholamine produced by the adrenal medulla.

Action: Direct agonist at α-, β$_1$-, and β$_2$- receptors, increased glycogenolysis, lipolysis, gluconeogenesis—leads to increased blood glucose and lactate.

Pharmacodynamics: instant onset, half-life 2min. Metabolized by MAO.

Indications: (1) cardiac arrest (asystole, VF, EMD), (2) anaphylaxis, (3) low cardiac output states, (4) bronchospasm.

Clinical use: (1) *cardiac arrest:* high dose. 0.5–1mg bolus iv (5–10mL of 1:10 000); (2) *anaphylaxis:* low to moderate dose. 0.5–2mL of 1:10 000 bolus iv; (3) *low cardiac output* states: bolus 0.5–2mL of 1:10 000 iv (1mL of 1:10 000) then infusion 0.03–0.2 micrograms/kg/min; (4) *bronchospasm:* 5mL of 1:1000 epinephrine nebulized.

- Administration by central line: extravasation causes skin necrosis.
- Infusions require continual arterial line blood pressure monitoring.
- With high-dose epinephrine extreme hypertension, CVA or MI may result. *Reserve bolus administration for the peri-arrest patient.*
- Monitor SVR: a vasodilator may be required.
- Myocardial oxygen demand is increased.
- Ischemia due to vasoconstriction at high doses may occur: lactic acidosis is common at moderate doses, but this usually reflects enhanced glycogenolysis and inhibition of pyruvate dehydrogenase (📖 p65).
- Serum lactate and glucose rises, particularly in diabetic patients: low glucose suggests hepatic ischemia which is a poor prognostic sign.
- Epinephrine is an effective bronchodilator and stabilizes mast cells: it is useful in the treatment of anaphylaxis and bronchospasm.

Milrinone 0.3–0.9 micrograms/kg/min

Bipyridine derivative that inhibits phosphodiesterase.

Action: potent inotropic and vasodilator effects.

Pharmacodynamics: half-life is 4h. Metabolism is hepatic, with 30% excreted unchanged in the urine.

Indication: low cardiac output state in the setting of raised SVR and/or pulmonary hypertension. Avoid in patients at risk of vasoplegia (📖 p190).

Clinical use: optimize preload. Milrinone is commonly started together with a low dose of norepinephrine to partially offset its vasodilator effect.

- Administration by central line, monitor with arterial line.
- May cause thrombocytopenia.
- Milrinone increases cardiac output by increasing contractility and decreasing afterload, reducing myocardial oxygen demand.
- Less risk of arrhythmias than other inotropes.

Dobutamine 3–10 micrograms/kg/min

Synthetic catecholamine.

Action: direct β_1-agonist (inotropy), small β_2 effect ($\downarrow$SVR) with minimal α- or DA receptor action. Metabolite of dobutamine is an α-antagonist.

Pharmacodynamics: half-life is 2min. Hepatic metabolism.

Indication: low cardiac output secondary to increased afterload.

Clinical use: as for dopamine. Reduce vasodilator infusions, as dobutamine acts like a combination of an inotrope and a vasodilator.

• Administration by central line, monitor with arterial line.
• Improvement in urine output and splanchnic perfusion secondary to increased cardiac output and splanchnic vasodilatation.
• Reduction in afterload reduces myocardial oxygen demand.
• Dose dependent and reflex tachycardia.

Dopamine 3–10 micrograms/kg/min

A catecholamine precursor to norepinephrine and epinephrine.

Action: α, β_1, β_2 and DA_1 agonist, and release of stored neuronal NA. At the low to middle of the dose range β and DA effects ($\uparrow$HR, contractility, $\downarrow$SVR at low doses) predominate. Above 10 micrograms/kg/min α effects predominate (increased SVR, PVR, arrhythmias).

Pharmacodynamics: fast onset, slow offset. Metabolized by MAO.

Indication: (1) low cardiac output states; (2) renal insufficiency.

Clinical use: Optimize preload, commence dopamine at 3 micrograms/kg/min and titrate upwards depending on BP/cardiac output. If no improvement at high doses reassess with a view to a second inotrope.

• Mixed α, β_1, β_2, and DA_1, seen by some as a disadvantage.
• Administration by central line: extravasation causes skin necrosis.
• Improvement in urine output is secondary to increased cardiac output rather than any direct effect on renal vasculature.
• Tachycardia and arrhythmias may occur.
• Systemic vasodilatation occurs at low doses.
• Pulmonary vasoconstriction may occur.
• Dopamine can reduce respiratory drive.

Dopexamine 3–10 micrograms/kg/min

A synthetic analogue of dobutamine with primary vasodilator action.

Action: potent DA_1, β_2 agonist ($\uparrow$CO, HR, and vasodilation). Little effect on α- and β_1-receptors. Inhibits norepinephrine uptake, potentiating norepinephrine effects.

Pharmacodynamics: half-life 6–10min. Hepatic metabolism.

Indication: low cardiac output secondary to increased afterload.

Clinical use: as for dopamine. Reduce vasodilator infusions, as dopexamine acts like a combination of an inotrope and a vasodilator.

• Administration by central line, monitor with arterial line.
• Improvement in urine output and splanchnic perfusion secondary to increased cardiac output and splanchnic vasodilatation.
• Reduction in afterload reduces myocardial oxygen demand.
• Dose dependent and reflex tachycardia, but less than dobutamine.

Pressors

Pressors cause vasoconstriction
- α_2- adrenergic stimulation increases SVR and PVR
- α_1- adrenergic stimulation ↑contractility without ↑HR.

Norepinephrine 0.03–0.3 micrograms/kg/min

Catecholamine produced by the adrenal medulla.

Action: direct α- agonist: potent vasoconstriction + β_1 effect = ↑BP.

Pharmacodynamics: immediate onset, half-life 2min. Metabolized by MAO.

Indication: hypotension because of low SVR in good to high CO states.

Clinical use: low-dose norepinephrine (0.03–0.06 micrograms/kg/min) is often started empirically in the well-filled patient with warm peripheries, where low BP and filling pressures are thought to be a result of profound vasodilation. Norepinephrine requirements may be very high (>1.0 microgram/kg/min) in severe sepsis.
- Administration by central line: extravasation causes skin necrosis.
- In hearts with borderline CO norepinephrine should be avoided or used in conjunction with another inotrope, for the reasons described.
- Norepinephrine increases afterload and contractility, resulting in increased myocardial oxygen demand.
- There is increased risk of vasopasm of arterial conduit resulting in ischemia, and rarely infarction.
- End-organ ischemia may result from the intense vasoconstriction.
- Norepinephrine is contraindicated in pregnancy.
- Great care must be taken in changing infusions in norepinephrine dependent patients as catastrophic falls in systemic pressures may in occur in the short time it takes to disconnect one pump and run a second infusion through.

Metaraminol (Aramine®) bolus 0.5–1.0mg iv

Potent synthetic sympathomimetic amine.

Action: direct α-agonist: potent vasoconstrictor + β_1 effect = ↑BP

Pharmacodynamics: metaraminol has a longer duration of action than norepinephrine. Immediate onset, half-life 4–5 min. Metabolized by MAO.

Indication: temporizing measure to treat hypotension.

Clinical use: boluses of metaraminol are sometimes given to improve blood pressure prior to institution of bypass or during patient transfer. If repeated boluses of metaraminol in the ICU achieve a good but not sustained response, an infusion of norepinephrine is indicated.
- Metaraminol increases afterload and contractility, resulting in increased myocardial oxygen demand.

Phenylephrine (40–180 micrograms/min)
Potent synthetic sympathomimetic amine.

Action: pure α-agonist: potent vasoconstrictor. Causes reflex decrease in heart rate. Tachyphylaxis (a rapid decrease in the response to the drug) may be seen after a few hours.

Pharmacodynamics: immediate onset, half-life 30–40min. Metabolized by MAO.

Indication: hypotension because of low SVR in good to high CO states.

Clinical use: low-dose phenylephrine may be started empirically in the well-filled patient with warm peripheries, where low BP and filling pressures are thought to be a result of profound vasodilation.
- Administration by central line: extravasation causes skin necrosis.
- In hearts with borderline CO phenylephrine should be avoided or used in conjunction with another inotrope, for the reasons described.
- Phenylephrine increases afterload and contractility, resulting in increased myocardial oxygen demand.
- There is increased risk of vasospasm of arterial conduit resulting in ischemia, and rarely infarction.

Vasopressin (Pitressin®) 2.4–8 units/h
Synthetic analogue of ADH.

Action: acts at V1 (arterial smooth muscle) receptors, not α-receptors. Also acts on V2 renal tubule receptors.

Pharmacodynamics: very rapid onset, half-life 10–20min. Metabolized in liver and kidneys.

Indication: hypotension because of low SVR in good to high CO states.

Clinical use: Vasopressin may be started empirically in the well-filled patient with warm peripheries, where low BP and filling pressures are thought to be a result of profound vasodilation. In patients with vasoplegia, addition of Vasopressin to norepinephrine or phenylephrine reduces the dose of catecholamines required to restore vascular tone, and may therefore avoid the adverse effects on end-organ perfusion associated with high dose catecholamine therapy.
- Administration by central line: extravasation causes skin necrosis.
- Vasopressin has no effect on adrenergic receptors: for the same improvement in systemic arterial pressure achieved by norepinephrine, there may be less adverse effects on splanchnic and renal perfusion.

Methylene Blue

Action: Blocks cGMP-mediated vasodilatation leading to rapid restoration of vascular tone in vasoplegic patients.

Pharmacodynamics: onset 5–10 minutes, half-life several hours. Renal excretion.

Clinical use: Bolus 2mg/kg, infusion 0.6mg/kg for 6–12 hours in patients with vasoplegia refractory to maximal pressor support.

Vasodilators

Nitroglycerin (NTG) 5–200 micrograms/min

Also known as glyceryl trinitrate (NTG), or trinitroglycerine.
Venodilator. Increases cGMP production.

Action: at low doses dilates veins reducing venous return to the heart, decreasing heart size and preload, stroke volume and cardiac output. This reduces myocardial oxygen demand. Dilates coronary vasculature reducing vasospasm, redistributing more flow to ischemic myocardium. This has an antiarrhythmic effect.

Pharmacodynamics: metabolized by liver and smooth muscle to nitrites. Half-life 1–3min.

Indications: (1) in many units NTG is started routinely as prophylaxis against myocardial ischemia and coronary spasm; (2) myocardial ischemia; (3) coronary and conduit vasospasm; (4) hypertension; (5) pulmonary hypertension.

Clinical use: NTG is routinely started at the lowest end of the range above and titrated against BP to maintain MAPs 70–75mmHg.

- Administration may be by peripheral line, sublingually, or topical NTG patches 5–15mg over 24h.
- NTG selectively reduces preload, except at high doses.
- NTG lowers PVR and is a useful adjunct in the treatment of pulmonary hypertension and right heart failure pre- and postoperatively.
- Nitrites, the metabolites of NTG, oxidize hemoglobin to methemoglobin: impaired oxygen transport characterized by elevated PaO_2 but poor SaO_2 may result if patients receive large doses of NTG over several days, or if renal and hepatic excretion is impaired.
- Tolerance can be avoided or treated by stopping NTG infusion for several hours.

Labetalol (1–4mg/min)

β-blocker with α-blocking properties and a vasodilatory effect.

Actions: like all β-blockers labetalol reduces BP by negative inotropic ad chronotropic effects. Contractility, stroke volume, cardiac output and heart rate are all reduced. SVR and diastolic pressure are largely unchanged. α-blocking effects prevent reflex vasoconstriction.

Pharmacodynamics: onset 3–5min, half-life 3h.

Indications: labetalol, like other β-blockers, should not be used in borderline or low cardiac output states to reduce heart rate. It is indicated for control of hypertension with satisfactory cardiac output, particularly hyperdynamic, hypertrophic, tachycardic hearts.

Clinical use: labetalol can be given as a bolus (0.25mg/kg/min iv over 2min with subsequent doses at 15min intervals) or as an infusion.

- AV conduction is slowed as β-blockers depress the AV node: complete heart block may be precipitated.

SNP (sodium nitroprusside) 0.3–10 micrograms/kg/min

Vasodilator. Converted to NO in vascular smooth muscle which increases cGMP production.

Action: venodilation reduces venous return to the heart, decreases heart size and preload, stroke volume, and cardiac output. Arterial vasodilation reduces afterload. Myocardial oxygen demands falls. At low doses the proportional decrease in preload is greater than the decrease in afterload. Reduces PVR.

Pharmacodynamics: half-life 1–2min. SNP reacts with hemoglobin to release highly toxic free cyanide ions (CN^-). Normally a hemoglobin molecule binds four cyanide ions to give cyanomethemoglobin which is non-toxic. Patients on high doses of SNP, or severe renal or hepatic dysfunction are at risk of cyanide and thiocyanate toxicity, where CN^- ions are no longer inactivated by binding with hemoglobin. CN^- inhibits cytochrome oxidase preventing mitochondrial oxidative phosphorylation, resulting in tissue hypoxia despite adequate PaO_2.

Indications: treatment of hypertension refractory to high-dose NTG.

Clinical use: infusions are started at the lower end of the dose range, with high dose NTG still running, and titrated against BP.

• Administration via a central line. Monitor BP with arterial catheter.
• Infusions should be tapered slowly to avoid rebound ↑SVR and PVR.
• Solution must be protected from light.
• *SNP toxicity:* tachyphylaxis, elevated mixed venous PO_2 (secondary to decreased cellular oxygen extraction), metabolic acidosis, fatigue, nausea, miosis, psychosis, hyper-reflexia, and seizures are signs of SNP toxicity. Discontinue SNP immediately. Ventilate with 100% oxygen. Treat with either sodium thiosulphate 12.5g iv slow bolus (mild or chronic SNP toxicity), or sodium nitrite (300mg iv slow push) and amyl nitrite (severe SNP toxicity).

Nitric oxide 0.05–50 parts per million

Naturally produced from L-arginine in endothelial cells: ↑cGMP in cells.

Actions: venodilation. Administration by inhalation results in selective pulmonary vasodilation and improvement in VQ mismatch, as it vasodilates areas of lung that are well ventilated. It is rapidly inactivated once it crosses the alveolar membrane, systemic effects are minimal.

Pharmacodynamics: half-life in blood 6s.

Indications: severe pulmonary hypertension, RV failure.

Clinical use: dilute NO is blended into the ventilator inlet gas. The lowest effective concentration should be utilized and responses monitored with a PA catheter 40ppm is maximal dose. Wean slowly.

• NO is not injected between the ventilator and the patient to avoid formation of toxic NO_2.

Epoprostenol (Flolan®) 3–50 ng/kg/min

• Synthetic analogue of prostaglandin (vasodilator, antithrombotic).
• *Actions:* administration by inhalation results in selective pulmonary vasodilation and improvement in VQ mismatch, as it vasodilates areas of lung that are well ventilated. It is rapidly inactivated once it crosses the alveolar membrane, systemic effects are minimal.
• *Pharmacodynamics:* half-life 20min: rebound hypertension.
• *Indications:* severe pulmonary hypertension, RV failure.
• *Clinical use:* nebulized into the ventilator inlet gas.

Antiarrhythmics

Potassium chloride (10–40mmol)

The myocardial cell membrane is highly permeable to potassium. The high concentration of potassium ions inside myocardial cells (140mmol/L) compared to low concentrations in extracellular fluid (4mmol/L) makes up the bulk of the resting cell membrane potential (📖 pp56–57).

Action: hyperkalemia (📖 p271) decreases the resting membrane potential and the intensity of the action potential. At high concentrations (>6.0mmol/L) this results in AV block, and reduction in the force of contraction. At concentrations >10mmol/L the heart arrests in diastole. Hypokalemia (📖 p270) increases the resting membrane potential resulting in increased excitability and arrhythmias such as atrial fibrillation.

Pharmacodynamics: 800mmol of K⁺ enters glomerular filtrate per day: most is reabsorbed in the proximal tubules and loops of Henle (📖 p69).

Indication: maintenance of serum K⁺ 4.5–5.0mmol/L postoperatively.

Clinical use: 10–20mmol in 50mL 5% dextrose can be administered by central line over 20min, or 40mmol in 1L 5% dextrose can be administered peripherally over 8h. **Never bolus:** can cause asystole
* Cardiac arrhythmias including asystole can result if infusion is too fast
* Respiratory and metabolic alkalosis exacerbate hypokalemia.
* Potassium should be administered cautiously in patients with renal impairment as hyperkalemia can quickly result.

Magnesium sulfate (1–2g)

The normal serum Mg²⁺ is 1.0mmol/L. Magnesium promotes cardiac electrical stability by affecting ion transport across membranes (📖 pp56–57).

Action: arrhythmias associated with magnesium depletion can be minimized with magnesium replacement.

Pharmacodynamics: renal excretion

Indication: Mg²⁺ may be given empirically to treat arrhythmias in cardiac surgical patients who are normally Mg²⁺ depleted.

Clinical Use: 1–2g magnesium sulfate in 50mL 5% dextrose may be given via central line over 20min, 1–2g MgCl may be given orally.
* <1% of total body magnesium is in the serum: intracellular levels do not correlate well with serum magnesium.

Calcium chloride (250–1000mg iv)

Calcium is an inorganic substance physiologically active only as Ca²⁺

Action: calcium plays an important role in excitation–contraction coupling. It is a positive inotrope and reverses myocardial depression.

Pharmacodynamics: calcium is incorporated into bone and binds to protein, heparin, and citrate.

Indication: hypocalcemia, hyperkalemia, massive blood transfusion (📖 p149), decreased myocardial contractility from calcium channel blockers, protamine, and peri-arrest.

Clinical use: calcium chloride should be given through a central line: peripheral administration can cause sclerosis of veins.
* Can cause severe bradycardia or complete heart block.

Amiodarone (150–300mg bolus iv)

Amiodarone is an iodinated benzofuran.

Action: increases the refractory period of all cardiac tissues: atria, ventricles, and conducting system. It reduces sinus node automaticity. It is a non-competitive α- and β-antagonist, with a vasodilatory action.

Pharmacodynamics: half-life is 20–100 days. Elimination is by hepatic metabolism. High lipid solubility results in tissue accumulation.

Indication: AF, ventricular and supraventricular tachycardia.

Clinical use: loading iv: 300mg in 50mL 5% dextrose over 1h followed by 900mg in 250mL 5% dextrose over 23h, then reducing dose of 600mg per 24h for 1 week, then 400mg per 24h for 1 week. Loading orally: 400mg tid for 24h, then 200mg tid for 1 week, then 200mg bid for 1 week. Maintenance dose is 200mg per 24h. Amiodarone should be discontinued after 4–6 weeks if the patient reverts to sinus rhythm to reduce the risk of toxicity.

- Arrhythmias including torsades, and hypotension can occur.
- Amiodarone is a negative inotrope: avoid in patients with poor LV.
- Amiodarone can cause hepatitis, pulmonary fibrosis, hypothyroidism or hyperthyroidism, neurologic and gastrointestinal problems. Liver, respiratory, and thyroid function should be monitored regularly.
- Amiodarone potentiates warfarin, digoxin, and diltiazem.

Digoxin (maintenance 62.5–250 micrograms od)

A glycoside derived from the foxglove plant.

Action: digoxin increases intracellular calcium by inhibiting Na^+, K^+- ATPase. Increased Ca^{2+} release from the sarcoplasmic reticulum resulting in increased force of contraction. Ventricular automaticity is increased, but atrioventricular conduction is decreased.

Pharmacodynamics: onset 30 min. Half-life 1.7 days. Renal excretion.

Indication: fast AF and supraventricular tachycardias.

Clinical use: adult loading dose is up to 1250 micrograms over 24h in iv increments of 125–250 micrograms. Maintenance dose is titrated by serum levels: 1–2.0nmol/L 6–8h post dose.

- Digoxin will slow the rate of these arrhythmias, not achieve cardioversion: its inotropic effect is particularly beneficial in poor LV.
- Digoxin toxicity results in arrhythmias including fast AF, VT, and VF, AV block, and GI and CNS symptoms.
- *Digoxin toxicity* is exacerbated by $\downarrow Mg^{2+}$, $\uparrow Ca^{2+}$, and $\downarrow K^+$, alkalosis and acidosis, renal failure and hypothyroidism, all of which can result in toxicity despite low serum digoxin levels. Treat by correcting electrolytes. Digibind® 1 vial (38mg) in 4mL water iv is an antidote.

Lidocaine (1mg/kg iv bolus)

Tertiary amine local anesthetic that blocks Na^+ channels.

Action: activity localized to ventricles decreasing automaticity. Lidocaine can convert ventricular escape rhythm to asystole.

Pharmacodynamics: duration 15–30min. Hepatic metabolism.

Indication: ventricular arrhythmias. Lidocaine has *no* atrial action.

Clinical use: overdose results in confusion and seizures, respiratory depression, and sedation, but very safe drug within therapeutic range.

Chronotropes

Chronotropes increase heart rate

- Pacing is a quicker, more easily reversible option than drug boluses and infusions for raising heart rate in most patients.
- β_1 stimulation leads to ↑contractility, heart rate, and conduction.
- *Muscarinic cholinergic* activity is predominantly parasympathetic.

Atropine (0.3–1mg iv bolus)

Atropine is a belladonna alkaloid.

Action: a competitive antagonist at muscarinic cholinergic receptors, reducing parasympathetic tone to 'reveal' underlying sympathetic tone.

Pharmacodynamics: almost instant onset. When given iv offset is 15–20min. When given im, sc, or po offset 4h. Renal elimination.

Indication: bradyarrhythmias, reduction of oral secretions.

Clinical use: normally given as in iv bolus, starting with 0.3 micrograms iv, repeated up to 1.0mg as necessary.

- Atropine can also be given im, sc, po, and via the ET tube.
- Low doses (<0.2 micrograms) can exacerbate bradycardia.
- Antimuscarinic cholinergic side effects include urinary retention, sedation and confusion.

Isoprenaline (0.01–0.3 micrograms/kg/min)

Synthetic catecholamine

Action: direct β_1 (↑contractility, conductivity, and heart rate) and β_2↑ (vasodilation and bronchodilation) effect. No α activity.

Pharmacodynamics: plasma half-life 2min. Hepatic metabolism by MAO, 40% conjugated, 60% excreted unchanged.

Indication: bradycardia unresponsive to atropine resulting in low cardiac output states (📖 p221), AV block and β-blocker overdose. Indications pretty limited as usually AV pacing or low-dose epinephrine can achieve similar results without associated vasodilatation.

Clinical use: give 2mg isoprenaline in 250mL 5% dextrose, at a rate of 0.02–0.3 micrograms/kg/h).

- Isoprenaline can be safely given through a peripheral line.
- Cardiac output is increased as a result of increased heart rate, contractility, and reduced afterload.
- An infusion gives a sustained improvement in heart rate that may not be achieved with atropine boluses.
- Peripheral vasodilation may result in hypotension: the combination of tachycardia, decreased diastolic time, increased contractility, and hypotension can precipitate myocardial ischemia because of the mismatch in myocardial oxygen supply and demand.

- Arrhythmias may be precipitated by the increased conductivity.
- Profound coronary vasodilation can theoretically result in diversion of myocardial blood flow from ischemic myocardium.

Inotropes with a chronotropic effect

The following inotropes also tend to result in an increase in heart rate, either as a result of β_1 effects, or as a result of reflex tachycardia associated with vasodilation:

- Epinephrine.
- Dopamine.
- Dopexamine.
- Dobutamine.

Diuretics

Key facts

- Diuretics cause net loss of sodium and water from the body by action on the kidney: their primary effect is to decrease Na^+ and Cl^- reabsorption from the filtrate: increased water loss is secondary.
- Diuretics act by: (1) direct action on the cells of the nephron (loop, thiazide and K^+- sparing diuretics) or (2) modifying the content of the filtrate (osmotic diuretics).

Loop diuretics

Furosemide, bumetanide (both sulphonamides).

Action: loop diuretics block reabsorption of electrolytes from the loop of Henle, increasing excretion of water and Na^+, Cl^-, K^+, Ca^{2+}, and Mg^{2+}. As much as 25% of the glomerular filtrate may pass out of the nephron resulting in an intense diuresis. Bumetanide is 40–60x more potent than furosemide. Both caused a transient vasodilation and ↓CO.

Pharmacodynamics: given iv onset is 30min, orally onset is 4–6h.

Indication: volume overload, pulmonary edema, hyperkalemia.

Clinical use: boluses iv or po, (10–120mg), or iv infusion (1–25mg/h).

- Loop diuretics cause ↓K^+, metabolic alkalosis (as a result of loss of H^+ and K^+ ions), and rarely ototoxicity.
- Allergic reactions occur in patients sensitized to sulphonamides.
- Although loop diuretics are used to convert oliguric to polyuric renal failure *the temporary increase in urine output has no prognostic effect on the progression of acute tubular necrosis.* In hypovolemic states loop diuretics may exacerbate acute tubular necrosis by provoking a diuresis, worsening hypovolemia, cardiac output, and renal ischemia.

Thiazide diuretics (potassium-depleting diuretics)

Bendrofluazide, bendroflumethiazide, indapamide, metolazone

Action: these have a moderate diuretic effect. They inhibit reabsorption of Na^+ and Cl^- in the distal tubule. Potassium excretion is significant.

Pharmacodynamics: onset 1–2h, duration 12–24h. Excreted by glomerular filtration and tubular secretion.

Indication: cardiac failure and hypertension.

Clinical uses: bendrofluazide po 2.5–5mg od. Indapamide 2.5–5.0mg od.

- Thiazides compete with uric acid for excretion, raising serum urate.
- Hypersensitivity reactions include pancreatitis and pulmonary edema.

Potassium-sparing diuretics

Spironolactone (aldosterone antagonist), *amiloride.*

Action: spironolactone blocks the sodium-retaining and potassium-secreting action of aldosterone in the distal tubules. It also reduces hydrogen ion secretion. Amiloride acts directly on sodium channels, preventing sodium uptake in the distal tubule.

Pharmacodynamics: spironolactone half-life 10min, but active metabolite has a half-life of 16h. Amiloride has a half-life of 24h.

Indication: prevention of hypokalemia. Ascites, pleural and pericardial effusions caused by congestive cardiac failure. Nephrotic syndrome.

Clinical uses: spironolactone 25–50mg od. Amiloride 2.5–5mg od (sometimes in conjunction with furosemide as Frumil® 5/40 or 2.5/20).

Osmotic diuretics

Mannitol (polysaccharide).

Action: pharmacologically inert substance which is filtered in the glomerulus but not reabsorbed by the nephron. In the proximal tubule passive water reabsorption is limited by the presence of the non-reabsorbable solute within the tubule, as is Na^+ reabsorption. There is a large increase in the amount of water excreted with a proportionally much smaller increase in the amount of Na^+ excreted. Unlike the loop diuretics, mannitol retains its efficacy even in low glomerular filtration states. In acute renal failure due to hypovolemic states where the glomerular filtration rate is reduced, and absorption of water and Na^+ in the proximal tubule is almost complete, the distal nephron is at risk of irreversible damage. Mannitol protects against this by increasing the volume of filtrate passing through the distal tubules. Mannitol is also a free radical scavenger. Because proportionally much less Na^+ than water is excreted, mannitol is not useful in treating conditions associated with Na^+ retention.

Pharmacodynamics: rapid onset, short half-life.

Indications: Prevention of renal failure secondary to hypoperfusion or hemoglobinuria, and treatment of cerebral and pulmonary edema.

Clinical use: Initial dose 12.5g to a maximum of 0.5g/kg iv. 12.5g is routinely added to the pump prime in some centers to maintain a diuresis on bypass.

- Mannitol initially expands intravascular volume: this may exacerbate congestive cardiac failure.
- Mannitol causes hypotension if administered too rapidly.

When should diuretics be given for oliguria?

- When you are reasonably confident that pre-renal causes, e.g., hypovolemia, hypotension, low cardiac output and post-renal causes such as Foley catheter problems or obstruction are not the cause, *and*
- Positive fluid balance will be detrimental to the patient now or in the near future, e.g., patient with borderline lung function, severe LV or RV dysfunction, obvious fluid overload.
- There are some broad rules of thumb:
  - Almost all patients need diuresis once they leave ICU.
  - Most ICU patients will do fine whether you give fluid or diuretic for low urine output, and it isn't worth a protracted debate. *But:*
  - Oliguric patients with good hemodynamic indices on minimal pressors can safely be diuresed early if extubation is a priority.
  - Oliguric patients needing large doses of pressor to maintain MAPs most likely need fluid to avoid renal malperfusion, and careful assessment of the underlying problem (pp184–185).
  - Septic (p239) and vasoplegic (p190) patients have high fluid requirements, and diuresis is rarely indicated in the acute phase.
  - Patients with SAM (p190) or LV hypertrophy should be diuresed very, very cautiously: sometimes a little fluid overload is safer.

EKG monitoring

Indications

All cardiac surgical patients should have a 12-lead EKG preoperatively, and daily 12-lead EKGs postoperatively, as well as EKG monitoring intra-operatively and for 48h postoperatively. This facilitates:
• Diagnosis of ischemia.
• Diagnosis of arrhythmias and conduction defects.
• Diagnosis of electrolyte disturbances.

Contraindications

There are no contraindications to electrocardiography.

Techniques

The electrodes and EKGs are shown in Fig. 5.12.

3 electrode system: this system is used for continual monitoring, e.g., during surgery. It utilizes three electrodes, placed on the right arm, left arm, and left leg. The limb leads are placed on the back of the shoulders and hips to avoid interfering with the operative field. Many modifications of the system exist to aid diagnosis of arrhythmias and ischemia.

5-electrode system: five leads, four each on one extremity and one chest lead placed in the anterior axillary line in the 5th intercostals space gives additional sensitivity for diagnosis of ischemia.

12-electrode system: three extremity leads and six chest leads allow a 12-lead EKG to be produced (three augmented leads are produced by combining the extremity leads). This is the most sensitive diagnostic EKG. It is not used for monitoring.

Common problems

Poor trace: ensure good electrical contact. Skin should be hair and oil free. Change adhesive electrodes for fresh ones.

Wandering baseline: Check electrical contact, untwist cables, make sure that patient is lying still.

Interference causing fine oscillations of baseline: electrical interference is caused by poor insulation and filtering. Check cable insulation, replace cable if necessary. Skeletal muscle tremor including Parkinson's disease can also cause interference: ensure patient is warm and relaxed.

Basic EKG interpretation

This is described on p212.

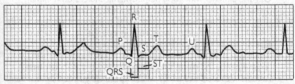

Fig. 5.11 Normal sinus rhythm.

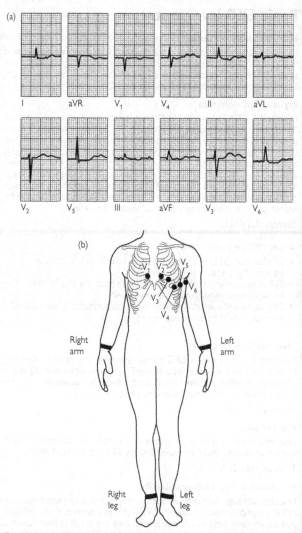

Fig. 5.12 (a) EKG readings and, (b) Electrode placement and 12 frontal plane axes for a 12-lead EKG.

Basic EKG interpretation

Normal sinus rhythm

Fig. 5.11, p210, shows normal sinus rhythm. Note the P wave, followed in 0.12–0.2s (3–5 small squares) by a QRS complex that lasts <0.12s (<3 squares), and which is followed by a T wave. The ST segment is flat and is at the isolectric point (the same level as the PQ segment).

Myocardial ischemia

Features: Fig. 5.13 shows an EKG trace typical of myocardial ischemia. Note how the ST segments are elevated. ST segment elevation in leads II, III and aVF reflects inferior ischemia (right coronary artery system), in leads V1–V6 reflects anterior ischemia (left anterior descending artery) and V4–6 suggests septal ischemia (posterior descending and circumflex arteries). New ST segment elevation as little as 1mm in these leads is significant and should be acted on (📖 p185). Note: ST segment is NOT well correlated with ischemia when conduction is abnormal as in left bundle branch block, complete heart block, or ventricular pacing.

Therapy: 📖 p185.

Acute MI or pericarditis?

- ST elevation (STE) in pericarditis is concave: in AMI it is flat or convex (Fig. 5.13a).
- STE in pericarditis is diffuse: in AMI it is in coronary distribution.
- PR depression in pericarditis, Q wave in AMI.
- T wave inversion only AFTER ST segments normalize in pericarditis, whereas in AMI it may coexist with STE.

Myocardial infarction

Features: Fig. 5.13 shows EKG traces typical of myocardial infarction. Note ST segment elevation followed by ST segment depression, Q waves (downwards deflection after the P wave rather than upwards) and later T wave inversion in the territories described.

Therapy: 📖 p185.

Pericarditis

Features: this is occasionally a feature of postoperative patients' EKGs at day 5 post surgery. Note concave upwards ST elevation in all leads.

Therapy: 📖 *p264.*

Hyperkalemia and hypokalemia

Features: although regular blood gas sampling should mean that hyperkalemia is never diagnosed as a result of EKG changes, patients in renal failure, and longer-term patients without arterial lines are at risk of hyperkalemia. Note the flattening of the P wave, tenting of the T wave, and widening of the QRS complex. The sine waveform heralds cardiac arrest. In hypokalemia U waves are a feature.

Therapy: 📖 pp270–271.

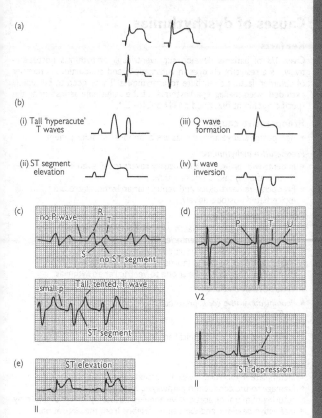

Fig. 5.13 (a) Possible morphology of ST segment elevation in acute MI. The commonest causes of ST segment elevation are not ischemia/infarction and ST segment elevation therefore has poor sensitivity for AMI but it's an important diagnosis to get right. Concave shapes are usually not AMI. (b) Temporal changes seen in acute MI. (c) EKG changes in hyperkalemia. (d) 'U' waves in hypokalemia. (e) Concave upwards ST segment elevation, characteristically seen in all leads in pericarditis (as opposed to coronary distribution specific ST segment elevation see in acute MI).

Causes of dysrhythmias

Key facts

Over 1/3 of patients develop supraventricular arrhythmias postoperatively, as a result of changes in automaticity and conduction. A number of common factors contribute to arrhythmias. These need to be rapidly excluded when managing arrhythmias at the same time as instituting the specific treatment described on 📖 pp216–231.

Preoperative causes

- *Age*: postoperative arrhythmias are commoner in older patients.

Preoperative arrhythmias:

- Patients with pre-existing AF usually revert to AF even if their initial rhythm after bypass is sinus rhythm.
- Preoperative heart block and ventricular arrhythmias are often exacerbated postoperatively.

Etiology of heart disease:

- Mitral valve disease associated with an *enlarged left atrium*.
- Patients with *dilated left ventricles* (ischemic cardiomyopathy, decompensated valvular heart disease).
- *Hypertrophic left ventricles* (aortic stenosis, hypertensive cardiomyopathy) are more prone to ventricular arrhythmias.

Intraoperative causes

- *Poor intraoperative cardioprotection.*
- Ineffective cooling.
- Inadequate cardioplegia.
- Incomplete electromechanical arrest.
- Ventricular distension.

Surgical procedure

- Incomplete myocardial revascularization.
- Damage to the conduction pathways during decalcification and suturing of mitral or aortic valve annulus, atriotomy, or ventriculotomy.
- Ineffective de-airing and exclusion of debris from the circulation.
- There is a 1–2% incidence of complete heart block requiring permanent pacemaker insertion after aortic valve replacement (📖 p263).

Postoperative causes

Cardiovascular

- Myocardial ischemia secondary to incomplete revascularization, coronary vasospasm, conduit kinking or occlusion, hypoxia, or high myocardial oxygen demand should be excluded as a cause of arrhythmias.
- Failure of valve repair or prosthesis.
- Hypovolemia.
- Pulmonary artery catheter (particularly if placed in RV).
- Less commonly, central venous catheter insertion.
- Intracardiac pacing wires.
- Endocarditis.
- Pericarditis.

Respiratory
- Hypoxia.
- Hypercapnia.
- Acidosis.
- Endotracheal tube irritation.
- Pneumothorax.
- Atelectasis.
- Pneumonia.

Electrolyte imbalance
- Hyperkalemia.
- Hypokalemia.
- Hypomagnesemia.
- Hypocalcemia.

Drug related (withdrawal/toxicity)
- β-blockers.
- Digoxin.
- Calcium channel blockers.
- Bronchodilators.
- Tricyclic antidepressants.
- Adrenergic and dopaminergic infusions are arrhythmogenic.
- Alcohol.

Metabolic
- Hyper- and hypothyroidism.
- Hypoglycemia.

Systemic
- Fever, hypothermia.
- Anxiety and pain predispose to tachyarrhythmias.
- Bradycardias are common when the patient is asleep.

Vagal stimulation
- NGT insertion.
- Gastric dilation.
- Intubation.
- Nausea and vomiting.

Mechanical
- Pericardial collections.
- Tamponade.
- Tension pneumothorax.
- Cold fluids injected into RA via central line.
- Chest contusion.

Lethal arrhythmias

Cardiac arrest in the monitored patient

- The ALS algorithms are on the inside front cover.
- Defibrillate VF or pulseless VT.
- Secure an airway.
- Hand ventilate with 100% oxygen at a rate of 10 breaths/min.
- Start external cardiac compressions at a rate of 100/min if defibrillation not possible or not indicated (EMD, asystole).
- Listen for bilateral breath sounds. Look for symmetrical expansion.
- Get iv access, check electrolytes, blood sugars, blood gases.
- Look for reversible causes: mechanical—cardiac tamponade, tension pneumothorax, massive PE, and metabolic—hypokalemia, hyperkalemia, acidosis, hypoxia, and hypovolemia and hypothermia.
- Give 10ml 1:10,000 epinephrine if no response

Ventricular fibrillation

Features: irregular, fine, sinusoidal trace (Fig. 5.14a). No cardiac output.

Therapy: immediate defibrillation. Do *not* delay defibrillation for *any* other procedures, e.g., intubation, cardiac massage, starting iv therapy.

- 3× shock 200J (biphasic, if monophasic defibrillator give up to 360J).
- Commence CPR.
- Give 1mg epinephrine iv (10mL of 1:10,000), repeat at 3min intervals.
- Repeat cycle.
- Give 1mg/kg lidocaine, correct acidosis and electrolytes.
- Emergency re-exploration is sometimes indicated for refractory VF in early postoperative period if surgical cause suspected (kinked conduit) or for institution CPB with a view to RVAD or LVAD support.

Pulseless ventricular tachycardia

Features: wide complex tachycardia (Fig. 5.14b). No cardiac output.

Therapy: treat as VF.

- Sometimes runs of VT are short and self-limiting. If recurrent these are best treated with lidocaine or amiodarone infusions, magnesium, and correction of acid–base and electrolyte abnormalities.
- Sustained and non-sustained VT may degenerate into VF.

Asystole

Features: flat EKG trace (Fig. 5.14c) or low amplitude fibrillation. No cardiac output.

Therapy: pace if possible (📖 p228). If not commence CPR immediately.

- If epicardial pacing wires are present pace immediately (📖 p228).
- Give atropine 1mg iv once, and epinephrine 1mg iv at 3min intervals
- Fine, low amplitude VF resembles asystole and may respond to electrical defibrillation: if in doubt defibrillate.
- An absolutely straight line suggests telemetry lead disconnection.
- Treat hyperkalemia (📖 p271) aggressively with 50mL 50% dextrose and 15 units insulin iv push.

Pulseless electrical activity (PEA)

Previously called electromechanical dissociation (EMD).
Features: no cardiac output despite EKG trace compatible with output.
Therapy: commence CPR immediately and try to pace if possible. Attempt pacing if epicardial wires are present.

Complete heart block

Features: wide complex < 35bpm (Fig. 5.14d) with no or poor cardiac output.
Therapy: pace if possible. Commence CPR if no cardiac output. Usually the patient will maintain some cardiac output and chest compressions are not necessary.

- If epicardial wires are present pace immediately (□ p228).
- If there is an adequate cardiac output do not commence chest compressions. Treat pharmacologically (see □ p206).
- If no cardiac output give atropine 1mg iv once, and epinephrine 1mg iv (10mL of 1:10,000) at 3min intervals until cardiac output restored.
- Transvenous pacing wires should be placed immediately if epicardial wires are not functional/present.

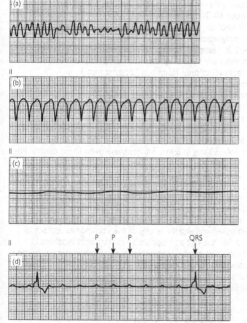

Fig. 5.14 Rhythm strips showing (a) VF, (b) VT, (c) asystole, (d) complete heart block.

Dangerous atrial arrhythmias

These arrhythmias are potentially dangerous in patients with: (1) borderline cardiac output, (2) stiff, non-compliant hypertrophic ventricles where reduced filling times lead to decreased stroke volumes, and (3) SAM (🔲 p190). *Loss of synchronized atrial contraction may reduce stroke volume by up to 30%.*

Atrial fibrillation and atrial flutter

Features: irregularly irregular usually narrow complex tachycardia. Atrial rate >380 in fibrillation, atrial rate <380 in flutter (Fig. 5.15).

Therapy: there are 2 options depending on the clinical status:

- *Synchronized DC cardioversion:* This is covered on 🔲 p224. It is indicated in two main groups of postoperative cardiac surgical patients:
  - Acute hemodynamic compromise
    The stable adequately anticoagulated patient (🔲 p262) who has not responded to appropriate arrhythmic and electrolyte management.
- *Pharmacological cardioversion:* This is indicated in hemodynamically stable postoperative patients.

Management of atrial fibrillation or flutter on ICU

- Correct hypokalemia: give 20mmol KCl in 50mL 5% dextrose via the central line over 10–20min, and repeat as necessary to obtain serum K^+ of 4.5–5.0mmol/L.
- Correct hypomagnesemia: give 1–2g $MgSO_4$ in 50mL 5% dextrose via the central line empirically if it has not already been given, as up to 60% of patients are hypomagnesemic postoperatively, and serum magnesium represents only 1% of total body stores.
- These two measures are usually sufficient to convert early AF.
- Correct hypoxia (🔲 p160) and acidosis (🔲 p170).
- Start weaning potentially arrhythmogenic infusions, e.g. isoprenaline.
- If the patient is hemodynamically compromised give 1 × 100J *synchronized DC cardioversion* (🔲 p224) increased by 50–100J increments to maximum of 360J in the anesthetized patient.
- Amiodarone 150–300mg in 50mL 5% dextrose over 1h via central line, followed by amiodarone 900mg in 250mL 5% dextrose over 23h via central line (🔲 p205) may achieve cardioversion in patients with good to moderate LV, and is first choice agent in most units.
- Digoxin 125 mcg in 50mL 5% dextrose over 20min via central line, repeated until rate control is achieved up to a maximum of 1250 micrograms in 24h, is preferable for rate control in patients with poor LV.
- Although β-blocker withdrawal is one of the commonest causes of postoperative AF, it is not appropriate to restart beta blockers in patients still requiring or very recently weaned from inotropic support.
- Overdrive pacing can work in atrial flutter (🔲 p230).
- Consider starting a therapeutic dose of low-molecular-weight heparin e.g. enoxaparin 1mg/kg sc bid in patients who have been in AF >24h, and who are not a bleeding risk (avoid heparin for the first few days after complex aortic surgery where normal coagulation is the cornerstone of maintaining hemostasis).

- The target INR for patients in chronic AF is 2.5–3.0, and warfarin should be commenced on the 2nd or 3rd postoperative evening for patients still in AF, with no bleeding problems.

Why treat atrial fibrillation and flutter?

These are not benign arrhythmias. In addition to the hemodynamic compromised described earlier:

- 15% of non-anticoagulated patients have intracardiac thrombus by TEE (usually in the LA appendage) within 48h of new AF.
- 30% of patients without an embolic event can be shown to have intracardiac thrombus within 72h of onset of AF.
- TTE has a much lower sensitivity than TEE for LA thrombus.
- 5% of non-anticoagulated patients undergoing DC cardioversion for AF will have an embolic event vs. 1% of anticoagulated patients.
- The rate of stroke in patients with AF under the age of 65 is approximately 1% per year, increasing to approximately 5% per year in patients over the age of 65.
- Although the natural history of AF following CABG is not well documented, non-anticoagulated patients with a history of angina or myocardial infarction have a 6–8% risk of stroke per annum.
- The risk of intracranial hemorrhage in anticoagulated patients is about 0.5% per year, increasing to about 1% in patients > 80 years.

Supraventricular tachycardia

Features: narrow complex regular tachycardia, rate 150–250bpm. It is sometimes difficult to distinguish between an SVT and atrial flutter.
Therapy: DC cardioversion as described for AF.

- Carotid sinus massage has been recommended to slow the ventricular response rate, because re-entrant rhythms involving the AV node may be interrupted in this way, and to aid diagnosis by revealing the atrial rhythm. Bear in mind that arteriopaths are at risk of cerebral emboli from carotid plaques dislodged in this way.
- Adenosine (3mg iv bolus increased by 3 mg increments and repeated at 2min intervals) produces a transient AV block. The half-life of adenosine is 10s which is sufficient to terminate a supraventricular tachycardia but will result in up to 10s of complete heart block.
- Calcium channel blockers (diltiazem 0.25mg/kg iv over 2min repeated 15min later) convert 90% of patients to sinus rhythm.
- Digoxin helps gain rate control in refractory SVT.

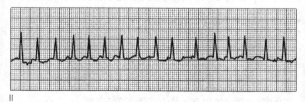

II

Fig. 5.15 Rhythm strip featuring atrial fibrillation: not the irregularly irregular QRS complexes with absent p waves.

Other dangerous arrhythmias

This section describes the management of VT in *hemodynamically stable* patients. If the patient has lost cardiac output (📖 p216) get help and follow the ALS algorithm on the inside front cover.

Ventricular tachycardia (pulse present)

Features: wide complex regular tachycardia, impaired cardiac output.

Therapy:
- If at any stage the patient loses cardiac output (📖 p216) start the ALS algorithm for VF/pulseless VT.
- Correct hypokalemia: give 20mmol KCl in 50mL 5% dextrose via the central line over 10min, and repeat as necessary to obtain serum K⁺ of 4.5–5.0mmol/L.
- Correct hypomagnesemia: give 1–2g MgSO₄ in 50mL 5% dextrose via the central line empirically if it has not already been given, as up to 60% of patients are hypomagnesemic postoperatively, and serum magnesium represents only 1% of total body stores.
- Correct hypoxia (📖 p160 and acidosis 📖 p170).
- Start weaning potentially arrhythmogenic infusions, e.g., isoprenaline.
- If the patient is hemodynamically compromised sedate with the help of an anesthesiologist and give 1 × 200J synchronized biphasic shock, and repeat if needed.
- Amiodarone 300mg in 50mL 5% dextrose over 1h via central line, followed by amiodarone 900mg in 250mL 5% dextrose over 23h via central line (📖 p205) may achieve rate control and is first choice agent in most units.
- Alternatively lidocaine 1mg/kg iv bolus, followed by an iv infusion of 4mg/min for 30min, 2mg/min for 2h, then 1 mg/min may achieve cardioversion.
- Look for and treat any evidence of myocardial ischemia (📖 p185).

Ventricular ectopy

Features: wide complexes that may occur occasionally or in couplets (ventricular bigeminy), may be unifocal or multifocal, and are usually followed by a compensatory pause.

Therapy: although ventricular ectopics occurring less than one per screen are usually benign, particularly if present preoperatively, in a small number of patients they reflect myocardial ischemia and may herald lethal arrhythmia.
- Look for signs of myocardial ischemia and treat accordingly (📖 p185).
- Correct hypokalemia: give 20mmol KCl in 50mL 5% dextrose via the central line over 10min, and repeat as necessary to obtain serum K⁺ of 4.5–5.0mmol/L.
- Correct hypomagnesemia: give 1–2g MGSO₄ in 50mL 5% dextrose via the central line empirically if it has not already been given, as up to 60% of patients are hypomagnesemic postoperatively, and serum magnesium represents only 1% of total body stores.

- Correct hypoxia (📖 p160) and acidosis (📖 p170).
- Atrial pacing at a rate greater than the ventricular rate may abolish ectopics and improve cardiac output, but does not address any underlying pathology.

Sinus or junctional bradycardia

Features: narrow complex, rate <60bpm. Impaired cardiac output.

Therapy: if epicardial pacing wires are present, pace immediately (📖 p228).
- Stop any infusions causing bradycardia, including amiodarone, β-blockers, and digoxin.
- Give a bolus of atropine (0.3 mg iv) repeated in increments up to 1mg.
- Start isoprenaline infusion (25mg in 250 mL 5% dextrose, at a rate of 0.01–0.3 micrograms/kg/min).

Second-degree heart block

Features: either Mobitz type I—PR interval increasingly prolonged with regularly absent QRS or Mobitz type II—PR interval constant with intermittently absent QRS (Fig. 5.16).

Therapy: a permanent pacemaker may be indicated (📖 p263): discuss with cardiologists if second degree heart block persists beyond post-op day 4.

Trifascicular block

Features: wide QRS complex (>0.12s or 3 small squares) and prolonged PR interval (>0.2s or 5 small squares) (Fig. 5.16).

Therapy: do not remove temporary pacing wires until the patient has been evaluated by a cardiologist. Hold off starting β-blockers. A permanent pacemaker is indicated if trifascicular block is associated with symptomatic pauses or other sinus irregularities.

Left bundle branch block

Features: wide QRS complex (>0.12s or 3 small squares). The ST segment cannot be interpreted: elevation or depression is *not* well correlated with ischemia in left bundle branch block.

Therapy: as for trifascicular block.

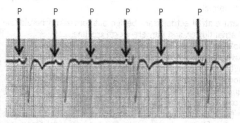

Fig. 5.16 Trifascicular block with Mobitz type II block. Note the wide QRS (left bundle block), prolonged but constant PR interval (which together indicate trifascicular block), and intermittently dropped QRS (Mobitz type II).

Benign arrhythmias

Sinus tachycardia

Features: sinus rhythm with a rate >100bpm. Rates >140 suggest SVT.

Therapy: although this is usually a benign response to sympathetic over-activity (pain, anxiety), it may be a compensatory response to poor cardiac output. Sinus tachycardia increases myocardial oxygen demand and reduces ventricular filling times. In hearts with stiff non-compliant ventricles characterizing preoperative AS, this may result in poor filling, decreased cardiac output and myocardial ischemia.

- Look for and treat the common underlying causes: pain, anxiety, pyrexia, gastric dilatation, hypercapnia, hypovolemia and anemia.
- Salbutamol nebulizers may be an unavoidable cause.
- If you are sure that the tachycardia is not compensating for poor cardiac output, and if the patient is not requiring inotropic support, and if the systolic BP is at least at pre-op values consider restarting at a low dose β- or calcium channel blocker if these were discontinued preoperatively. Short-acting drugs (metoprolol 25mg tid po) are safest.
- Inotropes, particularly epinephrine, dopamine, dopexamine, and dobutamine cause tachycardias. You may need to change or wean them.

Junctional tachycardia

Features: narrow complex tachycardia without P waves.

Therapy: junctional tachycardia is caused when junctional tissue has a faster intrinsic rate than the sinus node. Drugs slowing the sinus node should be stopped. Although it is a benign arrhythmia, loss of synchronized atrial contraction can reduce cardiac output by up to 30%.

- Stop digoxin and β-blockers.
- Attempt atrial or AV pacing.
- Consider metoprolol (25–50mg po tid) a short acting β-blocker, or diltiazem 60mg tid po to slow the junctional focus, with atrial or AV pacing if the underlying sinus rate is slow.
- Overdrive pacing may help establish synchronized AV contraction.

Atrial ectopics (Fig. 5.17a)

Features: P waves with a different morphology, associated with a longer than normal PR interval.

Therapy: premature atrial ectopics are benign but sometimes herald the onset of AF or atrial flutter, and they are worth treating.

- Correct hypokalemia: give 20mmol KCl in 50mL 5% dextrose via the central line over 10min, and repeat as necessary to obtain serum K^+ of 4.5–5.0mmol/L.
- Correct hypomagnesemia: give 1–2g $MgSO_4$ in 50mL 5% dextrose via the central line empirically if it has not already been given.
- Correct hypoxia (📖 p160) and acidosis (📖 p170).
- Give digoxin (125–250 micrograms iv over 1h, repeat up to a total of 1250 micrograms). Digoxin decreases the frequency of atrial ectopics and reduces the ventricular response rate if AF does develop.
- β-blockers decrease the frequency of ectopics.

1st-degree heart block (Fig. 5.17b)

Features: PR interval >0.2s (5 small squares).

Therapy: this is benign. In a patient that has undergone aortic valve surgery it suggests damage to the conduction pathways passing close to the aortic annulus. This often resolves over the weeks postoperatively as edema and hematoma settle. The patient warrants follow-up by a cardiologist as occasionally insertion of a permanent pacemaker is indicated, but unless first-degree heart block is accompanied by a new left bundle branch block or symptomatic bradyarrhythmias, temporary pacing wires can safely be removed on day 3/4.

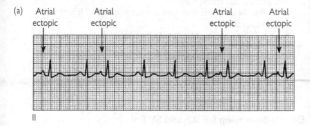

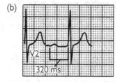

Fig. 5.17 Rhythm strips showing (a) atrial ectopics and (b) first-degree heart block.

Cardioversion

Key facts

Synchronized DC cardioversion is the treatment of choice for tachyarrhythmias compromising cardiac output, such as AF and SVT, and for AF refractory to chemical cardioversion.

Checklist for elective DC cardioversion

- Is it indicated?
  - Is the patient still in AF?
- Is it safe (📖 p262)?
  - Either AF has lasted <24h.
  - Or the patient must have had at least 6 weeks of formal anticoagulation.
  - Or a TEE excluding intra-cardiac thrombus.
- Is the patient ready?
  - The potassium should be 4.5–5.0.
  - The INR if anticoagulated should be >2.0.
  - The patient should have a valid consent form.
  - The patient should be starved for 6h.

DC cardioversion for AF and SVT

Patient should be anesthetized: some anesthesiologists prefer not to intubate, managing the airway with a bag and mask. You can either use adhesive external defibrillator pads which remain fixed to the patient until the procedure is completed, or hand-held paddles and gel pads. As soon as the anesthesiologist is happy:

- Expose chest.
- Place pads on chest in position shown in Fig. 5.18a: the aim is to direct as much of the current as possible through the heart.
- Place three EKG electrodes on the patient as shown, and connect to the fibrillator so that an EKG trace is visible.
- Switch defibrillator on and turn dial on to appropriate power setting (100J, 200J, 360J; Fig. 5.18c).
- *Press the SYNC button, and ensure that each R wave is accented on the EKG: failure to do this can mean that a DC shock is delivered while the myocardium is repolarizing, resulting in VF. Check that the SYNC button is on before every shock for AF.*
- If you are using hand-held paddles hold them firmly on the gel pads.
- Perform a visual sweep to check that no one is in contact with the patient at the same time as saying clearly, 'Charging. Stand clear'.
- Press the charge button.
- Press the shock button when the machine is charged.
- If the shock has been delivered successfully the patient's muscles will contract violently: anyone in contact with the patient will experience a large electric shock.
- Check the rhythm.
- If still AF press the charge button and repeat the sequence.

Complications of DC cardioversion

- Complications of general anesthesia (📖 p256).
- Systemic embolization (📖 p275, p278).
- Failure to cardiovert.
- Burns from incorrect application of gel pads.
- Muscle pain from involuntary contraction.
- Arrhythmias including asystole and VF.

Common pitfalls

Failure to deliver a shock: check that the defibrillator is switched on and adequately charged. Check that the correct power setting has been selected. Change the machine.

Failure to cardiovert: check the latest available serum potassium was 4.5–5.0. Check that the correct power setting has been selected. Replace gel pads with fresh ones. Reposition the patient on their side and the pads as shown and try two further shocks at 200J (Fig. 5.18). Don't start at too low a power setting: each shock leaves the myocardium less sensitive to further shocks. There is some evidence that 200J as the first power setting results in less myocardial damage and a better conversion rate than multiple shocks at lower power settings.

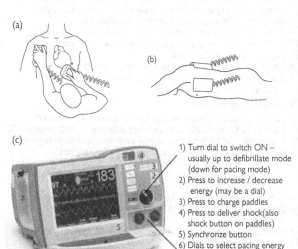

1) Turn dial to switch ON – usually up to defibrillate mode (down for pacing mode)
2) Press to increase / decrease energy (may be a dial)
3) Press to charge paddles
4) Press to deliver shock(also shock button on paddles)
5) Synchronze button
6) Dials to select pacing energy
7) Paddles housed on the sides

Fig. 5.18 Using defibrillators. (a) Correct positioning for defibrillation and cardioversion. (b) Alternative positioning for synchronized DC cardioversion. (c) Standard defibrillator console. 'On' dial may also be method of selecting energy level. © Zoll Medical Corporation.

Defibrillation

Key facts

- Defibrillation is the treatment of choice for VF and pulseless VT.
- *Biphasic defibrillators* cycle current direction every 10ms: the same amount of current (roughly 12Amps and 1500V) is delivered but with less energy (200J compared to 360J in older monophasic models) reducing the risk of burns and myocardial damage.

External defibrillation for VF and pulseless VT

Do not delay defibrillation for maneuvers such as intubation, massage, or administration of drugs.

- Expose chest.
- Place gel pads on chest in position shown in Fig. 5.18a: the aim is to direct as much of the current as possible through the heart.
- Switch defibrillator on (📖 Fig. 5.18c, p225) and turn dial on to appropriate power setting (200J for external defibrillation).
- Press charge button.
- If you are using hand-held paddles instead of adhesive external defibrillator pads, place them firmly on gel electrodes and hold.
- Perform a visual sweep to check that no one is in contact with the patient at the same time as saying clearly, 'Charging. Stand clear.'
- Press the red/orange shock button on the paddles.
- If the shock has been delivered successfully the patient's muscles will contract violently: personnel in contact with the patient may experience an electric shock.
- Check the rhythm: if VF charge again and repeat the sequence.
- If the rhythm changes to one compatible with an output check the pulse before proceeding further.

Internal defibrillation

- *Familiarize yourself early on with how to connect the internal paddles to the defibrillator console: it's different in most models, ICU nurses may not be familiar with how to do this, and an emergency resternotomy is not the time to be trying to figure it out.*
- In some models one of the external paddles disconnects at the handle, and this is the part that the internal paddle lead plugs into, in other models the internal paddles plug directly into the console.
- Switch defibrillator on (📖 Fig. 5.18c, p225) and turn dial on to appropriate power setting (30–50J for internal defibrillation) before you scrub.
- Hand out lead for internal paddles and connect them to defibrillator.
- Nurse will need to press charge button.
- Place concave surface of paddles squarely and firmly over LV and RV taking real care not to dislodge coronary anastomoses (placing the anterior paddle into the left pleura reduces the risk of damaging the LIMA to LAD) or pacing wires, or lacerate the myocardium (the paddles are relatively sharp edged) and press button on paddle handles to deliver shock (Fig. 5.19).

Common pitfalls

- *Failure to deliver a shock*: check that the defibrillator is switched on and adequately charged. Check that the correct power setting has been selected. Check that the SYNC button is *off* if you are trying to defibrillate VF. Change the machine and paddles.
- *Failure to defibrillate*: exclude causes of intractable VF, e.g., coronary ischemia, hypoxia. In internal defibrillation decompress the heart using massage (with the flows down if you're on cardiopulmonary bypass). If using external paddles in OR, inflate both lungs to ensure energy reaches the heart.

Internal cardiac massage and defibrillation

If the chest is open internal defibrillator paddles can be used. Shocks are given starting at 30J to a maximum of 50J. Remove the paddles with caution as rough contact with the myocardium may be enough to cause the heart to revert into VF. Internal cardiac massage should not be performed by inexperienced hands because of the risk of AV dehiscence, RV or LV rupture, or dislodging bypass grafts. The safest method is, standing on the patient's right, to carefully place your right hand under the ventricles, your left hand over the ventricles and compress carefully with the flat of your hands, not fingertips (Fig. 5.19c). One-handed massage is less effective and more likely to rupture the RV. If the patient is in asystole or complete heart block epicardial pacing wires can easily be placed, so that pacing can commence.

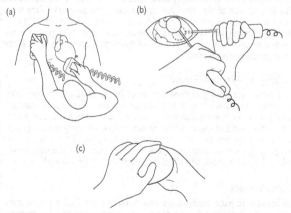

Fig. 5.19 (a) Correct positioning for defibrillation. (b) Correct positioning for internal defibrillation. (c) Correct positioning for internal cardiac massage.

Pacing overview

Key facts

- For maximum cardiac output the optimum heart rate in the immediate postoperative period is 90bpm, and the optimum rhythm is sinus.
- But arrhythmias and block are common, for the reasons described on 📖 pp214–215, and pacing is often required to optimize heart rate and rhythm.

Basics

Depending on the procedure and the patient's rhythm the surgeon may place temporary wires on the epicardium, prior to closing the chest. One or more atrial wires may be attached to the right atrial appendage, or the oversewn atrial cannulation sites. One or more ventricular wires may be attached to the epicardium of the right and sometimes left ventricle. Both sets of wires are brought out to the skin by passing them directly lateral to the xiphisternum, and normally sutured in place.

In most units the atrial wires are brought out to the right of the xiphisternum. The ventricular wires are brought out to the left of the xiphisternum. Be familiar with the convention at your unit.

Some surgeons prefer not to place any pacing wires, in order to avoid bleeding complications (📖 p259), if there is no evidence of bradycardia or heart block immediately post bypass. If the patient is bradycardic, with no evidence of abnormal AV conduction, some surgeons place atrial pacing wires, others prefer to rely on isoprenaline and atropine. Patients who have undergone valve surgery should have ventricular pacing wires inserted routinely because of the risk of developing complete heart block in the postoperative period.

Making a 'skin indifferent'

You need two pacing connections in order to pace a chamber: one indifferent and one active. If the surgeon has only placed one unipolar pacing wire (or the bipolar wire is not working) this will become the active. You need to create an indifferent. In an emergency place a green needle through the skin and attach to the pacing box. Otherwise insert an epicardial wire so that the bare wire is in contact with the skin, break off the straight needle, and attach the blunt end to the pacing box.

Pacing modes

It is possible to pace the atria, the ventricles, or both. Pacing can be *mandatory* or *asynchronous* (unaffected by any intrinsic rhythm), or demand. Demand pacing means that intrinsic action potentials are sensed and at a preset level are allowed to inhibit pacing potentials, so that the patient's own rhythm comes through. Sequential pacing means that both atria and ventricles are paced, to simulate the synchronized AV contraction of sinus rhythm. A list of modes is given as follows.

Temporary pacing modes (Table 5.3)

I   Chamber paced.
II   Chamber sensed.
III   Response to sensing.
A   Atrium.
V   Ventricle.
D   Dual chamber (both atrium and ventricle).
D   Dual effect (inhibits and triggers pacing).
I   Inhibits pacing.
O   No effect on pacing.

Table 5.3 Pacing modes

I	II	III	Description	Indication
A	O	O	Asynchronous atrial pacing	Sinus bradycardia
A	A	I	Demand atrial pacing	Sinus bradycardia
V	O	O	Asynchronous ventricular pacing	No ventricular rhythm, cautery
V	V	I	Demand ventricular pacing	Heart block
D	O	O	Asynchronous dual pacing	No ventricular rhythm, cautery
D	V	I	AV sequential, ventricular demand pacing	Suitable for most bradyarrhythmias.
D	D	D	AV sequential, dual chamber demand	

(a)

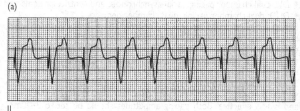

II

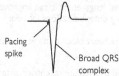

Pacing spike

Broad QRS complex

Fig. 5.20 Rhythm strip showing ventricular pacing.

Pacing

Atrial pacing

- *AOO*: asynchronous atrial pacing—useful if using electrocautery.
- *AAI* : Demand atrial pacing.

For effective atrial pacing normal AV conduction is required. It is ineffective during AF and atrial flutter. Pacing amplitude is 3–20mA. Indications include:

- Sinus bradycardia.
- Junctional bradycardia.
- Suppression of atrial and ventricular ectopics, if pacing is set at a slightly faster rate.
- Supraventricular and junctional tachycardia, and atrial flutter can be treated by overdrive pacing.

Ventricular pacing

- *VOO*: asynchronous ventricular pacing. Not often used because of the risk of VF if pacing spikes coincide with the T wave of intrinsic rhythm. Useful during surgery if patient has no underlying rhythm when electrocautery interferes with pacing.
- *VVI*: demand ventricular pacing.

For effective ventricular pacing set the pacing amplitude to 3–20mA. Ventricular pacing is much less effective than atrial and dual chamber pacing because of loss of synchronized AV contraction. Indications:

- Slow ventricular response rate to AF and atrial flutter.
- Any bradycardia with no atrial wires or failure of atrial pacing.
- Overdrive pacing of supra-ventricular tachycardia below.

Dual chamber pacing

- *DOO*: asynchronous dual chamber pacing. Caution as for VOO.
- *DVI*: dual chamber pacing, atrial asynchronous and ventricular demand.
- *DDD*: dual chamber pacing, dual chamber demand.

Effective dual chamber pacing requires atrial and ventricular pacing wires, but does not require normal AV conduction. Dual chamber pacing is more effective than ventricular pacing as synchronized AV contraction is maintained. This is particularly important in patients with hypertrophic ventricles where atrial contraction contributes up to 30% of cardiac output. It is less effective than atrial pacing at maintaining cardiac output because in ventricular pacing ventricular contraction starts from an abnormal focus and is less effective. Both pacing amplitudes should be set to 3–20mA. PR interval is set at 150ms: lengthening it can improve cardiac output by increasing ventricular filling time. Indications include:

- Complete heart block
- First- and second-degree heart block if the ventricular rate is slow.

Overdrive pacing

- This is occasionally used to treat supraventricular tachycardias. Select the maximum pacing output (20mA) and atrially pace at a rate 20bpm faster than the atrial rate (up to 600bpm!). When capture is achieved abruptly turn off the pacemaker: sinus rhythm may result.

Problems with pacing

Failure to pace—no pacing spikes: the pacing output may be too low: turn it up. The pacing wires may not be in contact with myocardium, the wires may be short-circuiting, the leads or contacts may be faulty, the box battery may be low. *Check all connections yourself.* Swap the pacing wires between active and indifferent port. Change the pacing leads, change the box. Create a skin indifferent (📖 p228) and try it with each of the epicardial wires in the active contact in turn. The EKG gain may be insufficient to show spikes: select a different lead or increase the gain. Use *transvenous pacing wires* to pace the pacing-dependent patient: in an emergency use *external pacing pads* (Fig. 5.18).

Failure to pace—pacing spikes present: pacing wires may be in contact with an area of high threshold, or out of contact altogether with the myocardium. Increase the output to maximum, swap the pacing wires or create a skin indifferent as described previously. Try an alternative mode of pacing.

Increasing threshold: in completely pacing-dependent patients it is important to check the pacing threshold daily. This is done by gradually decreasing the output until there is no longer pacing capture: the minimum output before loss of capture is the pacing threshold. Hematoma, edema, and scarring result in increased threshold. In pacing-dependent patients consider transvenous wires if threshold >10mA.

Oversensing: if the pacemaker senses T waves, or AF, demand pacing will be inhibited. Try increasing the sensing threshold or change modes.

Competition with patient's own rhythm: pacing can result in a dramatic decrease in cardiac output if it interferes with the patient's intrinsic rhythm. Use demand pacing, or try turning off the pacemaker altogether.

Pacing diaphragm: proximity of phrenic nerve causes diaphragm contraction: reduce output or use V pacing (A wires closer to phrenic nerve).

Removal of pacing wires

When the patient is no longer pacing dependent, usually by day 3 postoperatively, pacing wires are removed. It's usually safest to do this during daytime operating hours in case of bleeding complications. In anticoagulated patients the INR should be <2.5. Heparin should be discontinued until the APTT is <50. Patient should be recumbent. The wires should be untied if knotted in place, and any suture securing them removed. Apply firm pressure and pull the wires out smoothly. If much resistance is encountered pull wire taut and cut flush with the skin. Occasionally removal of pacing wires causes bleeding. Acute tamponade should be suspected in any patient who presents with hypotension following pacing wire removal (📖 p259). Some units leave one small mediastinal drain in until wires removed to avoid this problem.

Atrial electrogram

If the atrial pacing wires are attached to the two arm leads of a standard EKG (the leg leads remaining in the conventional position) a bipolar trace of atrial electrical activity (AEG) will be produced in lead I. This helps in the diagnosis of atrial arrhythmias.

Renal management

Key facts

- Cardiopulmonary bypass results in major changes in fluid distribution and renal function, moderated by pharmacological agents employed primarily for hemodynamic support (📖 p136).
- Most patients arrive in ICU 3–7kg above their preoperative weight, in a state of *total body sodium and water overload*, because of the fluid requirements driven by the changes described below.
- In a minority of patients correct fluid management is the difference between a satisfactory postoperative course and one complicated by multisystem failure. Basic fluid management is described on 📖 p238. The management of oliguria is outlined on 📖 p238. Diuretics are discussed on 📖 pp208–209. Renal pathophysiology and management is described in more depth here.

Renal effects of cardiopulmonary bypass

The period of low flow, non-pulsatile, hemodilute, hypothermic perfusion associated with bypass and the endocrine and CNS responses to major surgery have a complex series of effects on renal physiology.

- Activation of the renin–angiotensin system and aldosterone production results in sodium and water retention, and potassium excretion.
- ADH production stimulated by hypovolemia, nausea, and vomiting also causes vasoconstriction and water retention by increasing reabsorption of water in the distal collecting tubules.
- The stress response to surgery also results in elevated plasma cortisol, which contributes to sodium retention and potassium excretion.
- Complement, bradykinin, and kallikrein increase capillary permeability promoting shift of fluid to the interstitium from the vascular space.
- This is augmented by hemodilution as a result of blood loss, volume replacement given by the anesthesiologist to compensate for vasodilation at induction, and the 2L crystalloid pump prime. The reduced plasma oncotic pressure results in more movement of fluid into the comparatively high osmotic pressure interstitial space.
- Renal cortical blood flow is decreased by hypothermic vasoconstriction, but increased by hemodilution. During rewarming vasodilation of all capillary beds, not just renal, results in even greater fluid shift into the interstitium.

Etiology of renal failure

Renal dysfunction

- Creatinine >1.2mg/dL (126µmol/L), slightly lower in females.
- BUN >21mg/dL (urea >7.0 mmol/L).
- Creatinine clearance: normal is 90–130mL/min.

- *Preoperative risk factors*: age >75 years, creatinine >12.0 mg/dL, LV dysfunction, hypertension, diabetes, peripheral vascular disease, hypoperfusion as a result of diuretic therapy and vasodilators, sepsis, congestive cardiac failure, intrinsic renal damage caused by NSAIDs, contrast, aminoglycosides, diuretics, endocarditis, obstructive uropathy.

- *Intraoperative risk factors*: combined CABG and valve surgery, long bypass time, prolonged hypoperfusion, circulatory arrest.
- *Postoperative risk factors*: pre-renal—hypoperfusion. Many perfusionists routinely add 20g mannitol to the pump prime to protect the distal tubule and promote a diuresis. Vasoconstriction states; renal—sepsis, medications, hypoxia; post-renal—obstructive uropathy/foley catheter.

Preventing renal failure

There are a number of preoperative, intraoperative, and postoperative measures designed to reduce the risk of renal dysfunction.
- Preoperatively, ensure adequate hydration (+ acetylcysteine in patients with renal dysfunction) before undergoing procedures involving contrast for which the patient may be fasted for long periods of time
- Identify and discontinue where possible nephrotoxic medications, particularly NSAIDs and ACE inhibitors.
- Would the patient benefit from a period on the ICU preoperatively for optimizing with inotropic support and invasive monitoring? Consider stenting stenotic renal arteries (will need clopidogrel).
- Intraoperatively maintain adequate perfusion pressures (50–70mmHg).
- Postoperatively maintaining satisfactory cardiac output and optimizing intravascular volume is the most important factor in avoiding renal dysfunction (📖 pp186–187).

When should diuretics be given for oliguria?

- When you are reasonably confident that pre-renal causes, e.g., hypovolemia, hypotension, low cardiac output and post-renal causes such as Foley catheter problems or obstruction are not the cause, *and*
- Positive fluid balance will be detrimental to the patient now or in the near future, e.g., patient with borderline lung function, severe LV or RV dysfunction, obvious fluid overload.
- There are some broad rules of thumb:
  - Almost all patients need diuresis once they leave ICU.
  - Most ICU patients will do fine whether you give fluid or diuretic for low urine output, and it isn't worth a protracted debate. *But:*
  - Oliguric patients with good hemodynamic indices on minimal pressors can safely be diuresed early if extubation is a priority.
  - Oliguric patients needing large doses of pressor to maintain MAPs most likely need fluid to avoid renal malperfusion, and careful assessment of the underlying problem (📖 p234).
  - Septic (📖 p284) and vasoplegic (📖 p190) patients have high fluid requirements, and diuresis is rarely indicated in the acute phase.
  - Patients with SAM (📖 p190) or LV hypertrophy should be diuresed very, very cautiously: sometimes a little fluid overload is safer.

- Optimize preload by giving *colloid* to increase it aiming for an RAP of 12–16, a PAWP of 10–14, or an LAP of 12–16., remembering that in several conditions required filling pressures may be over 20mmHg (📖 p143).

The oliguric patient

Key facts

- Glomerular filtration rate and hence urine output is a sensitive measure of cardiac function. Most patients arrive in ICU in a state of *total body sodium and water overload*, which becomes more pronounced with the additional volume given as the patient warms and vasodilates.
- Patients with normal preoperative renal function should maintain a diuresis of at least *1mL/kg/h*: renal dysfunction is uncommon in these patients in the absence of other risk factors (🕮 p233).
- If called to treat oliguria: always start by asking yourself what the cause is—once you have ruled out important causes of oliguria, then you can start to think about whether you need to treat it.

Management of oliguria

Check that the Foley catheter is not the problem

- The urine catheter may be obstructed, bypassing, or malpositioned. Is the bed wet? Flush with 60mL saline—can you draw this amount back without difficulty? If not, or if the urine is bypassing the catheter, or if the bladder is palpable, change the catheter.

Optimize cardiac function

- Patients who were markedly hypertensive preoperatively may require high mean arterial pressures to maintain a satisfactory urine output.
- Start by assessing whether cardiac output is sufficient: if the patient is warm, well-perfused, with palpable distal pulses, good hemodynamic indices (CI >2.5L/min/m², SVO_2 >75%, MAPs >70mmHg, HR 60–80bpm, CVP 4–16mmHg) on minimal pressors then:
  - They are unlikely to be hypovolemic, or in incipient ATN (in the absence of other risk factors), so don't give fluid.
  - If the patient is not fluid overloaded, and will tolerate positive balance, don't give a diuretic, just watch for a couple of hours.
  - If positive fluid balance will be detrimental to the patient now or in the near future, e.g., borderline lung function, severe LV or RV dysfunction, obvious fluid overload, give 20–40mg furosemide iv.
- If cardiac output is not sufficient treat this first (🕮 p184), before giving diuretics, which can be harmful in low output or hypotension.
  - Remember that RV failure (🕮 p191), tamponade (🕮 p144), bleeding (🕮 p144), myocardial ischemia (🕮 p185), mesenteric ischemia (🕮 p275), ATN (🕮 p232), and sepsis (🕮 p239) may all present with oliguria.
  - *Optimize preload* by giving careful fluid challenges to achieve filling pressures of 14–16mmHg (🕮 p186).
  - *Optimize contractility* with inotropes: dobutamine (250mg in 50mL 5% dextrose at 3–6mcg/kg/min) is a good first-line choice: the diuresis normally seen within a few hours (🕮 p188).
  - *Treat any residual hypotension* with low-dose norepinephrine) 0.03 micrograms/kg/min) if patient likely requires higher MAPs.
  - *Treat acidosis, arrhythmias, hypoxia, anemia.*

• *If you do not see a response within an hour or two there is potentially a serious problem: get senior help whatever time it is.*

Loop diuretics

• Remember diuresis will exacerbate most low cardiac output states (📖 p184).
• If the patient is adequately filled and MAPs are satisfactory *give a loop diuretic*: 20mg of furosemide iv, and if there is no response give a further 40mg furosemide iv.
• A furosemide infusion (250mg furosemide in 50mL 5% dextrose at 1–10 mg/h) can be used instead of repeat bolus doses of furosemide.
• Loop diuretics do not prevent or directly cause acute tubular necrosis but they do have a beneficial effect in converting oliguric to polyuric renal failure (📖 p208), helping to prevent or relieve pulmonary edema.
• If the urine produced in response to diuretic challenges is concentrated, the patient is probably inadequately filled: give fluid bolus.

Osmotic diuretics

• Mannitol is an *osmotic diuretic* used during bypass: some centers use 15–25g in the pump prime. It may be indicated in the fluid-overloaded patient who has a depleted intravascular space as its oncotic properties mean that fluid is drawn back into the intravascular space. If urine output does not improve quickly there is a risk of causing pulmonary edema.

Treat the important problems associated with oliguria

The management of these complications is described on 📖 p236:
• Pulmonary and cerebral edema.
• Fluid overload.
• Hyperkalemia.
• Acidosis.
• Drug toxicity.

Further assessment and management

• If these measures fail to produce a satisfactory response a more accurate assessment of cardiac indices and underlying problems is required urgently. *In the first 48h after surgery a patient should never have several hours of very low urine output without senior assessment.*
• Most patients have *pulmonary artery catheters*: consider placing one if not already present to better evaluate left and right ventricular function, and optimize fluid status.
• A TEE will identify left and right ventricular dysfunction and tamponade.
• A CXR will show pulmonary edema, or hemothorax.
• *Hemodialysis* is indicated in the oliguric patient to avoid pulmonary edema indicated by deteriorating blood gases despite increasing respiratory support, hyperkalemia, and acidosis: it is not indicated purely for rising serum creatinine and urea in the first instance (📖 p236).

Management of renal failure

The management of oliguria is described on □ p234, and the pathophysiology of renal failure is described on □ p232. This section deals with the management of established oliguric renal failure.

Indications for renal replacement therapy

- Hyperkalemia.
- Acidosis.
- Pulmonary edema.
- Drug toxicity.
- Progressive uremia or uremia associated with pericarditis, encephalopathy, seizures, coagulopathy.

Key facts

The aim in established renal failure is firstly to avoid the potentially lethal complications of renal failure (hyperkalemia, acidosis, pulmonary and cerebral edema, severe uremia and drug toxicity), and secondly to avoid exacerbating the renal insult. Investigation of the underlying causes of renal failure is also important.

- Optimize hemodynamics to obtain higher MAPs (80–100mmHg), except in established anuria, where this is unlikely to improve function.
- Treat hypoxia aggressively.
- Aim for daily fluid balance of even to negative 500mL to avoid pulmonary edema in anuric patients.
- Remove the Foley catheter to avoid infection if the patient is anuric.
- Monitor electrolytes daily, and potassium and acid–base every few hours, avoid potassium supplements and medication that increases potassium levels (ACE inhibitors): treatment of hyperkalemia is described on □ p271, and acidosis on □ p170.
- Avoid nephrotoxic drugs (aminoglycosides, NSAIDs, ACE inhibitors) and monitor serum levels of drugs dependent on renal excretion (digoxin, antibiotics such as vancomycin and gentamycin).
- Essential amino acid diets are recommended for patients who are able to eat: patients on dialysis require high protein content (1.5g/kg/day) as dialysis results in negative nitrogen balance.
- Enteral and parenteral feeds can be similarly adjusted.
- Renal US, renal angiography may be indicated.

Hemodialysis and hemofiltration

There are two main techniques of renal replacement therapy used on cardiac ICUs: hemodialysis and hemofiltration. In both techniques access to the circulation is required and blood passes through an extracorporeal circuit that includes either a dialyser or a hemofilter.

- In hemodialysis blood flows along one side of a *semipermeable* membrane as a solution of **crystalloids is pumped** against the other side of the membrane, against the direction of blood flow.
- In hemofiltration **blood under pressure** passes down one side of a **highly permeable** membrane on the other side of which is a static crystalloid solution.

- In hemodialysis removal of solutes depends on diffusion: molecules move from high to low concentration, and smaller molecules move faster, so the amount of solute removed depends on its concentration in the dialysis fluid and on the size of the molecule.
- In hemofiltration removal of solutes with a molecular weight up to 20 000 depends on convective flow: all molecules are removed at a similar rate and virtually all ions are removed.
- In hemodialysis large molecules are not efficiently removed.
- In hemofiltration large molecules are so effectively removed that drugs such as heparin, insulin, and vancomycin may need to be replaced, and reduction in circulating inflammation mediators and pyrogens leads to a reduction in pyrexia and systemic inflammation.
- In hemodialysis controlled amounts of sodium and water are removed by creation of a transmembrane pressure gradient.
- In hemofiltration large amounts of salt and water are removed and must be replaced by an infusion of an appropriate amount of physiologic crystalloid into the distal port of the hemofilter.
- Hemofiltration has become an increasingly popular form of renalreplacement therapy for acute renal failure postoperatively, even though it is several times more expensive than dialysis. This is because the continuous nature of the process suits patients with multi-organ dysfunction. There are fewer of the dramatic swings in fluid balance and electrolytes that characterize dialysis. There are several variants.

Continuous arteriovenous hemofiltration (CAVH): this is the original and simplest form of filtration. The femoral artery and vein are cannulated, and blood passes though the hemofilter under arterial pressure alone. It is therefore less appropriate for patients with low cardiac output states. Prolonged arterial cannulation carries complications (📖 p173).

Continuous arteriovenous hemodialysis with filtration: because clearance rates are as low as 10ml/h with CAVH a dialysis circuit is added to the equipment, improving clearance rates at considerable cost.

Continuous venovenous hemofiltration (CVVH): an occlusive pump is incorporated into the circuit to drive blood so that venous cannulation is all that is required. This also allows control of blood flow and filtration rate. Clearance of up to 100mL/min can be achieved. This is the most commonly used system in intensive care units.

Continuous venovenous hemodialysis with filtration: some systems add hemodialysis to the CVVH circuit. Although there is a theoretical benefit it is rare that metabolic stability cannot be achieved with CVVH.

Management of the hemofiltered patient

- A double lumen catheter (Vascath or Mahurkar) is inserted into a central vein. The blood pump is set at 125mL/min and the hemofiltration rate to 25mL/min. The replacement fluid pump is programmed to balance the inflow and outflow of fluid to achieve a preset rate of fluid loss. The circuit is heparinized with an infusion of 200–1600 units per hour. Lactate is the commonest replacement anion, but in lactic acidosis a lactate-free replacement solution must be employed. Replacement of magnesium, calcium, phosphate, and bicarbonate is necessary. Profound hypotension is not uncommon when commencing hemofiltration.

Fluid management

Key facts

- Most patients arrive in ICU 3–7kg above their preoperative weight, in a state of *total body sodium and water overload*. The pathophysiology underlying this is discussed on ☐ pp106–107.
- Fluid management is directed at optimizing preload (☐ p186) without exacerbating interstitial edema, which tends to occur because of a generalized capillary leak syndrome (☐ p137).
- Success can make the difference between a short, uncomplicated postoperative course and the patient remaining on the ICU for weeks.

Maintenance crystalloid

Regimes vary widely between units. The principle is minimizing the additional sodium and water load, while maintaining intravascular volume. Standard protocols include:

- Normal saline or 5% dextrose at a rate equal to the previous hour's urine output.
- Dextrose saline at a rate of 50mL/h.

Colloid challenges

Colloids expand the intravascular space more effectively than isotonic crystalloid. To optimize preload by maintaining preset filling pressures colloid boluses in the form of either blood, blood products, or synthetic colloids should be given. The choice depends on the patient's hematocrit and whether bleeding required correction of coagulopathy with clotting products.

Fluid replacement options

Colloids, and blood most successfully, produce a more lasting expansion of intravascular volume than crystalloid, which rapidly enters the interstium.

Myocardial perfusion, particularly of the microvasculature, is improved by maintaining lower than normal hemoglobin concentration, which also reduces transfusion minimizing exposure to the associated complications. Transfusion has associated risks. But profound anemia reduces oxygen delivery, which can only be compensated for by increased cardiac output to a certain extent (Box 5.7), so patients are generally transfused to maintain Hb>8.0g/dL if indicated by symptoms, low SVO2, hypoxia or other issues.

Sepsis, SIRS and MOD

Key facts

- Sepsis is a systemic response to infection usually characterized by fever >38°C, tachycardia, and/or WCC>12x10⁹/L or <4x10⁹/L.
- Systemic inflammatory response syndrome (SIRS) is a pro-inflammatory state that does not include a documented source of infection.
- Sepsis and SIRS may lead to multiple organ dysfunction (MOD), and are associated with significantly increased mortality.
- The priorities of management are volume resuscitation, maintaining oxygen deliver, and end-organ support.

Post-operative sepsis

Patients with active endocarditis may present with clinical sepsis in the early post-operative period, but more commonly sepsis does not manifest until post-operative day 3. Signs include fever, rigors, leukocytosis or neutropenia; and may be less specific e.g. vasoplegia, deteriorating RV or LV function, poor oxygenation, renal failure or confusion. Signs may be subtle in elderly patients, immunocompromised or suppressed, and those on steroids. Examine the whole patient, and culture sputum, urine, blood, Common sources include:

- Pneumonia (📖 p268).
- Wounds (📖 pp284–285).
- Indwelling lines (culture, remove and replace) (📖 p175). Groin lines highest risk.
- Urinary tract infection (including after Foley removal).
- Endocarditis.

Empiric antibiotic therapy should be started with advice from infectious disease team as soon as patient has been cultured, and switched as soon as sensitivities are available; and supportive measures as for SIRS.

Systemic inflammatory response syndrome (SIRS)

- SIRS is defined as 2 or more of tachycardia >90bpm; tachypnea >20rpm; pyrexia >38°C; WCC>12x10⁹/L or <4x10⁹/L; without identifiable bacteremia and in the setting of a known cause of endothelial inflammation e.g. pancreatitis, ischemia, multiple trauma, hemorrhagic shock, immune mediated organ injury, or CPB.
- The pathophysiology is mediated by activation of complement, cytokine and clotting cascades, cell and humoral mediated immunity; increased intestinal permeability and translocation of bacteria and endotoxins may be an underlying cause.
- Metabolic acidosis, low output state and MOD are common features.
- Management includes:
  - Aggressive volume resuscitation: aim is to achieve normovolemia, increase cardiac output and O2 delivery.
  - Maintenance of O2 delivery by airway protection and ventilatory support, inotropic support of cardiac function, and avoidance of pressors to reduce splanchnic malperfusion.
  - End-organ support may include enteral, renal and hepatic support.

Gastrointestinal management

GI complications including upper and lower GI bleeding, ischemia, pancreatitis cholecystitis, and paralytic ileus are described in ⏛ Chapter 8. This section deals with routine management of the GI system on ICU.

Examples of enteral feeds

- *Standard feeds*: Osmolite, Nutrison standard.
- *Fiber enriched*: Jevity, Nutrison Multi Fibre.
- *High energy*: Nutrison Energy, Ensure Plus.

Pathophysiology

Ischemia

Splanchnic hypoperfusion may be caused by caused by emboli, low perfusion pressures on bypass, and low cardiac output states postoperatively, exacerbated by sympathetic vasoconstriction mediated by the CNS response to surgery as well as exogenous catecholamine administration in the form of drugs such as norepinephrine. Mucosal ischemia and mesenteric ischemia may result, characterized in its most severe forms by focal necrosis. Salt and water retention caused by activation of the renin–angiotensin system, capillary hyperpermeability and fluid loading results in mucosal edema. Morphine reduces gastric motility and positive pressure ventilation contributes to gastric dilatation.

Peptic ulceration

The majority of cardiac surgical patients share several risk factors for peptic ulceration: age, NSAID use, and smoking.

Ileus, nausea and vomiting

Ileus, anorexia, nausea, and vomiting are caused predominantly by opiate analgesia, and lack of mobility, exacerbated by the CNS effects of bypass. They are significant causes of morbidity in the ICU.

Table 5.4 Complications of enteral and parenteral nutrition

Enteral feed complications	Parenteral feed complications
Tube malposition, complications of insertion, blockage, kinking, occlusion, loss into GI tract	Catheter malposition, complications of insertion, blocking, kinking, occlusion, embolus air/thrombus
Aspiration pneumonia, diarrhea, constipation, distension, hyperglycemia	Substrate overload, hyperglycemia, hyperosmolarity, hyperammonemia
Infection around enterostomy	Catheter-related sepsis
Fluid and electrolyte disturbances, deficiency syndromes *rare*	Fluid and electrolyte disturbances, deficiency syndromes
ARDS secondary to aspiration	Abnormal liver function, intestinal atrophy and sepsis, respiratory compromise

Basic management

- NG tube insertion maintains gastric decompression during positive pressure ventilation, removes gastric contents minimizing the risk of aspiration, decreases acidity, and allows administration of oral medication and nutrition later in the ICU.
- Patients on CPAP benefit from prophylactic NG tube insertion, otherwise most units reserve NG tubes for patients requiring enteral nutrition, or evidence of gastric dilatation.
- Patients should be routinely started on motility agents and laxatives (such as senna 1 od and lactulose 10mL bid) once extubated, as these reduce the duration of ileus, improving nausea and constipation.
- All patients should receive omeprazole 20mg po od.
- Analgesia should be downscaled from intravenous and oral opiates to non-opiate analgesia such as acetaminohen 650mg po/pr/iv as soon as possible, to avoid ileus, constipation, anorexia, nausea, and vomiting.
- Avoid NSAID analgesia in elderly patients to avoid peptic ulceration.
- Give regular iv antiemetics to treat persistent nausea and vomiting.

Enteral and parenteral nutrition

- For satisfactory wound healing and convalescence a nutritionally balanced intake of approximately 2000–3000kcal/day is required. If the patient has not been extubated within 48h, or oral calorific intake is inadequate for other reasons, NG feeding should be started. If the GI tract cannot be used, total parenteral nutrition is an alternative. It is associated with more complications than parenteral nutrition (Table 5.4) and so every effort, including nasojejunal tubes and PEG placement, should be made to feed enterally.

Most enteral tube feeds come in sterile, 500mL and 1000mL packs, are nutritionally complete and provide 1kcal/mL. They are based on whole protein. Fiber-enriched feeds also provide 1kcal/mL but are thought to be better for patients who may require long-term feeding. They contain soluble soy polysaccharides, and fructo-oligosaccharides which remain undigested passing to the colon where they are fermented by bacteria into short-chain fatty acids which promote absorption of Na^+ and water, reducing diarrhea. These molecules are also probiotic. High-energy feeds contain 1.5 kcal/mL and are used in patients requiring reduced fluid input.

- Involve the pharmacist/dietician to make patient-specific feeds.
- Renal failure patients require high energy, low volume, and electrolyte feeds: Nepro provides 2kcal/mL and high protein content.
- High-fat-low carbohydrate feeds provide 55% of the energy content as fat: this is thought to reduce CO_2 production during respiration, and is designed for patients with severe respiratory compromise: there is no clear evidence of any benefit from these regimes.
- Drugs can be given by the NG tube being used for enteral feeding. Liquid preparations designed for oral administration should ideally be used as crushed tablets may block the tube: the feed should be stopped and the NG tube flushed with saline before and after administration of drugs.
- The therapeutic effect of warfarin is reduced by the vitamin K content in feeds: it is frequently necessary to increase the dose of warfarin.
- Phenytoin interacts with enteral feeds which should be stopped for 2h before and after phenytoin administration.

Neurological management

Stroke and other neurological sequelae of cardiac surgery are described on 📖 pp278–281. This section outlines routine neurological management on the ICU.

Pathophysiology

A large proportion of patients undergoing cardiac surgery can be shown by sophisticated cognitive testing to have sustained a neurological deficit, but in the majority this is not evident clinically. A minority of patients will suffer clinically obvious CVAs (📖 p278). A number of processes contribute to neurological dysfunction. Cerebral hypoperfusion as a direct result of low perfusion pressures, embolic occlusion of vessels, hypothermia, and hypoxemia is exacerbated by inhibition of cerebral autoregulation by anesthetic drugs. Alpha-stat management during cardio-pulmonary bypass helps counter this (📖 p124). Hyperglycemia is associated with a worse outcome of anoxic brain damage, perhaps due to the generation of oxygen free radicals.

Basic management

- Anesthetic levels are decreased towards the end of the operation, commonly by discontinuing inhaled anesthetic (e.g., halothane, isoflurane, nitrous oxide) and by starting continuous infusion of propofol (0.3–3mg/kg/h), fentanyl 1–10 micrograms/kg/h) or midazolam. This provides firstly adequate anesthesia for transfer and the first few hours on the ITU, and a basis for weaning anesthesia at a controlled rate.
- Sedation is obtained by using these anesthetic drugs at lower infusion rates or dexmedetomidine (Precedex ® at 0.2–0.7 mcg/kg/hr).
- Sedation covers a wide range of conscious states from almost wide awake to unresponsive: the ideal level of sedation is one where the patient is easily rousable from light sleep, able to obey simple commands, without anxiety or agitation.
- Effective sedation minimizes distress, ensures that invasive procedures are tolerated, allows the use of artificial ventilatory patterns, and helps control fits.
- Additional neuromuscular blockade may be required once the patient has reached the ICU: the main aim is to prevent shivering which can increase oxygen consumption by over 500% and exacerbate mediastinal bleeding, and to reduce respiratory compromise in the patient who is 'fighting the ventilator', e.g., vecuronium (0.05mg/kg) iv.
- Muscle relaxants have no impact on analgesia or awareness. It is critical to ensure that the patient has an appropriate level of anesthesia: give fentanyl, propofol, or midazolam.
- As anesthesia is weaned additional analgesia may be required, and a morphine NCA which can be converted to a PCA, and regular paracetamol, are routinely started.
- Remember when bolusing narcotics that even small doses can have a major impact on ventricular function: the scenario of the agitated patient that experiences cardiovascular collapse as a direct consequence of attempts at standard sedation is well recognized.

Assessment of neurological function

The following assessments are made on admission to the ICU and then every 4h for the first 24h, and then every 12h:

- Eye opening (spontaneous, to speech, to pain, not open).
- Movement (obeys commands, purposeful, withdraws to pain, abnormal flexion, abnormal extension, no response).
- Power (all four limbs) 5 normal, 4 against resistance, 3 against gravity, 2 with gravity, 1 muscle twitch only, 0 nil.
- Comprehension and orientation (to 'yes/no' questions).
- Sensation in main dermatomes.
- Assess pupil size and reaction to light.

The ICU patient with a new neurological deficit

- Around 1% of patients will have a postoperative CVA, and a similar number of patients experience seizures (with some overlap). Open heart cases (valve surgery), deep hypothermic circulatory arrest, and severe atherosclerotic aortic disease are the main risk factors, together with a previous history of stroke or seizure.
- The rationale for making an early neurological assessment prior to resedating patients is the narrow window available to intervene on acute intracerebral pathology.
- If a patient develops a new neurological deficit they should undergo urgent CT angiography of the brain to assess both the arterial tree and perfusion, as well as identifying intracerebral hemorrhage:
  - Hemorrhage is relatively uncommon, and should be treated by correcting any coagulopathy. Mass effects may require hemicraniotomy.
  - Embolic problems are more common—intra-arterial thrombolysis or embolectomy is very occasionally possible within a window of a few hours after the ischemic event.
  - Most commonly no acute pathology is seen on the first CT scan, and the management is directed at providing MAPs of 90–100mmHg instead of 65–75mmHg, which may be associated with an immediate improvement in some neurology. This maneuver is not safe until intracranial bleeding is ruled out by CT scan.
- The rare patients who fail to regain consciousness after weaning sedation should undergo EEG: a significant proportion are in undetected status epilepticus and require anticonvulsant therapy (☐ p283).
- The intubated seizing patient may be effectively treated with propofol, but phenytoin is the first-line and mainstay of treatment.
- Management of stroke and seizures after the first postoperative day or so is covered in more detail on ☐ p283.

Placing arterial and venous lines

Arterial cannula

Set-up
- Usually prepacked kit contains: 20-gauge cannula (use a 16-gauge in the femoral artery if later IABP insertion is anticipated), connectors and three-way tap, guidewire, 2mL 1% lidocaine, 5mL syringe, blue needle, 10mL sterile saline, skin prep, gauze swabs, small drape, suture.
- Explain the procedure to the patient if appropriate.
- For radial artery cannula insertion place the forearm on a pillow so that the wrist is dorsiflexed, for femoral artery insertion lie the patient flat (if obese, tape or have someone hold stomach out of the way).
- Prep the skin and infiltrate local anesthetic with blue (22-gauge) needle.

Landmarks
- Radial artery: between tendon of flexor carpi radialis and head of radius.
- Femoral artery: lies midway between the anterior superior iliac spine and the symphisis pubis.

Technique
- Prepare and check equipment. Sterile gloves.
- Palpate pulse between 2 fingers for 2–3cm.
- Pass cannula slowly at 45° into skin watching for arterial flashback.
- Once the cannula is *in situ*, aspirate and flush via the three-way tap.
- Ask nurse to place wrist on backboard to stabilize, and connect to transducer—check the trace is arterial.
- Suture femoral arterial line in place with 3/0 silk.
- *Transfixion technique:* the cannula is passed through both artery walls, the needle completely withdrawn, and the cannula then withdrawn slowly until flashback occurs, at which point it is advanced into the artery.

Partial transfixion technique: the cannula is advanced until flashback stops, and the needle withdrawn while holding the cannula steady, which is then advanced into the artery.

Non-transfixion: the cannula is advanced carefully in 0.5mm increments until flashback is seen, at which point the catheter is carefully slid off the needle in the artery.

Guidewire
A guidewire is useful where it is possible to get flashback, but difficult to advance the catheter up the artery.

Central venous catheter

Set-up
- Usually prepacked kit contains: appropriate central venous catheter, enough three-way taps for all individual lumens, 10mL 1% lidocaine, 10 mL syringe, a blue (23-gauge) needle and a green (21-gauge) needle, 20mL saline, 2 or 3/0 silk on a large handheld needle, 11 blade scalpel, skin prep, sterile drape, gauze swabs.
- You also need US probe with sterile bag if this is to be utilized.
- Sterile gloves and gown, and enough drapes to cover whole patient.

- Explain the procedure to the patient if appropriate (sign consent).
- Ask a nurse to set up pressure transducer and connection tubing.
- Patient's EKG and pulse oximetry should be continually monitored.
- Ensure that there is adequate light, a space behind the bed which you can work in, and that it is possible to place the bed in Trendelenburg.

Landmarks

- *Central approach to internal jugular vein:* apex of triangle formed by clavicular and sternal heads of sternocleidomastoid muscle, aiming the needle towards the opposite nipple.
- *Posterior approach to internal jugular vein:* point where line drawn horizontally from the cricoid cartilage to the lateral border of the clavicular head of SCM, aiming needle towards sternal notch.
- *Anterior approach to internal jugular vein:* medial border of sternal head of sternocleidomastoid, aiming needle towards ipsilateral needle.
- *Sublcavian:* advance the needle at 45° to the junction of outer and middle 1/3rd of the clavicle, then direct needle towards sternal groove.

Technique

There are numerous techniques.

- Prep and drape the patient so that all landmarks are exposed.
- Infiltrate local anesthetic around the planned puncture site.
- Spend 2–3min laying out the equipment in the order of use, secure three-way taps to central line and turn to closed position.
- Ask the nurse to place the bed in 10–20° of Trendelenburg.
- Ballot the internal jugular vein, or under US guidance using aseptic technique and a green needle on a 10mL syringe enter the skin at 45°.
- On aspirating venous blood remove the syringe but leave the green needle *in situ* as an exact marker of position, depth, and direction.
- An alternative is to use a 23G catheter over a needle: the needle is withdrawn and connection tubing attached once the catheter is in the vein, so that confirmation that this is venous not arterial can be obtained by direct manometry, prior to vessel dilatation: the guidewire is placed down the catheter once this is done.
- Take the large-bore hollow needle attached to the 10mL syringe and using the green needle as a guide cannulate the internal jugular vein.
- Aspirate 3–5mL of blood when there is flashback and then remove the syringe leaving the wide-bore needle *in situ*.
- Pass the guidewire down the wide-bore needle, watching for ectopics, and keeping hold of it at all times.
- Once an adequate length of wire is in place, remove the needle over the wire, and apply pressure to the vein.
- Make a 3mm nick in the skin over the wire with a scalpel.
- Pass the dilators over the wire into the vein.
- Remove the dilators, apply pressure, and pass the central venous pressure cannula over the wire into the vein up to about 15cm.
- The wire normally protrudes through the brown (proximal) lumen which should therefore be left open.
- Aspirate, flush, and close all lumens, suture the catheter to the skin.
- Check that there is a satisfactory venous trace.
- CXR to identify pneumothorax.

PA catheter, pericardiocentesis

PA catheter

Set-up if there is no PA catheter sheath already in situ:
- As for central line insertion (📖 p244).
- PA catheter sheath.

Set-up if there is a PA catheter sheath in situ:
- PA catheter plastic sleeve, PA catheter, 3 × three-way taps, connectors, 10mL syringe, 20mL saline flush, sterile gloves and gown, sterile drapes, skin prep, 2 or 3/0 silk suture on a large hand-held needle.
- Position patient as for central line insertion.
- Continual EKG and pulse oximetry monitoring is mandatory.
- A manometry line flushed and zeroed.
- Depending on the monitoring system being used, connection leads and box.

Technique
- Using aseptic technique insert PA catheter sheath in the manner described for central venous catheter insertion (📖 p244).
- Connect PA catheter to LED light source as per instructions and check LED functions and the balloon inflates and deflates.
- Flush all lumens with saline.
- Attach and zero the manometry line.
- Place tip of PA catheter through folded plastic sleeve (don't unravel it until the PA catheter is completely through), and into the PA sheath, connect sheath to sleeve and unroll the sleeve over the length of the PA catheter: is it now possible to continue without aseptic technique.
- Pass the PA catheter through the PA catheter sheath, into the SVC, and RA, holding the PA catheter so that it is concave to the patient's left.
- The pressure trace should show pressures for the changing vessels and chambers appropriately for every 10cm or so that the catheter is advanced.
- Once the tricuspid valve is crossed and an RV pressure trace is visible inflate the balloon.
- Pass the PA catheter further until either a wedge trace is achieved (📖 p176), or the length is >60cm.
- If no wedge trace is obtained, deflate the balloon, withdraw the catheter to about 30cm, inflate the balloon, and try again.
- Once a wedge trace is obtained, deflating the balloon should reveal the PA trace. If this is not the case deflate the balloon and withdraw the catheter a few mm and try again.
- Obtain a CXR to confirm satisfactory position.

Pericardiocentesis

Used, usually by cardiologists under fluoroscopic guidance, to relieve acute pericardial tamponade. Most surgeons favor a subxiphoid incision or even a resternotomy in early postoperative period as effusions are rarely simple and amenable to drainage through narrow-gauge catheters.

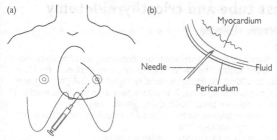

Fig. 5.21 Technique of pericardiocentesis.

Set-up
- Pericardoicentesis needle or catheter, 10mL 1% lidocaine, 10mL syringe, a blue needle and a green needle, 20mL saline, 2 or 3/0 silk on a large handheld needle, 11 blade scalpel, skin prep, sterile gauze.
- Sterile gloves, gown, and drapes.
- Explain the procedure to the patient where appropriate.
- Ensure patient has continual EKG monitoring.
- Fluoroscopy or echo guidance mandatory in elective setting.

Landmarks
1/2cm below and to the left of the xiphoid, aiming at 45° to skin, pointing at left shoulder or nipple.

Technique (Fig. 5.21)
- Prep and drape the skin, infiltrate local anesthetic and make a 3mm nick in the skin 0.5cm immediately to the left of the xiphoid tip.
- Insert the needle applying continuous aspiration aiming at 45° to skin, pointing at left shoulder or nipple, keeping an eye on echo/screening monitor (or EKG if no imaging available) as the needle is slowly advanced: if there are ectopics or changes in the ST segments stop and withdraw the needle a few mm.
- When in contact with the pericardium, 'pop' the needle a few mm into the pericardial space.
- If EKG changes, this indicates contact with the myocardium and the needle should be withdrawn slightly into the pericardial space where no ST segment elevation should be seen.
- When in the pericardial space, aspirate fluid.
- If the tamponade is successfully reduced, RAP should be decreased, cardiac output should increase and pulsus paradoxus should disappear.

Complications
- Cardiac puncture, laceration of a coronary artery, air emboli, arrhythmias, hemothorax, pneumothorax, infection.

Chest tube and cricothyroidotomy

Chest tube insertion

Set-up

- 28F intercostal drain, underwater seal containing water to up to mark, connection tubing, line clamp, Roberts or other instrument for blunt dissection, 20mL 1% lidocaine, 10mL syringe, blue (23G) and a green (21G) needle, 20mL saline, 2 or 3/0 silk on a large handheld needle, 11 blade scalpel, skin prep, sterile drape, gloves, gown, gauze.
- Explain the procedure to the patient if appropriate: recheck side on X-ray and sign consent form.
- Ensure continual monitoring of pulse oximetry.
- Position the patient at 45° with the arm abducted.

Technique

- Typical site for insertion is 5th intercostal space in the midaxillary line.
- It may extend anteriorly to the anterior axillary line.
- Prep and drape the skin. Infiltrate site for tube insertion with local anesthetic ensuring anesthesia at all layers down to and including parietal pleura, and the periosteum of the ribs posterior to the incision.
- A 2cm transverse skin incision is made and the intercostal space is dissected bluntly. Place purse-string suture now.
- The pleura is opened using blunt-tipped instrument introduced over the superior aspect of the ribs, and a finger placed into the pleural space to make sure there are no adhesions.

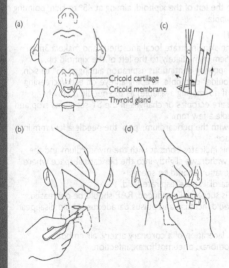

(a)

(b)

(c)

(d)

Cricoid cartilage
Cricoid membrane
Thyroid gland

Fig. 5.22 Technique of cricothyroidomy.

- A chest tube is then passed bluntly into the pleural space, being guided superiorly for a pneumothorax and basally for a hemothorax.
- The drain is connected immediately to an underwater seal: ask the patient to cough while you hold the drain and watch for air bubbles in the underwater seal to confirm correct placement. Secure the drain.
- A pigtail can be placed using the same landmarks but employing a Seldinger technique for simple effusions and pneumothoraxes.

Complications

- Misplacement: subcutaneous, intraparenchymal.
- Trauma to other structures: diaphragm, spleen, liver, heart, aorta, lung parenchyma, intercostal arteries (entry sites too low, posterior or trocar used instead of blunt dissection).
- Surgical emphysema, wound infection, empyema, pain.

Cricothyroidotomy

Emergency need for a surgical airway

- Major maxillofacial injury.
- Oral burns.
- Fractured larynx.

Need for tracheal toilet in the extubated patient.

Set-up

- Minitracheostomy, size 6.0 ET tube or 12G cannula in emergencies.
- Artery forceps, 20mL 1% lidocaine, 10mL syringe, blue (23G) and a green (21G) needle, 20mL saline, 2 or 3/0 silk on a large handheld needle, 11 blade scalpel, skin prep, sterile drape, gloves gown, gauze.
- Explain procedure to the patient where appropriate. Sign consent.
- The trauma patient's C-spine should be immobilized.

Landmarks

- The cricoid membrane is a small diamond-shaped membrane palpable just below the prominence of the thyroid cartilage.

Technique (Fig. 5.22)

- Prep and drape.
- If the patient is conscious and maintaining their own airway, infiltrate local anesthetic using aseptic technique.
- Stabilize the thyroid cartilage with the left hand.
- With your right hand make a 2cm transverse incision (smaller for minitracheostomy) through the skin overlying the cricothyroid membrane, and then straight through the cricothyroid membrane.
- Now turn the scalpel blade 90° within the airway so that it acts as a temporary retractor.
- Place an artery forceps through the incision and open it, remove the scalpel and insert a size 6.0 ET tube.
- Suction the tube, secure, and connect to a source of oxygen.
- Some minitracheostomy kits use the Seldinger technique: aspirating air freely is a sign that the needle is in the trachea and that a guidewire can be gently passed down the lumen.

Management of chest drains

Technique of insertion is described on ☐ p248. This section describes the types of chest drainage systems available, and basic protocols for managing chest drains.

Types of drainage system

Underwater seal

Underwater seal drains used to consist of three bottles connected by tubing, the third bottle providing suction control determined by the depth the connection tube penetrated below the water level in the bottle. Now most hospital wards have reliable high-volume, low-pressure wall suction, which means that simple, lightweight, single underwater seal bottles can be used instead of the cumbersome three-bottle systems. The system has to be kept upright.

- Underwater seals are suitable for any condition requiring chest drainage.
- They can be used with or without suction.
- Suction is usually 2–5kPa.

Heimlich valves

The Heimlich valve is a one-way flutter valve within rigid tubing. It can be connected to a standard chest drain. The system allows air and fluid out of the chest cavity, but prevents both from entering. The system has to be open to air, which makes collecting liquid effluent more difficult.

- Heimlich valves are usually considered in patients with a permanent air leak for whom surgery is not appropriate, and for whom the main goal of therapy is discharge to home or palliative care.

Portex bag

- The Portex bag was designed as an ambulatory chest drainage system. It consists of a Heimlich valve within a drainage bag which has a capacity of about 1500mL, and can be emptied intermittently. This drainage system cannot be connected to suction.
- These drains are indicated in patients with chronic pleural collections, in whom surgery is not appropriate.
- As the systems are airtight, an air leak is a contraindication.

Suction

Almost all conditions can be safely managed by an underwater seal system without suction, but suction helps to reinflate the acutely collapsed lung, and improves drainage of fluid. There is a huge range in surgeons' preferences for suction protocols: the following points represent commonly used protocols.

- 1kPa = 7.5mmHg = 10cmH$_2$O.
- Suction should be high volume, low pressure: approximately 2–3kPa.
- Blocked suction tubing, or a blocked filter at the wall is the equivalent of clamping the drain: have a low threshold for suspecting either.
- Most surgeons put most thoracic drains on suction for 24–48h: the exceptions to this are patients with pneumonectomies who are not placed on suction.

- Ventilated patients cannot generate their own negative intrapleural pressures and therefore all chest drains in these patients, with the exception of post-pneumonectomy drains, should be placed on suction.
- Some surgeons do not routinely place their thoracic patients on suction postoperatively unless an early CXR, requested for all patients, shows that the lung has not fully re-expanded.
- Some surgeons prefer to delay suction by 6h or so in patients who have undergone chemical pleuradesis.
- It is usually safe for a patient with an underwater seal on wall suction to mobilize off-suction for brief periods.
- Discontinue suction in extubated patients after 24–48h when the lung is fully inflated on CXR, and there is no air leak (the drain does not bubble when the patient coughs).
- Suction is unlikely to secure expansion in the lung that has been collapsed chronically: it is most effective in the immediate postoperatve period.

Clamping drains

More patients have died as a result of clamped drains than unclamped drains. The practice of clamping chest drains during transfer is a dangerous one. It reveals a failure to understand how a modern underwater seal drain works, as well as reflecting outmoded practice that dates back to the time of tuberculosis, when drain bottles contained caustic sterilizing fluid that could drain back into the patient if lifted above the level of the chest during transfer. The only indications for clamping a chest drain are:

Post-pneumonectomy

The post-pneumonectomy chest drain is usually clamped for an hour at a time, and unclamped briefly to allow blood to drain. Leaving the drain unclamped risks causing mediastinal shift towards the pneumonectomy side, and cardiovascular compromise. The drain is usually removed on day 1 postoperatively.

Massive hemothorax or effusion

If more than 1500mL of fluid is drained immediately on insertion of a chest tube, and the patient appears hemodynamically compromised as a result of drainage, it is appropriate to clamp the drain for a brief period. In massive hemothorax the effect is to attempt to tamponade the bleed, buying a little time to organize surgical exploration. In a massive effusion this allows time for the lung to expand without re-expansion pulmonary edema, and to reduce mediastinal shift caused by rapid drainage.

Decision-making in long-term drains

Occasionally a surgeon may decide to see if a patient with a chronic effusion or air leak can manage without a drain, by clamping the drain. Tension pneumothorax may result from doing this in a patient with an air leak. Such patients must be observed frequently for any sign of respiratory or hemodynamic compromise, surgical emphysema, or radiological evidence of lung collapse, and if any of these occur, the drain must be unclamped. If the patient tolerates the clamp for 24h it is usually possible to remove the drain.

Complications

Normal postoperative course

This is an overview of the expected postoperative course for uncomplicated cardiac surgical patients.

First 6h

- Myocardial function often deteriorates over the first 6h (📖 p136).
- Inotropic support may increase during the first 6h.
- Pacing may be required.
- Many patients are extubated within 6h.
- A diuresis of at least 1mL/kg/h is usual.
- Mediastinal drainage should decrease steadily.
- Insulin requirements increase.
- Prophylactic antibiotics are continued.
- Aspirin is given 75–325mg po or via NG tube.
- Preoperative antianginals are discontinued.

Day 1

- Inotropes are weaned.
- Most patients are extubated.
- Large chest drains removed after 3h of consecutive zero drainage.
- Post drain removal CXR is taken.
- The patient is transferred from ICU and mobilized.
- The patient may have a PCA.
- Routine oral medication is commenced (aspirin 75–325mg od, furosemide 40mg od, preoperative statin, paracetamol 1g qid, lactulose 10mL bid, senna 2 tablets, and LMWH, e.g., enoxaparin 40mg od s/c.
- Patients who require formal anticoagulation are started on warfarin.
- Patients should be sitting out of bed, and start eating and drinking

Day 2

- Monitoring lines (arterial, central venous, and urinary catheters) are removed.
- The patient is transferred to the ward and should be walked.
- PCA should be discontinued.
- Insulin sliding scales are discontinued and normal antihyperglycemic regimens commenced if the patient is eating and drinking.

Day 3

- Anticoagulation should be therapeutic for mechanical valves: start iv heparin if this is not the case.
- If there are no contraindications remove temporary pacing wires and small mediastinal drain if kept (📖 p231).

Day 4

- Patient should complete a satisfactory stairs assessment with a physio.
- All blood results and imaging should be returning to normal values.
- Adequate pain control should be possible with regular paracetamol and occasional oral opiate analgesia.
- The patient should have passed stool.

Days 5–7
- The patient should be ready for discharge home.
- Weight should be back to baseline, and diuretics may be discontinued in the patient with good LV and no fluid overload.

Routine tests
Protocols vary: this is a common standard.

Blood tests
CBC, coagulation studies, electrolytes on day 1, day 2, day 3, day 5, and day 7.

EKG
1–2h post-op, 12h post-op, and day 2 post-op.

CXRs
Daily if chest drains are present on suction, immediately post-drain removal, and day 2, 4, and 7 thereafter.

TTE
Day 5 for valve surgery patients, particularly mitral valve repairs.

CT angiography
If renal function permits, for all ascending, arch, and descending aortic repairs.

Rounds
Patients should be seen twice a day. In the morning review the blood results and CXRs. For formal rounds:
- Make sure you have a nurse or physician assistant with you.
- Make sure someone writes a summary including problem list and plan in the patient's chart.
- Ask the patient if they are experiencing any problems.
- Establish whether they are mobilizing appropriately, eating and drinking. and have adequate pain control.
- Check the chart for: (1) temperature, (2) BP trends, (3) oxygen saturations, (4) weight, (5) fluid balance and mediastinal drainage if these are still being monitored.
- Feel pulse, look at most recent EKG and telemetry.
- Look at JVP and ankles.
- Look at wounds, check for sternal mobility.
- Listen to heart sounds in valve patients.
- Listen to chest in all patients, and check most recent CXR.
- Check diabetic charts for blood sugar control, and review all medications.
- Review the previous day's blood results and overall trends.
- Make a clear problem list, a clear plan and follow-up.

Overview of complications

See Table 6.1–6.3.

Table 6.1 Complications of cardiac anesthesia (see 📖 pp87–99)

Procedure	Complication
Induction	Hemodynamic instability, myocardial ischemia, malignant hyperpyrexia, allergic reactions
Intubation	Loss of airway control, aspiration, damage to teeth/crowns, damage to oropharynx, damage to vocal cords, malposition of ET tube
Ventilation	Atelectasis, air trapping, chest infection
Radial and femoral catheters	Peripheral ischemia, superficial sepsis, hematoma, local neuropathy
Central venous line	Pneumothorax, carotid artery puncture, brachial plexus injury, hemothorax, hematoma, arrhythmias, malplacement, kinking, loss of guidewire into heart
PA catheter	As for central line, also: pulmonary artery rupture, complete heart block ventricular arrhythmias, tricuspid valve damage
Urinary catheter	Urinary tract infection, bacteremia, inflation of balloon in prostatic urethra →rupture, misplacement PV
TEE	Damage to oropharynx, esophageal rupture

Table 6.2 Complications of bypass

System	Complications
Cannulation	Atheromatous emboli (CVA), aortic dissection, peripheral ischemia or neuropraxia (femoral/axillary cannulation), selective perfusion head and neck arteries due to malplacement of cannula, damage to right atrium, IVC and SVC tear, damage to coronary sinus, damage to RCA and SA node. Hemodynamic instability. Massive air embolus
Cardiovascular	Fluid retention, peripheral edema, decreased myocardial compliance, myocardial stunning, ischemia-reperfusion injury
Respiratory	Perivascular edema, reduction in effects of surfactant, decrease in FRC, and compliance, atelectasis, increased physiological shunts, ARDS
Renal	Acute renal failure, decreased renal perfusion, sodium and water retention, hemoglobinuria
Hepatobilary	Jaundice, fulminant hepatic failure, acute pancreatitis
Gastrointestinal	Gastritis, peptic ulceration, mesenteric ischemia, increased permeability to endotoxins
CNS	CVA, cognitive deficit, anoxic brain injury, seizures
Hematological	Microemboli, activation coagulation and complement cascades; DVT and PE are unusual

Table 6.3 Complications of specific cardiac operations

Operation	Complication
Median sternotomy	Re-exploration for bleeding, sternal wound infection, pseudoarthrosis, dehiscence, brachial plexus injury, pain, keloid scar
Resternotomy	Trauma to right ventricle or aorta and catastrophic hemorrhage, injury to patent grafts causing ischemia or intractable VF
Thoracotomy	Rethoracotomy for bleeding, wound infection, seroma, damage to nerve to serratus, loss of mobility, chest infection, hemothorax, prolonged air leak, paraesthesia
Any cardiotomy	AF, cardiac tamponade, pericardial effusion, aortic dissection, CVA, phrenic nerve injury, mediastinitis
CABG	Graft occlusion (early or late), steal syndromes, ischemia, leg wound infection, edema from LSVG harvest, pleural effusion on side of IMA harvest, hand ischemia and neuropraxia if radial artery harvest
AVR	CVA, heart block requiring permanent pacemaker, paraprosthetic leak, prosthetic valve endocarditis, prosthesis failure
MVR	CVA, heart block, inadvertent occlusion of Cx artery or coronary sinus, AV dehiscence, paraprosthetic leak, prosthetic endocarditis, valve thrombosis, SAM
Thoracic aorta repair	CVA, paraplegia from spinal ischemia, peripheral limb and end organ ischemia

Consent

The following complications should be specifically described when obtaining informed consent from patients for cardiac surgery:

- Death (calculate percentage risk from Euroscore or STS score 📖 inside front cover).
- Stroke (1–2% for coronary artery bypass, 2% for calcified aortic valve surgery, 5% for prior CVA or concomitant carotid artery surgery).
- Re-exploration (1–2%).
- Arrhythmias (usually AF) 30%.
- Permanent pacemaker (1–2% for valve surgery).
- Deep sternal wound infection (0.5% in routine cases, 1–3% in diabetics, active smokers, obese patients).
- Superficial wound infections (10%).
- Chest infections (5% in routine cases, 10% in active smokers).
- Peptic ulcer disease (1–2% in routine cases with no previous history).
- Acute renal failure requiring dialysis (<1% in cases with no previous history of renal impairment).
- Prosthetic endocarditis (1–2%).
- Prosthesis failure (see 📖 p366).
- Paraplegia in thoracic aortic surgery (📖 p436).

Hypotension and tamponade

Hypotension

Hypotension on ICU is covered on 📖 pp142–143. Cardiac tamponade can cause sudden or gradual onset of hypotension up to several weeks after surgery and needs immediate treatment (📖 p150). There is a large differential diagnosis for hypotension (see Box 6.1) but the commonest causes once the patient has left ITU are:

- Hypovolemia.
- Arrhythmias.
- Change in drugs (stopping inotropes, recommencing antihypertensives).
- Vasovagal (removal of drains, vomiting, micturition syncope, postural).

Box 6.1 Causes of hypotension after leaving cardiac ITU

Cardiovascular
- Hypovolemia—bleeding, polyuria.
- Arrhythmias: heart block, sinus bradycardia, fast AF and flutter, VT.
- Ischemia, perioperative MI, congestive heart failure.
- Cardiac tamponade.
- Prosthesis or repair failure.

Respiratory
- Severe hypoxemia.
- Acute hemothorax, tension pneumothorax.
- Massive PE.

Gastrointestinal
- GI bleed, pancreatitis, acute GI pathology.

Neurological
- CVA.

Drug induced
- Withdrawal of inotropes too quickly.
- Recommencing antihypertensives too quickly.
- Amiodarone, ACE inhibitors (even if not given for 24h), Mg.
- Overdose of opiates, benzodiazepam, digoxin.

Metabolic and endocrine
- Electrolyte abnormalities unlikely on their own to cause low BP.
- Hypothyroidism, addisonian crisis, hypoglycemia, ketoacidosis.

Infection
- Sepsis.

Diagnosis and basic management

Go and see the patient. The causes of hypotension are listed in Box 6.1. Is the patient in cardiac tamponade?

- Get the patient into bed and sit at 45° initially.
- Secure iv access, give 500mL colloid over 5–10min (250mL if the patient is known to have poor LV).

- Give 100% oxygen.
- While the fluid is given assess pulse rate and rhythm, look at JVP, assess the recent trends on the chart and assess response to the fluid bolus. Gradual hypotension and tachycardia, combined with negative fluid balance suggest hypovolemia. A high JVP suggests either fluid overload, congestive heart failure, or cardiac tamponade.
- Get monitoring: EKG, pulse oximetry, and automatic NIBP.
- If good response to fluid, give more.
- If no or slow response to fluid resuscitation, and basic management of arrhythmias (📖 pp262–263) get help.
- Arterial blood samples can be tested at the bedside for hypoxia, hypercapnia, acidosis, ↑glucose, ↓glucose, ↑K⁺, ↓K⁺, ↓Hb.

Late cardiac tamponade

Some patients have pericardial effusions postoperatively which normally resolve without causing cardiac tamponade. In about 5% of patients these effusions increase in size, and may cause tamponade. Late tamponade may present with ill-defined symptoms of malaise, lethargy, chest discomfort, and anorexia with or without the classical findings listed in Box 6.2.

Box 6.2 Clinical findings in late cardiac tamponade

- Progressive hypotension and tachycardia
- Raised JVP, pulsus paradoxus, ↑peripheral edema.
- ↑Creatinine and ↓urine output.
- Muffled heart sounds and pericardial rub are non-specific post-op.

Causes

The causes of late cardiac tamponade are:
- Intrapericardial bleeding, e.g., following removal of pacing wires (prevented in some centers by leaving a small mediastinal drain in until after pacing wire removal), coagulopathy, or anticoagulation.
- Serous effusions due to hypervolemia, or post-cardiotomy pericarditis.

Diagnosis

Any of the physical signs listed in Box 6.2 may be present, together with an enlarged cardiac silhouette on the PA CXR. Confirmation is by urgent TTE or by TEE if views are inadequate. The location of the effusion should be described as well as the depth (anything >2cm is significant, but remember that large chronic effusions may not cause tamponade, while small acute ones may). Cardiac tamponade is present if there is RV diastolic collapse.

Management

- Secure iv access and give volume to restore BP.
- Place patient NPO, start 15min obs, and monitor with telemetry.
- The definitive management is urgent aspiration—pericardiocentesis for late simple effusions (>4 weeks) or subxiphoid pericardial window for bloody or loculated effusions (📖 p490). Within one or 2 days of surgery the management is urgent resternotomy (📖 p150).

Chest pain and ischemia

Chest pain

Chest pain is common after cardiac surgery, but it normally reflects the effects of a median sternotomy, rib retraction, and drains. Taking a careful pain history should help differentiate between the causes of chest discomfort listed in Box 6.3.

Box 6.3 Causes of postoperative chest pain

Dull, central ache
- Myocardial ischemia (usually brought on by exertion).
- Cardiac tamponade (📖 p143, p259).
- Pericarditis (classically soreness rather than ache).
- Peptic ulcer disease, esophagitis (worse on leaning forward and hot drinks, better with antacid), rarely pancreatitis.

Pain on movement
- Musculoskeletal pain, wound infection, unstable sternum.
- Chest drains.

Pleuritic pain
- Chest infection.
- Pneumothorax.
- Chest drain *in situ*.
- PE.

Diagnosis

Take a careful history and examine the patient. A CXR will demonstrate most lung pathology and a 12-lead EKG should help identify myocardial ischemia or pericarditis. Review previous medical history for peptic ulcer disease and the drug chart for NSAID use. Consider a TTE for persistent chest discomfort that is neither ischemic nor musculoskeletal in origin to exclude late cardiac tamponade presenting atypically, and a CT chest to identify mediastinitis if the patient has other evidence of infection.

Myocardial ischemia

Myocardial ischemia on ICU is covered on 📖 p185. Presentation later after cardiac surgery with myocardial ischemia may be due to factors listed in Box 6.4.

Box 6.4 Causes of post-op myocardial ischemia

- Incomplete revascularization.
- Early graft occlusion (usually related to technical issue).
- Vasospasm of arterial conduits (unusual once patient has left ICU).
- Trauma to native coronaries at or near annulus during valve surgery.
- Hypotension.
- Arrhythmias.
- Hypoxemia, profound anemia.

Diagnosis

Take a history: focus on dull pain related to exertion (ischemic) vs. sharp, positional, or pain worse on coughing. The physiotherapists may report bradycardia on exercising. A 12-lead EKG will confirm the presence of myocardial ischemia. Cardiac enzymes (CK-MB and troponin I and T) are often raised postoperatively, but serial measurements showing a continued or large rise suggest ongoing myocardial ischemia. The definitive investigation is cardiac catheterization to identify coronary obstruction.

Management

In patients with poor native vessels where incomplete revascularization was all that was possible, medical treatment is the mainstay. In patients with normal coronary arteries who underwent valve surgery, and in patients thought to have undergone complete revascularization, ongoing ischemia may need ICU management (🕮 p185), otherwise:

• Ensure the patient is on aspirin 325mg od po.
• Ensure patients with radial artery grafts, or total arterial revascularization are given calcium channel blockers (diltiazem 60mg three times a day po) if BP will allow.
• Consider re-starting preoperative antianginal medication.
• Discuss indications for angiography with surgeons and a cardiologist.

Perioperative myocardial infarction

Box 6.5 contains the criteria for diagnosis of primary MI. Perioperative MI is difficult to diagnose because the patient may be unable to give a good history, or to distinguish between cardiac and non-cardiac chest pain; postoperative EKGs contain many non-specific changes, and heart block may mask ST changes; and because cardiac enzymes are usually raised postoperatively. New Q waves are diagnostic after the fact.

Box 6.5 Diagnostic criteria for myocardial infarction

In the setting of symptoms suggestive of acute coronary syndrome:
• EKG shows ST segment elevation: STEMI.
• No ST elevation, but elevated CK-MB (2 × normal) and troponin positive: non-Q wave or NSTEMI.

Causes

Graft occlusion (🕮 p303) causes infarcts but up to 80% of perioperative infarcts are supplied by patent grafts. The causes of MI in these cases are incomplete revascularization, inadequate myocardial protection, emboli, and vasospasm.

Diagnosis and management

These signs suggest perioperative MI, which normally manifests on ICU:
• Hemodynamic compromise associated with:
  • ST depression, new Q waves (new T wave inversion is a common finding in postoperative EKGs and probably does not reflect MI) and a significant increase in CK-MB beyond usual postoperative levels.
• Regional reduction in wall motion on echo.

Management is described on 🕮 p185.

Late arrhythmias

Atrial fibrillation

This protocol can also be used to treat multiple ventricular ectopics. Go and see the patient! If the patient is hemodynamically stable reassure them: AF happens to 1 in 3 patients after cardiac surgery. If patient is hemodynamically compromised (because of fast rate, hypertrophic LV following AVR for AS) organize DC cardioversion (📖 p224). Treat with:

• 10–20mmol KCl via central line to bring serum K^+ to 4.5–5.0mmol/L.
• 10–20mmol $MgSO_4$ via central line empirically.
• Restart β-blocker if this has been stopped, even if ↓BP.
• 300mg amiodarone over 1h via central line if mod to good LV.
• Followed by 900mg amiodarone over 23h iv, then oral dose.
• If poor LV give 250 micrograms digoxin iv over 30 minutes instead, and repeat digoxin to a maximum of 1500 micrograms, or until rate controlled.
• If no central access give potassium orally (e.g., 4 × tablets Sando-K) or peripherally (20mmol in 500mL N saline over 4h).
• Give magnesium sulfate orally.
• Load amiodarone orally (400mg three times a day for 24h).
• If the patient has longstanding AF and cardioversion is unlikely, digoxin may help gain rate control.
• Patients in AF should be on a LMWH and aspirin to prevent formation of mural thrombi, stroke, and PE.

Risk factors for atrial fibrillation postoperatively

• Age.
• Preoperative AF.
• Hypokalemia.
• β-blocker withdrawal.
• Inotropes especially dopamine, dobutamine, and isoprenaline.
• Digoxin toxicity can cause fast AF.
• Sepsis, especially chest infection.

Management of AF refractory to medical therapy

It is important to re-establish sinus rhythm in patients with new AF after cardiac surgery. Although AF is perceived as a largely benign arrhythmia, patients have a five fold increase in the incidence of neurological events postoperatively. 15% of patients in AF have been shown by TEE to develop mural thrombus within 48h (📖 p219). Long-term warfarinization is associated with a 0.5% pa incidence of intracranial hemorrhage (📖 p219).

• If a patient has been in constant AF for >36h but <72h despite optimal medical treatment they should undergo DC cardioversion under TEE guidance (📖 p224).
• If a patient has been in constant AF for over 72h, but has not been anticoagulated, they should be sent home on warfarin with a target INR of 2–2.5 and a reducing dose of amiodarone (200mg tid po 1 week, 200mg bid po 1 week, 200mg od po 4 weeks), reviewed in clinic

at 6 weeks and if they are still in AF they should be DC cardioverted, or if in sinus stop warfarin and amiodarone.
- If the patient is in paroxysmal AF a DC cardioversion is likely to have only temporary success: warfarinize and reassess in 6 weeks as described earlier.
- It is occasionally appropriate to attempt DC cardioversion for established AF in patients who have not been anticoagulated, providing that no mural thrombus can be identified on a TEE immediately prior to DC cardioversion.

Bradyarrhythmias

The diagnosis of bradycardias is explained on 📖 pp217 and 221. The commonest causes of bradycardias after cardiac surgery are:
- Drugs: β-blockers, calcium channel blockers, amiodarone, digoxin.
- Heart block, particularly post valve surgery.
- Patient's normal resting heart rate (e.g., fit, young patients).
- Hypoxia (late sign).

Management

Go and assess the patient: are they sitting up comfortably having tea, or are they unresponsive?
- If unresponsive follow the arrest protocol (inside front cover).
- Look for pacing wires and connect them to a functioning box (📖 p228).
- In an emergency give atropine 0.5 mg iv and repeat up to 3mg in total.
- In an emergency it is possible to pace externally (Fig. 5.18).
- If the patient is comfortable simply stop any iv amiodarone or digoxin, stop calcium channel blockers and β-blockers.
- Check electrolytes and blood sugar and treat accordingly.
- Get a 12-lead EKG to exclude new heart block or ischemia.
- Heart block postoperatively normally resolves within 3–4 days as hematoma and edema around the conducting pathways settle, and electrolyte abnormalities are stabilized, but if this does not happen discuss the patient with the cardiologists with a view to a pacemaker: they will usually request an event recorder or 24h tape.
- If a patient waiting for permanent pacemaker insertion needs anticoagulation use iv heparin.
- If a patient is transferred from ICU with no or minimal underlying rhythm, always make sure they are monitored with telemetry, and that you check the pacing thresholds daily (📖 p231). If these start to rise, the patient needs a permanent pacemaker or temporary transvenous pacing wires.

Indications for permanent pacemaker post-op
- Complete heart block.
- Mobitz type II heart block.
- Bradycardia <40bpm, associated with congestive cardiac failure, pauses >3s, or symptoms.
- Symptomatic bifascicular or trifascicular block.
- First-degree heart block in isolation is not an indication for a PPM.

Other cardiac problems

Hypertension

Once antihypertensive infusions such as NTG and propofol are discontinued, and myocardial function recovers from the insult of surgery, BP normally returns to preoperative levels. Preoperatively most patients have high BP controlled with a variety of oral medication including antianginals, most of which are discontinued in the perioperative period. Hypertension becomes a feature of most patients by day 3 postoperatively if appropriate drugs are not started. To treat hypertension restart preoperative antihypertensives at a lower dose, bearing in mind the following considerations:

- Patients should not need antianginals, e.g., nitroglycerin, isosorbide mononitrate, or nicorandil, and these are normally discontinued.
- ACE inhibitors (ramipril 2.5–10mg od po nocte) are started routinely in most patients for secondary prevention, and used in patients with poor LV to reduce afterload.
- ACE II inhibitors (losartan 40mg bid po) are used in patients where the dry ACE inhibitor cough is problematic.
- ACE inhibitors are not restarted in patients with hypotension or impaired renal function, but this may be reviewed when the patient is seen in outpatients.
- Start β-blockers, e.g., metoprolol 12.5–75mg po bid for secondary prevention, arrhythmia prophylaxis, and BP control.
- Patients with radial artery grafts are usually on a calcium channel blocker (diltiazem 60mg od po for 6 weeks) to prevent vasospasm.
- In patients with tachyarrhythmias and good LV function, β-blockers are the first-line treatment for hypertension, but calcium channel blockers can also work well in this context.

Pericarditis

Pericarditis post-cardiotomy (also known as post-pericardiotomy and Dressler's syndrome) affects about 5% of patients. It is commoner in young patients. It may occur within a week of surgery or be delayed by several months.

Diagnosis

- The classical findings are constant chest pain that is sore rather than dull, pyrexia, and a pericardial rub.
- Malaise, lethargy, myalgia, and arthralgia often feature.
- WCC, ESR, and CRP are often raised.
- Pericardial and/or pleural effusions may be noted on CXR and echocardiography.
- ST segments are elevated concave upwards in all leads.

Treatment

- Give NSAIDs (ibuprofen 400mg tid po for 6 weeks).
- Prednisolone (10mg od po) has been used successfully in cases refractory to NSAIDs. Associated pericardial effusion should be treated as appropriate (📖 pp259, 265).

Pericardial effusion

Many patients have small pericardial effusions postoperatively which resolve without causing cardiac tamponade. In about 5% of patients these effusions increase in size. If the patient is not hemodynamically compromised by cardiac tamponade (🕮 p259), these effusions may be treated by starting or increasing diuretic therapy.

* Most patients are already on furosemide 40mg po od, and this may be increased in increments up to 80mg po bid.
* If this fails to correct edema and effusions, consider adding spironolactone 25mg po od (a potassium-sparing diuretic which is particularly effective in the setting of ascites) or a short course of bumetanide 2mg od po for 72h or metolazone 5mg od po for 72h (these are thiazide diuretics which are effective at reducing refractory fluid overload but can impair renal function).
* Correct hypoalbuminemia by securing a dietician review to assess nutrition and prescribing protein food and drink supplements (cartons of Fortisips, Fortijuice, or Ensure with every meal) or NG feeding.
* Cardiac tamponade must be actively excluded and, if present, treated (🕮 p259).

Constrictive pericarditis

Constrictive pericarditis complicates about 0.1% of cardiotomies, and is a late sequelae of up to half of cases of post-cardiotomy syndrome. A hemorrhagic pericarditis progresses over a matter of months to years to a thickened, fibrotic, and frequently calcified pericardium that tamponades the heart (🕮 p488). Other risk factors include mediastinal irradiation and postoperative hemopericardium. The diagnosis and management is described on 🕮 pp488–489.

Complications of valve surgery

See Table 6.4.

Table 6.4 Overview of the complications of valve surgery

Complication	Mechanical valve	Bioprosthetic valve
Infective endocarditis	0.5% within 30 days, 2% at 5 years.	0.2% within 30 days, 2% at 5 years
Prosthesis failure	Negligible	Aortic 30% at 15 years, mitral 60% at 15 years
Bleeding problems	2% of patients will have a major bleeding episode pa. Mortality 1.3% pa Thromboembolism: 2% pa	Bleeding events rare, thromboembolism 1% pa Annual stroke rate lower than for mechanical valves
Heart block	13% transient. 2% permanent. Uncommon in MVR	13% transient. 2% permanent. Uncommon in MVR
Survival	No difference	No difference

Infective endocarditis

Infective endocarditis complicates 0.2–0.5% of mechanical valve replacements within 30 days of surgery, 2% at 5 years, and 1% pa thereafter. The figures for tissue valves are similar, but slightly less at 30 days. Prosthetic endocarditis is described on 📖 p418.

- Blood cultures should be taken in any valve patient with a temperature >36.5°C more than 3 days postoperatively.
- Standard advice regarding antibiotic prophylaxis for invasive procedures should be adhered to from day 1 after surgery, not just following discharge: bladder catheterization should be covered by one dose of gentamicin 120mg im, for example.
- Any potential source of bacteremia should be treated aggressively: infective endocarditis can result from iv cannula cellulitis, superficial wound infections, urinary and respiratory tract infections, and most commonly infections related to arterial and central venous catheters.

Paraprosthetic leak

Incidental paraprosthetic leaks occur in about 2% of aortic valve replacements and 1% of mitral valve replacements. Paraprosthetic leaks within 30 days of surgery are usually either the result of the sewing ring being poorly seated within a calcified, irregular annulus; or the result of a suture cutting out of the annulus. Wash jets, the regurgitant jets typical of the valve mechanism, may be mistaken for paravalvular leaks.

- Late paravalvular leaks are usually associated with endocarditis, in which case they almost inevitably require surgical repair after treatment with antibiotics.
- High-velocity paravalvular leaks may cause hemolysis (📖 p289) severe enough to be an indication for valve replacement.
- If neither hemolysis or infective endocarditis is present, the management of the paravalvular leak depends on the degree of hemodynamic compromise: small leaks that do not progress can be treated conservatively for many years.

Prosthesis failure

Structural problems, not associated with thrombosis, endocarditis, hemolysis or hemorrhage, may necessitate valve replacement.

- Structural failure of mechanical valves is rare: the few valves that have had a higher than expected incidence of problems, such as the silver-coated sewing ring of the Silzone valve, have been withdrawn.
- Bioprostheses last longer in the aortic position and older patients than in the mitral position and younger patients (📖 p366): a 70-year-old having bioprosthetic AVR is very unlikely to experience bioprosthesis failure, whereas a 50-year-old has a roughly 50% lifetime risk of prosthesis failure.
- Patients are reviewed yearly, either by the cardiologists or by the surgeons, with a TTE to identify and monitor valve failure.
- The indications for surgery for structural failure of a bioprosthesis are similar to those for native valves (📖 pp376, 342, with a higher threshold for intervention according to the risk of reop surgery).

Bleeding and thromboembolism

Thromboembolic events include TIA and stroke. Valve thrombosis is obstruction of the mechanism of the prosthesis due to thrombus.

- The incidence of thromboembolism is the same in patients with tissue valves as it is in appropriately anticoagulated patients with mechanical valves: 1–2%% per patient per year. Patients with mechanical valves have a higher stroke risk because there is a 1–2% pa risk of major hemorrhagic event including strokes associated with anticoagulation.
- Valve thrombosis is most commonly due to inadequate anticoagulation because of poor compliance, changes in other medication and illness: 95% of cases of valve thrombosis therefore occur in mechanical valves.
- Smaller aortic valves may be at higher risk than larger valves.
- Patients with prosthetic valve thrombosis may present with angina, pulmonary edema, poor peripheral perfusion and systemic embolization, and acute hemodynamic compromise. TTE, TEE, fluoroscopy or CT may be needed to show failure of one or both leaflets to open.
- Thrombi <5mm that are not obstructing the valve orifice or mechanism may be treated with formal anticoagulation alone. Thrombolysis is rarely effective in chronic organized thrombus: the treatment is emergency reoperative valve replacement with a bioprosthesis.

Complete heart block

About 15% of patients undergoing isolated mitral or aortic valve replacement suffer transient heart block postoperatively, and so most surgeons routinely place temporary epicardial pacing wires.

- Heart block normally settles after 3–4 days as hematoma and edema resolves: persistence beyond this should be discussed with a cardiologist in case a PPM is indicated (📖 p263).
- About 1% of valve surgery patients will require permanent pacemaker insertion (📖 p263); this is a day case procedure and should not delay discharge, but may be postponed until the INR is <1.5.
- The preoperative risk factors for PPM are not well defined but probably include preoperative heart block and heavily calcified valves.

Respiratory complications

Chest infection

Incidence of pneumonia after cardiac surgery varies from 2 to 20%. The variation in incidence reflects variation in diagnostic criteria.

Diagnosis

A history of cough with purulent sputum, or purulent secretions aspirated from the ET tube, suggests chest infection. Pyrexia, bronchial breath sounds, reduced air entry, leukocyte neutrophila, raised CRP, and signs of consolidation on CXR confirm the diagnosis. Sputum culture may yield sensitivities of causative organisms. In the dyspneic, hypoxic patient perform arterial blood gases to guide immediate management.

Management

There is no good evidence that preoperative physiotherapy helps to prevent chest infection after surgery. The single most important intervention is to prevent patients with active chest infections undergoing surgery: any elective patient with a current cough (dry or productive), temperature, clinical signs of chest infection, neutrophilia, or suspicious CXR should be deferred for a fortnight and then reassessed. Other risk factors include active smokers, or patients who have stopped smoking within the last 6 weeks, patients with COPD, obesity, patients requiring prolonged ventilation, and patients who aspirate, particularly those recovering from stroke or with a vocal cord paresis.

- Physiotherapy helps patients expectorate, preventing mucus plugging.
- Effective analgesia is important to allow patients to cough.
- Culture sputum and blood, bronchoscope intubated patients.
- Empiric antibiotic cover varies between institutions but ciprofloxacin 250mg bid po provides good Gram −ve and +ve cover until organism sensitivities are known. Treat aspiration pneumonia with iv cefuroxime 1g tid and iv metronidazole 500mg tid.
- If the patient requires oxygen (PaO$_2$ <8.0kPa on room air) humidifying it reduces the risk of mucus plugs, and makes secretions easier to shift.
- The hypoxic, tachypneic, tiring patient on maximal respiratory support should be reviewed urgently by a senior for reintubation.

Pulmonary embolism

Postoperative PE is rare (<2% of cases) because bypass results in residual heparin effect, hemodilution, thrombocytopenia, and platelet dysfunction; and LMWH and TED stockings are used universally. The diagnosis and management is discussed in more detail on pp476–477.

Vocal cord problems

The incidence after cardiac surgery is probably about 1–2%. Patients present with hoarseness, breathlessness, difficulty phonating and expectorating, and coughing after drinking. These patients should be placed NPO to minimize risk of aspiration pneumonia, be reviewed by an ENT surgeon (vocal cord injection may be required) and undergo a speech and swallow assessment.

Exacerbation of COPD

The incidence of COPD in cardiac surgical patients is about 5%.

- Most studies show that mild to moderate COPD is not associated with a significant increase in postoperative complications, mortality, or length of stay.
- Severe COPD and preoperative steroid use has an associated incremental mortality of around 2% following cardiac surgery, with significantly poorer medium- and long-term outcomes.
- Ensure that all patients are routinely prescribed regular postoperative nebulizers (saline 5mL prn, salbutamol 2.5–5mg 4 times a day prn and becotide 500 micrograms 4 times a day prn) which also reduce risk of mucus plugging.
- β-blockers may safely be recommenced, but beware of starting β-blockers for the first time in patients with asthma or severe COPD.
- In hypoxic patients with COPD give maximal oxygen by CPAP if necessary and monitor blood gases: do *not* restrict oxygen for fear of reducing hypoxic respiratory drive, as in the acute setting hypoxia is a far more important complication than problems due to hypercapnia.

Pleural effusion

Up to 40% of patients undergoing cardiac surgery develop pleural effusions which may be unilateral or bilateral. IMA harvesting is associated with a higher rate of ipsilateral pleural effusions: up to 75% of patients are affected. It is unclear if pleurotomy at the time of IMA harvest, or taking pedicled rather skeletonized IMA, increase the risk of pleural effusion.

Diagnosis

Often asymptomatic. Dyspnea, pleuritic chest pain, decreased air entry, dullness to percussion suggest pleural effusion. It may be difficult to distinguish between consolidation and effusion on a CXR, but a meniscus is suggestive of pleural effusion and an air–fluid level diagnostic of a hydropneumothorax. If in doubt US or chest CT will quantify the size of the effusion and locate a safe area and direction for drainage.

Management

- Small pleural effusions can be treated with increasing diuretic therapy (furosemide 40–80mg bid).
- Large pleural effusions (>3–4cm deep on US) should be drained with a pigtail catheter (📖 p249) if late or a formal chest drain (📖 p248) if early and likely to be predominantly blood and clots.
- Leave the drain in on suction until <100mL drains in 24h.

Phrenic nerve paresis

Phrenic nerve paresis after cardiac surgery is common, although it may not manifest clinically. Although direct trauma particularly during IMA harvest, traction from the sternal retractor, SVC cannulation, and diabetic neuropathy have all been suggested as causes, the single most important factor is probably cold injury from slush placed in the pericardial cradle for topical cooling. Unilateral injury is of limited importance in patients with good respiratory function. Diagnosis and management of bilateral phrenic nerve palsy is discussed on 📖 pp748–749.

Renal complications

Acute renal failure

The etiology, diagnosis, and management of renal failure on ICU is described on 📖 pp232–238. Patients with elevated creatinine and urea who have returned to the ward should be weighed daily and have daily serum electrolytes monitored. If renal markers deteriorate:

- Insert a urinary catheter and commence hourly fluid balance chart.
- Recheck the drug chart for and stop nephrotoxic medication, e.g., ACE inhibitors, NSAIDs, and antibiotics such as teicoplanin and gentamycin.
- Actively look for and exclude relative hypotension, hypovolemia, sepsis, and delayed cardiac tamponade as reversible causes.
- If the patient is hypovolemic stop diuretic therapy and hydrate carefully. If fluid overloaded give 80mg iv furosemide.
- Ask yourself if the patient needs readmission to ICU for central venous monitoring and inotropic support.

Refractory peripheral edema

The pathophysiology underlying the state of fluid and salt overload in most patients is described on 📖 pp106–107. In most patients this corrects with a large diuresis, encouraged with loop diuretics, over the first few days postoperatively, but in a minority significant fluid overload persists. If patient weight remains >3kg above preoperative weight:

- Check serum electrolytes and treat appropriately (following sections).
- Check albumin and treat with daily protein supplements if low: this will take days to weeks to correct.
- If edema is refractory to furosemide increased to up to 80mg po bid, consider a stat dose of bumetanide (2mg po) or metolazone (5mg po) which may be repeated if creatinine is not elevated.
- Spironolactone 25–50mg po od is a potassium-sparing diuretic that is effective for management of ascites and pleural effusions.
- Consider fluid restriction of 1500mL per 24h.
- Treat symptomatically with TED stockings and elevation of legs.
- Unilateral peripheral edema may be caused by DVT, cellulitis, extravastion of iv fluids, stroke, hematoma, and saphenous vein harvest.

Hypokalemia

Hypokalemia (K^+ <4.0) is common and as it predisposes patients to arrhythmias, such as AF and digoxin toxicity it should be treated. Hypokalemia is normally caused by diuretic therapy, insulin sliding scales, diarrhea and vomiting, steroids and poor nutrition. Acute severe hypokalemia (K^+ <3.0) in postoperative cardiac patients may result in life-threatening arrhythmias. It can be recognized by small or inverted T waves, depressed ST segments, prolonged PR interval, and U waves on the EKG (Fig. 5.13d).

- Educate the patient about which foods are rich in potassium (bananas, prunes, apricots, tomatoes, orange juice) and ensure availability.
- Change furosemide to co-amilofruse 5/40 or 2.5/20 which contains furosemide (either 40mg or 20mg) and amiloride (5mg or 2.5mg) which is a potassium-sparing thiazide diuretic.

- Add oral potassium supplements up to 160mmol daily (1 tablet of Sando K^+ contains 20mmol of K^+, 1 tablet of Slow K^+ which is better tolerated by most patients contains 12.5mmol KCl).
- If a central line is in place give 20mmol KCl in 50–100mL of 5% dextrose over 20min to 1h. Never give a bolus of KCl.
- If it is necessary to use a peripheral line place a maximum of 40mmol of potassium in 1L 5% dextrose running at a maximum of 125mL/h.
- Monitor KCl daily, and avoid discharging the patient home on a combination of potassium supplements and potassium-sparing diuretics as rebound hyperkalemia will be a risk.

Hyperkalemia

Hyperkalemia (K^+ >5.0) is seen in the setting of renal failure, tissue necrosis, and potassium-sparing diuretics and supplements. Acute hyperkalemia (K^+ >6.0) can cause life-threatening ventricular arrhythmias. EKG changes that herald myocardial dysfunction are flattened P waves, wide QRS complexes, tenting of T waves, and in peri-arrest hyperkalemia a sine wave appearance (Fig. 5.13c).

- Treat the patient with EKG changes as an emergency.
- Give 50mL of 50% dextrose containing 15U of Actrapid insulin as an infusion over 10–20min, repeating as necessary, checking blood sugar and K^+ after each infusion (use blood gas machine).
- Give 10mL calcium gluconate 10% iv over 2min, repeat.
- Calcium Resonium or Kayexalate® enema binds K^+ and removes it from the body.
- Dialysis should be urgently considered in patients with refractory hyperkalemia despite these measures, irrespective of renal function.

Hyponatremia

Hyponatremia (Na^+ <135mmol/L) occurs in fluid overload where patients have been given 5% dextrose fluid maintenance over long periods rather than normal saline, as a result of diuretic therapy, diarrhea and vomiting, renal failure, cardiac and liver failure, and SIADH (syndrome of inappropriate ADH secretion). Profound hyponatremia will lead to confusion and fits as a result of potentially life-threatening cerebral edema. Assess the patient for dehydration or edema, and measure urine osmolality and urinary sodium. SIADH is diagnosed by finding concentrated urine (sodium >20mmol/L) in the setting of hyponatremia; or hypo-osmolar plasma (<260mmol/kg), and low serum cortisol without hypovolemia.

- If the patient is edematous restrict daily fluid intake initially to 1.5–1.0L.
- Stop thiazide diuretics, but continue loop diuretics.
- If dehydrated give 1L normal saline iv over 8–12h.
- SIADH occurs in 1–2% of cardiac surgery patients as a result of increased secretion of vasopressin (or ADH) and should be treated by a combination of fluid restriction for several days. Loop diuretics, and sodium supplements may help.

Disturbances of acid–base balance

These are discussed on 📖 pp168–171.

Gastrointestinal symptoms

Abdominal pain

Distinguishing between peritonitic and colicky pain is particularly difficult in elderly, sedated, or confused patients following cardiac surgery. Classic signs of peritonitis, and localizing signs are frequently not present despite major intra-abdominal pathology. Take a full history, note recent drug regimes, examine the patient, and request CBC, biochemistry, LFTs, amylase, CRP, blood gases, abdominal plain film, and erect CXR in the first instance. Stool and blood cultures should be taken.

Differential diagnosis of post-op abdominal pain
- Constipation or paralytic ileus.
- Wound pain, muscular pain from coughing.
- Myocardial ischemia, lower lobe pneumonia.
- Peptic ulceration.
- Pancreatitis.
- Gallbladder pathology including cholecystitis, biliary colic.
- Small and large bowel obstruction.
- Ischemic bowel.
- Perforated viscus (chest tubes, TEE, ischemia).

Constipation

Failure to pass stool by day 4 postoperatively is not uncommon. Constipation may be caused by reluctance to use a bed pan, lack of privacy, immobility, pain on straining from wounds or anal fissures, dehydration, poor nutrition, inadequate dietary fiber, opiate analgesia, iron supplements, tricyclic antidepressants, and spinal anesthesia. Treatments are:

- Bulking agents, such as increasing dietary fiber with bran or dried fruit, methylcellulose 500mg tid, all of which increase stool bulk and decrease transit time.
- Stool softeners such as liquid paraffin, glycerin suppositories 1–2 od pr and phosphate enemas 1–2 od pr.
- Osmotic agents such as lactulose 10–20mL bid or magnesium hydroxide 50mL per 24h po, which should be taken with plenty of water.
- Stimulants such as senna 1 tablet bid po, bisacodyl 5–20mg nocte po, sodium docusate 60mg od po, co-danthramer 50mg po od, which should not be used in the long term as tolerance develops.

Diarrhea

Liquid stools may be caused by preoperative conditions such as inflammatory bowel disease or irritable bowel, or acute GI pathology including ischemic bowel and GI bleeding, but is more commonly due to inappropriate prescribing of laxatives, antibiotic therapy, digoxin, and cimetidine.

- Pseudomembranous colitis is caused by overgrowth of *Clostridium difficile* following antibiotic therapy, particularly with cephalosporins: send stools for culture and treat positive *C. diff* toxin diarrhea with either oral metronidazole (400mg tid) or oral vancomycin (125mg qid).

Nausea and vomiting

This affects up to 75% of patients. It predisposes to increased bleeding, incisional hernias, aspiration pneumonia, reduced absorption of oral medication, impaired nutrition, and metabolic abnormalities such as hypokalemia. Causes include:

- Bypass, prolonged surgery, anesthetic agents, e.g., etomidate, ketamine, N_2O, intraoperative and postoperative opioids, spinal anesthesia, gastric dilatation from ineffective bag and mask ventilation CPAP.
- Postoperative ileus, bowel obstruction, constipation, gastric reflux, peptic ulceration or bleeding, medications including many antibiotics, NSAIDs, opiates, statins, pancreatitis, sepsis, and hyponatremia.

Treat by withholding opiate analgesia (use regular paracetamol and NSAIDs if no contraindications), starting regular antiemetic, e.g., ondansetron, adding a second with different mechanism of action if needed, mobilizing patient. Treat ileus, monitor and correct fluid and electrolyte losses.

Classification of antiemetics

- Combination of two different types of antiemetic increases efficiency.

Antidopaminergic agents
- Active against emetic effect of opiods. Sedative. Extrapyramidal side effects—avoid in Parkinson's disease.
- E.g., prochlorperazine 12.5mg im, droperidol 1–1.25 mg iv, metaclopramide 10mg iv/im/po tid.

Antihistamines
- Sedation, tachycardias, hypotension with iv injection.
- E.g., cyclizine 50mg im/iv/po tid.

Anticholinergics
- Active against emetic effect opioids. Sedation, confusion, dry mouth
- E.g., hyoscine (scopolamine) 0.3–0.6mg im.

Antiserotonergics
- Lowest side effect profile of all antiemetics. Effective in chemotherapy nausea. Quite useful for postoperative nausea and vomiting.
- E.g., ondansetron 1–8mg po/iv/im tid, granisetron 1mg po/iv tid.

Paralytic ileus

Paralytic ileus occurs in up to 5% of patients after cardiac surgery. It may share features with small bowel obstruction, including nausea, vomiting, constipation, absent bowel sounds, and dilated loops of gas-filled bowel on abdominal plain film: usually patients are pain free, and passing flatus.

- Possible causes include gastric distension from ineffective bag and mask ventilation or CPAP, splanchnic and mesenteric ischemia, venous congestion, pseudomembranous colitis, drugs particularly opiates, other GI pathology including peptic ulceration, cholecystitis, and pancreatitis.
- Pass an NG tube to decompress the stomach and consider a flatus tube.
- Stop opiates and contributing drugs, and mobilize patients if possible.
- Put the patient NPO and give normal saline 80–125mL/h iv.
- Prolonged ileus and pseudo-obstruction may necessitate colonoscopy.

Gastrointestinal complications

Serious gastrointestinal complications occur in about 2% of patients following cardiac surgery, with previous history of GI pathology, age, severe atherosclerosis, or vascular disease all risk factors. The diagnosis is more difficult in postoperative, sedated, confused, and elderly patients, but the management is much the same as in non-surgical patients. Half of these patients undergo laparotomy: the mortality is up to 20%.

Upper gastrointestinal bleeding

Upper GI bleeding is most commonly caused by peptic ulcer disease, followed by gastritis, esophageal varices, esophageal tears and occasionally trauma to the esophagus or oropharynx from intubation with NG tubes, and TEE probes. Peptic ulceration risk after cardiac surgery is increased by the stress of major surgery, anticoagulation, NSAIDs, coagulopathy, and splanchnic hypoperfusion.

Diagnosis
- Hematemesis (may be via NG tube) more commonly occult.
- Melena, or positive fecal occult blood (FOB) test (guaiac).
- Abdominal pain, peritonism, hypotension, tachycardia.
- Drop in Hb (1g/dL per unit of blood lost) may be only evidence.

Prophylaxis
- Prophylaxis with omeprazole 20mg po od or omeprazole 40mg iv infusion over 2h should be given to patients with a history of peptic ulcer disease, gastritis, or hiatus hernia.
- Start NG feeding patients that fail to extubate early: 10mL h NG feed offers gastric protection reducing translocation of endotoxin.
- Avoid NSAIDs in patients with any history of dyspepsia or elderly.

Management
- Secure iv access with two large gauge (grey or brown) cannulas in the antecubital fossa, or use a Swann sheath if present for rapid volume replacement (a triple lumen is insufficient as it is long and narrow).
- XM 4 units of blood
- Transfuse blood to bring the Hb back to 8–9.0g/dL, titrating the rate of transfusion against BP, pulse, and CVP if available.
- Check coagulation and correct any coagulopathy.
- Discuss with gastroenterology with a view to esophagogastroduodenoscopy (EGD) ± injection of bleeding points.
- In patients on warfarin for mechanical valves restart heparin (APTT 50–70) once active bleeding subsides or has been treated.

Lower gastrointestinal bleeding

Lower GI bleeding is characterized by fresh rectal blood, but may require passage of an NG tube or even EGD to exclude an upper GI source. Common causes are mesenteric ischemia, infective colitis including *C. difficile*, angiodysplasia (Heydes' syndrome when associated with aortic stenosis), and bleeding from colonic polyps. Mesenteric angiography may be necessary to identify the lesion before surgical resection.

Mesenteric ischemia

Mesenteric ischemia may be caused by global hypoperfusion due to low cardiac output states, high doses of pressors, atherosclerotic embolism, thromboembolism, and associated with sepsis, DIC, or HITT. It presents on the ICU as worsening metabolic acidosis, failure to absorb NG feeds, and abdominal distension. Awake patients may complain of severe abdominal pain, nausea, and vomiting. Diarrhea which may initially be bloody is often present. Bowel sounds are absent. Peritonism is a late sign suggesting perforation. Diagnosis on clinical grounds is difficult in the paralyzed and ventilated patient. Contrast CT or angiography is useful. Definitive management is laparotomy and resection of infarcted segments with or without primary anastomoses. Not infrequently infarcted areas of bowel are so widespread that surgery is 'open and close' only.

Bowel obstruction

Small and large bowel obstruction post cardiac surgery is most commonly due to adhesions from previous surgery, followed by incarceration of hernias (inguinal, femoral, epigastric, incisional). Rare causes include occult carcinoma and pseudo-obstruction. Small bowel obstruction, which requires urgent general surgical review and surgery if not resolved within 24–48h, is characterized by colicky abdominal pain, nausea, vomiting, and distended loops of small bowel on abdominal X-ray (central valvulae conniventes cross the entire lumen of bowel which measure >6cm in diameter). Large bowel obstruction may usually be managed conservatively for longer.

- Place the patient nil by mouth, pass a NG tube.
- Start iv fluids (normal saline 1L with 40mmol K^+ over 8–12h.
- Discuss with general surgery.
- Reassess for signs of peritonism every few hours, check all labs daily.

Pancreatitis

A transient small rise in serum amylase is seen in over 1/3 of patients, pancreatitis occurs in 1%. It is caused by splanchnic hypoperfusion, but systemic emboli, prolonged use of vasopressors may contribute and activation of inflammatory pathways on bypass also contribute. Preoperative actors such as steroid use, gallstones, alcohol abuse, and hyperlipidemia are less important. Any patient with abdominal pain should have a serum amylase check. Complications of pancreatitis include shock, ARDS, renal failure, $\downarrow Ca^{2+}$, and DIC. Management is conservative:

- Give colloid to replace third-space fluid, with hourly fluid balance.
- Give morphine.
- Inotropic support is required in severe cases.
- Discuss with general surgeons.

Cholecystitis

This has an incidence of up to 1:200 after cardiac surgery, with patients presenting up to 2 weeks after surgery with fever, nausea, abdominal pain. Diagnosis is by US, and treatment is medical (iv fluids, nil by mouth, and antibiotics). The etiology is ischemic injury and cholecystectomy is often indicated.

Liver failure

Hepatic failure

Approximately 10% of patients develop mild hepatic dysfunction after cardiac surgery with a transient rise in liver enzymes and bilirubin. Fulminant hepatic failure, which complicates <0.1% of cardiac surgery patients with no known preoperative hepatic dysfunction, has a mortality of about 80%.

Etiology

- *Preoperative dysfunction*: hepatitis, cirrhosis, biliary obstruction.
- *Hemolysis*: blood transfusion, haematoma, paravalvular leak, glucose 6-phosphate dehydrogenase deficiency, prolonged bypass, excessive use of pump suckers.
- *Hepatocellular injury*: exacerbation of preoperative disease, low cardiac output states, splanchnic ischemia, prolonged high-dose pressors (causes splanchnic hypoperfusion), right heart failure, hepatotoxic drugs (acetaminophen, halothane, antiretrovirals).
- *Cholestasis*: intrahepatic (hepatitis, hepatocellular necrosis, cholestasis, parenteral nutrition, sepsis, drugs including opiates), and extrahepatic (biliary tract obstruction).

Diagnosis

Fulminant hepatic failure is acute hepatic failure occurring within 8 weeks of exposure to the insult, and complicated by hepatic encephalopathy. In addition to increases (in the high thousands) in AST, ALP, LDH and several-fold increase in σ-GT and bilirubin. Features of hepatic failure include:

- Jaundice: secondary to conjugated hyperbilirubinemia.
- Hepatic encephalopathy.
- Coagulopathy: secondary to ↑PT, ↓platelets and platelet function, DIC.
- Ascites.
- Sepsis, including increased susceptibility to fungal infections.
- Acid–base disturbance: commonly metabolic acidosis due to ↑lactate.
- Metabolic derangements: commonly ↓Na.
- Hypoglycemia due to glycogen depletion.
- Cerebral edema and raised intracranial pressure.
- Hepatorenal and hepatopulmonary failure.
- Reduced systemic vascular resistance.
- Arrhythmias including VF.

Management

Modest elevations in liver enzymes and bilirubin are usually transient and benign: no action other than reducing hepatotoxic medication is usually required. Management of fulminant hepatic failure is mostly supportive:

- Check blood glucose frequently and replace as indicated.
- Renal failure requires dialysis.
- Cardiovascular support requires PA catheter insertion and inotropes.
- Give empirical antibiotic prophylaxis.

Hepatorenal failure

Hepatocellular failure is commonly complicated by renal failure. This is attributed to:

- ↑peripheral vasodilation.
- ↑renal vasoconstriction.
- Resulting in ↓GFR and oliguria.

If there is no clear primary cause of renal failure, this is called hepatorenal syndrome. Evidence from transplantation suggests that the renal failure is entirely secondary to liver failure as the renal failure improves both after liver transplantation, and after transplantation of the affected kidney into an individual without liver dysfunction. The renal dysfunction is proportional to the severity of hepatocellular failure, and acute tubular necrosis may supervene. Therapy is supportive: careful management of filling and systemic vascular resistance. Dialysis may be required for refractory acidosis, hyperkalemia, and fluid overload.

Hepatopulmonary syndrome

Hepatocellular failure is less commonly complicated by hypoxemia, as a result of abnormal ventilation–perfusion ratios and diffusion capacity. This is attributable to:

- ↑ intrapulmonary vasodilatation.
- ↑PVR.
- Failure of oxygen to diffuse as readily into the centre of dilated vessels.
- ↑CO limiting the time for gas exchange.

Stroke

The incidence of stroke in cardiac surgery is about 1–2% for CABG, 2–3% for valve. Patients with one or more risk factors have a much higher incidence of stroke: this affects consent and operative planning.

Risk factors for stroke
- Increasing age (>80 years risk of CVA 3–5%).
- Diabetes.
- Previous history of stroke or TIA (increases risk three-fold).
- Carotid artery atherosclerosis.
- Perioperative hypotension.
- Calcified or very atherosclerotic ascending aorta.
- Calcified aortic or mitral valve.
- Left-sided mural thrombus.
- Cardiotomy.
- Long duration of CPB, DHCA.
- Postoperative AF.
- Failure to give antiplatelet therapy postoperatively.

Etiology

Embolic
- Microemboli, debris from operative field.
- Mural thrombus.
- Debris from valve excision, particularly calcified aortic valve.
- Septic emboli from endocarditis.
- Trauma to aorta from cannulation and clamping.
- Air embolism.
- Carotid atheroma.

Hemorrhagic
- Heparinization on bypass.
- Postoperative warfarinization.

Cerebral hypoperfusion
- Carotid and vertebral artery stenosis, dissection.
- Hypotension.
- Circulatory arrest (long period or insufficient cooling).
- Raised intracranial pressure.

Hypoxia
- Profound hypoxia before, during or after bypass for >3min.

Clinical features

Most neurological deficits are apparent once sedation has been weaned (i.e., within 24h), but 1/3 of strokes occur several days postoperatively. Any deficit resolving within 24h is called a transient ischemic attack (TIA). Clinical features include:
- Failure to regain consciousness once sedation has been weaned.
- Hemiplegia (middle cerebral artery or total carotid artery occlusion).

- Initial areflexia becoming hyperreflexia and rigidity after a few days.
- Aphasia, dysarthria, ataxia, inadequate gag reflex, aspiration.
- Visual deficits, unilateral neglect, confusion.
- Persistent, marked hypertension, hypercapnia.

Diagnosis

The aim is to establish a definitive diagnosis, establish a cause to guide appropriate secondary prevention, and establish a baseline of function to help plan long-term rehabilitation, or withdrawal of therapy.

- Carry out a full neurological examination (cognitive function, cranial nerves, and tone, power, reflexes, and sensation in all four limbs).
- Modern contrast head CT will show infarcts within 2h (older scanners may not pick up lesions until they are 2–3 days old). You must distinguish between hemorrhagic and ischemic CVAs (1 in 10 are hemorrhagic): MRI is necessary to image brainstem lesions.

Prevention

Carotid endarterectomy

The single most important preoperative intervention is identifying significant carotid artery disease. All patients with a previous history of stroke or TIA, or with a carotid bruit should undergo Doppler ultrasonography of their carotids. Some surgeons Doppler all patients over the age of 65, and all patients with other severe extracardiac arteriopathy.

- Patients with a stenosis of their internal carotid artery <75% have a greater risk of stroke from carotid endarterectomy than they have from cardiac surgery alone, and their carotid disease should be left.
- Patients with a stenosis of >75% but <99% of their internal carotid artery and a history of TIA or stroke have a lower risk of stroke if they undergo carotid endarterectomy (or stenting in suitable subjects).
- Generally the overall risk of death or stroke seems lowest if carotids are treated after cardiac surgery, rather than before or as a combined procedure, which also avoids the problem of needing to stop the antiplatelet medication required after carotid stenting.

Operative technique

- Maintain MAPs 80mmHg in patients at risk of ischemic strokes.
- Selection of cannulation sites can be guided by intraoperative US of the ascending aorta, which identifies diseased plaques at risk of embolization, and is much more accurate than digital palpation.
- Meticulous removal of debris from the operative field in open heart (especially aortic valve surgery) surgery, exclusion or air from all arterial lines, and thorough de-airing is a key part of stroke prevention.
- 'No touch' technique in coronary artery bypass grafting (🕮 p321).
- Systemic cooling provides some additional cerebral protection.
- Limiting use of pump suction reduces microemboli.

Postoperative measures

- Aspirin (and clopidogrel after CEA) and BP control.
- Again, maintain MAPs >80mmHg.

Management of stroke

Initial management

- Assess the airway, breathing, and circulation (🕮 inside front cover).
- If the patient is unable to maintain their airway insert a Gudel airway, bag and mask ventilate with 100% O_2, and call anesthesia.
- Monitor BP, but do not attempt to correct high pressures as these are critical for adequate cerebral perfusion.
- Monitor oxygen saturations.
- Secure iv access and give colloid if indicated.
- If the patient is able to maintain their own airway and is not hemodynamically compromised, explain what has happened and reassure.
- Perform a full neurological examination.
- Put the patient NPO if there is no gag reflex.
- Send complete blood count and chemistry, and coagulation.
- Send blood cultures if there is any history of endocarditis, pyrexia.
- Get an EKG (identify AF, heart block, or other causative problem).
- Request an urgent CT head to identify emboli/hemorrhage.
- Unless there is a strong suspicion that the stroke is hemorrhagic, aspirin should be continued, as it has a negligible effect on the outcome of hemorrhagic stroke, but a small positive effect on the outcome of ischemic stroke.

Hemorrhagic stroke

Hemorrhagic stroke (including subarachnoid and subdural hemorrhage and intracranial bleeds) should be suspected if there is a history of head injury, or major coagulopathy. CT confirmation of diagnosis should be obtained urgently as early neurosurgical management may be indicated. If the patient is being warfarinized for a mechanical valve prosthesis the risk of causing an embolic event by reversing anticoagulation (with vit K, FFP, or clotting factors) is <0.02% for each day that the patient is not anticoagulated. The risk of rebleeding is greatest within the first 24h. Anticoagulation should be stopped, and coagulopathy corrected. Restart anticoagulation within 1–2 weeks if the patient is stable.

Embolic stroke

Aim for MAPs 80–100mmHg to improve perfusion. Request TTE to identify source.

Longer-term management

Medical treatment

Cardiothoracic patients are not candidates for thrombolysis: recent major surgery is one of the exclusion criteria. Aspirin reduces death and dependency by 13 patients per every 1000 treated. There is no evidence that LMWH, unfractionated heparin, or warfarin improves outcome.

Secondary prevention

Aspirin, ticlopidine, dipyridamole, and clopidogrel reduce recurrences (relative risk reduction of about 13%). Warfarin and heparin reduce recurrence embolic strokes in AF.

Ventilation

Patients with severe strokes, particularly those involving the basilar artery territories, may need intubation and ventilation for respiratory failure resulting from several causes:
• Abnormal patterns of respiration including apnea, Cheyne–Stokes.
• Loss of protective pharyngeal reflexes leading to aspiration.
• Failure to clear secretions.

Weaning ventilation, including criteria for weaning and extubating, are discussed on 📖 pp164–165. There are three general approaches to weaning:
• Spontaneous breathing trials (SBT).
• Pressure support ventilation (PSV).
• Synchronized intermittent mandatory ventilation (SIMV).

Spontaneous breathing trials can be performed with the patient either on or off the ventilator, and usually involve a T-piece and humidified supplemental oxygen. SBTs last from 30min to 2h. Positive pressure support or CPAP is usually added. In SIMV the mandatory ventilation rate is reduced so that the patient has to increase spontaneous breaths. Tracheostomy (📖 p166) is useful in selected patients to improve comfort but does not increase the speed of weaning from ventilation, which can take weeks to months.

Intubation for apnea complicating stroke is a poor prognostic sign; most deteriorate neurologically, and few of these patients are successfully weaned from ventilation. Intubation primarily for airway protection has a more successful outcome. The majority of patients can be weaned from ventilation, but aspiration pneumonia may complicate recovery.

Feeding

Protective pharyngeal reflexes are impaired in stroke. The decision to remove a tracheal tube and to commence oral feeding is based on standardized swallow assessments, usually carries out by a speech and language therapist (SALT). NG feeding is mandatory until these tests are passed. Feeding is then graduated, starting with thickened fluids and progressing to solids.
• Swallow assessment consists of giving a decannulated patient who is alert and able to sit upright, consecutive teaspoons of water followed by a glass of water: the patient fails if at any stage they fail to actively swallow, or if it results in coughing, spluttering, or gurgly voice.
• The dye test consists of placing a small amount of blue dye in the mouth of the patient with an ET or tracheostomy tube *in situ*: the patient fails if dye is then found in bronchial secretions on suction.
• Videofluoroscopy (modified barium swallow) is the gold standard for diagnosis of continuing aspiration.
• A PEG (percutaneous endoscopic gastrostomy) tube is usually required for long-term feeding in a nursing home environment.

Mobilizing

Structured neurophysiotherapy and intensive nursing is vitally important in preventing complications such as pressure sores, strictures, constipation, and aspiration pneumonia as well as maximizing early return of function.

Neurological complications

Confusion

Confusion is common post-operatively. It is often obvious, with a disoriented, uncooperative, or hallucinating patient. Frequently, confusion is not overt, consisting of inactivity, quietness, slowed thinking, and labile mood, and it is only spotted by relatives or nursing staff. Actively assess whether the patient is oriented in time, person, and place. Perform a quick mini mental state examination if you are still unsure.

Management

- If the patient's behaviour poses a physical danger to himself or others, it may be necessary to sedate as first-line management: haloperidol 2.5mg may be given up to a total of 10mg in 24h po, im, or iv, but if the patient remains disturbed 2.5–5mg of midazolam should be given iv, and the patient placed under close observation.
- Beware of sedating the hypoxic or hypotensive patient as this may trigger a cardiorespiratory arrest.
- Treat respiratory failure (📖 p268) and low BP (📖 p258).
- Reassess the drug chart: stop opiates and benzodiazepines.
- Correct metabolic abnormalities.
- Alcohol withdrawal is diagnosed from a history of chronically high alcohol consumption often with raised σ-GT, combined with psychomotor agitation postoperatively. It can be treated with diazepam 5–10mg tid po/pr: haloperidol lowers the seizure threshold so is not first line therapy for confusion in these patients.
- Perform a neurological examination to look for focal neurological deficit and consider head CT to exclude stroke.
- Reassure patient and relatives: confusion is common, almost always reversible, and it is not a sign that the patient is 'going mad'.

Common causes of confusion

- Sleep deprivation, ICU psychosis.
- Medication (particularly benzodiazepines, opiates, anticonvulsants).
- Stroke, 'post-pump' (micro air emboli).
- Hypoxia, hypercapnia.
- Shock.
- Sepsis.
- Alcohol withdrawal.
- Metabolic disturbances (↓glucose, Na$^+$, pH, ↑Ca^{2+}, Cr, urea, bilirubin).
- Post-ictal.
- Pre-operative dementia.

Seizures

Seizures may be generalized (loss of consciousness with or without tonic-clonic features, absence seizures, atonia) or partial (localized to part of one hemisphere). Causes of seizures include:

- Physical: stroke, intracranial bleed, cerebral air emboli, septic emboli

- Metabolic: withdrawal of alcohol, anticonvulsants or benzodiazepines, (↓↑glucose, Na⁺, pH, Ca²⁺, ↑Cr, urea, bilirubin), tricyclic antidepressants, lidocaine toxicity.

Management
Status epilepticus is any seizure lasting >30min, or repeated seizures without intervening consciousness. Treat by securing the airway, give oxygen, suction if required, diazepam 10mg iv (or PR) over 2min, and then 5mg/min until seizures stop or respiratory depression occurs, then start phenytoin 15mg/kg iv up to 50mg per min if seizures continue. Most seizures are self-limiting: start regular phenytoin as prophylaxis and look for an underlying cause.

Peripheral nerve injuries

Brachial plexus injury
This is caused by indirectly by sternal retraction, and directly by trauma when placing central lines. It presents as paresthesia and weakness in the C8–T1, and if severe C6–C7. Formal diagnosis is by EMG studies. It can be avoided by placing the sternal retractor as caudally as possible and opening it slowly. Treatment is physiotherapy, with referral to a pain service for chronic pain unresponsive to analgesia.

Horner's syndrome
Ptosis, meiosis, anyhydrosis, and enophthalmosis resulting from damage to the sympathetic nerve supply to the eye at any stage from its journey from the central nuclei and spinal cord to post-ganglionic fibres via the stellate ganglion. Inadvertent damage during central line placement, carotid endarterectomy, harvest of the very proximal IMA, and stroke may cause this syndrome. Treatment is symptomatic.

Recurrent laryngeal nerve palsy
This may occur as a result of IMA harvesting, trauma to the arch of the aorta, e.g., from cannulating, trauma to the nerve in the neck from internal jugular vein cannulation, pressure injury from a malpositioned ET cuff, and cold injury. It presents as hoarseness and breathlessness after extubation. Patients should be seen by an ENT surgeon (📖 p268).

Phrenic nerve palsy
This is discussed on 📖 pp269, 748–749.

Sympathetic dystrophy (radial and saphenous nerve)
Injury to these nerves when harvesting conduit usually results in paresthesia (over the anatomical snuff box in radial nerve injury and over the medial malleolus and ankle in saphenous nerve injury). Occasionally this is associated with increasing pain, swelling, and trophic changes (hair loss, shiny skin). Sympathetic dystrophy is difficult to treat: it may respond to NSAIDs such as ibuprofen, regular analgesia, or amitriptyline for intractable neuropathic pain.

Ulnar nerve injury
Failure to protect the arms with padding intraoperatively may lead to ulnar nerve paresis from pressure injury to the ulnar nerve as it passes round the medial epicondyle of the elbow.

Wound infections

Deep sternal wound infection

The incidence of deep sternal wound infection is reported at 0.5–5%. As up to 75% of wound infections present after discharge from hospital, the incidence is frequently under-reported. Risk factors include:

- *Preoperative*: age, diabetes, obesity, smoking, steroid therapy, COPD.
- *Operative*: paramedian sternotomy, bilateral pedicled mammary artery harvest, prolonged surgery, poor surgical technique (including excessive bone wax and cautery to the periosteum, inaccurate placement of sternal wires, poor aseptic technique).
- *Postoperative:* re-sternotomy for bleeding, multiple transfusions, mediastinal bleeding, prolonged ventilation, and impaired nutrition.

Deep sternal wound infection (DSWI) definition

The Centers for Disease Control and Prevention (CDC) define DSWI as infection in tissue deep to the subcutaneous layers *and* either positive cultures, macroscopic/histological evidence, symptomatology, *and* pus.

Diagnosis

- Fever.
- ↑WCC, positive blood cultures.
- Sternal 'click' (ask the patient to cough, or turn their head left and right while feeling for movement in the sternum).
- Serous or purulent discharge, wound dehiscence.
- Pericardial effusion.
- CXR may show fractured or migrating sternal wires.
- CT may show evidence of non-union, pus, and osteomyelitis.

Prevention

- *Preoperative*: weight reduction in obese patients, reducing steroid therapy, optimizing respiratory function, screening for and treating MRSA. Shaving patients in the holding area and not the night before results in lower numbers of skin organisms.
- *Operative:* meticulous aseptic and operative technique. Separate leg and sternal wound instruments (sharing increases the incidence of *E. coli* sternal wound infection).
- *Postoperative*: appropriate antibiotic prophylaxis. One dose must be given on induction to ensure peak blood levels by the time of incision. Wash hands between examining every patient (alcohol rinse has been shown to be more effective than soap and water at reducing cross-infection).

Management

- A cough lock may reduce pain and reduce the impact of dehiscence.
- Iv antibiotics (teicoplanin 400mg od + tazocin 4.5g tid).
- Vacuum dressing.
- Surgical debridement and rewiring may be necessary.

Rewiring for sternal wound infection

This is never undertaken lightly. Patients may have multiple organ dysfunction as a result of sepsis, tissues are friable, and surgery often takes place at a time when adhesions are maximal (4–6 weeks postoperatively). The principles are the same as for an elective resternotomy (□ p346). Ensure that the patient has appropriate antibiotics on induction, a radial arterial and central line. Devitalized tissue is debrided back to bleeding margins, including the sternal edges which need to be undermined sufficiently to place sternal wires. All pus is evacuated from the pericardium, paying great care to anastomotic lines, any of which may be involved in infection. Send pus and bone for culture to guide treatment and detect osteomyelitis. Often primary closure cannot be achieved due to extensive debridement: options include pectoralis major advancement flaps, transrectus abdominus muscle (TRAM) flaps, and rarely omental flaps. Plastic surgeons should be involved for these. There are many alternative closure techniques:

- Standard closure: residual osteomyelitis may flare into repeat infection.
- Betadine washout: adjunct to all techniques, of no proven benefit.
- Robicek closure, sternal bands or plates to improve stability.
- Irrigation systems: used in refractory cases, or for prosthetic material.
- Sternectomy and pec major or omental flap, most commonly staged with vacuum dressings: eradicates most persistent infections.

Superficial wound infection

The CDC defines SWI as infection involving only skin and subcutaneous tissue *and* either purulent drainage, positive cultures, or symptoms. The incidence of superficial sternal wound infection is about 3–5%, open saphenous vein harvest site infection up to 25%, and superficial radial wound harvest site infection about 2%. Diagnosis is usually based on local cellulitis or discharge. Swab the wound, take blood cultures if pyrexial. Management includes:

- Antibiotics, e.g., ciprofloxacin 500mg bid po for 1 week.
- Incision and drainage of any fluctuant areas.
- Vacuum dressing for deep wounds with large amounts of pus.
- Monitoring for any signs of deep sternal wound infection.

Brief guide to antibiotic cover

- Sternal wound and radial artery wound infections are most commonly caused by Gram +ve organisms, and leg wound infections are caused predominantly by Gram −ve organisms.
- Gram +ve organisms (e.g., *Staphylococcus*, *Streptococcus*, and *Clostridium* spp.) are sensitive to penicillins.
- Gram −ve organisms (pseudomonas, *E. coli*, enterobacter, *Klebsiella*, *Shigella*) are sensitive to ciprofloxacin (500mg bid po: oral absorption better than iv).
- Broad-spectrum antibiotics with good Gram −ve and Gram +ve cover include cefuroxime 750–1.5g iv tid.
- MRSA wound infection should be treated with teicoplanin 400mg iv or im bid for two doses then od, or vancomycin 1g bid, both of which are nephrotoxic.

Wound complications

Sternal instability and sterile dehiscence

Sterile sternal instability and dehiscence is usually due to poor surgical technique, or 'cheese-wiring' of sternal wires through a soft, osteoporotic sternum. The incidence is 1–2%. The patient complains of excessive costochondral pain and 'clicking' on movement, and instability may be palpated when the patient coughs. This may be managed either conservatively with prophylactic antibiotics and support dressings, or with elective sternal rewiring. If it does not become infected, an unstable sternum eventually forms a cartilaginous flexible union or pseudoarthrosis. An unstable sternum is a risk factor for prolonged ventilation and chest infections in the postoperative period.

Sternal dehiscence

Sternal dehiscence presents similarly to abdominal wound dehiscence:
• Serosanguinous discharge from the wound on days 3–5 postoperatively.
• ↑WCC.
• Sudden opening up of wound on coughing, straining.

Get the patient back into bed, reassure them, cover the wound with sterile saline soaked gauze, give the patient 2.5mg im morphine, and put them NPO. Take microbiology swabs. Most patients should be debrided and rewired under general anesthetic. Occasionally, wires have cheese-wired through a soft sternum, e.g., patients are managed conservatively with vacuum dressings and cough-locks.

Hypertrophic and keloid scars

Midline incisions have a tendency to form raised, red hypertrophic scars. Keloid scars (where the lumpy scar tissue exceeds the margin of the scar) are common in patients of African descent. There is no known way of avoiding these unsightly scars, apart from attempting to minimize the length of the sternotomy incision, or considering submammary incisions. Topical silicone gel dressings worn for up to 24h a day for several months will reduce the prominence of hypertrophic scars, but they can relapse when the dressings are abandoned. Keloid scars do not respond to surgical excision, but referral to a plastic surgeon is indicated if the patient is unhappy with the cosmetic result, as steroid injections may offer some improvement.

Sternal wires

Sometimes patients complain of prominent sternal wires. This is commonest in very thin patients. If the sternum is stable, sternal wires may be removed. This should be done under general anesthetic with appropriate invasive monitoring: even a simple removal of sternal wires can turn into an unexpected resternotomy. If the patient is unhappy with just one or two wires make sure you mark them with the patient preoperatively. These can be removed through stab incisions.

Complications of thoracotomy incisions

Post-operative pain is more challenging in thoracotomy patients compared to sternotomy patients (📖 pp648–649), and may progress to chronic post-thoracotomy neuralgia. Wound infections are uncommon and usually respond to appropriate antibiotic therapy. Lung herniation is seen more often with anterior thoracotomies where serratus and lattissimums dorsi do not cover the intercostal spaces which are further apart than they are more posterolaterally: this is diagnosed clinically (pain and protrusion of soft mass on coughing), and confirmed by CT, and can be treated by revision of the incision using a mesh closure. Avoid this by minimizing rib retraction, and a layered closure involving muscle, and circumferential rib sutures.

Hematological complications

Heparin-induced thrombocytopenia (HIT)

HIT occurs in about 5% of patients receiving heparin (5.5% of patients on bovine heparin, 1.0% with porcine heparin). It is characterized by formation of complement-mediated heparin-dependent IgG platelet antibody. It occurs after 5–10 days after initiation of heparin therapy, or after the first dose of heparin in patients with previous exposure to heparin within the last 3 months.

Diagnosis
- Decrease in platelet count by over 30% to <150 × 10^9/L, or by over 50%.
- *And* positive serology for HIT antibodies
- Heparin-induced thrombocytopenia and thrombosis (HITT) occurs in about 20% of patients with HIT and is characterized by major thrombotic episodes, and has a mortality of about 30%
- Patients may show tachyphylaxis to heparin, as well as bleeding complications; and thrombotic sequelae such as strokes, DVT, PE, peripheral, and splanchnic ischemia.
- Two assays:
  - Screening ELISA assay for antibodies against heparin-platelet factor complex which is more likely to have false positive than
  - Confirmational serotonin release assay (SRA).

Treatment
- Discontinue all heparin therapy, including heparinized saline flushes.
- If it is at all possible, delay any surgery requiring bypass until HIT antibodies are undetectable, and then follow standard heparinization, but do not use heparin in the postoperative period.
- If it is impossible to delay bypass surgery then danaparoid and iloprost are alternatives to heparin with the major disadvantages that they cannot be reversed after bypass, and require specialized assays.
- Hirudin, iloprost, danaparoid, argatroban, and warfarin are alternative anticoagulants to heparin in the postoperative period, and should be used in patients with HITT.

Disseminated intravascular coagulation (DIC)

DIC is extremely rare during bypass but may occur postoperatively as a complication of sepsis, transfusion reaction, drug reaction, transplant rejection, and aortic aneurysm surgery. It is characterized by widespread activation of coagulation, resulting in the formation of intravascular fibrin, fibrin degradation products, consumption platelets and clotting factors, and ultimately thrombotic occlusion of vessels. Patients may present with bleeding from indwelling venous lines, wounds, and minor abrasions.

Diagnosis
There is no single diagnostic test. The following findings suggest DIC:
- Sudden fall in platelet count to <100 × 10^9/L.
- Bleeding and/or thrombotic complications.
- ↑APTT, PT, INR.
- ↑fibrin degradation products.
- ↓fibrinogen in severe DIC.

Management

The key is to treat the underlying disorder. Bleeding patients should receive FFP, platelets, blood, and cryoprecipitate as indicated by coagulation screens. Patients with thrombosis should be heparinized.

Excessive heparinization

Management depends on whether the patient is bleeding (see 📖 pp145, 150). In the stable patient, who is not bleeding, simply stop the heparin infusion and recheck APTT in 4-6 hours. Heparin may be reversed rapidly with protamine (25–50mg iv) or FFP. The complications of protamine are described on 📖 pp116–117; the complications of transfusion are described on 📖 pp148–149.

Excessive warfarinization

Management depends on whether the patient is bleeding, and why they are warfarinized:

- If the INR is <6.0 and the patient is not bleeding simply omit warfarin and recheck INR daily, restarting warfarin once the INR is within target range. Check for evidence of liver dysfunction (📖 p276), and common contributing factors such as right heart failure (📖 p191), and drug interactions which elevate INR in patients on warfarin (e.g., amiodarone, cephalosporins, ciprofloxacin, tylenol, omeprazole).
- Check medications for interactions that may be causing INR to increase, e.g., amiodarone, antibiotics
- If the INR is >6.0 give 10mg vit K im.
- If the patient is bleeding give FFP (📖 p145).
- If the patient has a mechanical valve the risk of thromboembolic events when anticoagulation is reversed is about 0.02% per day: anticoagulation with heparin or warfarin should be recommenced within 1–2 weeks once any bleeding complications have resolved.

Hemolysis

Transient hemolysis manifesting as mild hematuria on arrival in ICU is most commonly due to cardiopulmonary bypass (📖 p95, p103, p104). Persistent or late hemolysis may be due to small, high velocity paravalvular leaks (📖 p266), is not uncommon in VAD patients (📖 p499), and may be a manifestation of transfusion reactions (📖 p148) or drug toxicity.

Hemolysis is diagnosed by increased presence of reticulocytes, hemoglobinuria, and frequently raised LFTs, and bilirubin. Management is supportive: keep the patient hydrated and avoid nephrotoxic and hepatotoxic agents to reduce the risk of renal and hepatic compromise, transfuse if indicated. Severe, refractory cases due to paravalvular leaks may require redo surgery.

Ischemic heart disease

Pathophysiology

Key facts

- Stenotic coronary artery disease (CAD) is narrowing of the coronary arteries caused by thickening and loss of elasticity of the arterial walls (atherosclerosis). The pathological changes are described on 📖 pp72–73.
- Stable plaques are mostly responsible for the lesions seen on angiography and stable angina: MI is due to unstable plaque rupture and thrombosis: 50% of MIs occur distal to angiographically 'normal' vessels.

Morphology

In patients with symptoms that warrant coronary angiography:
- 40% have three-vessel disease (3VD), 30% two-vessel disease (2VD).
- 10–20% have a significant stenosis of the left main stem (LMS).
- 95% with one completely occluded vessel have a significant stenosis in at least one other vessel.
- The ostia of large arteries and sites of branching are usually involved.
- Diffuse distal disease is less common.
- Occasionally a segment is intramyocardial: on angiography these segments are straight, free of branches, and usually free of disease.

Structural and functional changes

Coronary artery stenoses progress with time, in severity and distribution. Rate of progression is variable, and regression of lesions has been observed. Over a 2-year period, 50% of patients develop new significant lesions. Stenoses of 50% of cross-sectional area limit coronary flow reserve (the increase in blood flow that occurs to match increased myocardial oxygen demand 📖 p22). Coronary blood flow at rest is reduced by stenoses of 90%. At its most severe CAD results in vessel occlusion.

Left ventricular dysfunction: LV function may be abnormal in systole or diastole, during exercise or at rest. In normal people, global LV systolic function improves with exercise. In patients with CAD, areas of localized regional wall motion appear during exercise. These areas can be demonstrated as myocardial perfusion defects. If CAD is severe enough, these areas become confluent and global systolic LV function falls, sometimes so profoundly that exercise causes hypotension. This is reflected by EKG changes. Early diastolic function, which is energy dependent, is eventually impaired: filling times increase as does LVEDP. Dysfunction at rest is a result of irreversible scarring or hibernation (📖 p28, pp74–75).

Symptoms

Exertional angina: this is common. It results from reduction of coronary flow reserve, and the severity depends on the mismatch between myocardial oxygen supply and demand, i.e., both the severity of the CAD and the amount of work the myocardium is required to do. It is graded according to severity (Box 7.1) (see also 📖 p2 for more details).

Dyspnea: graded in the same way as angina (see Box 7.1). A number of mechanisms contribute. Acutely, transient systolic, and/or diastolic LV dysfunction results from worsening myocardial supply:demand mismatch caused by increases in preload, afterload, hypotension, or exertion. LV dysfunction leads to ↑LVEDP, causing sudden elevation in pulmonary venous pressure, detected by pulmonary venous baroreceptors which result in the sensation of dyspnea. Orthopnea results from the sudden increase in preload on lying flat. Paroxysmal nocturnal dyspnea is due to pulmonary edema, and poorly understood changes in respiratory drive.

Nausea: parasympathetic stimulation results in nausea and vomiting.

> **Box 7.1 New York Heart Association (NYHA) class**
> - Class I: asymptomatic.
> - Class II: symptoms causing slight limitation of ordinary activity.
> - Class III: symptoms causing marked limitation of ordinary activity.
> - Class IV: symptoms occurring with mild activity, or briefly at rest.
>
> Angina lasting >15min at rest is 'unstable angina'.

Unstable angina: this term, which covers a multitude of syndromes all of which reflect an adverse prognostic turn, applies to patients with severe and persisting angina. It is most commonly caused by non-occlusive thrombus at the site of an unstable plaque. Unstable angina normally recurs as either another episode of angina or as an acute MI. Patients can be divided into low-, medium-, and high-risk categories depending on the duration of their angina, severity of symptoms, presence of EKG changes, and hemodynamic compromise.

Acute coronary syndrome (ACS)
- This includes unstable angina, NSTEMI, and STEMI.
- Unstable angina is differentiated from NSTEMI by raised cardiac enzymes (CK-MB or troponin) that are present in NSTEMI.
- STEMI is differentiated from NSTEMI by EKG changes.

Non-ST segment elevation MI (NSTEMI): this is closely related to unstable angina. The key difference is severity, characterized by the presence of CK-MB and troponin I and T, in NSTEMI. Troponin correlates to short-term mortality in patients with ACS: in one study <2% of patients with troponin I levels of 0.4–1.0ng/mL were dead 42 days after presentation, compared to 7.5% with troponin I levels >9.0ng/mL.

ST segment elevation MI (STEMI): this is caused by acute total or sub-total vessel thrombotic occlusion (🕮 p72). Patients with severe proximal LAD lesions are particularly at risk of large MIs. In patients with symptoms severe enough to warrant coronary angiography 10% have an acute MI within 1 year and 30% have an acute MI within 5 years. Hospital mortality of STEMI is 7–10%, and can be predicted by size of infarct, reserve in the adjacent viable myocardium, and the number of prior MIs.

Death: overall survival for a group of patients with clinically evident CAD is 75% at 5 years after starting medical treatment.
- In 1VD the survival is the same as normal (unless proximal LAD).
- For 2VD the 5-year survival is 75%, lower if LV function is impaired.
- In 3VD the 5-year survival is 50%, lower if LV function is impaired.
- Tight, symptomatic LMS disease has a 2-year survival of 50%.

The evidence for CABG

Key facts
CABG has been compared to medical therapy, percutaneous transluminal coronary angioplasty (PTCA), and stenting (bare metal and drug-eluting), in randomized controlled trials (RCTs) and large registries.

Key studies
- *CABG vs. medical therapy*: 3 large RCTs—Veterans Administration (VA), European Coronary Surgery Study Group, and Coronary Artery Surgery Study (CASS); 4 smaller ones (Texas, Oregon, and 2 New Zealand studies), and several large registries.
- *CABG vs. PTCA*: 9 large RCTs: BARI, EAST, GABI, Toulouse, RITA, ERACI, MASS, Lausanne, CABRI.
- CABG vs. PCI: 13 large RCTs: SYNTAX, ARTS, SoS, AWESOME, ERACI II, SIMA, Diegler. Several large registries, e.g., Hannan et al.
- *PCI vs. medical therapy*: large RCTs, e.g., COURAGE, and meta-analyses.

Problems with the data
- RCTs and their meta-analyses are the 'highest' form of evidence as biases inherent in registries are eliminated, but problems include:
  - Patient selection in most early studies excluded individuals >65 years, women, and high-risk patients such as those with multi-vessel or left main disease, resulting in study populations that were not representative of clinical practice, and dominated by patients least likely to benefit from CABG, e.g., 60% of CASS patients had 2VD.
  - Medical and surgical treatment have changed since early RCTs.
  - Large numbers of patients crossed over to the intervention arms.
  - Limited follow-up (<5 years) under-represents benefits of CABG.
  - Combined endpoints give equal weight to death and reintervention.
- Registries may better reflect 'real-world' practice, but:
  - Non-randomized data cannot account for all confounders influencing both choice and outcome of a treatment strategy so two different patient populations are being compared, not just two treatments.

CABG vs. medical therapy
These trials form the basis of later studies but are of largely historical interest as only one trial used arterial grafts (CASS), and in only 14% of patients, newer methods of cardioprotection were not used, ASA, statins and ACE inhibitors were not standard, β-blockers were used in <50% of patients, and up to 50% of medical patients crossed over to surgery:
- Median survival for LMS was 13.3 years with CABG vs. 6.6 years without.
- Median survival for proximal LAD disease was 13.1 years with CABG vs. 6.2 years with medical therapy.
- Patients with worse LV gained most survival benefit from surgery.
- There was no difference in MI, and survival converged after 12 years because of SVG occlusion and medical patients crossing over to surgery.

CABG vs. PTCA

These studies had similar flaws to CABG vs. medical studies. The primary problem was that patients in whom survival had already been shown to be better with CABG than medical therapy were not included (only 5% of patients with multivessel disease at participating centres were enrolled: half did not meet the inclusion criteria (which excluded LMS disease), and most that did were not randomized—so the study populations were biased to PTCA and unrepresentative of clinical practice:

- 5-year survival was similar for CABG (89.3%) and PTCA (86.3%).
- Diabetics had much better survival with CABG than PTCA.
- By 1 year 20% of patients randomized to PTCA required CABG.
- At 5 years the reintervention rate was 7× higher with PTCA.

CABG vs. PCI

SYNTAX

- 1800 'all-comers' including LMS and multivessel disease randomized plus registry of 1300 ineligible patients, planned 5-year follow-up.
- Death at 3 years double in PCI patients (11% vs 4.5% in CABG patients, p=0.03).
- In the tercile of patients with the lowest SYNTAX (coronary complexity) scores death and MACCE was the same for PCI and CABG.

The Arterial Revascularization Therapies Study Group (ARTS) trial

- 1205 patients with multivessel disease.
- No difference was detected at 1 year in MACCE.
- There was a higher rate of repeat revascularization in the stenting group (16.8%) compared to the CABG group (3.5%).

Stent or Surgery (SoS) trial

- 988 patients with multivessel disease.
- There was a higher rate of repeat revascularization in the stenting group (21%) compared to the CABG group (6%).
- 3× more deaths in PCI group (CABG 0.8% 30-day mortality).
- No difference in cognitive function at 1 year.

Coronary angioplasty with stenting vs. coronary artery bypass in patients with multiple-vessel disease (ERACI II) trial

- 450 patients were randomized to stent or CABG. 40% 2VD.
- This trial is the only one to show an increased risk of death at 1 year in the CABG group (8%) vs. the stent group (3%), but the annual volume at participating centres only averaged <60 CABG total.
- Repeat revascularization was higher in the stent group (17%) compared to the CABG group (5%).
- There was no difference between the groups for MACCE.

PCI vs. optimal medical therapy

COURAGE randomized 2287 patients with significant CAD and ischemia: at median follow-up of 4.6 years there was no difference in MACCE (death, MI, stroke, hospitalization for unstable angina). 30% of medical patients vs. 20% of PCI needed revascularization. Only 30% were 3VD, and LMS was excluded. Most meta-analyses report similar results.

Indications for CABG

Key facts

Surgery is for prognosis or symptoms. The indications are adapted from consensus guidelines published in 2009 and 2010 (references on □ p825).

Classification system for recommendations

- Class I: conditions for which there is evidence and/or general agreement that a given procedure is useful and effective.
- Class II: conditions about which there is conflicting evidence:
- II a: weight of evidence/opinion is in favour of usefulness/efficacy.
- II b: usefulness/efficacy is less well established by evidence/opinion.
- Class III: conditions for which there is evidence and/or general agreement that a given procedure is not effective and may be harmful.
- **Level of evidence:** A, multiple RCTs or meta-analyses; B, single RCT or non-randomized studies; C, consensus, small/retrospective studies.

Stable angina

See Table 7.1.

Table 7.1 Indications for revascularization in patients with lesions suitable for both and low predicted surgical mortality

Revascularization	Subset of CAD	Class	Level
For prognosis	Left main >50%	I	A
	Proximal LAD >50%	I	A
	2VD or 3VD with ↓LVEF	I	B
	Large area ischemia (>10% LV)	I	B
	1VD without proximal LAD and without >10% ischemia	III	A
For symptoms	Any stenosis >50% with limiting angina or equivalent on OMTx	I	A
	Dyspnea/CHF and >10% LV ischemia supplied by vessel with >50% stenosis	IIa	B
	No limiting symptoms with OMTx	III	C

Indications for CABG vs. PCI	CABG	PCI
1VD or 2VD—non-proximal LAD	IIb C	I C
1VD or 2 VD—proximal LAD	I A	IIa B
3VD simple disease, full functional revascularization achievable with PCI, SYNTAX score <22	I A	IIa B
3VD complex lesions, incomplete revascularization achievable with PCI, SYNTAX score >22	I A	III A
LMS (isolated or 1VD, ostium/shaft)	I A	IIa B
LMS (isolated or 1VD, distal bifurcation)	I A	IIb B
LMS + 2VD or 3VD, SYNTAX score <32	I A	IIb B
LMS + 2VD or 3VD, SYNTAX score >33	I A	III B

Acute coronary syndromes

NSTEMI

Mortality is high, and similar to that for STEMI patients after the first month. NSTEMI patients are a heterogeneous group. Aims of revascularization are: (1) symptom relief and (2) prognosis. RCTS show early invasive strategy reduces severe recurrent ischemia, and need for hospitalization and reintervention, with reduction in mortality and MI in medium term.

- Choice of PCI or CABG depends on the severity and distribution of CAD (similar to Table 7.1), and predicted risk of surgery.
- The optimal timing of surgery and PCI is different: early PCI provides greatest benefit in ACS, but benefit from CABG is greatest when patients can undergo surgery after several days of medical stabilization.

STEMI

Primary PCI in setting of STEMI in experienced centres within 6–12h after symptom onset provides better angiographic and clinical outcomes than fibrinolysis, which remains an important alternative because of variability in access to PCI. There is a limited role for CABG in acute STEMI:

- In cases of unfavorable PCI anatomy or PCI failure, emergency CABG involving STEMI should only be considered when a very large myocardial area is in jeopardy and surgical revascularization can be completed before this area becomes necrotic (3–4h).
- Like NSTEMI—outcomes with CABG improve the more time elapses between the acute event and surgery. In the absence of persistent pain or hemodynamic compromise waiting 3–7 days is recommended.
- Surgery is indicated but associated with very high mortality for mechanical complications of STEMI including free wall rupture, ischemic VSD and papillary muscle rupture.

Heart failure and CABG

The indications for revascularization for CAD in the setting of CHF are similar to those outlined in Table 7.1, but the operative mortality is increased which impacts on aspects of the decision to operate:

- Patients without demonstrated viability are unlikely to benefit from revascularization and high-risk surgery should therefore be avoided.
- Patients with severely dilated LV have a low likelihood of showing improved LVEF even the presence of substantial viability (🕮 p28).
- MRI is the standard imaging technique to assess myocardial anatomy, regional and global function, viability, infarct size, and transmurality.
- In patients with LVEF <35% and predominantly anginal symptoms, CABG is recommended over PCI for significant LMS, LMS equivalent, and proximal LAD disease with 2VD or 3VD.
- In patients with LVEF <35% and predominantly heart failure symptoms (no or mild angina) CABG can be considered if there is viability, with aneurysmectomy if there is a large LV aneurysm (🕮 p348).

Redo CABG

PCI is mainstay of therapy, but redo CABG may be indicated for patients with several diseased grafts, reduced LV function, several chronic total occlusions in absence of patent LIMA to LAD graft, or severe symptoms/ischemia despite optimal medical therapy (🕮 pp342–347).

When not to operate

Key facts

- ACC/AHA guidelines identify several scenarios where there is evidence that CABG is likely not to be efficacious, or likely to do harm.
- If you remember that you are operating for symptoms and/or prognosis, then lack of a benefit in one area places a great deal of scrutiny on your rationale for operating for the other.

Anatomy

CABG is not indicated in borderline coronary stenoses (50–60%) diameter in locations other than the LMS without demonstrable ischemia on non-invasive testing, or for insignificant (<50% diameter) stenoses.

Asymptomatic patients

The aim of surgery in these patients is to improve prognosis. Surgery is only beneficial in asymptomatic patients at high risk of MI or death (☐ p296) because of severity of lesions, i.e., in severe LMS disease, LMS equivalent, or proximal LAD disease.

- Take a careful history: ischemia may present as epigastric discomfort; arm, neck, or jaw pain; or dyspnea rather than angina.
- Beware of the patient with dyspnea as their predominant symptom rather than angina. Documenting the presence of ischemia by exercise EKG, echocardiography, or thallium scan (☐ p28), carefully assess ventricular dysfunction (systolic and diastolic) and take care to rule out non-cardiac causes of their dyspnea.
- In very elderly patients, or patients with severe comorbidity, who are unlikely to see a survival benefit from surgical revascularization, lack of symptoms is a strong argument for not operating—you risk decreasing quality of life, without an incremental increase in length of life. This scenario sometimes arises when CAD is identified during the work-up for another procedure, e.g., hip replacement. Think carefully: PCI may be the most reasonable approach.

Patients with chronic stable angina

Patients with 1VD or 2VD not involving proximal LAD stenosis who (1) have mild symptoms that are not necessarily due to myocardial ischemia or, (2) have not received an adequate trial of medical therapy, and have only a small area of viable myocardium or no demonstrated ischemia on non-invasive testing should not be offered surgery, as it is unlikely to have any prognostic or symptomatic benefit.

Patients with unstable angina/NSTEMI

Unstable angina is best managed initially by medical treatment. The risk of CABG, which is performed for prognostic and symptomatic indications described in Table 7.1, decreases with distance between the acute event and surgery: waiting 48–72h if the patient has no ongoing signs of ischemia, on iv heparin, NTG, and an IABP if necessary, is the best strategy.

Patients with acute MI

Primary reperfusion >12h after the start of an evolving ST-segment MI without evidence of ongoing ischemia is high risk and has no survival benefit. In the patient with cardiogenic shock post acute MI, the most reasonable surgical strategy may be ECMO or a temporary VAD (📖 pp496–501) rather than CABG.

Patients with poor LV and no ischemia

Operative mortality for isolated CABG in selected patients with chronic severe LV dysfunction is around 5%, compared to patients with preserved LV function where it is 1–2%. Long-term survival is poorer. However, selected patients with severe LV dysfunction and CAD still derive significantly more benefit from surgical revascularization than they do from PCI or medical management, in terms of symptoms, freedom from revascularization and survival. Patients with poor LV being considered for CABG should have: (1) *severe, obstructive CAD* with (2) *adequate targets, and* documented evidence of (3) *ischemia* and (4) *viability*.

- If dyspnea and other failure symptoms predominate over angina then the benefits of CABG are less clear: it is a relatively high-risk strategy compared to PCI or medical management (📖 p493), with debateable prognostic or symptomatic benefit.
- Patients with severely dilated LV have low likelihood of showing improvement in LVEF, even if they have large areas of viability: concomitant ventricular restoration (📖 p495) may have a role in ameliorating symptoms of heart failure, or in end-stage ischemic cardiomyopathy assist devices (📖 p496) and transplantation (📖 p504).

Patients post failed PCI

CABG is not indicated if there is no evidence of ischemia, or if PCI was abandoned simply because of target anatomy. The absence of reflow after PCI is not an indication for CABG.

- If you are called to cath lab to be confronted by a patient who has been undergoing chest compressions for more than just a few minutes, first establish whether the primary issue is tamponade (surgery indicated if pericardiocentesis not possible) or ischemia, and what the patient's baseline comorbidity and functional status was.
- Emergency CABG has high mortality in this situation: it is often more reasonable to place the patient on ECMO or a temporary assist device (📖 pp500–501) rather than performing CABG.

Elderly patients

Age per se is not a contraindication to surgery. The normal life expectancy of an octogenarian is about 6 years. Look carefully though for factors such as porcelain aorta, end-organ dysfunction that might push the balance in favour of PCI.

Small or occluded distal vessels

Angiographic appearances may be deceptive (vessels with tight proximal stenoses may just be underfilled), and in the majority of cases it is possible to place a graft at operation.

Planning coronary artery surgery

Key facts

There are different ways of performing almost every element of a CABG. Several factors are taken into account when planning a CABG to provide minimum morbidity and mortality, and longest graft patency and life expectancy.

History

Document:

- Age, frailty (extreme age/frailty may favour PCI, or fewer grafts).
- Severity and nature of symptoms: anginal type symptoms usually predominate, whereas patients presenting with predominantly heart failure type symptoms (e.g., dyspnea) may need further evaluation.
- Number and timing of previous MIs impact risk and timing of surgery.
- Coronary anatomy, LV function, valvular heart disease.
- Previous PCI and operations.
- Risk factors for perioperative mortality including renal dysfunction, pulmonary dysfunction, peripheral vascular disease, strokes.
- Risk factors for wound infections including smoking history, diabetes, steroid use, significant involuntary weight loss, malnutrition.
- Saphenous vein stripping, DVT, chest wall radiation, dominant hand.

Examination

- A targeted clinical examination is carried out to screen for:
- Obesity, pectus deformities, previous surgery.
- Presence of other cardiovascular problems such as poorly controlled hypertension, arrhythmias, valvular heart disease, carotid artery disease, peripheral vascular disease, evidence of heart failure.
- Varicose veins, venous ulceration.
- Allen's test (📖 p7).
- Respiratory pathology.

Blood tests

- Standard screening tests are described on 📖 pp8–9. A FBC, clotting, serum electrolytes, LFTs, and group and save are routinely performed.

CXR

A PA CXR is used to assess:

- Pulmonary pathology.
- Evidence of heart failure.
- Calcification of the ascending aorta.
- Method of closure, if previous sternotomy.
- Rarely mediastinal masses.

Cardiac catheterization

Coronary angiography

Coronary angiogram should not be >6 months old. The objective of CABG is to achieve complete revascularization.

- All stenoses >50% in diameter in all coronary artery vessels should be bypassed: ideally there should be good distal run-off.
- If the right coronary artery is non-dominant it is not grafted.
- Similarly, small, short branches in the left coronary circulation are not always grafted.
- Some surgeons elect not to bypass branches that are very close to arteries that will be revascularized, arguing that the myocardium will be adequately supplied by nearby arteries.
- Most surgeons will only bypass the more significant vessel of two vessels that communicate distal to a stenosis.
- A significant LMS lesion means that all major coronary arteries in the left system need revascularization.
- If there is a distal stenosis in addition to a proximal LAD or LMS stenosis it may necessary to either bridge the distal lesion so that the whole length of the LAD is supplied, or revascularize both segments with either a jump graft or two separate grafts.
- Lesions in the mid portion of important vessels are sometimes bridged, to provide supply proximally and distally.

Cardiac catheterization
- Ventriculography is usually performed in the absence of renal dysfunction or haemodynamic instability giving an estimate of LV function and regional wall motion abnormalities, and MR (📖 p22).
- Gradient across the aortic valve can be assessed by measuring LV and aortic pressure either simultaneously or by pull-back.
- Right heart catheterization should be performed in patients with very poor LV function to quantify pulmonary hypertension.

Echocardiography

All patients undergoing coronary artery bypass surgery should undergo preoperative TTE to identify valvular heart disease (e.g., ischemic MR) and accurately quantify LV function.

Myocardial perfusion studies

The principles of myocardial perfusion studies, which include MRI, technetium scans, stress echocardiography, and PET scans, are described on 📖 p28. These are requested to determine whether myocardium is akinetic as a result of irreversible scarring from myocardial infarction (in which case there is no benefit from revascularizing the vessel supplying that territory), or as a result of hibernation or stunning (in which case there is a benefit to be gained from revascularization) (📖 p297).

Carotid artery duplex

These are performed in patients that give a previous history of stroke or TIA, have carotid bruits, or have evidence of severe polyarteriopathy.

CT scan

Increasingly routinely performed in patients over the age of 75 years to identify aortic calcification that may change intraoperative strategy, and occult pulmonary and mediastinal pathology.

Conduit selection

Key facts

Choice of conduit is determined by the quality of the available conduit, the suitability of the targets, and the age and comorbidity of the patient (Table 7.2).

Table 7.2 Approximate conduit patency rates

Conduit	1-year patency	Late patency rates
Left internal mammary artery	98%	90% at 10 years
Right internal mammary artery	96% to LAD, Cx 80–90% to RCA	90% at 5 years
Radial artery	Highly dependent on target coronary	
Right gastroepiploic artery	95%	90% at 3 years
Right inferior epigastric artery	90%	Not known
Long saphenous vein	80–90%	50% at 10 years
Short saphenous vein	Not known but probably similar to LSV	
Cephalic vein	<60%	
Saphenous vein (stored)	40%	

Internal thoracic arteries

LIMA to LAD graft: this is the mainstay of CABG as it provides better survival and freedom from MI, symptoms and PCI than SVG to LAD.[1] Over 90% of LIMA to LAD anastomoses are patent 10–20 years postoperatively, and late graft occlusion is uncommon. Stenoses, which occur in 5–10% of LIMA to LAD anastomoses, do not usually progress to occlusion. Free LIMA to LAD graft has a patency rate slighter lower than pedicled LIMA. The excellent patency of mammary artery grafts is probably due to endothelial cell function, which seems to help resist atherosclerosis, and grafting to the LAD or Cx territory which has a larger run-off than the RCA territory.

BIMA vs. LIMA (see also 🕮 p321): bilateral internal mammary artery (BIMA) shows better long-term patency than LIMA + SVG and may improve symptom-free survival (this is difficult to judge from retrospective studies which do not adjust for all the confounders that affect choice of conduit), but most studies, including recent randomized data, show double the risk of deep sternal wound infection. For that reason most surgeons avoid BIMA in obese, diabetic, current smokers, or older patients. The in-situ RIMA will only reach proximal right-sided or very proximal left-sided lesions. 'T' grafting free RIMA off the LIMA allows the RIMA to be grafted to the more distal Cx and PDA sequentially (🕮 p321). The in-situ RIMA may be anastomosed to the LAD, and the LIMA to the Cx system. Alternatively, the in-situ RIMA may be passed through the transverse sinus to the Cx system, where bleeding or torsion may be difficult to address, but this minimizes problems posed by RIMA crossing the midline at future sternal re-entry.

Skeletonized vs. pedicled IMA: skeletonizing the IMA (🕮 p320) facilitates sequential and distal grafting, and may help reduce deep sternal wound infection particularly where BIMA is used. Patency is comparable to pedicled LIMA at 10 years.

Relative contraindications to LIMA
- Previous radiotherapy to the left chest.
- Atherosclerotic or stenosed left subclavian artery (could use free graft).
- Emergency surgery for cardiogenic shock.

Relative contraindications to BIMA
- Diabetes, particularly females.
- Obese patients, particularly females.
- Current smokers, COPD, or other respiratory impairment.
- Immunocompromised patients, long-term high-dose systemic steroids.

Radial artery grafts

Patency rates of radial artery grafts (📖 p316) are dependent on the distal vessel: patency rates exceed 90% at 1 year and 80% at 5 years, but are much lower if the stenosis being bypassed is <70%, has poor run-off, or is a right-sided vessel—in these situations radial patency has been shown to be lower than SVG. Occluded or thread-like arterial grafts are found where the stenosis being bypassed is <70%. The radial is much more muscular and prone to spasm than the IMA.

Saphenous vein

SVG has an early patency rate of 80–90% and a 50% patency rate at 10 years. Late patency is about 80% when it is used to bypass the LAD which has a large run-off. Patency may be reduced by excessive manipulation during endoscopic harvest. Stenosis is caused by:

Thrombosis: this is the commonest cause of early graft failure, and is usually due to technical factors. Endothelial cell loss and exposure of the basement membrane predisposes to graft thrombosis by causing accumulation of platelets, fibrin, and thrombus on the luminal surface. Thrombosis also occurs in heavily atherosclerotic areas. When antiplatelet therapy is not used up to 10% of grafts occlude within a few weeks of surgery.

Anastomotic narrowing: this occurs proximally in about 20% of vein grafts at 1 year, and distally in about 50% of patients at 1 year, and may be due to technical factors, atherosclerosis, or intimal hyperplasia.

Intimal hyperplasia: this diffuse thickening of the intima, occurs almost universally in vein grafts, and appears to be a remodelling process that approximates the vein lumen to that of the distal arterial lumen. This diffuse narrowing is detectable in most SVGs angiographically at 1 year.

Fibrous atherosclerotic plaques: these begin to develop in vein grafts 3 years postoperatively and are present in most vein grafts by 10 years. They are responsible for flow-limiting stenoses. They are related to damage to the graft endothelium as a result of harvest and insertion into a high-pressure arterial system, and the patient's tendency to develop atherosclerosis. Aggressive cholesterol management can slow this process. Vein graft atherosclerosis differs from native vessel disease: it is diffuse, and plaques are superficial, friable with overlying mural thrombus.

Reference

1. Loop et al. Influence of the IMA graft on 10 year survival and other cardiac events. NEJM 1986; 314:1–6.

Off-pump versus on-pump CABG

Key facts

CABG can be carried out with cardiopulmonary bypass (on-pump or ONCAB), or without (off-pump or OPCAB). Most surgeons perform CABG on-pump: the advantages of a still, clear operating field, myocardial protection, and hemodynamic and respiratory control, outweigh many of the disadvantages of bypass (🕮 p106). Improvements in methods of stabilizing the heart have led to some surgeons adopting OPCAB to avoid the complications of cannulation and cardiopulmonary bypass.

The evidence

Randomized controlled trials

Over 50 RCTs of off-pump versus on-pump surgery have been published, mostly underpowered to detect a difference in stroke or mortality, with some showing reductions in postoperative atrial fibrillation, transfusion requirements, inotrope requirements, ventilation times, length of hospital and intensive care unit stay, and cost compared to on-pump coronary artery surgery. Some of the problems outlined on 🕮 p294 apply to these studies: additionally the off-pump learning curve may impact trial results from less experienced trial centers.

• In the largest RCT reported to date, the ROOBY (Randomized On/Off Bypass) investigators randomized 2203 patients undergoing urgent or elective CABG. Unlike the majority of off-pump trials, poor LV, advanced age and acute coronary syndromes were not exclusion criteria. Vessels <1.1mm or diffuse disease were exclusion criteria.

• At 1 year the composite outcome of death, MI, or any revascularization after 30 days, was significantly higher in the off-pump group, as was death from cardiac causes. Patency of both saphenous and LIMA grafts was lower in the off-pump group. No difference was seen in renal failure, reop for bleeding, stroke, or cognitive function.

• No RCTs have shown a difference in 30-day mortality or stroke: Van Dijk et al., Puskas et al., and Angelini et al. did, however, show a significant reduction in transfusion requirements, serum markers of myocardial damage, and a cost saving with off-pump surgery in low-risk patients in trials that randomized 281, 197, and 401 (2 pooled randomized controlled trials) patients respectively.

Meta-analyses

A large, recent meta-analysis including 86 trials containing 10716 patients found increased mortality with off-pump CABG (3.7% vs. 3.1%, p=0.04), and fewer distal anastomoses with off-pump. No differences in MI or stroke was seen.

Registries

Several retrospective analyses of large registries, on the other hand, have demonstrated a statistically significant difference in postoperative mortality and stroke. Differences in outcome may be due to patient selection as it isn't possible to control for all confounding variables in retrospective studies, even with risk adjustment.

- Hannan et al. compared over 13 000 off-pump and 35 941 on-pump patients operated on between 2001–2004.
- The off-pump group had lower risk adjusted mortality fewer strokes less respiratory failure postoperatively but there was no difference in 3 year mortality.

Summary

Mortality: recent data from a large RCT and meta-analysis shows increased operative mortality with OPCAB compared to ONCAB.

Stroke: no RCTs have looked at 'no-touch' technique versus CPB. Randomized trials have not shown a difference in stroke rates. The majority of retrospective analyses have shown reduced rates of stroke in off-pump (2%) versus 1% in on-pump CAB: may be due to patient selection.

Postoperative MI: no difference in the incidence of postoperative MI has been shown, but fewer cardiac enzymes are released in OPCAB.

Incomplete revascularization: ROOBY trial found significantly fewer grafts performed than planned in the off-pump group.

Graft patency rates: ROOBY trial found a third higher incidence of at least 1 occluded graft at 1 year (37% vs. 29%), reduced SVG patency (77% vs 88%), and fewer excellent LIMA grafts (89% vs 93%).[1]

Length of stay: length of hospital and ICU stay depend on several non-patient related variables. ROOBY showed no difference in length of ICU/ hospital stay, or time on a ventilator.

Renal failure: retrospective studies have shown reduced rates of renal failure in OBCAP patients, but not seen in ROOBY.

Bleeding, transfusion, and resternotomy: these have been shown to be reduced in OPCAB, in some but not all randomized and retrospective studies. No difference in any of these was seen in ROOBY trial.

Atrial fibrillation: the prevalence of postoperative AF in OPCAB patients is lower according to some retrospective and randomized studies.

Current indications for OPCAB surgery

- OPCAB is a suitable alternative to CPB in experienced centers. Combined with a 'no touch' or anaortic technique (📖 p321) it is the first approach for patients with a very atherosclerotic or calcified aorta, and may be associated with much reduced risk of stroke in a broader patient population.

Reference

1. Shroyer AL, Grover FL, Hattler B et al. On-pump versus off-pump coronary-artery bypass surgery. N Engl J Med. 2009;361:1827–37.
2. Moller CH, Penninga L, Wettersley J et al. Off-pump versus on-pump coronary artery bypass grafting for ischaemic heart disease. Cochrane Database Syst Rev. 2012;3:CD007224.
3. Hannan EL, Wu C, Smith CR et al. Off-pump versus on-pump coronary artery bypass graft surgery. Circulation. 2007;116:1145–52.

Open saphenous vein harvest 1

The anatomy of the long saphenous vein is described on 📖 p55. Assessing the conduit is described on 📖 p7, and complications of saphenous vein harvest are described on 📖 pp283 and 285.

Indications

- Suitable for the majority of patients undergoing CABG.
- Occasionally a segment is required unexpectedly if a coronary vessel is inadvertently damaged during non-CABG surgery, or for salvage grafting if the patient fails to come off bypass.
- Short segment may be used in patch repair in carotid endarterectomy.

Contraindications

- Overlying sepsis.
- Multiple large varicosities in the LSV itself.
- Deep venous insufficiency in that leg.
- Previous DVT in that leg.
- Inadequate diameter lumen.

Technique

The aim is to obtain the required length of conduit and close the wound before the heparin is given to minimize bypass time and hematomas.

Options for saphenous vein harvest

- Open technique starting at ankle.
- Open technique starting at groin.
- Closed technique using vein stripper.
- Endoscopic harvest.
- Short saphenous vein harvest.

Prepping and draping

The legs and groin should have been shaved in the anesthetic room. Shaving on the ward the night before surgery results in increased rates of wound infection. The legs are prepped after the trunk. Prep the area of the incision first, then from clean areas to dirty. Leave the groin until last. An unscrubbed assistant lifts the legs so that you can prep the undersurface. If a diathermy plate is on the buttocks, take care not to use so much prep that it dribbles down onto the plate as this can result in diathermy burns. Finally ask the assistant to spread the legs so that you can prep the groin. Lower the prepped legs so that the feet can be draped, making sure the medial malleolus is in the operative field.

Surface anatomy

Surface anatomy of the long saphenous vein

The long saphenous vein runs between the following points (Fig. 7.1a):
- 1cm above and anterior to the medial malleolus.
- 4cm posterior to the medial border of the patella.
- 2cm below and 1cm medial to the mid-inguinal point.

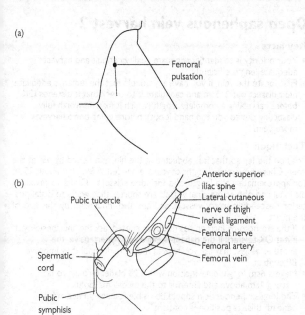

Fig. 7.1 (a) Incision for long saphenous vein harvest in the groin. (b) Instruments on the saphenous vein set: (i) McIndoe scissors, (ii) Metzenbaum scissors, (iii) Mayo scissors, (iv) DeBakey forceps, (v) Mosquito clips (vi) Dunhill clips, (vii) Ligaclip applicator.

Open saphenous vein harvest 2

Key facts

- Your priority is to identify adequate quality conduit and harvest adequate length efficiently.
- First locate the vein, if you have any doubts that the lumen is adequate next dissect out 2–3cm and cannulate it to check that it distends OK **before** harvesting a complete length (which it may be worth fully dissecting out so you can hand it out), before going on to harvest more vein.

Technique

Position the leg so that it is abducted at the hip, and flexed by 45° at the knee. Check how many lengths of vein are needed. A length is about 25cm (or approximately the length of a McIndoe scissors). Grafts to proximal diagonal and obtuse marginal vessels are shorter than grafts to distal posterior descending artery vessels, and are also influenced by the size of the heart.

- If the sternotomy incision has not been started, ask the anesthesiologist if it is OK to start: if the patient is extremely hypertensive, the anesthesiologist may ask you to wait momentarily until they improve BP control.
- Make a 6cm longitudinal incision with a 23 blade, through to fat, starting 1cm above and anterior to the medial malleolus.
- The long saphenous vein should be visible running immediately beneath this: its position is constant.
- If you can't see the vein spread the soft tissue with a McIndoe scissors until it comes into view: if you see muscle/ligament you are too deep.
- Keeping in the plane of the vein, pass one blade of a curved Mayo scissors over the vein, separating the fascia and skin off the vein. Lifting the scissors up, away from the vein, divide the skin cleanly.
- Rapidly follow the vein up the leg in this way so that the required length of vein is exposed.
- Assess the lumen as you go: if it narrows markedly follow it 2–3cm to see if it increases, and check that surgeon is happy with the lumen. Anything <0.5cm or >1cm is probably not useable.
- Your next priority is to ensure that you have a length ready to use.
- The most distal length has fewest branches: using blunt dissection with the McIndoe scissors carefully free the vein from surrounding fascia, so that the side branches are revealed.
- Taking care not to avulse the side branches pass the jaws of a mosquito clip with a 3/0 silk or Vicryl tie underneath the side branch, and put three careful throws flush with the long saphenous vein.
- Ligaclip the leg end of the sidebranch and divide it.
- Proceed up the leg. As soon as one length is free, insert a tester into the most distal end, placing an artery clip across the vein distally.
- Inflate the vein with saline or heparinized blood, compressing it distally between a thumb and forefinger, to see if there are any leaks.

- If there is a leak from an untied side branch place a mosquito clip on the end of the side branch and tie it off flush with the vein.
- If there is a hole in the vein, from a varicosity or avulsed side branch, this needs to be repaired with 6/0 Prolene (Fig. 7.4).
- Dissect out the rest of the vein in the same way, check for leaks, and check that the surgeon is happy with the length, place a Dunhill on the vein proximately, and cut both ends.
- Place a Redivac drain if the patient is very overweight or there is a flap.
- Close the legs with continuous 1/0 Vicryl to deep fascia and 3/0 Vicryl or Monocryl on a curved needle, using subcuticular stitch (Fig. 7.2c).
- Clean the leg, dress the wound with Mepore and bandage the leg firmly, but not too tightly, from ankle to thigh (Fig. 7.2a).

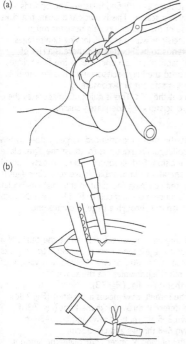

Fig. 7.2 (a) Repairing the vein. (b) Tying in the tester.

Open saphenous vein harvest 3

Key facts

- Harvesting conduit quickly and efficiently is a key skill that is frequently left to the most junior members of the team to perform unsupervised.
- Doing it well means the difference between a pain-free patient, who mobilizes quickly and has an angina-free interval of several years after surgery; and a patient who fails to mobilize because of pain and wound infections, and may experience resternotomy for bleeding within hours or graft occlusion within months.

Incision

The aim is to make the cleanest incision so that skin edges are not macerated, keeping directly over the vein to avoid creating a flap. The cleanest incision is made with a fresh scalpel, e.g. a 23 blade, but most surgeons compromise, using a Mayo scissors as they find it faster. The options are:

- Make the entire incision with a scalpel. This is quick and clean, but risks creating a flap if the course of the saphenous vein deviates much.
- Make multiple small skin incisions with a scalpel, leaving skin bridges (Fig. 7.3). This is fast and tends to heal better, but there is a risk of avulsing small branches of saphenous vein underneath the skin bridges.
- Cut down using a scalpel onto the Mayo scissors, which is held in the tunnel above the vein. This is safe but time consuming.
- Use the Mayo scissors to cut the skin. This is quick but macerates the skin edges unless the Mayo scissors are adequately sharp.

Exposure

One of the first things that the more experienced surgeon does when asked to help out a junior colleague in trouble is to adjust the light, place a retractor, and widen the incision. Bad exposure makes an easy operation difficult, and a difficult one almost impossible. Make sure your light is adequate at all times. Use a self-retaining retractor in the thigh and in fat patients. Remember that it is much more difficult to find the vein through a small, ineffective incision, than it is through a large, accurate one.

Surgical knots

These are a cornerstone of surgery. Loose ligatures can be the cause of a resternotomy for bleeding, and suggest the surgeon is unlikely to progress to tying coronary anastomoses with 8/0 Prolene. There are a variety of ways of tying surgical knots but the principles are the same:

- Put down each throw so that it lies flat (Fig. 7.3).
- One throw followed by the same throw makes a slip-knot (Fig. 7.3c).
- One throw followed by a different throw locks the knot (Fig. 7.3b).
- In braided suture put down 3–5 alternate throws and cut 2–3mm.
- In monofilament, put down 6–8 throws and cut 0.5cm.
- Lay each throw down with your index finger controlling the amount of tension you place on the knot most securely: too much tension can pull the tissue off the wound and too little leads to loose ligatures.

(a)

(b)

(c)

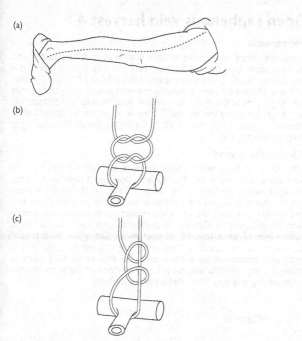

Fig. 7.3 (a) Saphenous vein incision. (b) Surgical knots: lying throws flat.
(c) Slip knot.

Open saphenous vein harvest 4

Hemostasis

If you are unsure of your ties, transfix both ends of the saphenous vein stumps before tying them. If you can see a vein end, ligate it even if it is not actively bleeding: when venospasm wears off and BP rises it will start to bleed. There is no point in inducing thermal burns by trying to cauterize bleeding points at the skin edge: the best solution is to approximate the skin edges by closing the wound. The key is to get the leg closed before heparin is given, if possible. Good bandaging technique (firm not tight) helps hemostasis (Fig. 7.4).

Closing the wound

Use 2/0 or 1/0 Vicryl on a curved needle, taking bites 1–1.5cm long and 1cm apart, as shown in Fig. 7.4c, to bring deep fascia together securely. Always sew into the fascial layer, not just the fat which will not support sutures. Avoid button-holing the skin in thin people by making sure that the needle is parallel to the skin. Use a straight handheld, or curved needle with 3/0 Monocryl or Vicryl to close the skin with a subcuticular stitch, making bites of about 1cm, 0.5 cm apart. Avoid putting too much tension on sutures as this causes ischemia: too little may result in the wound separating postoperatively. If this happens use interrupted 4/0 Prolene to repair. If using monofilament put at least six throws on the knots to avoid it unravelling, and bury it to avoid a stitch granuloma.

Do's and don'ts

Do's

- Do handle the vein *minimally*: intimal damage is less.
- Do stay close to the vein: it makes dissecting it out much easier.
- Do use sharp Mayos: crushing the skin impairs wound healing.
- Do preserve the saphenous nerve: it minimizes sympathetic dystrophy postoperatively as well as improving wound healing.
- Do use toothed forceps on skin: non-toothed crush the skin.
- Do ensure good hemostasis: hematomas cause wound infections.
- Do close the skin firmly, but not under tension: healing is better.
- Do evert the skin edges: healing and scars are better.

Don'ts

- Don't handle the vein with forceps: they damage endothelium.
- Don't tie to close to the vein: narrowing and kinking results (Fig. 7.4f).
- Don't tie too far away from the vein: clots may form (Fig. 7.4e).
- Don't create skin flaps: cut perpendicularly onto the vein (Fig. 7.4a).
- Don't tether the skin: this makes painful and ugly scars.
- Don't bandage too loosely: hematoma and edema will result.
- Don't bandage too tightly: this causes ischemia and poor healing.

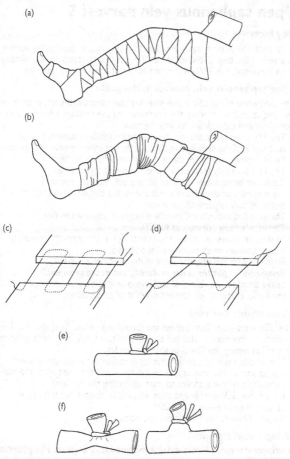

Fig. 7.4 (a) Correct methods of bandaging. (b) Incorrect method of bandaging. (c) Correct path of skin sutures. (d) Incorrect path of sutures. (e) Correct way of tying side-branches. (f) Incorrect way of tying side-branches.

Open saphenous vein harvest 5

Key facts

If the distal LSV in both legs is unsatisfactory in calibre or quality, the saphenous vein in the thigh is dissected out. If this is unsatisfactory, or has already been harvested, the SSV will give one length of conduit from each leg.

Long saphenous vein harvest in the groin

The landmarks of the LSV in the groin are less constant: the key is to make an oblique incision of adequate length starting over sapheno-femoral junction (SFJ), and extending it slightly medially.

- The SFJ is located at the mid-inguinal point (halfway between bony landmarks of the symphysis pubis and the anterior superior iliac crest).
- Extend the incision from there slightly medially for 8–10cm.
- The LSV is usually located in a plane between layers of fat.
- If it is not immediately obvious, place a self-retaining retractor in the wound, and using blunt dissection with a curved Mayo scissors systematically explore the incision.
- The vein lies within fat: if muscle is exposed you are too deep.
- The vein is most constant at the SFJ.
- Several branches can mimic the LSV: they are either much smaller, or follow courses much more medial or lateral.
- Follow it with the Mayo scissors as described on 📖 p312.
- *Remember to put the tester in distally, not at the groin end!*
- Leave an adequate stump of saphenous vein to tie proximally so that the femoral vein is not compromised at all by ligatures.

Short saphenous vein

The SSV runs from 2cm behind the lateral malleolus, over the Achilles tendon, up the back of the calf to the popliteal fossa. The most difficult part of harvesting the SSV is positioning the leg.

- The simplest way to position the leg is to flex the knee, use a towel clip to anchor the foot drapes to the table, and then adduct at the hip exposing the lateral aspect to start, abducting the hip later.
- Identify the SSV distally and then proceed to dissect out the SSV in exactly the same way as the LSV.
- Stop just before the SSV enters the popliteal fossa.

Using a vein stripper

A stripper is simply a 1cm metal ring, mounted at an angle on a long handle (Fig. 7.5). This method is quicker than conventional harvest as there is no long incision to close, but real care should be taken to avoid avulsing small branches and damaging the endothelium with too much traction. Three lengths of vein can be removed quickly, and with only small skin incisions to close this is a fast technique that improves wound healing and mobilizing. The drawback is a slightly higher rate of avulsed side branches requiring repair on the LSV, and which can cause leg hematomas.

- Expose the saphenous vein at the groin and ligate it proximally.
- Place a 0/0 silk suture distally in the vein and cut it long.

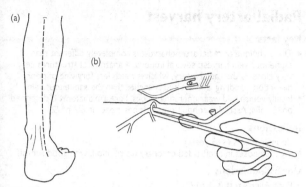

Fig. 7.5 (a) Short saphenous vein incision. (b) Using the vein stripper to harvest LSV.

- Pass the suture and the vein through the ring end of the stripper and pass the stripper down the vein until you meet resistance with skin tethering caused by a branch.
- Make a 1.5cm incision down onto the stripper where it has come up against a branch, and pass the stripper and vein up through the incision.
- Remove the vein from the stripper and the incision, and ligate and divide the branch, which is usually easily visible.
- Continue as far as necessary and test the vein in the usual manner.

Endoscopic vein harvest

There are several systems available, e.g., Vasoview, and they offer different approaches to the various aspects of endoscopic vein harvest:

- The saphenous vein is identified just above the knee about two finger breaths posterior to the medial patella.
- The subcutaneous space is created by blunt dissection anterior to the vein initially by digital dissection, then using balloon inflation with gas insufflation to maintain the subcutaneous space.
- Dissection is carried out with long-handled, blunt or 'U'-tipped instruments: side branches are clipped and divided with diathermy.
- Similar techniques have been used for radial artery harvest.
- While a large non-randomized study of endoscopic vs open vein harvest[1] showed lower patency rates in endoscopic vein grafts at 12–18 months, several of the participating centers were low-volume units, and equipment has moved on several iterations. A recent much larger study showed no increase in repeat revascularization at 4 years.[2] Certainly morbidity from leg wounds including infection is much less with endoscopic harvest: and in many countries, particularly with established physician assistant programs (the learning curve is longer than most surgical trainees spend on many units), it is the technique of choice.

References

1. Lopes RD, Hafley GE, Allen KB, et al. Endoscopic versus open vein-graft harvesting in coronary-artery bypass surgery. *N Engl J Med.* 2009;**36**:235–44.
2. Dacey LJ, Braxton JH, Kramer RS et al. Long-term outcomes of endoscopic vein harvesting after coronary artery bypass grafting. *Circulation.* 2011;**123**:147–53.

Radial artery harvest

Key facts

- The technique of radial artery harvest is completely different than saphenous vein harvest: several important anatomical structures lie very close to the radial artery, which is much less forgiving of poor dissection, handling, and avulsed branches than the saphenous vein.
- Ideally you should wear operating loupes. Forearm anatomy is described on 🕮 p54. Assessing conduit pre-op is described on 🕮 p172.

Indications

- Young patients (<65 years).
- Tight stenoses in a left-sided coronary distribution, with good run-off.

Contraindications

- Poor Allen's test (🕮 p172).
- Unsuitable targets (🕮 p303).

Technique

Make sure that the anesthesiologist is aware that radial artery will be harvested, and that they are clear which side: the radial artery catheter must be inserted on the contralateral side.

- Make sure there is an arm-board and an additional diathermy plate.
- Prep and drape the arm, once the patient has been draped (Fig. 7.6).
- Make an incision, just through the dermis, from the radial pulse at the proximal palmar crease to 1cm distal to the brachial pulse, straight or following the hairline (Fig. 7.6) using a 23 blade.
- With the cautery on coagulation at 50 divide the fat.
- Avoid dividing the superficial cephalic vein and the cutaneous nerves.
- Take great care at the wrist where the radial is very superficial.
- Avoid touching the radial artery at all times and keep wetting it with verapamil solution to minimize vasospasm.
- Proximally cauterize down onto the belly of brachioradialis (BR) and divide the filmy fascia that attaches it to flexor carpi ulnaris (FCU).
- If you continue to cauterize along the tendon of FCR, there is minimal risk of inadvertently damaging the radial artery.
- Place a self-retainer carefully between BR and FCU exposing the radial artery in the proximal forearm.
- Using a McIndoe scissors carefully divide the fascia overlying it all the way down to the distal forearm, as far as the proximal palmar crease.
- With the McIndoe scissors perpendicular to the artery, spread the fascia around the artery gently to expose all the side branches.
- Clip them flush with the venae comitantes alongside the radial artery.
- Holding the venae comitantes not the artery itself, divide the side branches on the FCU side using diathermy on 30–40.
- Now lift the radial artery up gently, Ligaclip, and divide the side branches that run beneath it. Then divide those on the FCR side.
- This becomes more difficult in the distal wrist where the plane of dissection is less clear and the radial artery much smaller.
- Continue proximally beyond the first muscular branch to FCR, but stopping at least 1cm distal to the origin of the radial artery.

- Now perform the intraoperative version of Allen's test: place a bulldog clip in the middle of the radial. If you cannot see or feel a pulse distally, or if pulsatile blood does not emerge from a needle placed distally, the collateral palmar circulation is not adequate and you must not divide the artery.
- If the test is satisfactory place an arterial clip proximally and distally, divide the artery with a knife, and place a mosquito clip or marker stitch to mark the proximal end.
- Transfix and tie both radial artery stumps with 3/0 silk or nylon.
- Place a 16G Redivac drain in the wound and secure it.
- Close the deep fascia with 3/0 Vicryl and the skin with 3/0 Monocryl.
- Dress and bandage firmly and place the Redivac drain on suction.
- There should be minimal drainage in the drain at the end of the case.
- The radial artery can be stored in a variety of solutions, e.g., verapamil 30µmol/L heparinized blood: some surgeons prefer the fascia to be divided with a Potts scissors and the artery distended.

Structures at risk during radial artery harvest

- Ulnar artery at its origin.
- Median nerve throughout its length.
- Superficial radial nerve throughout its length.
- Lateral antebrachial cutaneous nerve.
- Palmar cutaneous branch of the median nerve.
- Superficial dorsal branch of the radial nerve.

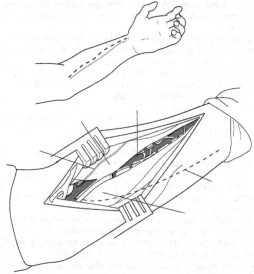

Fig. 7.6 Incisions for radial artery harvest and structures at risk.

LIMA harvest

Key facts

- A LIMA to LAD anastomosis is the most important aspect of CABG.
- Internal mammary artery can be harvested as a *pedicle* (with a strip of fascia, muscle, fat, and internal mammary veins intact), or *skeletonized* (removed without any other tissues attached).
- The pedicled method, which is used most commonly used, is described here, and the skeletonized technique described on 📖 p320. The LIMA anatomy is described on 📖 p54.

Indications

Used for LAD, or where RIMA is anastomosed to LAD, the LIMA can go to diagonal or Cx lesions (📖 p321).

Relative contraindications

- Inadequate flow.
- Salvage surgery.
- Previous radiotherapy to the chest wall.
- Left subclavian stenosis.

Technique

Good exposure is particularly important. The underside of the chest wall should be just above the surgeon's eye level. Some surgeons sit down to take the LIMA so that the assistants taking other conduit are not disadvantaged by the table being fully raised. After the median sternotomy, with the pericardium open or closed, place the mammary retractor in the incision and open it.

- Open the parietal pleura, or keep it closed by dissecting it off the chest wall (keeping it closed may reduce postoperative pleural effusion, and offer benefits in terms of postoperative lung function).
- If the lung obscures the view you can either pack it down with a large wet swab, or ask the anesthesiologist to reduce the tidal volume.
- Identify the LIMA. This is easiest proximally.
- Note how it curves medially, proximally.
- With the diathermy on 60 dessicate, make one tramline 3–5mm medial to the medial mammary vein, from the manubriosternal junction to the xiphisternum. Some surgeons tramline the lateral side too.
- Turn the diathermy down to 30, and holding on to the parietal tissue with the DeBakeys for countertraction, use a combination of diathermy and blunt dissection with the flat of the diathermy blade to work the LIMA pedicle off the chest wall.
- Side branches are limited to the rib spaces: it is easiest to get into the plane of dissection where the LIMA overlies the ribs.
- Clip the side branches flush with the LIMA and divide them at the chest wall with cautery: some surgeons do not use clips at all.
- Now, using diathermy, divide the parietal pleura on the lateral aspect of the LIMA pleura to free the pedicle from the chest wall.
- Applying countertraction, divide the side branches and fascia so that the proximal portion is freed from the chest wall, to the 1st rib.

- Give full-dose heparin, and check hemostasis.
- 2min after the full dose of heparin is given, place a clamp over the distal stump, divide the mammary at the bifurcation, check that there is good pulsatile flow from the mammary and then place a large Ligaclip over the distal end. Flow often improves during the time between initial harvest and LAD anastomosis.
- Wrap the mammary in a small swab soaked in papaverine, and place it in the pleura for later use. Tie the distal stump with 2/0 Vicryl.

Tips and pitfalls of LIMA harvest

- If you cannot visualize the mammary, look and feel for pulsations.
- Always maximize exposure: sometimes a few extra turns on the retractor and tilting the table away make a difficult section easy.
- If the LIMA is very stuck, use minimal diathermy: it is easiest to get into the right plane proximally, but safest to do so distally.
- If your pedicle is too narrow you'll spend most time trying to control bleeding from the mammary veins.
- Freeing the mammary proximally, as far as the subclavian vein, gives additional length and reduces the risk of it kinking.
- Packing bleeding and returning 5min later can allow you to see.
- If you can't control bleeding using pressure and fine suction, give the heparin, wait 2min, and place two bulldogs either side of the bleeding point so that you can see more clearly.
- Never clamp the mammary before heparinizing: it may thrombose.

Structures at risk during LIMA harvest

Form proximal to distal:
- Subclavian vein (avoid this—it is very difficult to reach to repair!).
- Phrenic nerve proximally where it is close to the LIMA, or more distally when you divide the pleura.

LIMA too short

- Skeletonizing, harvesting an additional inch or so proximally, and opening the pleura to drop it under the lung all give more length.
- If you injure the LIMA it is rarely possible to adequately repair it: if the injury is proximal consider using it as a free graft.
- Never leave the LIMA under tension: the graft will fail in the early post-op period, with potentially fatal anterior wall ischemia.

Poor flow

- Poor flow. Some surgeons advocate discarding the LIMA if flow <20mL/min, but others will use even low flow as long as it is pulsatile.[1] Low flow may have several causes:
  - Distal to bifurcation, or includes more vasospastic distal portion: just divide proximal to bifurcation and soak in papaverine.
  - Dissection: look for hematoma, and use proximal segment.
  - Spasm: usually improves with topical papaverine.
  - Tip crushed by scissors: use sharp instruments!
  - Avoid injecting papaverine: it has pH <4 and may damage intima.

1. Hata M et al. Clinical results of coronary artery bypass grafting with use of the internal thoracic artery under low free flow conditions. J Thorac Cardiovasc Surg 2000; 119:125–9.

RIMA harvest

Key facts

- This can be taken as a pedicle, but is more commonly taken skeletonized to avoid compromising wound healing if the LIMA has also been harvested.
- An additional reason for taking it skeletonized is the extra length needed to reach most potential targets.
- Anatomy of the RIMA is described on 📖 p58. Patient selection is described on 📖 p302.

Indications

Any patient undergoing CABG.

Contraindications

- Avoid bilateral mammary harvest in obese, diabetic females as it increases the risk of deep sternal wound infection (DSWI).
- Severe COPD, as BIMA and cough predisposes to sternal non-union.

Technique

Reverse the mammary retractor, so that it can be used on the right. If the LIMA has been taken it, do not divide it.

- Open the pleura and identify the RIMA.
- With the diathermy on 25–30, make a small nick in the parietal pleura adjacent to the mammary vein.
- Use a combination of blunt dissection with the flat of the blade and diathermy, free an area of pleura from the mammary, and continue the length of the RIMA. The easiest way to do this is to pull down very firmly on the pleura where it has been opened up and then use the diathermy in as short bursts as possible to extend the incision.
- The underside of the length of the RIMA should be left exposed.
- If you do this correctly you should hardly see the mammary veins.
- Now, still using blunt dissection, extend the plane between the RIMA and the chest wall: the best way of doing this is to pull very gently on the adventitia that is left on the underside of the RIMA and use the flat of the diathermy blade (without using the cautery) to work between the upper side of the RIMA and the chest wall.
- The best place to start this dissection is overlying the ribs where there are no side branches (side branches occur in the intercostals spaces).
- Place small Ligaclips flush with the RIMA and the chest wall on individual sidebranches, and divide the branches with a Potts scissors.
- Again, more care is required as it is easy to avulse the side branches.
- Continue so that the RIMA is free from xiphisternum to the 1st rib.
- Give heparin.
- 2min after the full dose is given, divide the mammary, check the flow, ligate both ends, and wrap the RIMA in a small swab soaked in papaverine.
- Incise the pleura so that the RIMA can be brought out to the RCA or through the transverse sinus to the left-sided coronary circulation.

Pitfalls in right internal mammary harvest

- Avoid damaging the mammary veins. Clipping them causes them to become congested, and obstruct the view even more.
- The RIMA has a shorter proximal course than the LIMA (📖 p58).
- Always take the RIMA to the bifurcation: the maximum length of RIMA is almost always used.

Total arterial revascularization

Total arterial revascularization (TAR) eliminates vein grafts, using various combinations of LIMA, RIMA, radial artery, and occasionally gastroepiploic artery to perform CABG. The rationale is driven by the observation of superior patency of arterial grafts compared to SVG (📖 p302). A large number of configurations are used, primarily reflecting constraints of length and availability of arterial conduit; the impact of target (distal run-off and lesion severity) on radial artery patency; competitive flow; and the desire to eliminate the need for aortic manipulation (anaortic or 'no touch' technique), to minimize the risk of stroke.

Anaortic or 'no-touch' technique

- This is associated with mortality and stroke rates <0.5% in several series, and may be the strongest reason for OPCAB versus ONCAB.
- Surgery is off-pump to eliminate need for aortic cannulation.
- Proximal aortic anastomoses are eliminated by:
  - Using the *in situ* RIMA to graft the RCA and proximal PDA (this can be a struggle for the *in situ* RIMA to reach without tension), or the LAD (with LIMA being used for Cx lesions), or the proximal Cx and OMs via the transverse sinus.
  - Using RIMA as a 'T' graft off the LIMA allowing multiple sequential grafts of more distal circumflex and PDA territories. While this allows maximum versatility, the risk of compromising the LIMA to LAD anastomosis is not negligible.
  - Using radial loop grafts off the *in situ* RIMA to reach distal targets.

Evidence supporting this approach

Although patency rates superior, evidence of resultant clinical benefit less impressive. It's unfortunate that none of the largest registry studies or RCTs have focused on anaortic TAR, as this likely provides the most benefit in terms of freedom from death or stroke after revascularization. The most widely cited study in support is the Cleveland Clinic 10000 patient registry study[1] which does not control for multiple key confounding variables, or identify which reoperations were for graft failure as opposed to valve surgery, progression of native disease, etc.), and does not show survival benefit in several patient subgroups. There are several RCTs: 10-year results expected in 2015.

Reasons for low uptake

TAR represents <15% of CABG in US, because it is a technically more demanding and time-consuming procedure, with short-term complications more compelling in clinicians' minds than unclear long-term benefits.

Reference

1. Lytle BW et al. Two internal thoracic artery grafts are better than one. *J Thorac Cardiovasc Surg* 1999; **117**:855–72.

Alternative conduit

Key facts

- The gastroepiploic artery as a pedicled graft and the inferior epigastric artery as a free graft have both been used as arterial conduit when more conventional options are not available.
- The contraindications to using these conduits are abdominal surgery, previous radiotherapy in the area, severe peripheral vascular disease, or evidence of end-organ ischemia.
- Cephalic vein and splenic artery have been used rarely.

Right gastroepiploic artery harvest

- Pass an NG tube to decompress the stomach.
- Extend the median sternotomy incision, dividing the linea alba from the xiphoid to halfway above the umbilicus.
- Divide the triangular ligament of the liver, and retract the liver superiorly and to the right (Fig. 7.7) and pull the stomach into view.
- The right gastroepiploic artery (RGEA) runs along the greater curvature of the stomach from the duodenum towards the cardia.
- Dissect off the RGEA clipping and dividing the side branches in the way described for the radial artery, working from the pylorus until sufficient length is achieved.
- Inadvertent diathermy burns to the stomach mucosa should be oversewn with non-absorbable monofilament, e.g., Prolene.
- Make an opening in the diaphragm medial to the IVC.
- Pass the pedicle either anterior or posterior to the duodenum and stomach, depending on where there is least distortion, through the diaphragmatic opening into the pericardial cavity.
- The RGEA is normally anastomosed to the distal RCA or PDA.

Inferior epigastric artery harvest

- The right inferior epigastric artery should be harvested if the LIMA is used, to avoid ischemic changes to the skin.
- Make a paramedian incision beginning at the level of the umbilicus along the lateral border of rectus abdominus, ending 2–3cm above the inguinal ligament (Fig. 7.7).
- Divide the anterior rectus sheath and retract the muscle laterally.
- Mobilize the artery with the venae commitantes as described for the radial artery (Fig. 7.6).
- Divide the artery and its pedicle proximally at its origin from the external iliac artery where it may be calcified, and distally where it bifurcates.
- Mark the distal end with a marker stitch or hemostat.
- Store it in a solution of verapamil in 30µmol/L heparinized blood until it is required.

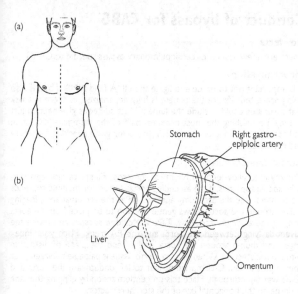

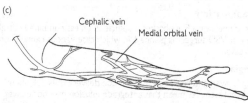

Fig. 7.7 (a) Incisions for right gastroepiploic artery harvest (RGEA) and right inferior epigastric artery harvest. (b) Exposure of the RGEA. (c) Cephalic vein.

Splenic artery

The splenic artery is exposed through a midline extension of the median sternotomy, as described for the RGEA. The lesser peritoneal sac is opened to gain access to the artery which travels along the superior margin of the pancreas. The spleen has a collateral blood supply from the left gastric artery, so splenectomy is not required.

Cephalic vein

• The cephalic vein can be harvested through an incision running from the anatomical snuff-box, over the lateral aspect of the forearm to the bicipital aponeurosis, using the open technique described for saphenous vein harvest (📖 p306).

Conduct of bypass for CABG

Key facts

There are a few aspects of cardiopulmonary bypass specific to CABG.

Heparinization

It is important not to divide and ligate the LIMA (and RIMA if that is also being harvested) before the patient is fully heparinized, as there is a risk that thrombus could occlude the lumen. Most surgeons give heparin just as they are finishing the most proximal part of the mammary dissection and spend the 2min after the heparin has being given checking mammary bed hemostasis

Aortic cannulation

The key is to allow enough room for the cross-clamp, cardioplegia cannula, and all top ends. If the ascending aorta is short, or multiple top-ends are planned, free the ascending aorta as far as the proximal arch. Placing a sling around the aorta allows gentle traction to be placed on the aorta bringing more length into view. Take a McIndoe scissors and divide the adventitia lying between the aorta and the PA trunk. Place your index finger and thumb around the aorta, and extend the plane of dissection with blunt dissection. When minimal or no tissue is palpable between your fingers pass a Sem C-clamp from right to left underneath the aorta and pull a wet tape through. Place this on gentle traction by clipping the tape underneath the horizontal bar of the sternal retractor.

Venous cannulation

A two-stage cannula or a Ross basket is sufficient, unless combined mitral valve surgery or VSD surgery is planned, in which case venous cannulation should be bicaval.

Cardioplegia

Cardioplegia is given anterogradely. Retrograde delivery is useful when:
- Tight proximal stenoses mean that antegrade infusion may not deliver complete cardioprotection, or to maximize cardioprotection in the very hypertrophied, ischemic, or dysfunctional LV.
- Cardioplegia is given antegradely initially, and then retrogradely at intervals. Once each distal anastomosis is performed cardioplegia may be given directly down the vein graft as well as retrogradely.
- If you are using a single-clamp technique, you can complete proximal anastomoses while giving retrograde.

Venting

The heart is normally vented by either an aortic root vent, usually a 'Y' connector on the cardioplegia cannula, or by an LV apical vent. When vessels are occluded aortic root venting may not be enough to keep the coronaries free of blood during the distal anastomosis.

Single clamp technique

Clamp time may be minimized by completing all distals first, removing the cross-clamp, and applying a side-biting clamp for the proximal anastomoses. In the single-clamp technique the cross-clamp remains *in situ* and a side-biting clamp is not used for the proximals which can be performed after each distal anastomosis, or at the end prior to removal of the clamp. The primary advantage of the single-clamp technique is less risk of stroke from repeated manipulation of the aorta.

Alternatives to cardioplegic arrest on bypass

As the heart remains perfused these techniques mean that it is sensible to try to restore flow to the areas affected by the most important stenoses first. The top-ends are usually performed after (or in some cases before) each distal anastomosis, and the heart allowed a period of perfusion before moving onto the next distal anastomosis.

Beating heart on bypass

Cardioplegia is not given, and the heart is not arrested. Instead stabilizers used in OPCAB are used to position the heart once it is on bypass, and distal anastomoses carried out in the normal fashion (📖 p328). Useful where aortic calcification precludes clamping but not cannulation.

Intermittent cross-clamp fibrillation

This is one of the oldest forms of cardioprotection, popular before the development of potassium-based cardioplegia. An increased understanding of ischemic preconditioning (📖 p75) and the adverse effects of cardioplegic arrest (📖 p74) have led to revived interest in this technique. The principle is based on the fact that a brief period of ischemia (<20min of cross-clamping) is readily reversed by perfusion with normal blood. The few randomized studies comparing this technique with cardioplegic arrest show no difference in mortality, stroke, or postoperative indices of ventricular function. Repeated cross-clamping of the aorta does not appear to be associated with increased risk of stroke in elective patients with no risk factors for peripheral vascular disease.

Indications: there is little objective evidence to support specific recommendations: it is a safe and useful alternative to cardioplegic arrest. The surgeon must, however, be able to reliably complete a distal anastomosis in <15min.

Technique: cardioplegia is not given, and the heart is fibrillated so that the distal anastomoses can be performed. This is carried out under moderate hypothermia (32°C). To prevent LV distension the aorta must be cross-clamped as soon as the heart is fibrillated. The sequence is:
- Fibrillator applied to heart.
- Flows down.
- Cross-clamp on and flows back up.
- Heart positioned.
- Distal anastomosis performed: must take <15min.
- Fibrillator removed as anastomosis completed.
- Anastomosis tested.
- Heart defibrillated.
- Flows down.
- Cross-clamp off and flows back up.
- Proximal anastomosis performed with side-biting clamp.

Positioning the heart on bypass

Key facts

- Positioning the heart is key to performing efficient and effective distals.
- It's always easier if the heart is adequately drained—always check the RA and RV are decompressed and your vent is on before lifting the heart, and again if the distal coronaries are obscured by blood flow.

Positioning the heart for the LAD and diagonals

- Slide your right hand under the heart, palm up.
- Lift the ventricles and rotate them slightly anticlockwise so that the LAD comes into view. This maneuver can be used before bypass to inspect the vessels without too much hemodynamic compromise.
- With your left hand use a DeBakey forceps to pack one or two large wet packs underneath the heart, holding it in position.
- Stay sutures should not be necessary.

Positioning for intermediate and OM vessels

- Slide your right hand under the heart palm up.
- Swap to small dry pack in your left hand, hold the apex firmly, and lift the heart right up, twisting the ventricles anticlockwise.
- Now pack one or two large wet packs underneath the heart using a DeBakey's in your right hand, and ask your assistant to place their right hand, thumb down across the left ventricle holding it in place.
- If you have two assistants, one can hold the heart from the left side of the table, standing to your left side at the patient's right shoulder.
- Letting the right pleura down sometimes helps exposure.
- Positioning the table head up, and rotating it towards you also helps.
- Inspecting the OM system before bypass is possible, but it causes rapid hemodynamic compromise, and most surgeons do not do it routinely.

Positioning the heart for the RCA vessels

- Using a DeBakey tuck a small dry pack down behind the LA appendage into the oblique sinus.
- With your left hand pull the acute margin of the heart slightly towards the head so that you can see the tip of the pack.
- Using the DeBakey drag the pack towards the IVC; this rotates the heart exposing the distal right and PDA vessels.
- An assistant can hold the acute margin using a small dry pack.
- Sometimes stay sutures are necessary to improve access.
- Positioning the table head down and rotating it away from you helps.

Stay sutures

Superficial stay sutures can be used simply to hold the vessel walls open and retract epicardial fat. Deeper stays straighten out the vessel and occlude flow. Superficial stay sutures, normally 3/0 Ethibond, are placed in the epicardial fat parallel to the arteriotomy, and fixed with rubber-shod clips. Deeper 1/0 or 2/0 Prolene is passed perpendicularly into the myo-cardium 1cm away from the coronary artery and out on the other side, and anchored with clips.

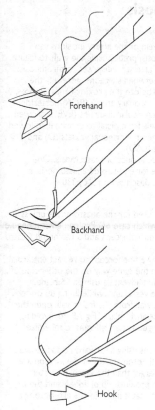

Forehand

Backhand

Hook

Fig. 7.8 Different ways of mounting the needle in the needle driver needed for coronary distals.

Vein distal anastomosis

Key facts

- Flaps or asymmetry in either the vein or the artery incisions can reduce the lumen of the anastomosis, predisposing the graft to failure. Handling the intima of the vein or artery predisposes to thrombosis.
- Although there is large variation between surgeons, generally the distal anastomoses are performed before the proximal anastomoses, in the following order: distal right coronary artery (RCA)/posterior descending artery (PDA)/lateral ventricular branches (LVB), followed by the obtuse marginal (OM) vessels from distal to proximal, followed by the intermediate vessel (Int), then the diagonal vessels (D) and finally the left anterior descending (LAD).
- There is also a wide variation in techniques of anastomosis. One simple technique is described here for end-to-side anastomosis: a variation on the same technique is described on 🕮 p330.

Technique

Double-ended 8/0 or 7/0 Prolene is used for the anastomoses unless the coronary vessel is very calcified, in which case 6/0 Prolene gives a needle with slightly greater durability. Fine microforceps and a ratcheted Castro needle holder are used (Fig. 7.8).

- Position the heart (🕮 p326). Using a fine forceps to retract epicardial fat with your assistant retracting in the same way on the other side of the vessel, clear the vessel of fat and adventitia using a 15 blade.
- Carefully identify the centre of the vessel and, while lifting up on the epicardial fat to separate the back wall from the front wall, open the vessel carefully using either a 15 or an 11 blade, Fig 7.9 (a), avoiding trauma to the back wall (some surgeons turn off vent to minimize this).
- Extend the incision in both directions using a forward Potts followed by a backwards Potts scissors, so that the apexes of the incision are cleanly cut and the incision is 2/3 larger than the vessel diameter.
- Prepare the vein by cutting off the proximal tip obliquely and then incising the heel by about 2mm, so that it matches the arteriotomy, Fig 7.9 (b).
- Suspend the vein by the toe using either a mosquito clip or a fine DeBakey in your assistant's left hand. They follow the suture with their right.
- Place a rubber-shod bulldog clip on the free needle.
- Start two stitches from the heel, pass the needle outside to in on the vein, backhand. Your next stitch is inside to out on the arteriotomy two stitches from the heel, backhand (Fig 7.10).
- Continue outside to in on the vein moving clockwise, inside to out on the artery moving anticlockwise until you are one or two stitches past the heel, on the outside of the arteriotomy.
- Wet the sutures with saline and gently pull on the both ends of the suture while your assistant brings the vein down with slight countertraction onto the arteriotomy, until the suture is taut and

all loops are taken up. If the arteriotomy is very friable put in fewer stitches before bringing the vein down.

- Now holding the vein taut so that the toe of the vein meets the toe of the arteriotomy, pass the needle outside to in on the vein and inside to out on the artery, forehand. The first stitch should be done in two passes, but after that it is possible to stitch both vessels in one pass.
- At the toe change the needle to backhand, and suture the toe in two passes, to ensure that you do not catch the back wall of the artery. A hook shot is an alternative (Fig. 7.8).
- Continue forehand to the start of the anastomoses: the first stitch after the toe is usually easier in two bites, but after that most stitches can be done in one pass—just retract the epicardium so you can see your stitches are full thickness and not catching the back wall.
- Take up the slack in the anastomosis without purse-stringing it.
- Tie the anastomoses: use a slip-knot and then lock it with eight throws.
- If you break the suture while tying it, and there is not enough left to do an instrument tie, the safest thing is to redo the anastomoses.
- Test the anastomosis by injecting heparinized blood, saline, or cardioplegia down the graft, noting how much resistance (there should not be much if the target vessel is >1.5mm), checking that you can see the artery and the myocardium perfusing distally and noting any leaks.
- Take particular care when repairing leaks at the toe, as catching the back wall of the artery here will effectively occlude the anastomosis.
- It is easiest to anastomose the toe before the heel when carrying out PDA grafts: start inside to out on the vein forehand, outside to in on the artery, moving down towards the heel on the diaphragmatic side of the anastomosis, then change needles and complete the toe backhand working anticlockwise forehand to complete the anastomosis.

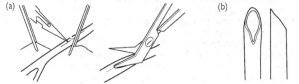

Fig. 7.9 (a) Creating the arteriotomy. (b) Preparing the vein.

Arterial distal anastomosis

Key facts

- The vein can be stretched or gathered slightly to match the size of the arteriotomy, but arterial conduit is not so forgiving, and the size match needs to be exact.
- To achieve this most surgeons do not prepare arterial conduit in the same way as venous conduit: they leave a large hood of excess artery which can be cut to size halfway through the anastomosis. The technique described here is for arterial grafts, but it can just as easily be used for venous grafting (but there is no need to shape the hood).

Technique

Preparing pedicled LIMA: make a V-shaped incision in the pleura, taking care to avoid the phrenic nerve. Bring the LIMA through from the pleural space and make sure that it is not twisted. Measure the length against where you want to graft the LAD and divide the LIMA accordingly. Blood flow should reflect the perfusion pressure: there should be a strong, horizontal stream of blood. If this is not the case it is advisable to use other conduit. Anchor the LIMA, so that the shiny parietal pleura is uppermost, by clipping it to the side towels. Using 90° scissors divide the fascia in front of the LIMA for 1–1.5cm. Next, staying in the midline, open the front of the LIMA. If the lumen looks particularly narrow, or if there are multiple side branches, continue a little lower.

Preparing skeletonized RIMA: cut the RIMA flush with the Ligaclip to get maximum and check the flow as earlier. Divide the front of the vessel in the midline as described for the LIMA.

Preparing the radial: either cut the distal end obliquely and incise it just as described for the saphenous vein, or create a hood that can be shaped to size later as described for the LIMA

- Distal anastomosis technique suspend the arterial conduit a few inches from the coronary artery.
- Make the arteriotomy as described on 📖 p328.
- Using double-ended 8/0 Prolene pass the first stitch forehand inside to out on the heel of the conduit, forehand outside to in on the arteriotomy, bring the arterial conduit down after.
- Place one needle on a rubber-shod bulldog, and then do three or four stitches forehand on the farside of the arteriotomy inside to out on the conduit, outside to in on the coronary artery, finishing outside on the conduit.
- Next swap the rubber-shod bulldog onto the other needle, and suture the other side of the arteriotomy backhand.
- Continue, swap to forehand, round the toe, just as described on 📖 p329, to the beginning of the anastomoses and tie it down.
- Check the anastomosis by either injecting the conduit with blood, or in the case of pedicled conduit, releasing the bulldog clamp temporarily. Replace the clamp or all cardioplegia will rapidly be washed out.

Troubleshooting the bleeding distal

- It's a bit depressing to find your distal anastomosis leaks, but it should be possible to sort it out without compromising the anastomosis.
- Always recheck distals with the clamp off, before weaning from bypass, as they can be difficult to fix with the heart full and beating.
- If bleeding is too much to clearly see, you can occlude the graft with a bulldog, or go down on the pump flow for 1min at a time.
- Position the heart as for the distal anastomosis, and squirt saline over the anastomosis to localize the bleeding point.
  - Side branch: usually safest to fix with a figure-of-8 stitch using 8/0 Prolene as a Ligaclip may distort the anastomosis, and if you need to remove it for any reason can destroy the integrity of the hood.
  - Dog-ear: fix poor spacing with 7/0 Prolene figure-of-8 full-thickness bites on conduit and arteriotomy.
  - Loose suture: use a fine nerve hook to carefully pull up the suture (which should stop the bleeding) and pass a 7/0 Prolene through the loop. Take a partial thickness bite adjacent to it across the conduit and arteriotomy taking care not to narrow the anastomosis with a fresh 7/0 Prolene and tie securely. Now tie the free end of this 7/0 to the 7/0 in the loose loop, so that the loop forms part of the knot (Fig. 7.10) which will secure the whole anastomosis.
  - Tear: do a partial thickness figure-of-8 bite using 8/0 Prolene parallel to the anastomosis in the conduit then in the coronary and tie.
  - Sometimes taking the tension off the anastomosis by suturing the divided the epicardial fat together, without constricting the anastomosis is sufficient.
- Deciding whether to give protamine is a fine judgment: often times bleeding is due to needle holes and raw surfaces and resolves, but if it doesn't you may need to use an off-pump stabilizer to get access.

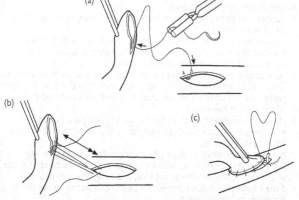

Fig. 7.10 (a) First stitch. (b) Parachuting the vein down. (c) Stitching the near side.

Jump or sequential grafts

Key facts

- Sequential grafts are useful when there is insufficient conduit to graft every artery individually. Any conduit, including LIMA can be used.
- The most distal anastomosis should be to the target vessel with the best outflow; otherwise preferential flow to the proximal anastomosis puts the distal anastomosis at high risk of failure.
- Avoid mixing arterial and venous conduit in 'T' or 'Y' grafts: competitive flow down the vein can cause early failure of the arterial conduit.

Advantages

- Using sequential grafts increases the number of arteries that can be revascularized by a single length of conduit from one to two or three.
- The number of proximal anastomoses and hence the need to handle the aorta is reduced, and may even be eliminated by using the IMAs to sequentially graft all targets.
- Patency rates of venous grafts may be increased, because of the augmentation of outflow.

Disadvantages

- Larger regions of myocardium are jeopardized if the conduit fails.
- LIMA to LAD flow may be compromised by 'Y' or 'T' grafts proximal to the LIMA to LAD anastomosis.

Technique

Take your time to measure and orientate the distended conduit correctly with the heart full: it may help to use a marker pen to mark the conduit where you plan to open it. Open the conduit transversely if it lies across the coronary artery, or longitudinally if it will lie parallel to the coronary artery (Fig. 7.11). For transverse incisions, the length of the incision should not exceed 2/3 of the diameter of the conduit, or the conduit will be flattened by the anastomosis. If using IMA or radial skeletonize the portion to be used in the side-to-side graft.

- Position the conduit 1cm away from the arteriotomy in the position that it will eventually lie in.
- Starting one stitch away from where you want the conduit to meet the heel of the arteriotomy, pass the suture from outside to in on the conduit and place a rubber-shod bulldog on the other end.
- Now suture inside to out on the arteriotomy, two stitches from the heel.
- Continue two stitches past the heel, then parachute the conduit down gently, check that there are no crossed stitches or loops, and take up all the slack in the suture.
- Most of the following stitches can be done in one pass: continue with the same suture along the nearside of the vessels to the toe and finishing on the far side.
- It is sometimes easier to start side-to-side anastomosis in the way described on 🕮 p328: i.e., suturing outside to in on the conduit, inside to out on the arteriotomy at the heel, and tying down immediately.
- If the conduit is small, a transverse incision reduces the risk of the anastomosis constricting it.

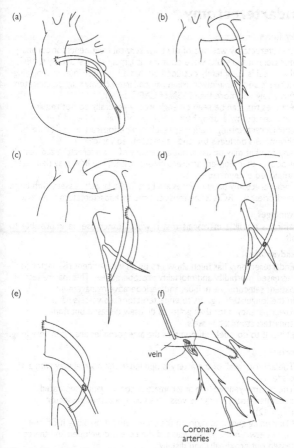

Fig. 7.11 Types of bypass graft. (a) Vein graft to the LAD, proximal anastomosis to aorta. (b) LIMA to LAD. (c) 'T' graft: LIMA to LAD with free RIMA anastomosed to LIMA proximally and diagonal distally (common combination is the RIMA anastomosed to diagonal or OM with PDA as a sequential. (d) Sequential graft LIMA to LAD and diagonal. (e) Sequential vein graft to LAD and diagonal with proximal anastomosis to aorta. (f) Technique of performing sequential vein graft.

Endarterectomy

Key facts

- Endarterectomy was one of the early surgical treatments for coronary disease, but as results were poor it was largely superseded by CABG.
- If a vessel is completely occluded but has a large distribution supplying ischemic and viable myocardium, an endarterectomy may be indicated (probably not more than 2–5% of CABG cases).
- Arteries that can be seen on angiography generally do not require endarterectomy as they have a true lumen that can be grafted: endarterectomizing them may result in a perioperative MI if acute thrombosis occludes the endarterectomized vessel.
- Any conduit may be used, but as patency of endarterectomized vessels is poorer than non-endarterectomized vessels, the IMA may be better employed elsewhere.
- Endarterectomy patency rates are best in the largest vessels, with large territories: the RCA is the most commonly endarterectomized vessel.

Advantages

Grafting is possible in vessels that it would otherwise be impossible to graft.

Disadvantages

- Endarterectomy has been shown to be an independent risk factor for increased morbidity and mortality postoperatively. This may reflect patient selection, technique, and perioperative management.
- In the longer-term, grafts to endarterectomized vessels have lower patency rates than grafts to diffusely diseased but non-endarterectomized vessels.
- Difficult to do safely off-pump as the arteriotomies are often very long.

Technique

- The anterior wall of the artery is opened in the normal way with a 15 blade.
- The creamy-yellow, firm atheromatous core is gently separated circumferentially from the vessel wall using a curved dissector (Fig. 7.12).
- Maintaining gentle tension on the core, without breaking it off, the plane between the vessel wall and the core is developed and the core teased out proximally and distally.
- Usually it is possible to extract the atheroma for several centimeters as far as the distal branches, and it should be seen to taper—confirming that distal branches have been adequately endarterectomized.
- Once the atheroma has been removed, conduit can be anastomosed to the vessel walls in the usual manner.
- If the endarterectomy breaks off, it may be necessary to extend the arteriotomy far enough to continue the endarterectomy: a vein patch may be needed to close a long arteriotomy which can then be grafted with arterial or venous conduit.
- Some surgeons routinely perform a long endarterectomy with vein patch.

Postoperative management

Because of the damage to the coronary intima, these anastomoses are much more prone to acute thrombosis postoperatively (5% risk of post-operative MI in recent series, down from up to 25% in historic series) and aspirin should be given early. These patients are either anticoagulated for 2–3 months postoperatively, or maintained on aspirin and clopidogrel. Some surgeons start heparin as soon as mediastinal drainage is <50mL/h.

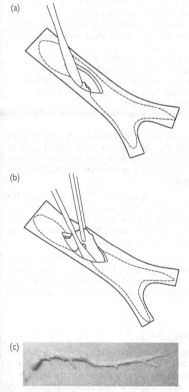

Fig. 7.12 (a) The endarterectomy plane is developed. (b) Atheroma is teased out. (c) Endarterectomy specimen—note tapered ends. Fig 7.12c reprinted with permission from Fukui, T, Takanashi, S, Hosoda, Y (2005) Coronary endarterectomy and stent removal in patients with in-Stent restenosis, *Ann Thorac Surg*;**79**:558–63. Copyright © The Society of Thoracic Surgeons.

Positioning the heart in OPCAB

Key facts

- The LAD and diagonal vessels are easiest to access, the RCA can cause problems with bradycardia, and the Cx vessels are more challenging to access particularly if close to the AV groove.
- Positioning the heart for off-pump surgery is a balance between achieving good exposure and maintaining hemodynamic stability.
- Certain maneuvers, particularly compressing the long axis of the heart, cause AV valve incompetence. The heart tolerates lifting and rotating well as long as compression and distortion are avoided.
- Opening the pleura widely improves positioning as the heart can be rotated further without compressing it, and **gradual movements** allow the heart to compensate.
- Reflex tachyarrhythmias may develop as a result of low CO: this makes the distal anastomoses much more difficult, and along with extrasystoles and rising PA pressures are an early warning of ischemia.
- Communication between surgeon and anesthesiologist is key to successful off-pump surgery (📖 pp98–99).

Exposure

Incision: usually a sternotomy for multi-vessel grafting, although left and right thoracotomy approaches are also used for more limited grafting. A limited skin incision is cosmetically appealing but reduces exposure and increases the amount of manipulation of the heart required for good access particularly for PDA grafting.

Pericardium: this is widely incised, with an extended 'T' inferiorly, extended down to the IVC, avoiding the phrenic, to maximize exposure. Placing a line of three stay sutures parallel to and just above the left phrenic, and pulling up on them (place the in the self-locking OPCAB retractor) brings the whole anterior surface of the heart completely into view.

Tape and snare: a broad tape (or a small pack) (Fig. 7.13b), is fixed to the posterior pericardium between the right and left superior pulmonary veins with a 0/0 Ethibond, which is then snared. Traction on the tape and the snare serves to lift the apex of the heart, and is particularly useful for Cx and PDA territory grafts.

Stabilizers

There are a variety of stabilizing adjuncts.

Suction devices: there are two types. The first is a cup-shaped device that is placed on the apex of the heart to position and stabilize. The second is a two-pronged foot, the prongs being placed either side of the segment of artery being grafted, to stabilize that region of heart. Both suction devices have a flexible arm that can be adjusted, and then tightened to make it rigid, and clips by which them can be attached to the sternal retractor. Some systems require a custom retractor. The connection tubing to the suction has a tap that can be turned on and off by the surgeon. The devices may be disposable, but reusable ones are available.

Pressure stabilizers: these are simple rigid systems that can be set up so that a metal plate stabilizes the area being grafted by pressing down on it. They do not stabilize as well as the suction devices, and tend to cause more hemodynamic compromise. Because they are less bulky than suction stabilizers, these devices have more of a role in mini-thoracotomy coronary surgery, and they are reusable so reduce cost.

> **Pitfalls of using stabilizers**
> - It is possible to damage the descending aorta and esophagus if stay sutures are placed too deep in the pericardium.
> - The phrenic nerve is at risk when opening the pleura widely.
> - Compressing and distorting the heart reduces cardiac output: although blood pressure may be maintained with pressors, the patient becomes increasingly acidotic.
> - Too high suction causes myocardial bruising.

Positioning the heart for LAD and diagonal vessels

Lift the ends of the tape either side of the heart up and left towards the head, pull the snare downwards, and apply the pronged suction to the segment of artery that is to be grafted (base on lower bar of retractor).

Positioning for the intermediate and OM vessels

Lift the ends of the tape upwards and to the left, allowing the heart to rotate to the right into the right pleural space, facilitated by opening the right pleura widely. It is usually necessary to stabilize the apex, and rotating the table to the right usually improves access. Apply the pronged suction (base usually on lower bar of retractor).

Positioning the heart for distal RCA and PDA

Lift the tape up and to the left, stabilize the apex with a suction cup and rotate the table towards the left and put it head-down.

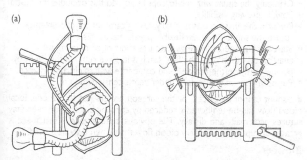

Fig. 7.13 (a) Positioning the heart for the LAD using two suction devices.
(b) Positioning the heart for the LAD using stay sutures and a pericardial sling.

Distal anastomoses off bypass

Key facts

- The distal anastomoses may be performed before the proximal ones or after: measuring the conduit when the proximal end has been performed first is slightly more difficult, but the advantage is that blood supply is immediately restored once the distal anastomosis is complete.
- It is usual practice to graft the LAD first to restore blood supply to the anterior wall and septum. Occasionally if the LAD provides the sole collateral blood supply to an occluded RCA it may be preferable to graft the RCA first, to reduce ischemia when the LAD is being grafted.
- The same suture techniques described on ☐ p328–31 can be used in off-pump surgery, although taking bites inside to out on the coronary is easier than outside to in if a shunt is used.
- Early recognition of ischemia (rising PAPs, extrasystoles, bradycardia, and ST-segment changes) is crucial to allow adjustments to be made, avoiding critical decompensation.
- Do not inject saline down completed vein grafts: its acidic pH can cause arrhythmias and hemodynamic disturbance.

Shunts

Using a shunt diverts blood from the operative field while ensuring that coronary blood flow is disrupted for the minimum amount of time. This is particularly valuable when performing the anastomosis to the RCA as ischemia in this territory leads to bradycardia and hypotension. If the lumen of the coronary artery is >1.2mm in diameter, a disposable shunt can usually be inserted once the arteriotomy has been created. The shunt consists of a flexible 1–2cm round-ended tube, with a tag that ensures that it doesn't migrate into the coronary vessel (Fig. 7.14). They are usually available in a range of sizes (1.0mm, 1.5mm, 2.0mm, and 2.5mm).

- Using two fine forceps, insert one end into the proximal part of the arteriotomy, then bend the shunt so that the other end can be inserted into the distal part of the arteriotomy.
- Clamping the shunt with the forceps as you do this occludes the blood flow, improving visibility.
- Perform the anastomosis normally, taking care not to inadvertently suture the shunt—the thin flexible plastic makes this a risk.
- Start leaving sutures loose two sutures short of completing the anastomosis, then once the final stitch is in place remove the shunt by pulling gently on the tag: it should come free with minimal resistance.
- Put both ends of your suture under gentle tension and tie.

If a shunt cannot be placed, or the surgeon prefers not to use one, local blood flow can be temporarily reduced by applying bulldogs or deep stay sutures proximally and distally. The obvious disadvantage is that there is greater disruption in coronary blood flow than when a shunt is used.

Blowers

Intermittent suction with a fine tip is useful when there is minimal blood flow. When blood flow into the operative field is constant a blowing device provides a less obtrusive means of improving visibility. Blowing devices now blow humidified CO_2 which dissolves readily, reducing the risk of air embolism. Humidification prevents tissues drying out. The strength of the jet of CO_2 is usually controlled by adjusting the outlet valve on the gas cylinder. The normal setting is 4–8L/min. The amount of humidification can be controlled by adjusting the setting of the pressure bag, and by adjusting the inflow in the operative field. It is best to only direct the blower onto the tissues intermittently as prolonged exposure may result in macerating the tissues.

Pitfalls of shunts and blowers

- It is possible to damage the vessel endothelium with repeated attempts to insert a shunt, which very occasionally may result in acute thrombosis of the vessel requiring revision of the anastomosis. If a smaller shunt will not easily enter the vessel, occlude the proximal vessel with a bulldog or a silastic loop.
- If the CO_2 is not humidified then the blower effectively desiccates the endothelium, again predisposing to early thrombosis.
- Always make sure you can see your needle tip relative to the shunt: if you suture the shunt inadvertently just carefully pull the suture back out and redo: if you only recognize this at completion of the anastomosis, it is usually possible to pull the shunt out enough to cut it free from the stray suture with a Potts scissors or an 11 blade.
- A shunt does not restore normal blood supply: it reduces the lumen that blood can flow through and occludes side branches, so ischemic changes can still result if anastomoses are not completed efficiently.

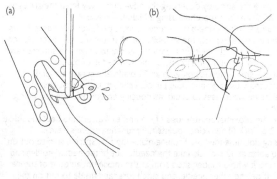

(a)   (b)

Fig. 7.14 (a) Inserting the shunt. (b) Removing the shunt.

Proximal anastomoses to aorta

Key facts

- Although it is possible to perform the proximal anastomoses before the distal anastomoses, before or after institution of bypass, most surgeons perform them after completion of the distal anastomoses: this gives maximum flexibility to decide where the distal anastomosis is.
- They can be carried out with the cross-clamp still on, which reduces the number of times the aorta is side-clamped, reducing the risk of stroke, but prolonging the cross-clamp time (single-clamp technique).
- Alternatively the cross-clamp is removed after the last distal is performed and the proximals are carried out using a side-biting clamp.
- Using the Heartstring device allows a hand-sewn proximal anastomosis to be carried out without any clamp in place.
- Correct orientation and length is key to graft longevity.

Technique

There are a variety of ways of performing this anastomosis. One method is described here. It is important to orientate the proximal anastomoses so that the conduit follows the most natural path, and is not kinked. It is also vital to measure the conduit accurately: if it is cut too long it is very likely to kink, and if it is cut too short both anastomoses will be under tension and thrombose early. Correct orientation is shown in Fig. 7.15. Taking wider bites of aorta than conduit around the heel, and wider bites of conduit than aorta at the toe produces the ideal 'cobra head' (Fig. 7.15).

- Look at the distal anastomosis while injecting blood or saline down the conduit, to establish the best way of orienting the conduit.
- Still injecting the conduit, after warning the perfusionist, place some occlusion on the venous line to fill the heart, to assess length.
- Divide it obliquely, keeping its orientation; if it is small conduit incise the heel 2–3mm, and fix it to the side-towels using a mosquito.
- Next, having palpated the aorta to avoid atheromatous plaques, prepare the aorta by dissecting the adventitia away from the area you plan to site your top-ends, using a McIndoe scissors.
- If you are using a side-biting clamp, ask the perfusionist to drop flows temporarily and apply the side-biter so that it is securely in place, and the toe of the clamp is flush with the aorta: too high and sutures catch on it, too low and the operative field will be full of blood.
- Make a 4mm stab incision with an 11 blade and create a round aortotomy using a 4mm hole punch, which must be kept clean of debris between uses to avoid introducing emboli into the ascending aorta.
- For the proximal anastomosis of circumflex vessels, the heel should lie at 2 o'clock (if 12 o'clock points towards the patient's head).
- Using double-ended 6/0 Prolene make the first stitch inside to out on the aorta at 12 o'clock, take the needle out of the needle-holder and secure it with a rubber-shod so that the maximum amount of suture is left on the other needle, and stitch forehand inside to out on the conduit, starting two stitches before the heel, at about 8 o'clock.

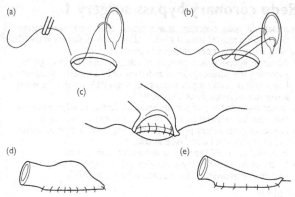

Fig. 7.15 (a) First stitch. (b) Second stitch. (c) After parachuting down.
(d) A satisfactory 'cobra head'. (e) An unsatisfactory one.

- Continue forehand outside to in on the aorta at 1 o'clock.
- Make even, full-thickness bites about 1mm from the edge of the
  conduit, 2mm from the edge of the aorta, and match the size of the
  conduit to the aortotomy so that a 'cobra-head' is produced.
- When you reach 6 o'clock on the aorta parachute the conduit down
  by pulling alternatively on the ends of the suture, and on the conduit
  to take up any loops: getting round to 6 o'clock makes the last stitches
  before you tie the anastomoses much easier, as they are not hidden by
  the vein, and can be done forehand.
- Check that there are no loops or crossed stitches.
- Change needles and suture the nearside forehand, from outside to in
  on the vein, and inside to out on the aorta in one pass, except for the
  first stitch which is better done in two passes.
- Tie down, and place a bulldog clamp across the conduit if there is not
  one already.
- For grafts to the right coronary system start at the toe of the conduit
  so that it lies at 12 o' clock, and for grafts to the LAD and diagonal
  vessels place the heel at 4 o'clock on the aorta (Fig. 7.15c).
- Remove the side-biting clamp if one is on, and prick the conduit to
  de-air it before removing the bulldog clamps: there should a full 'cobra
  head' rather than a flattened one, and no kinks or twists in the conduit.
- To repair any leaks from top ends, ask the perfusionist to 'go down on
  flow' and suture from conduit to aorta (backhand if necessary) usually
  as a figure-of-8.

Redo coronary bypass surgery 1

Numbers of redo coronary artery bypass operations have decreased steadily from a peak of around 25–30% of all coronary surgery in the 1980s to <5% today. This is probably due to several factors:

- Advances in operative technique including the use of arterial grafts extending the patency rates of grafts: use of BIMA is associated with a lower rate of redo surgery than use of single IMA, which in turn has a lower rate of reoperation than no IMA.
- Better understanding of primary revascularization strategy leading to less need for reoperation to graft untreated native vessel lesions.
- Advances in secondary prevention including the now near universal use of aspirin, statins, and ACE inhibitors.
- Increased use of PCI to treat native and conduit stenosis.
- Better understanding of who benefits and who does not benefit, leading to narrowing of the indications for redo CABG.

Etiology

In the 1960s and 1970s, the early period of CABG, the indications for redo surgery was early graft failure, which occurred in almost 1/3 of patients, and progression of atherosclerotic disease in non-grafted vessels, which occurred in >1/2 of patients. Improvements in operative technique and decision-making meant that by the 1980s, the commonest indications had changed: 92% of cases were for late graft failure, and reoperation for progression of atherosclerosis in non-grafted vessels was rare. Risk factors for redo CABG include:

- No use of IMA in original operation.
- Incomplete revascularization in original operation.
- Young age.
- Normal LV.
- 1VD or 2VD.
- Poor control of hypertension, hypercholesterolemia, smoking.

Pathophysiology

The pathophysiology of ischemia is similar to that in unoperated patients, but the underlying pathology is highly variable (□ p303). In the majority of patients presenting with ischemia within a year of coronary artery surgery, the grafts are patent: ischemia is attributable to incomplete revascularization. Late presentation is due to SVG atherosclerosis: patients with stenoses in conduits subtending the LAD do particularly poorly.

Indications for reoperation

The mortality of surgery is increased in reoperation: the mortality in UK and US national registries for primary CABG is 1–2% compared to 5–8% for redo CABG. The higher mortality is due to increased rates of postoperative infarction and reflects:

- More advanced age.
- Poorer LV function and more severe distal and diffuse disease.
- More aortic atherosclerosis and peripheral vascular disease.
- Atherosclerotic vein grafts prone to embolize when handled.

- Risk presented by resternotomy.
- Risk of compromising patent graft to LAD territory in resternotomy.
- Difficulty in securing myocardial protection with patent LIMA to LAD.
- Less adequate conduit availability.
- Hypoperfusion if arterial conduit used to replace stenotic vein graft.

ACC/AHA guidelines for redo CABG

Class I

- CABG should be performed in patients with prior CABG for disabling angina despite optimal non-surgical therapy (if angina atypical objective evidence of ischemia should be obtained. (*Level of evidence: B.*)
- Coronary bypass should be performed in patients with prior CABG without patent bypass grafts but with Class I indications for surgery for native vessel CAD (LMS, 3VD). (*Level of evidence: B.*)

Class IIa

- Coronary bypass is reasonable in patients with prior CABG and bypassable distal vessel(s) with a large area of threatened myocardium by non-invasive studies. (*Level of evidence: B.*)
- Coronary bypass is reasonable in patients who have prior CABG if atherosclerotic vein grafts with stenoses >50% supplying the LAD or large areas of myocardium are present. (*Level of evidence: B.*)

There are no randomized controlled trials of redo surgery versus PCI or medical intervention, all data is based on retrospective cohort analyses.

- There is little difference in 5-year survival between operated and non-operated patients with stenotic vein grafts.
- Late vein graft stenoses >50%, supplying either the LAD territory or large areas of myocardium are associated with a worse survival if managed medically.
- There is probably no survival benefit from reoperation in patients with patent LIMA to LAD grafts, and they should be offered PCI if suitable.
- Reoperated patients achieve better symptom control than medically treated patients.
- PCI has good results in early vein graft stenoses, native coronary disease, and anastomotic strictures, but is much less successful at treating late atherosclerotic vein graft stenosis.
- The 5-year survival after redo CABG is just over 75%, the 10-year survival is just under 50%.
- Emergency redo surgery has a high mortality.

Summary of indications for redo CABG

1 Viable myocardium.
2 Supplied by stenotic vessels.
3 With suitable distal targets.

Redo coronary bypass surgery 2

Key facts

The surgeon must have a complete understanding of the native coronary anatomy, the bypass graft anatomy, and the relationship of major structures to the sternum, as well as a plan for conduit selection. This requires:
- Old coronary angiograms as well as one within 6 months.
- Previous operation notes, confirmed by clinical examination.
- Chest CT in all patients: CT angiography if renal function permits.

Preoperative planning

Patent LIMA to LAD anastomosis.

Review the indications for surgery (📖 p343). This makes resternotomy potentially hazardous: if the LIMA is damaged before the heart is on bypass the result may be intractable VF, and has implications for myocardial protection (📖 p347).

Right ventricle or atrium, aorta or grafts adherent to sternum

This can only be reliably identified with a CT or MRI scan, which is the rationale for obtaining one in all reop patients to assist planning.
- *Very high risk:* e.g., aneurysmal aorta, patent LIMA or SVG adherent to midline of sternum: safest strategy may be to fully heparinize, cannulate peripherally, and go on bypass prior to sternal re-entry. Cooling gives the option of circulatory arrest in case of catastrophic bleeding but requires strategy for LV venting in case of fibrillation (📖 p346). Left and right lateral thoracotomy approaches, or mini-thoracotomy to aid dissection before sternotomy, are useful alternatives.
- *High risk:* e.g., right ventricle or dilated atrium adherent to sternum: peripheral arterial cannulation (5000U of heparin and tell perfusionist to flush cannula every 10min) with exposure of peripheral vein in readiness for cannulation if bypass required emergently is good option that allows mediastinal dissection without heparinization.
- *Moderate risk:* e.g., patent grafts but all well away from sternum on CT: consider dissecting out peripheral vessels prior to sternotomy, and ask to have coronary shunts in the room.

Before induction of anesthesia

External defibrillator pads must be placed on the patient: you will not be able to use internal defibrillator paddles effectively until the heart is fully mobilized. Shave groins. If you are using axillary cannulation ensure the anesthesiologist sites a radial artery cannula in that arm (to detect hyperperfusion) *and* on the opposite site. Long cases need axillary or femoral A-lines as vasoconstriction often leads to damping of radial lines.

Prepping and draping

Ensure that both groins, axillae, and legs are fully prepped and readily accessible. Mark all scars. Take the lines from the perfusionist.

Incision

If the patient has a markedly hypertrophic scar, excise it. Otherwise make your incision in the line of the original scar whether or not it is precisely in the midline. Making a fresh incision risks creating a patch of ischemic tissue between the two scars that will be slow to heal, and will leave two unsightly scars.

Resternotomy

- Remove the sternal wires by pulling on them with the heavy needle holder and cutting one side of the loop so that the wire in its entirety is pulled out: alternatively leave them *in situ* and use them as a guard, preventing the sternal saw from lacerating the RV.
- The upper table of the sternum can be sutured with No. 5 Ethibond, then used as countertraction during sternotomy, and dissection afterwards: or a Lanes tissue holder may be applied to the xiphisternum.
- An oscillating saw is used for resternotomy, and the sternum must be lifted up, but not pulled laterally, to avoid tearing adherent RV.
- The safest technique is not to saw completely through the posterior table in the first pass: rotate a forceps handle to open up the anterior table and divide the posterior table carefully with a Mayo scissors.

Dissection

It is difficult to predict how dense adhesions will be, but as a rule of thumb they become maximally dense up to 2–3 months after surgery, decreasing very gradually after that. Adhesions are most dense where there has been previous dissection, anastomosis, and cannulation sites. Diathermy and scissors are used. A 'no touch' technique is used around vein grafts to avoid dislodging atheroma and thrombus.

- Lifting up very gently on the left sternal edge, so as not to tear adherent RV or induce hemodynamic compromise, and staying close to bone, begin to free the mediastinal tissues from the chest wall using either cautery or a curved Mayo scissors.
- Place a sternal retractor once enough sternum is free and tension on all underlying structures has been relieved by dissection.
- Free the heart in the following order: diaphragmatic border (there is normally a plane of dissection here) left heart border, right heart border, aorta, right atrium.
- Cannulate and go on bypass, before continuing dissection of the apex, and finally the base of heart if necessary for grafting.
- Take great care to stay in the right plane, staying superficial to epicardial fat, avoiding 'skinning' the aorta (dissecting deep to the advential layer), and taking particular care round the thin-walled right atrium.

Redo coronary surgery

Dealing with a patent LIMA to LAD is discussed on 📖 p347. Generally the original vein grafts are left alone, and handled minimally to avoid causing atheromatous emboli. The distals are performed in the usual manner: some surgeons anastomose to the stump of the original vein graft if there is no distal stenosis, and it is the vein graft itself which is occluded. The proximals are usually performed onto the hoods of the original vein grafts, as these are softer than the atheromatous aorta. There is a body of opinion that vein grafts should be replaced by vein grafts: one study reported a 20% incidence of hypoperfusion when LIMA was used to replace stenotic vein graft to the LAD.

Problems specific to redo surgery

Key facts

- Immediately life-threatening problems include aortic injury on sternal re-entry, and damage to patent grafts particularly the LIMA to LAD.
- Potentially very major problems include laceration of the right atrium or ventricle on sternal re-entry, subadventitial degloving of the aorta, and problems associated with peripheral cannulation (🕮 p120).
- Potential problems requiring pre-planning are lack of conduit; failure to arrest the heart; lack of room on the aorta to cannulate, clamp plegia, vent and perform proximals; and lack of sites to graft distally.

Injury to aorta on sternal re-entry

Spectacular bright red bleeding and rapid hypotension of you and patient.

Management

- Give heparin, tell anesthesiologist and perfusionist, get senior help.
- Likely impossible to effect a rapid primary repair as no access, because the sternum is still not fully divided and freed from mediastinum.
- Primary aim is to control bleeding, go on bypass and cool enough to stop circulation so you can dissect aorta free and repair it. Two options:
  1 Apply pressure to bring sternal edges together: if this seems to stop bleeding you have a short period of time to cannulate groin.
  2 If this doesn't work one salvage maneuver is to place large Foley catheter into where you think the hole is, blow up balloon with 5–10mL saline, and pull back gently which may tamponade bleeding without occluding ascending aorta. Cannulate peripherally and cool down.

Avoiding this scenario

- Always get and review the pre-op CT scan: choose re-entry and cannulation strategy based on proximity of aorta. Patients at very high risk of this injury should be heparinized, cannulated, and cooled in readiness for circulatory arrest, which makes this kind of injury much less likely and relatively easy to deal with if it does happen.
- Dividing the posterior table with the Mayo scissors rather than sternal saw (or using a thoracotomy/VATS to dissect the aorta free prior to sternal division) reduces the risk of this injury.

Injury to patent LIMA or SVG

Notable for impressive bright red bleeding, ST segment changes, and VF.

Management

- Give heparin, tell anesthesiologist and perfusionist, get help.
- You may be able to effect a rapid primary repair, but commonly you cannot see to sew because of bleeding and adhesions.
- Usually possible to place a coronary shunt in the damaged conduit.
- Alternatively hook the cardioplegia line up to a catheter, place it pointing distally in conduit and ask the perfusionist to give continuous blood down it, while occluding any proximal bleeding segment with your finger or bulldog.
- Priority is then to go on bypass to minimize ischemic insult.

Avoiding this scenario
- Review all pre-op coronary angiography so that you can select re-entry and mediastinal dissection strategy appropriately (see earlier).
- There is almost no reason to dissect out the LIMA in a reop: the further you are away from it, the less likely you are to injure it.

Major injury to right ventricle or right atrium
Impressive amounts of very dark blood, hypotension.

Management
- Straightforward if you are already heparinized and cannulated: go on bypass (you will need vacuum assist to prevent airlock and ensure adequate drainage) and complete enough dissection to effect a repair with multiple pledgetted horizontal mattress 4/0 Prolene sutures.
- If you are not cannulated, management is more challenging:
  - Stop retracting and hold chest together to prevent further tearing.
  - Give heparin.
  - Expose and cannulate femoral artery.
  - Place a pump sucker in the RV and go on "suction bypass".
  - Meanwhile cannulate the femoral vein and switch to fem–fem bypass, with vacuum assist, and proceed as previously described.

Avoiding this scenario
- Choose your re-entry strategy based on careful evaluation CT or MRI.
- In high-risk cases one option is to cannulate, but instead of going on bypass exsanguinate patient into the pump prior to resternotomy to decompress the RV, transfusing back as soon as dissection is complete.
- Always pull up not laterally on sternum until RV is free of adhesions.
- Take particular care when freeing the RA: it may be necessary to leave a small cuff of pericardium attached to the atrium.

Problems with myocardial protection
- A patent LIMA is an asset, not a problem: there is no need to dissect this out and occlude it. Your options are:
  - Cardioplegic arrest required: cool the patient to 28°C and give intermittent retrograde and antegrade cardioplegia. The LIMA will run cold blood, protecting the heart and maintaining arrest.
  - Perform mitral and or coronary surgery with the heart beating or fibrillating. If there is even mild AI a large LV vent is needed.
- Retrograde cardioplegia largely avoids the need to figure out ways of giving cardioplegia down old vein grafts: give antegrade cardioplegia down new ones as you construct them.

What to graft
- Many surgeons replace all vein grafts older than 5 years.
- Replace vein grafts with >50% stenosis feeding viable myocardium.
- Epicardial scarring may make target location difficult.
- Existing grafts provide a guide: blind dissection is sometimes needed.
- The principles are the same as first-time surgery with two exceptions:
  - An occluded vein graft can be replaced with an arterial graft.
  - A moderately stenosed vein graft should be replaced with a vein graft to avoid postoperative hypoperfusion, even in the LAD territory.

Left ventricular aneurysm

Morphology

The definition of a LV aneurysm and the difference between that and other types of LV scars is controversial. LV aneurysms are a result of MI: coronary disease is frequently confined to the LAD system. They are well demarcated, transmural, fibrous scars, devoid of muscle tissue, and much thinner than normal myocardium. 85% are located anterolaterally, near the apex of the heart. Only 5–10% are posterior, and these are mostly false aneurysms. Externally pericardium is often densely adherent. Internally, trabeculae are replaced by smooth fibrous tissue, and mural thrombus is often attached to the wall. The thrombus sometimes calcifies, as may the overlying pericardium.

Structural and functional changes

LV aneurysms once occurred in up to 50% of survivors of large MIs, but this percentage is falling largely thanks to thrombolysis and angioplasty. Within 1 week of a large MI wall thinning and LV dilatation may be visible on echocardiography or ventriculography. Fibrous tissue takes at least 1 month to form. The LV wall is mostly composed of necrotic muscle tissue in the days after an MI, and this is when it is at greatest risk of rupture. Hyalinized fibrous tissue eventually replaces the muscle tissue. During systole the involved segments of wall are either immobile (akinetic) or bulge outwards (dyskinetic). If >20% of the LV wall is affected, non-aneurysmal portions of the LV also increase in size and thickness in response to the additional workload. True posterior aneurysms are associated with ischemic MR. RV function may be impaired as a result of a dyskinetic ventricular septum, pulmonary hypertension, and the tamponading effect of an enlarged LV.

- *Intractable VT* occurs most commonly in patients with poor LV, particularly where the ventricular septum is involved.
- *Postinfarction LV free wall rupture* occurs in about 10% of patients with acute infarction, and accounts for up to 20% of early deaths. It generally occurs between 1–7 days post infarction, and is usually a gradual process that begins with small endocardial tears, progressing to a haematoma which dissects through the necrotic myocardium resulting in sudden tamponade.
- *False LV aneurysm* occurs after postinfarction LV rupture when the pericardium is densely adherent to the epicardium. A slowly enlarging hemopericardium or false aneurysm eventually results, with a narrow mouth and a strong tendency to rupture, unlike true LV aneurysms.
- *Left ventricular remodelling* occurs after MI: even in the absence of scarring LV geometry changes and dilatation occurs, and is associated with progression of symptoms and poor prognosis. Surgical ventricular remodelling (SVR) is designed to address this and has been shown to improve ejection fraction and symptoms (□ p495).

Symptoms

Patients may have angina because of coronary artery disease, and classically complain of shortness of breath, persisting long after the MI. Up to 1/3 of patients have symptoms related to VT. Although most LV aneurysms contain thrombus, thromboembolic complications are rare.

- The size of the aneurysm and the functional characteristics of the remaining ventricle are major determinants of outcome.

Indications for surgery
- Symptomatic aneurysms.
- False aneurysms.
- Repeated thromboembolic events.
- Post infarction LV rupture.
- Coronary artery disease that fulfils the criteria for surgery (📖 p296).

Results of surgery
Early mortality after LV aneurysm repair, with or without CABG, is 5–7%, a substantial improvement on mortality rates of up to 20% a few decades ago. The improvement in survival is due to better myocardial protection, an emphasis on concomitant CABG, better protection against embolization, and treatment of VT. Following surgery: 1-year survival is 85%, 3-year survival is 75%, 5-year survival is 65%, although some centre report 5-year survivals as high as 88%.

The STICH trial
- The Surgical Treatment for Ischemic Heart failure study (STICH) hypothesized SVR when combined with CABG would decrease death and hospitalization from CHF compared to CABG alone.
- Patients enrolled if they had CAD amenable to CABG and EF <35%.
- 499 randomized to medical therapy + CABG, 501 to medical therapy, CABG + SVR (1200 patients randomized to CAG vs. medical therapy to look at second hypothesis concerning CABG vs. medical treatment)
- Jones et al.[1] found that adding SVR to CABG did not improve mortality, symptoms, or hospitalization for CHF compared to CABG alone in these patients.
- Several problems with the methodology that impact its conclusions were pointed out in a response by Buckberg & Athanasuleas[2] which can be summed up by their premise that the study examined the wrong operation in the wrong patients by the wrong surgeons:
  - Wrong operation: in previous reports a 40% reduction in LV size is needed for benefit, STICH planned a minimum reduction of 30%, but final data shows a mean reduction of only 19% in LV volumes.
  - Wrong patients: initial inclusion criteria required LV volume documented >60mL/m^2 and >35% akinesia, which changed in the final study to 'documented LV anterior wall dysfunction' with only 38% of patients having echo measurement of LV volume, and only half of patients having documented LV akinesia or scar.
  - Wrong surgeons: study proposal required 10 cases per center and 5 per surgeon to participate with strict outcome criteria, which changed to only 5 per surgeon and looser outcome criteria.

References
1. Jones RH et al. Coronary bypass surgery with or without surgical ventricular reconstruction. *NEJM* 2009; **360**:1705–17.
2. Buckberg GD & Athanasuleas CL. The STICH trial: Misguided conclusions. *J Thorac Cardiovasc Surg* 2009; **138**:1060–4.

Left ventricular aneurysmectomy

Key facts

- There are two main techniques: the classic technique is excision of the aneurysm and linear closure, and the *Dor procedure* involves patch closure or 'endoaneurysmorrhaphy', remodeling the ventricle (📖 p495).
- In both techniques the set-up is as described for CABG, including harvesting conduit if bypasses are planned (📖 p324–325). Particular care is taken to minimize handling the heart, in order to avoid dislodging mural thrombus.
- Myocardial protection is key particularly where LV function is compromised . Anterograde and retrograde cardioplegia is given. The heart is vented through a right superior pulmonary vein or root vent.

Linear closure

- After opening the LV loose thrombus is removed.
- The incision is extended round the aneurysm leaving a rim of scar tissue.
- The LV is irrigated to clear any residual thrombus.
- The edges of the incision are brought together so that the LV is distorted as minimally as possible, and the incision is closed using Teflon strips to buttress interrupted horizontal 0/0 Ethibond mattress sutures, followed by a second layer of continuous sutures (Fig. 7.16).
- It is important to avoid suturing any portion of the LAD.
- Before completely closing off the incision, the heart is de-aired: the perfusionist occludes the venous line to fill the heart and the anesthesiologist inflates the lungs to evacuate air from the pulmonary veins air can be removed by aspirating the LV apex in the standard manner.
- The distal anastomoses are then performed as described on 📖 p328.
- This technique is used to treat post-infarction LV free wall rupture.

Patch reconstruction

The aneurysm is incised but not excised. The recommended incision is in the thinnest portion of the aneurysm, parallel to the interventricular groove. A continuous purse-string (Fontan) suture using 2/0 Prolene is run along the line of demarcation of between the scar and the contractile myocardium (Fig. 7.16). A patch of PTFE which is sometimes backed with pericardium, measuring about 2 × 3cm, is then sewn into place, incorporating the purse-string suture and the heart is de-aired in the same way described above. The aneurysm is closed over the patch to reinforce it. The distal coronary anastomoses are then performed as described on 📖 p328. The LV cavity is often sized using a shaped balloon inflated with saline to a volume 50–60 × BSA.

Mitral valve surgery

Mitral valve repair (papillary muscle repositioning with a sling around the papillary muscles, together with some form of annuloplasty) or replacement can be carried out via the ventriculotomy if indicated, although a standard left atriotomy approach after closure of the aneurysm approach is more familiar to most surgeons.

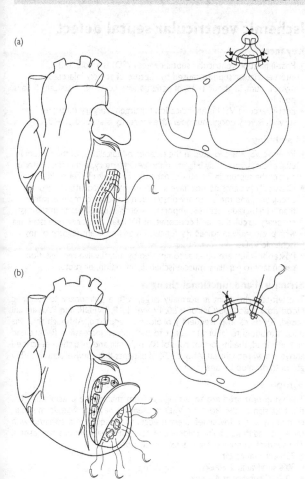

Fig. 7.16 Aneurysmectomy. (a) Linear closure. (b) Patch closure.

Postoperative management

Postoperative management is similar to CABG patients, with considerations for ventricular function which is likely to be particularly poor in the immediate postoperative period. Many patients will benefit from IABP, and may be on infusions of milrinone or dobutamine for several days after surgery. Patients with mural thrombus should be anticoagulated for at least 3 months after surgery.

Ischemic ventricular septal defect

Key facts

- Post-infarction ventricular septal defect (VSD) is a hole in the interventricular septum caused by rupture of acutely infarcted myocardium, in about 1–2% of patients with acute MI, classically 5 days post MI.
- Post-infarction VSD is an indication for urgent surgery (untreated survival is very poor), but operative mortality is around 30–40%.

Morphology

- Ischemic VSDs are located in the anterior or apical area of the septum in 60% of cases, caused by infarcts in the LAD territory, and in the posterior part of the septum in 20–40% of patients as a result of inferior MI.
- Classically patients do not have a well-developed collateral coronary circulation, and the coronary obstruction is usually complete, rather than a high-grade stenosis. Important stenoses usually exist in the right coronary circulation, and concomitant RV infarction or severe ischemia with profoundly impaired RV function is an important feature of any ischemic VSDs.
- Posterior VSDs are often accompanied by mitral valve regurgitation secondary to papillary muscle ischemia, infarction, or rupture.

Structural and functional changes

The left-to-right shunt is normally large, with a pulmonary to systemic blood flow ratio (Qp/Qs) of >2.0. PAWP, LAP, LVEDP, and PAP are all raised. RV function is frequently profoundly impaired. Although this was once attributed to failure to adapt to the sudden increase in RV preload and afterload, the important role of RV ischemia and infarction described above is now recognized. About 40% of patients that survive ischemic VSD go on to develop LV aneurysms.

Symptoms

The symptoms are hard to distinguish from that of the precipitating MI: the first sign of the ischemic VSD is usually a new pansystolic murmur, commonly at the lower left sternal edge, and frequently associated with the signs and radiographic evidence of new pulmonary venous congestion. The survival without surgery is extremely poor:

- 75% survival at 24h.
- 30% survival at 2 weeks.
- 10–20% survival at 4 weeks.

Indications for surgery

Because of the poor survival, post-infarction VSD is almost invariably an indication for operation. The best results are for surgery performed after the acute phase in patients with a good cardiac output, no pulmonary hypertension or edema, and satisfactory renal function, but emergency surgery is indicated for the vast majority of patients who present with cardiogenic shock and severe pulmonary edema.

Results of surgery

- Hospital mortality after VSD repair is about 40%.
- 5-year survival is about 50%.
- 10-year survival is about 30%.

Ischemic ventricular septal defect repair

Key facts

Preoperative management and assessment is critical: these patients are usually extremely unwell. If a PA catheter and IABP have not already been inserted, this should be done immediately. If stable enough the patient should undergo coronary angiography prior to transfer to the OR.

Set-up

- Open the pericardium to one side, and harvest a patch for later use.
- Bicaval cannulation with arterial return to the ascending aorta. Caval tapes: the patient is cooled to 30°C.
- Retrograde cardioplegia is often used as an adjunct to antegrade cardioplegia administered via the aortic root
- The LIMA is not normally used. Rapid institution of full cardiopulmonary bypass followed by speedy revascularization is the priority: saphenous vein graft can be taken much more quickly without delaying bypass, and while the VSD repair is effected.

Technique

There are two main techniques (primary repair and infarct exclusion) that are used, depending on the area infarcted. Primary repair is the most popular technique. The septum is usually approached via the LV.

Anterior VSD: the incision is made in the infarcted surface of the antero-lateral LV. The defect in the septum is usually immediately beneath the incision (Fig. 7.17a). The defect is not resected. A patch repair with PTFE, autologous or bovine pericardium is carried out so that the whole of the LV aspect of the septum is covered (Fig 7.17c). Infarct exclusion excludes the LV cavity from the infarcted myocardium by suturing a larger patch so that it extends all the way to the non-infarcted endocardium of the antero-lateral LV wall. Pledgetted horizontal mattress sutures of 2/0 Prolene are placed so that the pledgets are on the RV side of the repair, and sutures occupy the non-infarcted myocardium. Sutures must be placed quite close together. If it is possible to close the incision in the LV wall primarily this is done with interrupted horizontal mattress sutures of 0/0 Prolene placed across four layers of pericardium or PTFE felt trips (Fig. 7.17), and reinforced with continuous 2/0 Prolene over and over stitch. Otherwise a patch closure should be carried out.

Apical VSD: apical VSDs are usually associated with apical infarction: the apex of the heart is amputated if the VSD is immediately adjacent to the apical infarction (Fig. 7.17b). The defect, and effectively the VSD is closed primarily using interrupted horizontal mattress sutures of 0/0 Prolene placed across four layers of pericardium or PTFE felt trips (Fig. 7.17b), and reinforced with continuous 2/0 Prolene over and over stitch.

Posterior VSD: these are more difficult to repair. The apex of the heart is elevated with stay sutures, or a suction cup. A vertical incision is made

(a)

(b)

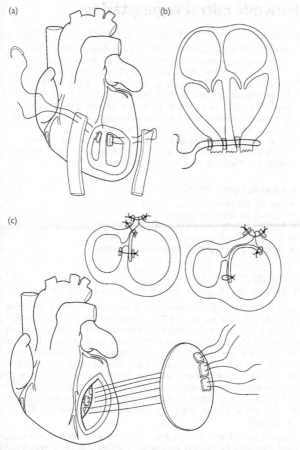

(c)

Fig. 7.17 (a) Anterior VSD repair. (b) Apical VSD repair. (c) Posterior VSD repair.

in the infarcted posterior wall of the LV, parallel to the PDA. The VSD is resected and a patch attached to the LV aspect of the remaining non-infarcted septum as described *previously* (Fig. 7.17a). Depending on how much of the free RV and LV wall is infarcted, the options for closure are patch closure of the RV, primary closure of the LV buttressed by an external patch, or infarct exclusion.

Ischemic mitral regurgitation

Key facts

- Ischemic MR is MR caused by ischemic heart disease, rather than MR co-existent with ischemic heart disease: the management and outcomes of ischemic and non-ischemic MR are very different.
- Chronic ischemic MR is usually Carpentier type IIIb (🔲 p400) due to *posterior leaflet restriction* from displacement of posteriomedial papillary muscle due to inferior LV ischemia. Anterior ischemia tends to result in symmetrical annular dilatation (type I MR). Both should be repaired with rigid, down-sized complete rings.
- Acute, new MR following an MI may be type II (prolapse) due to *papillary muscle rupture*. This usually requires replacement rather than repair, and is associated with high operative mortality.

Causes of ischemic MR

- Annular dilatation (type I).
- Papillary muscle rupture (type II)—acute.
- Papillary muscle necrosis (type II).
- Changes in configuration of the LV (type IIIb).
- Global and segmental LV dysfunction (type IIIb).

Morphology

The morphology of acute ischemic MR differs from that of chronic MR.

Acute ischemic MR: MR is a common complication of acute MI. Moderate to severe MR is present in up to 20% of patients in the first few days after an MI. It is a predictor of mortality. Acute ischemic MR is rarely caused by papillary muscle dysfunction: it is much more commonly due to LV systolic dysfunction preventing full leaflet coaptation. When papillary muscle rupture does occur, it may be partial or complete resulting in flailing of both anterior and posterior leaflets. In 75% of cases the posteromedial papillary muscle is ruptured, and in 25% of cases the anterolateral. The difference is probably due to the dual supply of the anterolateral papillary muscle (LAD and Cx vs. single supply of the posteromedial PM (PDA or Cx) (🔲 p46).

Chronic ischemic MR: this is type IIIb (restriction of normal leaflets) caused most commonly by papillary muscle displacement due to LV dysfunction and/or dilatation, or type I MR due to annular dilatation. Type IIIb is localized to the P3 area, due to the more common involvement of the supporting posteromedial papillary muscle in infarction.

Structural and functional changes

Papillary muscle rupture presents as an acute event, resulting in acute cardiogenic shock associated with raised LAPs, raised RVEDP, and pulmonary edema. The pathophysiology of acute MR is described on 🔲 p401. The course of chronic ischemic MR is similar to that described on 🔲 p400, but the degree of MR varies depending on LV function and preload.

Symptoms

Acute ischemic MR presents a few hours to weeks after an MI with pulmonary edema, hypotension, and an apical pansystolic murmur which is frequently absent in complete papillary muscle rupture. Chronic ischemic MR presents in much the same way as MR of other etiology (📖 p401). The survival of papillary muscle rupture without surgery is poor:

• 25% of patients survive 24h after complete papillary muscle rupture.
• 70% of patients survive 24h after partial papillary muscle rupture.
• MR after MI is a strong predictor of mortality.

Surgery for ischemic MR

Indications for surgery

In chronic ischemic mild MR, full revascularization may be sufficient to improve valve function. Moderate to severe chronic ischemic MR should be treated with mitral repair at the time of CABG. Patients with severe LV dysfunction and LVEDD >7.5cm gain little clinical benefit from conventional surgery and should be considered for medical management, ventricular assist device, or transplant (📖 p494). Acute severe MR is an indication for urgent surgery.

Techniques of ischemic mitral surgery

The principles of mitral valve surgery are described on 📖 pp404–410. The aspects specific to the ischemic mitral valve are:

• Acutely unwell patients require preoperative insertion of an IABP.
• LIMA harvest may not be appropriate in the unstable patient.
• Retrograde cardioplegia is a useful adjunct in acute coronary occlusion.
• The distal anastomoses are performed before the mitral valve prosthesis is inserted to avoid lifting the heart with a rigid structure sutured to the annulus, which can cause AV dehiscence.
• The proximals can be performed before or after mitral surgery.
• MVR is indicated in total papillary muscle rupture: particular care must be taken with the ring sutures as the tissues are friable.
• Mitral annuloplasty with a rigid down-sized ring is preferable for type IIIb and type I MR (restricted and annular dilation), with secondary chordal cutting to P2 and P3 usually required to achieve a good surface of coaptation and a durable repair.

Outcomes of surgery

• Surgery for acute ischemic MR has a hospital mortality of up to 70%.
• Repair of chronic ischemic MR has a hospital mortality is 3–10% depending on comorbidity. Poor LV function, extensive coronary artery disease, previous anterior infarction, and advanced age are strong predictors of mortality.
• Multiple retrospective studies show variable benefit of mitral repair over replacement for ischemic MR, but the repair strategies were flawed (few surgeons were consistently using down-sized rigid annuloplasty rings or employing chordal cutting, and rates of residual and recurrent MR were relatively high). The NIH is currently conducting multicenter RCTs of repair vs. replace in severe ischemic MR, although with an echocardiographic rather than a clinical primary endpoint.

Risk of coronary surgery

Crude survival

Risk-adjusted outcome is a cornerstone of understanding the results of surgery, planning surgery and predicting operative mortality for individual patients. Without adjusting for risk, after isolated CABG:

- 30-day survival is 98%.
- 1-year survival is 97%.
- 5-year survival is 92%.
- 10-year survival is 81%.
- 15-year survival is 66%.

STS score and EuroSCORE

These are both weighted, additive scoring systems that give scores for a number of patient-related and surgical variables, that are added together to give an indication of an individual patient's risk of perioperative mortality. The EuroSCORE (inside front cover) is derived from analysis of a pan-European database of surgical patients. It improves on the earlier Parsonnet score, which was based on a North American patient database. The EuroSCORE produces a number that equals the predicted percentage mortality but tends to overestimate risk. The STS score is a little more complex but provides quite accurate risk prediction.

Hospital mortality

The variables most predictive of early hospital mortality are listed in Box 7.2. Other variables associated with 30-day mortality include recent STEMI, diabetes, end stage renal disease, valvular disease, and COPD.

> **Box 7.2 Key predictors of earlier hospital mortality**
> - Older age.
> - Female gender.
> - Previous CABG.
> - Urgency of operation.
> - Increasing LV dysfunction.
> - LMS disease.
> - Increasing extent of CAD.

Risk factors for death after isolated CABG

- Patient risk factors:
  - ↑ or ↓age.
  - ↑weight or ↑weight/height ratio.
- Symptoms of reversible ischemia:
  - CCSA class.
  - No angina.
  - Unstable angina.
- Cardiac comorbidity:
  - Mitral regurgitation.
  - Aortic regurgitation.
  - Chronic atrial fibrillation.
  - Ventricular tachycardia/fibrillation.
  - Cardiac pacemaker.
- Non-cardiac comorbidity:
  - BMI >30 or <20.
  - History of vascular disease.
  - History of cerebrovascular disease.
  - Previous vascular surgery (non-carotid).
  - History of smoking.
  - ↓FEV$_1$.
  - History of renal failure.
  - Renal dialysis.
  - Serum creatinine.
  - Hypertensive.
  - ↑grade of diabetes and age.
  - History of malignancy.
  - History of hepatic disease.
  - ↑triglyceride level.
- Left ventricular function:
  - Cardiogenic shock.
  - Clinical status.
  - ↓EF.
  - Date of operation.
  - Limitation by heart failure.
- Coronary disease:
  - 90% LMS.
  - ↑number of diseased systems.
  - 3VD.

Results of coronary surgery

Morbidity and survival

Risk factors for reduced survival after CABG are shown in Table 7.3. Postoperative complications are described on 🕮 pp253–290. The most significant complications of CABG are:
- Significant cerebrovascular event in 1–2%.
- Deep sternal wound infection in ~1–2%.
- Renal dysfunction (7%) requiring dialysis (1%).
- Resternotomy for bleeding 1–2%.
- Major GI bleed requiring EGD or surgery 1–2%.

Recurrent angina

Angina recurs in 40% of patients by 10 years postoperatively. The highest rates of recurrence are at 3 months postoperatively, related to incomplete revascularization and early graft occlusion, and 5 years postoperatively as a result of progression of coronary disease and graft stenosis. Patients who experience recurrent angina, however, have a similar survival to patients that remain symptom free. Use of the LIMA as conduit has a much better graft patency rate in the long term, which is not, surprisingly, very correlated to improved freedom from symptoms.

Myocardial infarction

Incidence of perioperative MI is about 2–5% depending on definition. Postoperative MI is a predictor of mortality.

Quality of life

There are a number of quality of life measures, but the most important factors are; (1) freedom from angina, (2) freedom from medication, hospitalization, and reintervention, and (3) preserved exercise capacity. Most surviving patients have a satisfactory quality of life which begins to decline 5 years after surgery, mirrored by the increase in recurrent angina. Returning to work is very dependent on a number of factors. <20% of patients with an older age at operation, lower educational standard, longer absence from work, lower income and more physical job preoperatively, longer and greater angina, peripheral vascular disease, greater alcohol intake, emergency operation, and who fail to attend a cardiac rehabilitation programme return to work. 80% of patients without those factors return to work postoperatively. The amount of medication taken by patients is usually lower postoperatively. Functional exercise capacity is generally improved more by CABG than by medical treatment for up to 10 years. The improvement depends on preoperative LV function, graft patency and completeness of revascularization, and is related to the maximal heart rate achievable during exercise.

Graft patency

The patency rates of various conduit are summarized on 🕮 p302.

Table 7.3 Incremental risk factors for death after primary CABG

Risk factors	Impact on survival		
	Early	Constant	Late
Coronary operations:			
Greater disease complexity (higher SYNTAX score)			•
Non-use of LIMA		•	•
Use of patch grafts			•
↑Ratio of distals to conduits	•		•
↑Coronary endarterectomies	•		
↑Proportion of distals to small vessels	•		•
Incomplete revascularization	•		•
Concomitant procedures:			
Left ventricular incision or plication	•		
Institutional experience:			
Low surgeon volume	•		

Reintervention

Non-risk-adjusted freedom from re-intervention after CABG is around 90–95% at 3 years (based on SYNTAX 📖 p295). Vein graft atherosclerosis is the commonest cause of reintervention, followed by progression of native vessel disease. More frequent use of LIMA to LAD anastomoses has reduced the frequency of reoperation and lengthened the interval between the first and the second coronary operation. The other main risk factor for reoperation is younger age.

Postoperative progression of native vessel disease

High-grade stenoses in native vessels tend to progress whether they are proximal or distal to the anastomoses. Low-grade stenoses distal to the anastomoses do not tend to progress, although there is some evidence that suggests the opposite is true if the graft is non-functioning. 25–50% of lesser stenosis in non-grafted arteries progress within 5 years. In vessels that were disease-free at the time of re-operation new lesions will be detected in 15% at 5 years.

Left ventricular function

Segments of the LV that were dyskinetic or akinetic preoperatively usually improve, even in areas of scarring post MI. This supports hibernation theory (📖 p75). The improvement is reflected in regional perfusion defects which are improved after CABG in >65% of patients. Where preoperative ejection fraction recovery is limited but still usual, failure to improve LV function normally reflects incomplete revascularization. Coronary flow reserve returns to normal, reflected by a return of the normal increase in ejection fraction in response to exercise.

Valve disease

General principles

Aortic valve disease

Mitral valve disease

Tricuspid and combined valve surgery

Minimally invasive valve surgery is described on 📖 pp466–467

Types of valve prosthesis

Choice of valve prosthesis is discussed on 📖 pp370–371.

Key facts

- Valve prostheses are either *mechanical* or *bioprosthetic* ('tissue').
- Tissue valves are mounted on a metal frame (*stented*), or supported by pig aorta and cloth (*stentless*). Stented most commonly used.
- Stented valves are either *porcine aortic valves* or *bovine* pericardium.
- *Homografts* are human cadaveric aortic roots, complete with aortic valves *in situ* (📖 p368).
- A *pulmonary autograft* is the patient's own excised pulmonary valve used in the Ross procedure (📖 p368).

Examples of mechanical valves

Over 50 models of mechanical valves exist, underlining the fact that no one design meets all the criteria of the perfect prosthesis. Examples of three main types are shown in Fig. 8.1:

- *Bileaflet valves:* best hemodynamic profile and lowest thromboembolic risk so most widely used today. Commonly inserted models include *CarboMedics* (radio-opaque titanium ring, carbon disks), *St. Jude Medical* (pyrolytic carbon, available with a range of expanded and reduced sewing rings, rotatable and non-rotatable, not radio-opaque).
- *Tilting disk:* largely superseded by bileaflet which have better hemodynamic profile, include *Metronic-Hall A770* carbon coated, disk rotable in sewing ring and *Bjork–Shiley*, carbon coated disk, titanium struts).
- *Ball-in-cage:* First prostheses with long-term durability. Not manufactured now. Higher thromboembolic rate, bulky prostheses. e.g., *Starr–Edwards* best known model.

Examples of tissue valves

There is a similar variety of choices of tissue valves shown in Fig. 8.2. Discovery of glutaraldehyde fixation in the 1960s by Alain Carpentier, followed by antimineralization led to second- and third-generation tissue valves with improved durability. There are two main types:

- *Stented valves:* these are the most commonly implanted, as they are easy to implant being mounted on metal struts with fabric sewing rings
  - *Porcine stented valves:* these are made of pig aortic valves, usually with the porcine non-coronary cusp (which is smaller in the pig) replaced with a coronary cusp to make the valve symmetrical. Examples include *Carpentier–Edwards 2625*, *Hancock (Medtronic)*. The Hancock II has an anticalcification agent added to the fixative. The sewing ring is scalloped to allow supra-annular implantation. *Mosaic (Medtronic):* collagen crimp and flexibility is preserved. So-called because a 'mosaic' of technologies used to increase durability
  - *Bovine stented valves:* these are made of bovine pericardium (equine occasionally used). *Perimount (CE 2700/CE Magna)*.

(a)

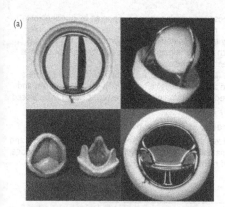

(b)

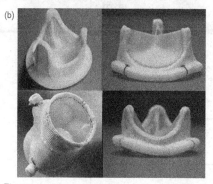

Fig. 8.1 (a) Clockwise from top left: St. Jude bi-leaflet, Starr–Edwards, Bjork–Shiley tilting disk, stented porcine bioprosthesis. Reproduced from Bloomfield P. (2002) Choice of heart valve prosthesis, *Heart*; **87**:583–9 with permission from BMJ Publishing Group Ltd. (b) The four main designs of bioprosthetic valve: porcine intra-annular valve; pericardial intra-annular valve; stentless porcine valve; supra-annular porcine valve. Reproduced from the *ESC Textbook of Cardiovascular Medicine*, with permission from Oxford University Press.

- *Stentless valves:* these are porcine valves supported by porcine aorta. The lack of a stent means they have a better hemodynamic profile, but are technically trickier to implant. The commonest type used is the *Freestyle*, which may be implanted in the subcoronary position as a valve replacement, as an inclusion root cylinder, or as a full aortic root replacement (📖 p390): hence 'freestyle'. *Toronto SPV:* stentless porcine valve. The aortic tissue is removed from all three sinuses and the valve is covered with a thin coat of polyester. It can only be placed in the subcoronary position.

Durability and freedom from reoperation

Figure 8.2 summarizes the main morbidity associated with tissue and mechanical valves, namely rates of thromboembolism and hemorrhage, including stroke, and rates of structural valve degeneration.

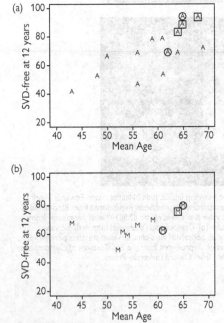

Fig. 8.2 (Continued)

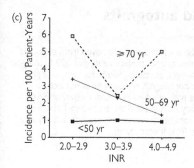

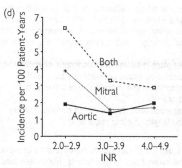

Fig. 8.2 Relationship between freedom from structural valve degeneration at 10 years, patient age, and type of valve implant (a: mitral, b: aortic): squares = pericardial valves, circles = third-generation porcine valves. Note how bioprostheses tend to fail earlier in the mitral position than in the aortic position. This reflects the fact that the mitral prosthesis must remain closed against systolic ventricular pressure, whereas the aortic prosthesis only has to remain closed against aortic diastolic pressure. Valves are thought to fail earlier in younger patients because of their greater hemodynamic demands compared to older patients. (c) INR specific incidence of all adverse events (thromboembolism, major bleeding, stroke) in patients with mechanical valves according to INR and valve position. (d) According to INR range and patient age.

Homografts and autografts

Key facts

- Homografts (aka allografts) are aortic roots removed from cadaveric human hearts and implanted as root replacements (📖 p390): the graft does not express MHC antigen as viable endothelial cells disappear within hours of implantation: allograft rejection does not occur.
- Pulmonary autograft is the patient's own pulmonary valve, originally implanted as a subcoronary AVR in the Ross procedure but now generally implanted as a root replacement (or very occasionally as a mitral replacement in the Ross II procedure).

Homografts

Homograft procurement

Valves are removed from disease-free cadaveric hearts, unsuitable for transplantation, of donors aged 6 months–55 years, up to 12h after death. The donor heart is procured using aseptic technique, preserved in cold Ringer's lactate solution, and packaged in a sterile plastic bag which is buried in slush.

- Homograft preparation takes place in a clean but not aseptic environment.
- The homograft block consists of all tissue between the base of the LV containing the anterior leaflet of the mitral valve and the aortic annulus, to the innominate artery.
- The coronary ostia are preserved with a small rim of coronary artery.
- The annulus is sized and the length of aorta recorded.

Homograft preservation

There are three main techniques for preservation, which aim to prevent bacterial colonization at the same time as preserving fibroblasts and endothelial cells. Cryopreservation has largely superseded antibiotic preservation. Homovital preservation is a recent development. After harvest the homograft block is stored in a culture medium that contains a low concentration of broad-spectrum antibiotics and stored at 4°C for 24h. The culture medium is changed and the tissue stored for a further 24h at 4°C. It can either be used at this time as a homovital graft or frozen in 10% fetal calf serum and 10% dimethylsulfoxide (DMSO) with controlled rate freezing (fall of 1°C per minute to –40°C) to achieve cryopreservation. This prevents the cellular damage caused by crystallization in conventional freezing processes. Once the homograft reaches –40°C it is transferred to nitrogen storage at approximately –195°C. Bacteriology and serology samples taken prior to storage must be reported clear before the homograft is used. Can be stored for up to 5 years.

Homograft preparation

The homograft is removed from the sterile foil container and placed in RPMI (Roswell Park Memorial Institute solution) with 10% DMSO. By DMSO is removed by serial dilutions and the graft is thawed and rinsed.

Advantages

- Where root replacement is indicated homografts are more pliable than Dacron composite valve replacements, and may be more resistant to infection (although there is little data to support this) so are favored in surgery for aortic valve endocarditis requiring root replacement where tissue is very friable and reinfection a significant risk.

Disadvantages of homografts
- Homografts are not as durable as mechanical valves, and may not be as durable as porcine or bovine valve replacement.
- Homograft aortic root replacement is a technically demanding operation (📖 p390) and the results are very dependent on the surgeon who requires experience in positioning the homograft in the correct anatomical position, dissecting out the coronary ostia and reimplanting them, and additional suture lines all of which carry an increased risk of postoperative bleeding and prolong the time for which the patient is on bypass, hence national mortality for aortic root replacement is ~7%, compared to ~1–2% for subcoronary AVR.
- Theoretical risk of transmitted infections: TB was transmitted in several cases before preservation and procurement protocols changed.
- Homografts are dependent on donor organ supply, which is falling.
- Homograft tissue is variable in quality, depending on the age of the donor, as well as the skill of the harvester: both the homograft aorta and the valve leaflets may be perforated, or buttonholed, and the tissue can be very friable.

Pulmonary autograft
Using the patient's own pulmonary valve to replace the aortic valve is known as the Ross procedure, after Donald Ross, the British surgeon who pioneered its use. The pulmonary valve is replaced with a pulmonary homograft (Fig. 8.7), which has a life expectancy of 15–20 years. The patient's own pulmonary valve in the aortic position has better life expectancy than bioprostheses, is resistant to infection, does not warrant formal anticoagulation, and most importantly 'grows' with the patient.

Indications for the Ross procedure (controversial)
- Young patients (<21 years).
- Older patients (up to 65 years) in whom an active lifestyle requires good hemodynamic function and contraindicates warfarin, if the surgeon can offer operative mortality <2% (comparable to simple AVR).

Contraindications to the Ross procedure
- Marfan syndrome and other connective tissue disorders.
- Rheumatic valve disease is viewed by some as a contraindication.

Disadvantages of the Ross procedure
The drawbacks are primarily related to the technical difficulty of both procedure and reoperation, and many more surgeons have been discouraged by the steep learning curve and abandoned the operation, than have managed to successfully adopt it as part of their repertoire. Mortality in one meta-analysis ranged from 1 to 7%. Reoperation for autograft dilatation is reduced by modifications where Teflon felt is used to buttress the proximal suture line. This procedure is described on 📖 pp388–389.

Choice of valve prosthesis

Key facts

- There is no strong data showing major long-term survival difference between mechanical vs. tissue valve in either aortic or mitral position.
- In patients >65 years a *bioprosthetic valve* will likely last the patient's lifetime, does not require long-term anticoagulation, and carries a ~1% annual risk of thromboembolic stroke; but valve failure becomes an increasing risk from 10–15 years depending on position and patient age.
- *Mechanical valves* last decades but ~15% will need explanting by 15 years because of endocarditis, pannus, or thrombosis; they require lifelong anticoagulation and have 3–4% *annual* risk of stroke or hemorrhage.

Disadvantages of bioprosthetic valves

Valve failure

Freedom from structural valve deterioration at 12 years in older patients is >90% with third-generation tissue valves such as the Carpentier–Edwards pericardial valves in the aortic position. Tissue valves last longer in the elderly as the hemodynamic demands on the valve are less: the chances of bioprosthetic AVR failure at 12 years is ~40% in patients 0–39 years, ~30% in 40–49 years, and ~10% in >70 years. (Lifetime risk of reoperation similarly highest for younger patients.) Tissue valves last less well in the mitral position compared to the aortic Fig. 8.2, and redo MVR is higher risk than redo AVR: hence the difference in age cut-offs in Table 8.1.

Hemodynamic profile

In smaller sizes (e.g., #19, #21) bioprostheses cause more flow obstruction than same size mechanical valves. *Stented* are more obstructive than *stentless* which are both more obstructive than mechanical.

Table 8.1 Relative indications and contraindications for valve types

	Mechanical	Tissue
Indications	Other mechanical valve (I)	<60 years (aortic)*
	>60 years (aortic)* <65 years (mitral)*	>65 years (mitral)*
	Other strong indication for anticoagulation	Younger patients who wish to avoid (IIa) or have contraindications to anticoagulation (I) Future pregnancy (IIb)
Contra-indications	Inability to comply with anticoagulation (bleeding disorder, social, e.g., IVDU, lack of access) Future pregnancy	Young patient where reoperation would carry high risk of mortality

* In the ACC/AHA guidelines age <65 years is an indication for mechanical AVR; but many feel this should be lower as newer bioprostheses last longer, and reoperation is safer now. I, balance of evidence supports; IIa conflicting evidence balance in favor vs IIb less established.

Calcification

Calcification of bioprostheses occurs in areas of greatest stress: the commissural regions of porcine valves, or the zone of flexion in porcine and pericardial valves, and preludes prosthesis failure. This may happen earlier in patients with renal failure, but the disadvantages of managing anticoagulation in these patients, and their shorter life expectancy, means bioprostheses are a reasonable choice in these patients.

Disadvantages of mechanical valves

Thromboembolic and hemorrhagic events

Without anticoagulation valve life-threatening thrombosis and thromboembolic events are inevitable. Even in an optimally anticoagulated patient (INR 2.5–3) the incidence of major thromboembolic events including stroke and hemorrhage is *still* 2–4% per year (higher in multiple valves and older patients). Bleeding problems (pericardial effusion, late tamponade) are more common postoperatively, and valve thrombosis is a later risk in patients not therapeutically anticoagulated (📖 p267).

Prosthetic valve endocarditis (PVE)

Mechanical valves may be at higher risk of infection than tissue valves during the first 3 postoperative months, but infection rates converge and are similar at 5 years. The cumulative risk of PVE is up to 3.1% at 1 year and 5.7% at 5 years. PVE is a class I indication for urgent valve replacement.

Choice of valve prosthesis in special groups

Younger patients

National registries show a trend towards implanting more tissue valves in younger patients (aged 40–60). This may reflect no long-term survival difference between mechanical and biological valves; lifetime stroke and bleeding rates >60% with mechanical valves; better durability of tissue valves; and fall in redo surgery mortality.

Pregnancy

Pregnant women have increased risk of mechanical valve-related thromboembolism: anticoagulation is vital. Warfarin, a teratogen, is contraindicated in the first trimester, and s/c heparin or i/v heparin should be administered instead, from initial attempts to conceive up until the beginning of the second trimester or delivery. So bioprostheses valves may be implanted in women of childbearing age, who will eventually need redo valve surgery.

Endocarditis

There is no data to suggest choice valve replacement impacts recurrence of endocarditis. Homografts have not been shown to give increased resistance to endocarditis, and they are less durable than porcine valves: their main advantage is being more forgiving to implant in very friable tissue.

Atrial fibrillation

AF is no longer an indication to implant a mechanical valve: concomitant ablation means 60% of patients will be in sinus rhythm at 1 year, obviating need for anticoagulation altogether if a bioprosthesis is implanted.

Small aortic root See 📖 pp392–393.

Pathophysiology of aortic stenosis

Key facts

- Incidence increases with age (rare <40 years of age, 2–3% >80 years).
- Etiology changes with age, although all end up as *calcific* in nature:
  - <70 years: *bicuspid* and *rheumatic* (📖 p78) commonest cause.
  - >70 years: *degenerative* commonest cause.
- Triad of symptoms (syncope, angina, dyspnea) reflect prognosis (Box 8.1).

Morphology

Calcium is deposited in the collagen framework of abnormal leaflets due to the shear stresses occurring with each cardiac contraction. Eventually the valve becomes a lumpy, rigid structure with a tiny orifice, calcification extending down the membranous septum and over the ventricular surface of the anterior mitral valve leaflet. 1–2% of people have a congenitally bicuspid aortic valve (right + left cusp fusion in >00%). shear stresses are greater and these valves calcify decades earlier. *Rheumatic disease* causes fibrous leaflet thickening, rolled leaflet edges, and fusion of commissures, and also results in accelerated calcific changes.

Structural and functional changes

The average decrease in the stenotic aortic valve is 0.1cm²/year. This occurs faster in degenerative and bicuspid stenosis than rheumatic stenosis. Major hemodynamic compromise does not occur until the valve is reduced to less than half the normal aortic valve area of 3–4 cm²; beyond this LV outlet obstruction rapidly increases. Turbulent flow in the ascending aorta may cause poststenotic dilatation.

- The LV hypertrophies in response to outlet obstruction.
- The number of myocytes is fixed at birth: hypertrophy is an increase in myofibrils, causing existing myocytes to become thicker, not longer.
- There are two types of ventricular hypertrophy: *concentric hypertrophy* which occurs in response to pressure overload, e.g., AS; and *eccentric hypertrophy* which occurs in response to volume overload, e.g., AI. Concentric hypertrophy maintains ventricular volume.
- There is also an increase in interstitial collagen, but not much fibrosis.
- Initially hypertrophy (increase in LV mass from 150 g/m² up to 300g/m²) allows generation of the high interventricular pressures required to maintain LVEF and CO through the stenosis, despite gradients >100mmHg: this is *compensated aortic stenosis*.
- *Laplace's law* T=Pr/2t: wall stress (T) is proportional to chamber pressure (P) and radius (r), and inversely proportional to wall thickness (t): concentric hypertrophy acts to normalize peak systolic wall stress.
- Eventually hypertrophy cannot compensate for increased wall stress, and the LV thins, dilates and EF falls: *low gradient low EF AS* (📖 p376).

Systolic function

- In compensated AS EF is preserved. Decompensated AS (*low gradient low EF AS*) occurs when systolic function (EF, LV fractional shortening, velocity of shortening) declines as a result of chronic afterload mismatch. *The transvalvular gradient falls (because cardiac output decreases) even though the valve stenosis is unchanged or worse* (📖 p376).

Diastolic function

- Diastole has an energy-dependent and a passive component (📖 p60). The passive component depends on normal compliance: this is reduced in AS. The time required for the energy-dependent phase is greater because of impaired myocardial relaxation, and decreased chamber compliance. LVEDP is increased, reducing diastolic coronary flow (📖 p62). Adequate LV filling is very dependent on 'atrial kick' and controlled rate (📖 p60). Patients may: (1) exhibit diastolic failure with PND, orthopnea and pulmonary edema even with normal EF, (2) decompensate if they go into AF, and (3) often take months to notice a symptomatic benefit after surgery

Coronary blood flow

In AS the myocardial oxygen supply–demand mismatch causes angina even in patients with normal coronary arteries, because of:

- Increased myocardial oxygen demand (increased muscle mass).
- Which outpaces compensatory increase in blood flow resulting in lower coronary blood flow per 100g of myocardium.
- ↑↑LVEDP reduces coronary perfusion during diastole.
- Increased systolic time reduces diastolic filling time.
- Decreased coronary vasodilatory reserve results in decreased coronary flow in exercise.
- Peripheral exercise induced vasodilatation reduces coronary perfusion.

Symptoms

Patients may be asymptomatic. Most present with any of the triad of angina, exertional syncope, and dyspnea. There is a 5% incidence of sudden death. Symptom onset is closely related to survival.

Box 8.1 Prognosis is predicted by symptoms in AS

- *Angina:* 50% of patients dead within 5 years without AVR, earliest symptom, due to O_2 supply–demand mismatch.
- *Exertional syncope:* 50% of patients dead within 3 years without AVR—due to combination of a relatively fixed CO which cannot respond to the drop in systemic perfusion pressures caused by exercise-induced peripheral vasodilatation.
- *Dyspnea:* 50% of patients dead within 2 years without AVR, late sign due to diastolic heart failure and/or congestive heart failure.
- *Sudden death* (5%) may be due to the increase in ectopy caused by impaired oxygen supply and changes at the cellular level, and complete heart block caused by calcification of conducting pathways.

Signs

- Slow rising, low amplitude pulse, occasionally with thrill at carotids.
- Sustained apex beat.
- Soft first heart sound, sometimes preceded by fourth heart sound, single heart sound if valve is calcified, ejection systolic murmur radiating from aortic area to right carotid.
- Soft early diastolic murmur (AI as leaflets become immobile).

Pathophysiology of aortic insufficiency

Key facts

- Commonest cause of isolated severe AI in West is aortic root/annular dilatation, followed by bicuspid valve, infective endocarditis, and rheumatic disease (📖 pp78–79).
- Acute severe AI is a surgical emergency.
- Chronic AI may be asymptomatic for years: symptoms include angina, exertional dyspnoea, and eventually cardiac failure.

Morphology

Pathology of any of the components of the aortic root can prevent leaflet coaptation, leading to AI:

- Annular dilatation (commonest cause in West), e.g., annuloaortic ectasia caused by cystic medial dilatation associated with connective tissue disorders such as Marfan syndrome, type A aortic dissection.
- Leaflet thickening/shortening due to rheumatic disease.
- Leaflet perforation (endocarditis).
- Calcification causing AS may also cause AI due to decreased leaflet mobility.

Structural and functional changes

Acute aortic insufficiency

Most commonly caused by endocarditis, aortic dissection, and trauma, this is a surgical emergency. There is no time for any of the adaptive changes that characterize chronic AI to develop and the sudden volume overload results in pulmonary edema as the filling pressure is increased in a non-compliant ventricle. Reduced coronary blood flow, low cardiac output, and hypoxia result in end-organ ischemia.

Chronic aortic insufficiency

Chronic AI is better tolerated than acute partly because of the following adaptive and maladaptive changes:

- AI leads to both volume overload, because of the regurgitant fraction, and pressure overload, because of the increased volume of blood ejected.
- Volume overload causes eccentric hypertrophy and LV dilatation.
- Pressure overload results in concentric hypertrophy: the same increase in myofibrils and interstitial collagen described in AS occurs in AI.
- Ventricular enlargement produces a larger total stroke volume (up to 20L/min), all of which enters the aorta during systole: this is compensated AI and the resultant increase in pulse pressure causes systemic hypertension and a large increase in LV afterload.
- LV compliance decreases and diastolic function is compromised as hypertrophy progresses.
- Eventually LV end-diastolic pressures and LAPs begin to increase: pulmonary hypertension and congestive cardiac failure is a feature of decompensated AI as well as acute AI.
- Finally as myocytes are stretched beyond their limit of effective contraction LV systolic function decreases, and the rate of increase LV end-systolic diameter accelerates to about 7mm per year.
- Coronary perfusion may be reduced for the same reasons as in AS.

Symptoms

Acute AI is characterized by cardiovascular collapse and the symptoms of pulmonary edema. Chronic AI is usually asymptomatic until LV function is significantly impaired. Symptoms eventually include angina (because of myocardial O_2 supply–demand mismatch caused by combination of increased O_2 consumption due to ventricular hypertrophy and contractility, and decreased coronary reserve caused by the fall in aortic–LV diastolic pressure gradient), effort dyspnea, and the symptoms of congestive cardiac failure. Fatigue may predominate.

Signs

- Large amplitude collapsing or 'water-hammer' pulse with a rapid upstroke.
- Quinke's sign: capillary pulsation visible in the nail bed.
- Corrigan's sign: visible pulsation in the neck.
- De Musset's sign: head nodding as a result of arterial pulsation.
- Duroziez's sign: 'pistol-shot' femorals.
- Sustained, laterally displaced apex beat.
- Single second heart sound, with third heart sound.
- Early diastolic murmur maximal at lower left sternal edge radiating to the apex and axilla.
- Ejection systolic murmur may be present.
- Late diastolic murmur (Austin Flint) from fluttering of the anterior mitral leaflet as it is hit by the regurgitant jet.

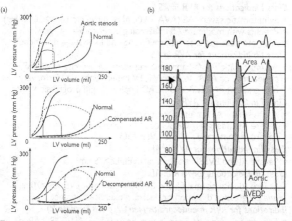

Fig. 8.3 (a) Pressure–volume loops in compensated AS and AI, and decompensated disease. (b) Cardiac catheterization tracing in aortic stenosis: note the difference in LV and aortic pressure which corresponds to the peak transvalvular gradient.

Timing of aortic valve surgery

Key facts

- Severe AS is defined as an aortic valve area (AVA) <1cm².
- If mean gradient >40mmHg then AS is severe, but *severe AS may be present at lower gradients* if the patient has poor LV function.
- The presence of symptoms or LV systolic dysfunction are both class I indications for AVR in both AS and AI.

Symptomatic aortic stenosis

The onset of symptoms in patients with AS is a poor prognostic sign (see Box 8.2). There is a 5% incidence of sudden death per year. Symptoms are most likely due to AS if AVA <1cm² or the transvalvular mean gradient >40mHg, and symptom onset in these patients mandates prompt AVR in all except very high-risk cases.

Low gradient, low EF (low flow) AS

There is a subgroup of symptomatic patients with transvalvular gradients of <40mmHg which fall into one of three main groups:

- Low gradient, low EF AS: severe AS results in ↓↓↓myocardial contractility with low gradient due to low cardiac output. Dobutamine infusion during echo or cardiac cath can help identify high risk candidates:
  - Positive *dobutamine stress test*: if cardiac output and transvalvular gradient increase in response to dobutamine, it suggests there is

---

Box 8.2 Indications for aortic valve surgery

Class I indications for AVR in AS
- Symptomatic severe AS (AVA <1.0cm² or mean gradient >50mmHg).
- Patients with moderate AS undergoing other cardiac surgery.
- Asymptomatic patients with severe AS and LV systolic dysfunction.

Class IIb indications for AVR in AS
- Asymptomatic AS and abnormal response to exercise (e.g., ↓BP, symptoms), or AVA <0.6cm²/VT, LV hypertrophy>/=15mm, very high gradient or calcification/CAD implying rapid progression risk.

Class I indications for AVR in AI
- Acute severe AI, symptomatic severe AI.
- Severe AI undergoing CABG or other valve surgery.
- Severe asymptomatic AI and LVEF <50%.

Class IIa indications for AVR in AI
- Severe AI and LVESD >55mm or LVEDD >75mm.

Class IIb indications for AVR in AI
- Severe AI with normal EF and LVESD >50mm or LVEDD >70mm *and* progressive dilatation or declining exercise tolerance.

Indications for AVR in endocarditis (see 🕮 p418 for details)
- Endocarditis and AI/AS resulting in heart failure, ↑LVEDP, LAP, or PAP (I), heart block, annular abscess, destructive penetrating lesion (I), recurrent emboli and vegetation despite appropriate antibiotics, fungal or other virulent organism (IIa), vegetation >10mm (IIb).

a true flow-limiting lesion in the setting of reversible ventricular dysfunction: surgery beneficial although higher risk than normal LV.
- In the irreversibly damaged LV there is no increase in transvalvular flow in response to inotropes, and (lack of *contractile reserve*) these patients present with high post-op mortality and worse survival.
- Pseudo AS: severe cardiomyopathy due to non-valvular cause, with only moderate or mild AS. The AVA increases during dobutamine stress testing. No benefit from surgery. CT or MRI can accurately quantify AVA and define abnormal myocardium.

Asymptomatic aortic stenosis

The majority of asymptomatic patients with severe AS have near normal life expectancy without AVR. Their 1–2% incidence of sudden death is less than the mortality of AVR, making it crucial to select only those patients at high risk of sudden death without surgery. Two techniques are employed: echocardiography and exercise testing. Asymptomatic patients with a transvalvular gradient >64mmHg have a 80% chance of becoming symptomatic within 2 years (hence an ACC/AHA IIb indication if surgery low risk). Exercise testing safe in asymptomatic patients, and can identify the presence of exercise-induced hemodynamic compromise which is an ACC/AHA IIb indication for AVR. The natural history of AS in asymptomatic patients with a positive exercise test is probably very similar to that of patients with exertional symptoms.

Aortic insufficiency

Acute severe AI is a surgical emergency. In infective endocarditis with lesser degrees of AI, the indications for early operation are annular abscess formation, new heart block, or evidence of heart failure (📖 p418).

Chronic aortic insufficiency

Even in severe AI it may be 10 years before symptoms become severe. The prognosis during this period is good: in severe chronic AI with preserved ejection fraction has an 80% 5-year survival. Surgery should take place before permanent LV dysfunction ensues: so surgery is often indicated in asymptomatic patients. Progressive LV enlargement or ↓LVEF heralds onset of symptoms and decompensation. AVR should therefore be carried out before LVEF <50%, LVESD >55mm, or LVEDD >70mm.

Elderly patients

The normal life expectancy for octogenarians is listed in Table 8.2. AVR in selected octogenarians has <5% operative mortality, and results in improved quality and length of life in patients with symptomatic AS.

Table 8.2 Normal life expectancy in octogenarians

Age (years)	Life expectancy	
	Males (years)	(Females (years)
70–75	12.2	15.3
75–80	9.5	11.9
80–85	7.1	8.9

Aortic valve replacement: set-up

Before you scrub
Note whether the coronary circulation is left or right dominant, and whether the left main stem is short. Is there AI (see below)? What is the size of the aortic root—small (📖 p392), aneurysmal (📖 p444).

Set-up
The patient is positioned and draped in the usual manner. Usually CO_2 insufflation on field, myocardial temperature probe, insulating pad.

Bypass
Standard cardiopulmonary bypass (CPB) at 32°C, two-stage venous cannula and standard aortic cannula (as distal as possible to provide adequate space for cross-clamp, aortic root vent, aortotomy, and proximal coronary anastomoses if planned). 4/0 Prolene purse-string for RSPV vent. Separate the PA from the aorta. Some surgeons tape the aorta.

Cardioplegia
Give anterograde cardioplegia to arrest the heart via a Medicut cannula: once the aortic root is opened further doses of cardioplegia are given with a handheld cannula (size 6 or 7 for LM ostia, size 5 or 5 balloon tip for RCA ostia) directly into each coronary sinus, and/or retrogradely.
- If there is AI the options are: (a) attempt to arrest the heart as described—can often obtain a good root pressure by lifting up on clamp and giving plegia rapidly despite AI—just need to ensure LV well vented so it does not distend; (b) fibrillate the heart on bypass, perform the aortotomy and give plegia directly into the coronary ostia; or (c) site a retrograde cardioplegia cannula and arrest heart with retrograde (takes a little longer). Retrograde plegia is useful routinely for AVR because:
  - Coronary ostia occasionally too difficult to cannulate directly.
  - Can continue to operate while giving retrograde cardioplegia.
- If the LMS is short be very careful not to push the handheld cardioplegia too far into the coronary ostia, as there is a risk of only protecting the LAD or the circumflex territory and not both.
- If the coronary circulation is right dominant give a larger amount of plegia into the right ostia, otherwise ratio of left:right plegia is ~2:1.

Venting
Any of the following routes can be used to vent the heart:
- Pump sucker placed retrogradely into the LV via the aortotomy (easy to place once aortotomy made but gets in the way a bit).
- LV apical vent (easy to place, but less easy to guarantee hemostasis).
- RSPV vent (sometimes less easy to place into LV, but out of the way and easy to secure hemostasis). Venting the PA also works.
- For de-airing it is safest to use aortic root vent until TEE free of air, rather than de-airing through the last suture of aortotomy closure.
- Prosthetic valves need the heart to eject to open and close: if you remove cross clamp before the heart has a rhythm the LV will distend:
  - Give hot-shot for 5–10min before you are ready to remove clamp.

- *Ensure* your LV vent is in place before starting aortomy closure, especially if patient cooled as may take long time to resume rhythm.
- Place an epicardial pacing wire before you remove the clamp.

Aortotomy

The goal of the aortotomy is to get close enough to the aortic valve to ensure good access, without getting so close that the RCA ostia and closure of the aortotomy are compromised. The choice of incision is dictated by any planned procedure on ascending aorta, the choice of prosthesis, the need for aortic root procedures such as enlargement, and concomitant CABG.

- Retract the fad pad overlying the aortic root.
- Separate the aorta from the PA, and carefully free the fat off the aorta proximally, taking care not to damage the RCA which arises close by.
- The standard aortotomy is made starting about 1cm from the sinotubular junction (~2 cm cephalad to the origin of the right coronary artery) starting at the uppermost point of the ascending aorta and extending one end of it proximally down towards the middle of the non-coronary cusp at the sinotubular junction, and the other end transversely (Fig. 8.4).
  - This incision permits aortic root enlargement and affords maximal exposure of the aortic valve (📖 pp392–393).
  - If in doubt make your aortotomy more distal rather than too proximal to avoid damaging the RCA ostia.
  - If you take the aortotomy too far into the NCC, it is more challenging to close it around the strut of a stented prosthesis, whereas if you do not take it far enough annular suture placement is a bit more difficult as you are effectively operating down a tunnel.
- A transverse aortotomy centred 15mm above the sinotubular junction extending round 2/3 of the aortic circumference gives adequate access to the aortic root without distortion: it is not easily adapted to aortic root enlargement.
- The aorta is transected about 15mm from the sinotubular junction (Fig. 8.4) which provides good exposure of the aortic root, but bleeding from the posterior aspect of the aortotomy suture line may be problematic: this incision is normally reserved for root replacement (📖 p390).

(a)   (b)

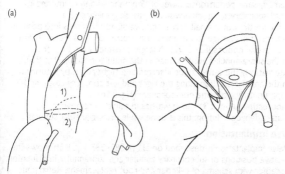

Fig. 8.4 (a) Oblique aortotomy and transverse aortotomy. (b) Extending the aortotomy.

Valve excision

Valve excision

The aortotomy is kept open using a Ross retractor or stay sutures. The first assistant's main role is to prevent stroke and perioperative myocardial infarction by ensuring all debris is removed using rough sucker with the guard removed. LV vent suction keeps the operative field blood-free.

- Use the McIndoe scissors to excise the valve leaflets by cutting along the edge of attachment: easiest to start at the non-coronary (NCC) and right coronary cusp (RCC).
- Scissors are used because the blunt tips will not perforate the aorta.
- Once the valve leaflets are excised use a rongeur, or a bone nibbler to remove calcium extending onto the aortic wall, the ventricular septum, and anterior mitral leaflet.
- Grasp each piece of calcium and gently remove with a twisting motion, using an 11 blade or McIndoe scissors to divide fibrous tissue.
- Leaving calcium predisposes to paravalvular leaks.
- Damage to the interventricular septum results in complete heart block.
- The area between the left and the NCC requires particular care, as it easy to perforate the aorta or the junction between the aorta and the ventricle here: if this happens the defect should be repaired before the valve is inserted.
- After the valve is excised run a finger round the inside of the annulus to detect residual calcium.
- Turn off vents and irrigate with cold saline which washes out any debris and affords topical cooling.

Sizing and preparing the valve

- Use the same make of sizer as the type of valve to be inserted: sizes vary between makes. The correct sizer is the largest one which passes with a bit of resistance into the LV. Always compare this with the sizes above and below. See ◻ p392 for patient–prosthesis mismatch (PPM).
- Although optimal aortic valve area depends on body surface area (◻ p392), a good rule of thumb is that valve sizes of 23mm and above offer good hemodynamic performance: valves of 19mm should only be inserted in small, sedentary adults: otherwise the intrinsic gradient is high.
- If the aortic root is small, forcing an oversized prosthesis into position will result in damage to the aorta and erosion of the annulus. There are several options (◻ p392). A larger prosthesis can be placed in the supra-annular position than in the annular position (Fig. 8.5), alternatively the valve can be inserted at a slight angle, by suturing it in the annular position along the right and left coronary cusps, and suprannularly along the non-coronary (Fig. 8.5b).
- Bioprostheses need 3 × 2min washes in saline to remove glutaraldehyde solution: this is done while placing annular sutures.

Valve implantation

- Valve implantation is described on ◻ pp382–383. Fig. 8.5b shows the relative positions of subcoronary annular and suprannular implantation, together with schema of cylinder and root replacement. Retrograde cardioplegia can be given while placing the sutures in the valve ring.

Closing the aortotomy

The commonest site of bleeding is at either end of the aortotomy, caused by either unrecognized tears in the aorta or incomplete closure. Avoid this by starting with a pledgetted mattress suture 2–3mm beyond the aortotomy at either end using 4/0 Prolene, and closing the aorta in one or two layers, using a simple running stitch meeting in the middle or horizontal mattress sutures which may be pledgetted (if fragile or very thin). Take care not to catch the back wall of the aorta (easy to do if the cross-clamp is close to the aortotomy) or the valve mechanism.

- Switch off the vents midway through the aortotomy closure otherwise the heart will be full of air by the time you finish.
- In small aortas the valve struts may prevent primary closure: use a diamond-shaped patch of pericardium and a 4/0 Prolene suture to close the defect a *patch aortoplasty* with several interrupted horizontal mattress sutures in the corners, and then running suture.

De-airing and evaluating valve

- Place the patient in Trendelenburg. de-airing is described on 🕮 p114.
- Assess TEE for residual AI, gradient, prosthesis function, other valves:
  - AI may be due to 'wash-jets' usually two parallel small jets normally seen with bileaflet valves; of no physiological consequence.
  - Paravalvular leaks due to suture holes may disappear after protamine, larger ones may need revision (🕮 p266).
  - Moderate gradient across small prosthesis common (🕮 p392).
  - New MR from aortomitral curtain if overly aggressive decalcification.

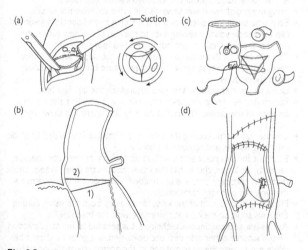

Fig. 8.5 (a) Excising the valve. (b) Aorta showing the relative position of 1) suprannular insertion and 2) subcoronary. (c) Cylinder implantation. (d) Root replacement.

Aortic valve implantation

Prosthesis selection is dealt with on ▭ p370, sizing is described on ▭ p380. Suture techniques can be divided into interrupted and semicontinuous.

Semicontinuous suture technique

Semicontinuous techniques require a non-absorbable monofilament such as 2/0 Prolene. One technique is described here: it can be used to implant prosthetic valves and homografts. With the assistant holding the valve, position the valve above the annulus and if not marked, mark the rough position of the commissures on the valve sewing ring. Suture underneath to above on the valve with the needle mounted backhand, and from above to below on the annulus with the needle mounted forehand.

- Take a single-ended 2/0 Prolene mounted forehand with a rubber shod on the cut end. Place the rubber shod under the retractor at 9 o'clock.
- Take a bite of the annulus from above down: usual place for starting is at the commissure between the right and the left coronary cusp.
- Next with the needle mounted back hand take a firm bite of the valve sewing ring from below up.
- Progress round the annulus and the sewing ring in an anticlockwise direction, spacing bites 2–3mm apart, with the assistant following so that all sutures are under tension to avoid you looping sutures, and so that the annulus is opened up by the sutures.
- If the prosthesis is held so that the area that you are suturing is always uppermost, even though both suture lines are progressing anti-clockwise, it looks as if they are progressing in opposite directions: this is why some surgeons call this a *counter-current* technique.
- Bring the prosthesis down towards the valve to maximize suture.
- Each time the suture becomes too short take an additional single-ended, clip the needle you are sewing with to the end of the new suture, cut just the needle off taking care not to create a loose remnant.
- You can only do this when the suture is on the upper aspect of the sewing ring: the first stitch with the new suture is into the annulus from above down.
- Use a leaflet retractor to separate sutures for the last few bites.
- Parachute the prosthesis down into position, by pulling alternately on each of the rubber shods and running the prosthesis down the sutures.
- Cut the stay stitch securing the valve to the valve holder with a 15 blade on a long handle, and remove the holder.
- Even out the sutures, tighten each in turn with a nerve hook checking carefully for loops, check that the valve mechanism opens freely, check that both coronary ostia are unimpeded, and then cut the sutures so that you can tie them comfortably.
- Place 8–9 throws so that the knot forms away from the valve, cutting the ends short so they do not interfere with the mechanism.
- As this is a semicontinuous technique it is sensible to maintain traction on the sutures either side of those being tied, but great care must be taken not to tear the proximal end of the aortotomy at this point by over-vigorous assistance.

Interrupted non-everting mattress suture

Interrupted sutures may be simple or horizontal mattress sutures (which may be everting or non-everting), with or without pledgets. Alternating color braided non-absorbable sutures such as 3/0 Ethibond are usually used. This technique is suitable for prostheses and homografts: horizontal mattress sutures tend to be used with prosthetic valves (everting in large annulus, non-everting in smaller, with pledgets where the annulus is very calcified or friable), and simple interrupted monofilament sutures for homografts. Either all the annular sutures are placed before putting any sutures through the prosthesis sewing ring (simpler), or each suture can be placed through the annulus and directly into the valve sewing ring.

- Take a double-ended 3/0 Ethibond with both needles mounted forehand hook, and a pledget mounted between them, and take a bite from below up on the annulus starting at the L/NCC commissure, repeating this 3mm away with the second needle and clipping both ends of the suture under tension to the drapes or valve holders, after making sure the pledget seats correctly and suture 'runs' freely.
- Repeat with the first stitch of the second suture 1mm away from the second stitch of the first suture, proceeding around the annulus and the valve sewing ring in an anti-clockwise direction. Usually easier to use a backhand from the middle of the RCC to the middle of the LCC from the right side of the table, or take forehand from the left side.
- Most surgeons alternate two colours of sutures and clip both ends of each suture together, some put a single throw on the sutures before giving them to the assistant, and others prefer to rely on the spacing on the valve sewing ring to tell which suture ends are the correct pairs.
- With the assistant holding the valve mounted on a holder, position the valve above the annulus. Note the number of sutures. Both ends of the double-ended sutures are placed through the valve sewing ring from below up. Securing the pledget above the annulus is what *everts* the annulus: this is bulkier than the semicontinuous technique and non-everting techniques. In the smaller annulus pledgets should be placed below the annulus, or not used.
- Make a rough estimate of how many sutures you'll need per commissure, to help you plan the spacing on the valve sewing ring.
- The assistant holds the sutures in their right hand once placed through the sewing ring to keep them under tension, and provide exposure.
- If for any reason a suture is cut before it has been placed through the valve sewing ring, a French-eye needle or standard green needle can be used to threat the loose end through the valve ring.
- When the suture ring is complete, gather the sutures together between two or three clips, and cut the needles off together, taking care not to lose any needles or to create any loose suture fragments.
- Wet the sutures with saline.
- Holding the sutures taut, parachute the valve into position, and complete implantation as described for semicontinuous technique: with braided sutures five throws is sufficient for each knot, and check each suture 'runs' before tying to avoid tying to the wrong suture, and leaving loose loops of suture below the annulus.

Stentless aortic replacement

Stentless aortic prostheses can be implanted in the subcoronary position which is described here, as a cylinder insertion or, in the case of the
Freestyle, implanted in the same way as an aortic homograft root replacement (📖 p390).

Subcoronary technique

The Medtronic Freestyle® needs to be trimmed before it can be implanted
using this technique, whereas the 3f is ready for use. The right and the left
coronary sinus are removed, the non-coronary sinus is left intact (Fig. 8.6).
If an oblique aototomy has been used, the non-coronary xenograft sinus
helps to buttress the closure.

* Transverse aortotomy. Excise and size the valve in the usual manner.
* Valves are sized according to the outside diameter of the prosthesis,
  as opposed to homografts which are sized according to the inside
  diameter. It is therefore not necessary to downsize: oversizing the
  stentless valves actually increases the gradient across the valve because
  of extra tissue occupying the orifice.
* It is particularly important to get the orientation of the prosthesis
  relative to the aortic root correct, as the patient's coronary ostia will
  be obscured if the orientation is incorrect: coronary arteries in the pig
  are closer together than in the human.
* The valve can be inserted using either interrupted or a semicontinuous technique, with or without pledgets: as the sewing ring
  is less rigid it is important to check that suture tension is constant
  throughout and that the sewing ring is not distorted.
* More so than for stented and mechanical prosthesis, the horizontal
  sewing ring means that sutures should remain in a flat plane on the
  aortic annulus, to avoid distorting the flexible sewing ring (Fig. 8.6c).
* The porcine aorta is attached to the patient's aorta using
  semicontinuous non-absorbable monofilament such as 3/0 Prolene
  (Fig. 8.6d) (3x single interrupted mattress sutures, one at each post, in
  the case of the 3f stentless valve).

Aortic root replacement technique

The additional dissection required to isolate the patient's coronary ostia
and create coronary buttons, and the additional suture lines required,
mean that this is a longer and more technically demanding operation than
subcoronary implantation. When the aortic root is dilated or distorted, it
is preferable to insert the Freestyle® as a root replacement. The coronary
ostia are closer together in the pig than they are in the human: when the
left coronary ostia of xenograft and patient are aligned, the right coronary
ostia in the xenograft is usually to the right of the patient's. It is usually necessary to extend the hole in the xenograft to match (Fig. 8.6), otherwise
implantation follows the steps described for homograft root replacement
on 📖 p386.

Cylinder implantation technique

This is described on 📖 p387.

Indications for stentless AVR
- Subcoronary: small aortic root, surgeon preference.
- Root replacement: see 📖 p390.

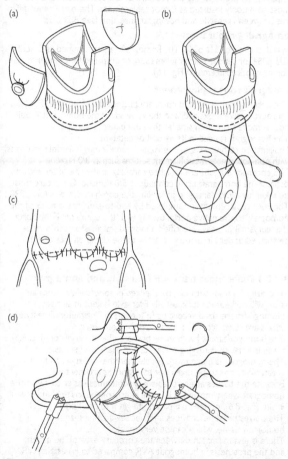

Fig. 8.6 (a) Preparing the Freestyle prosthesis. (b) Implantation of the stentless xenograft; (c) Placement of stitches on the aortic annulus; (d) Attaching the porcine aorta to the patient's aorta, with marker stitches and semicontinuous technique.

Homograft aortic replacement

Aortic homograft (also known as *allograft*), can be inserted in the same way as a Freestyle prosthesis as a subcoronary aortic valve replacement (📖 p384), as an inclusion cylinder (📖 p387), or as a root replacement (📖 p390). To preserve the architecture of the pliable homograft root, it is most commonly inserted as a root replacement. There are a few differences between Freestyle and homograft insertion (see Box 8.3).

Homograft preparation

This is described on 📖 p368. The homograft can be trimmed as described on 📖 p384 for subcoronary implantation, or prepared for cylinder implantation or root replacement (Fig. 8.6).

Homograft root replacement

• The aorta is transected and coronary buttons dissected free (Fig. 8.6).
• The aortic valve is excised, and the valve sized. the homograft should not be more than 3mm smaller than the patient's annulus.
• The homograft is used in its natural orientation.
• Implantation technique is an interrupted non-everting horizontal mattress, with non-absorbable monofilament sutures such as 3/0 Prolene.
• The coronary buttons are attached carefully to the site of the excised ostia of the homograft using continuous 5/0 Prolene. Great care must be taken to avoid damaging or kinking the coronary arteries (📖 p390).
• The root replacement is completed by end-to-end anastomosis of the homograft to the native aorta, usually with the clamp on: if the aorta is aneurysmal or heavily calcified a more distal anastomosis may be performed under circulatory arrest with the clamp off (📖 p435).

Box 8.3 Differences between Freestyle and homograft

• The size of homograft must be checked preoperatively as not all sizes will be kept in stock: usually Freestyle is kept in all sizes.
• Homografts are sized according to the internal diameter: Freestyle valves are sized according to the external diameter.
• The homograft must be carefully prepared before insertion (Fig. 8.6), there is a risk of damaging the aorta and the valve leaflets.
• The homograft is much more pliable than the Freestyle, and even greater care has to be taken not to distort its architecture.
• Because the tissues are so pliable it is sometimes easier to invert the homograft when implanting it in the subcoronary position and sew it *in situ* (Fig. 8.6), rather than parachuting it into position.
• The polyester fabric provides a firmer sewing ring than the homograft tissue, which can be very friable.
• There is less mismatch between the coronary ostia of the patient and the prosthesis in homograft AVR compared to Freestyle AVR.

Cylinder technique

- The homograft aorta is prepared by excising larger buttons of sinus aorta than in the root replacement technique. It is implanted in a similar way to the root replacement, but the native aorta is preserved so that the aortotomy can be closed directly (Fig. 8.6). This technique is used less commonly as there is a greater tendency to distort the valve geometry than with a complete root replacement technique.

Indications for homograft root replacement

- Infective endocarditis with root abscess requiring root replacement: not so much because of increased freedom from reinfection (which has not been shown in recent series), but because homograft is slightly easier to sew into friable tissue (particularly reop) than bio-Bentall, or Freestyle.
- Similar rationale for reop aortic root replacement—need to mobilize coronary buttons less extensively as homograft pliable.
- Surgeon preference is less common now as there is some data to suggest poorer durability of homografts compared to Freestyle root replacement.

The Ross procedure

Using the patient's own pulmonary valve to replace the aortic valve (pulmonary autograft) is known as the Ross procedure, after Donald Ross, the British surgeon who pioneered its use. The pulmonary valve is replaced with a pulmonary homograft. Rationale is discussed on 📖 p369.

Set-up and aortotomy

Some surgeons prefer no PA catheter. Aorto-bicaval cannulation (the RV is opened during the procedure so use of a two-stage cannula, may: (a) entrain air, and (b) result in poor venous drainage and a flooded field). Mark the pulmonary valve commissures before going on bypass.

Excising the PA root and preparing the aorta

- Assess the pulmonary valve by TEE, and then by direct visualization through small arteriotomy: large or multiple fenestrations, or bileaflet valves are not suitable for use as autograft.
- After clamping separate the PA from the aorta up to the bifurcation, and proximally as far as the area where they are fused adjacent to the right–left aortic commissure, just onto the RVOT muscle.
- Transverse aortotomy 1–2cm above commissures, transecting aorta if suitable for root replacement, and excising valve in standard way (📖 p380).
- Size valve using standard sizers, and place six stay sutures: three above each commissure, two above R&L coronary ostia, and one deep in NCC.
- Divide PA 1–2cm above the sinuses: there is no advantage to using the entire length of the PA as this has a tendency to dilate in the aortic position, and getting good exposure for a very distal pulmonary artery to homograft anastomosis is quite challenging.
- Divide fat between back of PA and LMS carefully staying close to PA.
- Open RVOT just below PA cusps, extending incision medially and laterally staying well away from cusps, keeping 3–5mm of muscle cuff, and staying in the natural plane between right and left ventricular septum posteriorly to avoid damaging the first septal artery which is located in the LV septum, and easily damaged during this dissection, compromising septal function and resulting in much of the morbidity associated with the procedure.
- The pulmonary autograft is sized and trimmed ready to be implanted.
- The aorta is transected and large coronary buttons mobilized (sharing the aortic wall equally between the buttons and annulus, and preserving pillars of native aorta).

Implantation of the pulmonary autograft

- Ideally <2mm difference between aorta and the pulmonary autograft.
- The pulmonary autograft is implanted in a similar fashion to the homograft root replacement described on 📖 p386 using semicontinuous 4/0 Prolene on RB1 and SH1 needles.
- Supporting the aortic annulus with a strip of Teflon felt or pericardium cut 1 size larger than the internal diameter helps prevent dilatation.
- If diameter of the aorta is larger than the PA this can be addressed either by bevelling the pulmonary trunk or by using interposition grafts.

Indications for Ross procedure
- Patient <21 years of age requiring AVR.
- Controversial: adults who do not wish to take warfarin in whom Ross can be performed with mortality close to that of isolated AVR.

Implantation of the pulmonary homograft

The PA can be anastomosed before the aorta as exposure is easier, or afterwards to reduce ischemic time: both are relatively straightforward full-thickness continuous 4/0 Prolene, except for the area around the infundibular septum where sutures must be partial thickness to avoid damaging the first septal branch of the LAD. Both suture lines can be buttressed with pericardial strips—bleeding is pressure dependent so ensure the anesthesiologist appreciates the need to keep systolics <100mmHg at all times to avoid major hemorrhage.

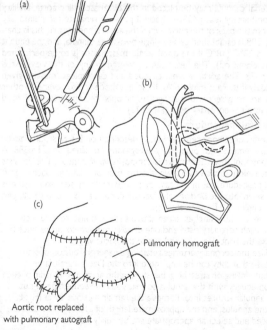

(a)

(b)

(c)

Pulmonary homograft

Aortic root replaced
with pulmonary autograft

Fig. 8.7 (a) Preparation of the aortic root and dissection of the infundibular septum. (b) Preserving the first septal branch of the LAD. (c) Completed Ross.

Aortic root replacement

Key facts

- Can be done using homograft, Freestyle porcine valve, pulmonary autograft (Ross), or most valved conduit (Bentall or bio-Bentall).
- Performed for annuloaortic ectasia/aneurysm where native valve cannot be preserved (spared), annular abscess, small aortic root (📖 p392).

Indications for root replacement

- Annuloaortic ectasia/aneurysm aortic root where valve cannot be preserved. Size cut-offs listed in more detail on 📖 p443.
  - Ascending 5.5cm asymptomatic incidental.
  - Ascending 5cm symptomatic.
  - Ascending 4.5cm Marfan (or symptomatic), bicuspid aortic valve.
- Infective endocarditis of the aortic root—annular abscess.
- Acute or chronic aortic dissection with aortic regurgitation (📖 p432).
- Small aortic root, to allow larger prosthesis than otherwise possible.

Set-up

The arterial cannula may be placed in the distal ascending aorta, axillary or femoral artery (📖 p433)—check! If possible separate the pulmonary trunk from the back of the aorta: when the aorta is aneurysmal this is challenging. CPB is established using a single two-stage cannula, and the patient cooled to 28°C (18°C if the distal aortic anastomosis is to be performed with the clamp off). The heart can be vented in any of the ways listed on 📖 p378. The aorta is cross-clamped and cardioplegia may be given antegradely if there is minimal AI. If there is moderate to severe AI other options are to arrest with retrograde, or open the aorta to give blood directly into the coronary ostia (📖 p378).

The Bentall procedure

Homograft aortic root replacement is described on 📖 p386, and aortic root replacement with pulmonary autograph is outlined on 📖 p388. A more commonly used alternative is composite valve conduit. This consists of a mechanical aortic valve sewn into the base of a tubular Dacron graft (Bentall procedure), or in the case of a bio-Bentall any stented prosthesis may be sewn into the bottom of a Dacron conduit at least one size larger, using a running 4/0 Prolene suture).

- Place six traction stitches: three above each commissure, two well above each coronary ostia and one deep in the non-coronary sinus to expose the root (Fig. 8.7), and excise the aortic valve.
- Mobilize the coronary arteries retaining a generous button of sinus aorta, so that they can be implanted into the Dacron graft later without kinking or stretching, but sharing the aorta at the nadir of each button equally with the annulus so that you have something to put your annular sutures into. Remove the remaining sinus aorta (Fig. 8.7).
- Size the annulus, and the approximate length of ascending aorta to be replaced and select an appropriate graft (usually size 26 or 28).

- Implant the composite graft using either of the techniques described for simple AVR on 📖 pp382–383. If tissues are friable, use interrupted pledgetted sutures (Fig. 8.7). In a bio-Bentall, annular sutures should be passed through the sewing ring of the conduit and the bottom 2mm of the conduit: it is this suture line that makes the join between graft and prosthesis hemostatic, not the 4/0 running Prolene.

- Next assess where the left coronary button sits, and create a 4mm hole in the graft with microcautery to which the left coronary button can be anastomosed with a 6/0 Prolene continuous suture line, which can be buttressed with a felt strip (starting halfway up the left side of the anastomosis forehand on the graft inside to out, outside to in on button, working past the heel and halfway up the right side before swapping ends of the suture). This is checked for hemostasis by applying a clamp distally and giving cardioplegia directly into the graft.

- The position of the right coronary button should be determined with the perfusionist filling the heart to avoid the proximal RCA kinking (suture with 6/0 Prolene starting halfway up the left side of the anastomosis forehand on the button inside to out, outside to in on the graft, working past the heel and halfway up the right side before swapping ends of the suture).

- In large aneurysms the coronary ostia may displaced so far laterally that an interpositional or Cabrol graft is required (📖 p445).

- Next shorten the distal end of the tube graft to match the distal aorta. Anastomose with continuous 4/0 Prolene (starting halfway up the left side of the anastomosis forehand on proximal inside to out, outside to in on distal, working past the heel and halfway up the right side before swapping ends of the suture). Tighten the suture line with nerve hooks, especially posteriorly where if bleeding occurs it will be most problematic to rectify. For the same reason, if there is a size mismatch cheat anteriorly not posteriorly.

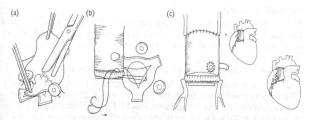

Fig. 8.8 (a) Exposure of the aortic root and creating coronary buttons. (b) Implanting the composite conduit. (c) Finished repair.

Small aortic root

Key facts

- The post-op gradient across an AVR depends on the valve size and CO: it is higher in small valves, large patients, tachycardia, hyperdynamic LV (hence β-blockers used to treat it).
- Post-op gradients are common, and it's probably sensible to minimize gradient by not implanting an AVR 'too small' for the patient's size.
- How small is 'too small' is quantified by *patient prosthesis mismatch (PPM)*, defined as indexed effective orifice area (IEOA)<0.85cm^2/m^2:
  - There is, however, no strong data to show difference in survival or symptoms according to whether patients have PPM.
  - This is partly because PPM tends to occur in patients with other risk factors for worse outcomes (females, obese, older patients).
- There are several options to avoid a high transvalvular gradient after AVR, in a patient at risk of this because of a small aortic root (Box 8.4).

Patient prosthesis mismatch

In vivo valve orifice area and body size are used to calculate IEOA: <0.8cm^2/m^2 results in a rapid rise in mean transvalvular pressure gradient during exercise, reflected by reduced LV mass regression postoperatively. No studies show strong evidence of worse survival or symptoms due to PPM. The consensus is that a 19mm valve should not be implanted in a large, active patient because of the large intrinsic gradient. Inserting the largest possible prosthesis may cause problematic annular erosion acutely or over time. Alternatives are listed in the Box 8.4: it is a question of balancing the theoretical disadvantages of moderate AS against the disadvantages of the surgical options.

Aortic root enlargement

The oblique aortotomy described on 🕮 p379 has the important advantage that it can be easily extended to allow aortic root enlargement, and can be easily closed with a patch enlargement. Root enlargements are either posterior (used mainly in adults) or anterior (used in children).

The Nicks procedure

The aortotomy incision is continued posteriorly through the NCC, onto the anterior leaflet of the mitral valve, and the roof of the LA is dissected away without opening it. Dividing the fibrous attachment of the aortic

---

Box 8.4 Options for small aortic root (simplest first)

Plan ahead: annular diameter <20mm on echo is likely to take only 19mm valve—will this be adequate? If patient very active or high BSA, or diastolic dysfunction, or low-grade low-EF AS—probably not.
- Implant mechanical valve (best hemodynamics for given size: but trading lifetime anticoagulation for a reduction in gradient).
- Suprannular stented valve (allows to upsize by one size).
- Stentless valve (slightly better hemodynamics than stented).
- Nicks root enlargement.
- Manougian root enlargement.
- Root replacement.
- Ross–Konno (enlargement via RVOT used in children only).

annulus in this way causes the edges of the aortotomy to open widely as there is little fibrous support. A 3–4cm wide teardrop-shaped patch of either pericardium or Dacron is shaped to fit the defect. Starting at the midpoint of the bottom of the incision the patch is sutured to the aorta, with or without Teflon pledgets (Fig. 8.8a). This must be done particularly carefully as this area is virtually impossible to access once the cross-clamp is removed. The valve is inserted in the usual manner, sewing it to the aortic annulus and the patch.

The Manougian procedure

This involves extending the aortotomy into the posterior commissure, between LCC and NCC into the interleaflet triangle, and onto the anterior leaflet of the mitral valve. The loose tissues of the triangle separate readily, and it is often but not always possible to enlarge the annulus sufficiently without having to divide the anterior leaflet of the mitral valve or enter the LA.

The Ross–Konno procedure

This is the Ross procedure (📖 p388) with anterior enlargement of the root.

Root enlargement using a homograft: Root replacement always allows a larger valve to be implanted: if even greater enlargement is needed (e.g., in reoperative surgery) the anterior mitral annulus may be divided. A homograft, complete with anterior mitral valve leaflet if necessary, is implanted in the subcoronary position, with closure of the roof of the LA with a pericardial patch, and pledget strips to buttress unsupported aorta. The NCC of the homograft is used to close the aortotomy and widen the aortic root.

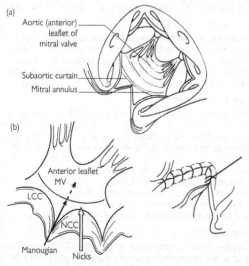

Fig. 8.9 (a) Extending the oblique aortotomy for root enlargement (Nicks procedure). (b) The Nicks and Manougian posterior root enlargement compared.

Valve-sparing procedures

There are a large number of procedures described for patients with morphologically normal aortic valves, but with AI caused by pathology affecting the sinotubular junction (STJ) or the aortic annulus (AA). The differences between and indications for the Yacoub (remodelling) and David (reimplantation) valve sparing procedures are described on 📖 pp446–447. The normal sinotubular junction, and annulus are described on 📖 p53.

> **Indications for valve-sparing procedures**
> • Normal AA and STJ: Commissuroplasty, leaflet plication.
> • Normal AA and ↑STJ: interpostion graft if sinuses do not need replacing (📖 p443).
> • ↑AA and ↑STJ: Yacoub or David procedure (📖 pp446–447) (Fig. 9.6c).

Normal AA and normal STJ

AI may be due to leaflet abnormalities (perforation, fenestration or prolapse) which can occasionally be satisfactorily addressed by primary repair and/or leaflet plication using 6/0 Gore-Tex or 7/0 prolene. Aortic commissuroplasty involves reducing the intercommissural triangle distance with horizontal pledgted mattress sutures. When AI is due to distortion of a sinus by Type A dissection (Fig. 8.10a, valve sparing options include sealing the dissected sinus with sutures or glue and replacing the ascending aorta with an interposition graft (Fig. 8.10e, and 📖 p444)—this is the preferred option; or a valve sparing root replacement (Fig. 8.10b) with coronary reimplantation which is technically extremely challenging in this context.

Normal AA and dilated STJ

This occurs in patients with aortic ectasia, which may be caused by connective tissue disorders such as Marfan, chronic hypertension, post-stenotic dilatation, and type A dissection. A simple interposition style graft can be placed, with or without a band of PTFE for additional support at the level of the STJ (Fig. 8.10e). It is not necessary to reimplant the coronaries.

Both AA and STJ enlarged

This is a feature of annuloaortic ectasia which is caused by connective tissue disorders such as Marfan. A number of modifications to procedures originally separately described by Magdi Yacoub and Tirone David exist. The main differences (see also 📖 pp446–447) between the various modifications are:
• How the size of aortic graft required is calculated.
• Whether an aortic annuloplasty is performed.
• Whether the aortic annulus is fixed circumferentially.
• Whether an inclusion cylinder technique is used.
• Whether and how pseudosinuses are created in the graft.

Checking competence

This can be assessed prior to completing the distal aortic anastomosis by holding the graft in the approximate anatomical position and filling it with saline, which should remain in the root. Formal assessment occurs with intraoperative TEE once the patient is off bypass.

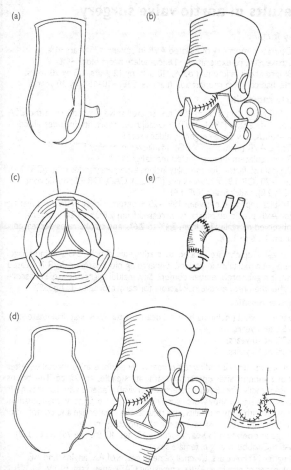

Fig. 8.10 (a) Cross-section of aortic dissection. (b) Creating pseudosinuses. (c) Resuspending the aortic valve inside the Dacron graft. (d) Valve-sparing surgery for true aortoannular ectasia with PTFE support of annulus. (e) Simple interposition graft.

Results of aortic valve surgery

Key facts

- Operative mortality of isolated AVR in patient <75 years ~1%.
- Stroke ~1%, re-exploration ~1%, complete heart block ~1%.
- Bioprosthesis failure (🕮 p366): 10–20% by 12 years, 1/3 by 20 years.
- Mechanical valve reoperation (pannus, SBE) ~10–15% by 20 years.

Early mortality

The following data is from 409 904 isolated valve procedures in the USA national database (1994–2003).[1,2] Unadjusted mortality includes all com-ers—reops, low EF, emergency, elderly, etc.:

- Single AVR (including CABG) unadjusted mortality 5.7%.
- Root replacement: unadjusted mortality 11.1%.
- Biggest risk factors for mortality include emergency (odds ratio (OR) 2.1), age >70 (OR 1.9), multiple valve (OR 1.6), CAD (OR 1.6) aortic root (OR 2.8), endocarditis (OR 1.6).
- Results improved between 1997–2006 despite sicker patient profile: for AVR predicted mortality increased from 2.8% to 3.2% whereas observed mortality fell from 3.4% to 2.6%, and stroke rates decreased from 1.5% to 1.3%.

Most early deaths are related to cardiogenic shock, CVA, hemorrhage. The higher mortality in patients undergoing bioprosthetic AVR is related to their higher preoperative comorbidity, including greater age. Euroscore weights the preoperative risk factors for early mortality (🕮 p358).

Late mortality

Overall survival (including hospital deaths) after AVR is approximately:

- 75% at 5 years.
- 60% at 10 years.
- 40% at 15 years.

Short-term survival is dictated primarily by perioperative mortality. After about 6 months after operation death rate steadies at ~2% pa. This begins to rise steadily after 5 years (late-term survival). Patients with bioprosthetic valves have significantly worse survival curves than patients with mechanical valves: as with early mortality, this reflects the greater age and comorbidity of this group. Other risk factors for late mortality include:

- ↑age at operation (30-day mortality 1% age 40, 8% age 75) (🕮 p358).
- Afro-Caribbean origin, female sex.
- Higher NYHA class, LV enlargement, grade of AR, angina, and AF.
- Number of previous AVRs, coexisting CAD, aneurysm, or LV structural abnormality.
- The operative myocardial ischemic time.

Complications of aortic valve replacement

The complications of cardiac surgery in general: rexploration for bleed-ing/tamponade (1%), perioperative MI (1%), deep sternal wound infection (1%), prolonged mechanical ventilation (2%), and organ dysfunction (5%)

are discussed in more detail on 📖 pp253–288. Complications particularly associated with AVR include:

CHB: permanent pacemakers are inserted for permanent CHB in about 1% of AVR patients. CHB results from trauma to the bundle of His after extensive debridement of calcium from the RCC/NCC junction (📖 p380). Worsens day 1–3, settles as edema improves.

CVA: the overall risk of CVA is about 2% for isolated AVR, increasing to 3% in combined AVR + CABG. CVA in AVR shares the same risk factors as in other cardiac surgery (📖 p278). Removal of all calcific debris from the operative field and thorough de-airing help prevent CVA.

Prosthetic endocarditis: mechanical valves are at slightly higher risk of endocarditis up to 3 months after surgery; the risks even out by 5 years. Homografts once thought lower risk, not supported by data. The cumulative risk of prosthetic valve endocarditis is about 1% at 1 year and 3% at 5 years post AVR. Early endocarditis (within 3 months of surgery) is usually hospital acquired: organisms are commonly staphylococci and Gram −ve cocci. Late prosthetic endocarditis usually results from a transient streptococcal bacteremia. The mortality is up to 60%.

Thromboembolism: the rate of valve thromboembolism is roughly 1–2% per year (📖 p267): the rate in adequately anticoagulated mechanical valves is similar to that in prosthetic valves. *Valve thrombosis* rare emergency: cardiovascular collapse, venous congestion and systemic embolization normally acute, but may be insidious. The management is iv heparin. If the thrombus is >5mm thrombolysis or reop tissue AVR is indicated.

Paraprosthetic leak: major paraprosthetic leak is uncommon (📖 p266). It is caused most commonly by prosthetic endocarditis (late), and less commonly by technical errors in insertion (early). Patients present with hemolytic anemia, and if severe, CCF. The treatment is surgery. If the area of dehiscence is small and there is no evidence of sepsis, one or two interrupted sutures may suffice. Otherwise redo AVR is indicated.

Prosthesis failure (📖 p366): failure of mechanical valves is almost exclusive to strut failure of a particular Bjork–Shiley tilting disk valve, withdrawn in 1986. Bioprosthetic AVR failure is <10% at 10 years in the over 70s, but closer to 30% in the 40–50-year age group (📖 p366). Degenerative failure in cryopreserved homograft AVR is between 5–10% at 10 years.

Reoperation for any reason: the risk of reoperation is highest in the first 6 months post AVR due to prosthetic endocarditis and paravalvular leak. It falls to about 1% a year where it remains for mechanical valves. The risk also falls initially in bioprosthetic valves, but begins to rise rapidly after 10–12 years due to structural degeneration.

Improvement in symptoms and LV function

90% of patients are NYHA class I or II, 5–10 years following AVR. Completely normal LV mass is rarely achieved, but where LVEDP was low preoperatively, LV mass returns to near normal values. Where LVEDP was raised preoperatively this does not happen.

References

1. Rankin JS. Amiodarone and cardiac surgery. *J Thorac Cardiovasc Surg* 2005; **131**:547–57.
2. Brown JM et al. Isolated aortic valve replacement in North America comprising 108,687 patients in 10 years. *J Thorac Cardiovasc Surg* 2009; **137**: 82–90.

Pathophysiology of mitral stenosis

Key facts

- Commonest valve lesion in developing countries.
- Usually caused by rheumatic valve disease: results in commissural fusion, leaflet thickening and calcification, and chordal fusion.
- Well tolerated with long asymptomatic interval.

Morphology

The commonest cause of MS is rheumatic fever: the disease process causes leaflet thickening and calcification, commissural and chordal fusion. Isolated MS occurs in 40% of all patients presenting with rheumatic heart disease, and 60% of patients with MS give a history of rheumatic fever. The ratio of female to male patients with this pathology is 2:1. Congenital malformation of the mitral valve occurs rarely (📖 p638).

Structural and functional changes

The cross-sectional area of the normal mitral valve is 4.0–5.0cm². Narrowing of this area to <2.5cm² means that a pressure gradient must be generated across the mitral valve in diastole in order to expel blood from the LA into the LV. This results in elevation of LA and pulmonary venous pressures. LA enlargement, AF, and thrombus formation result from chronic LAP overload. Pulmonary hypertension results from passive transmission ↑LAP, pulmonary vasoconstriction and irreversible pulmonary vasculature remodelling. Pulmonary edema occurs when pulmonary venous pressure is greater than plasma oncotic pressure. At rest, MS is usually asymptomatic, but any increase in transmitral flow rates (e.g., due to hyperdynamic circulation) or reduction in the diastolic filling period, e.g., tachycardia will result in an increase in the pressure gradient, resulting in dyspnea. Severe MS may have a low gradient in patients with a low CO.

Symptoms

The first symptoms of dyspnea in these patients are usually precipitated by exercise, sexual intercourse, emotional stress, infection, pregnancy, or rapid AF, because in the increase in the pressure gradient across the mitral valve described earlier. Recurrent chest infections are characteristic. Hemoptysis is caused by chest infections, pulmonary infarction, acute pulmonary edema, and rupture of small pulmonary vessels. Systemic embolism is frequent, particularly in AF.

Signs

- Decreased amplitude pulse, AF.
- 'Tapping' apex beat.
- Left parasternal heave due to RV hypertrophy.
- Thrill due to paplpable opening snap.
- Loud first heart sound, an opening snap loudest at lower left sternal edge.
- Presystolic murmur, delayed mid-diastolic murmur.

Pathophysiology of mitral regurgitation

Key facts

- Commonest valve lesion with incidence around 2%.
- Describe using *Carpentier's pathophysiological triad* (see Table 8.3):
  - *Leaflet dysfunction*: leaflet motion either I normal, II excessive, or III restricted (IIIa restricted opening, IIIb restricted closure).
  - *Lesion*: problem with MV apparatus, e.g., chordal elongation or rupture, leaflet perforation, annular dilatation, papillary muscle rupture.
  - *Etiology*: degenerative, ischemic, rheumatic, endocarditis, DCM.
- Mitral *prolapse* is systolic billowing of leaflets into the LA ± MR.
- MR causes dyspnea, CHF, AF, stroke, pulmonary hypertension.

Morphology

- The mitral valve consists of annulus, leaflets, chordae tendineae; papillary muscles; and the LV wall (Fig. 2.5). Disease involving these parts results in reduced leaflet coaptation leading to MR, described using Carpentier's pathophysiological triad (Table 8.3) and *segmental valve nomenclature* (🕮 p45).

Etiology

- *Degenerative disease* is commonest cause in West (incidence 2%):
  - Causes prolapse (type II MR) due to chordal elongation or rupture.
  - Histology shows *myxomatous degeneration*.
  - Spectrum from single-segment prolapse in small valve (*fibroelastic deficiency*) to multisegment prolapse in giant valve (*Barlow's*).
- *Ischemic MR* is usually due to chronic LV dysfunction and posterior displacement of papillary muscle (type IIIb) with normal leaflets; papillary muscle rupture can cause acute type II MR after MI.
- *Endocarditis* causes type I MR (leaflet perforation).
- *Dilated cardiomyopathy* causes type I MR (annular dilatation).

Table 8.3 Carpentier's pathophysiological triad

Leaflet dysfunction		Lesions	Etiology
CARPENTIER'S CLASSIFCATION OF MR AC	Type I	Leaflet perforation	Endocarditis
		Annular dilatation	Dilated cardiomyopathy, ischemic cardiomyopathy
	Type II	Chordal elongation/rupture, papillary muscle elongation	Degenerative disease (FED or Barlow's)
		Papillary muscle rupture	Ischemic cardiomyopathy
	Type IIIa	Commissural fusion, leaflet calcification, chordal fusion	Rheumatic disease
	Type IIIb	Papillary muscle displacement, LV dilatation	Dilated cardiomyopathy, ischemic cardiomyopathy

- *Rheumatic disease* results in type IIIa MR with restricted leaflet opening due to calcification and commissural fusion.
- *Systolic anterior motion* (📖 p191) results in MR + LVOTO.
- *Congenital*, e.g., cleft mitral valve, *connective tissue disease*, e.g. Marfan.

Structural and functional changes in chronic MR

Whatever the mechanism resulting in reduced leaflet coaptation, the pathophysiological changes progress through one or more of three stages: acute MR, chronic compensated MR, and chronic decompensated MR.

- *Acute MR* results in *LV volume overload* at end diastole, i.e., ↑preload, and ↓afterload due to the regurgitant pathway into the LA.
- The combination of ↑preload and ↓afterload means that a larger volume of blood is ejected from the LV.
- Because a large volume of ejected blood enters the LA rather than the aorta, forward stroke volume, and hence *cardiac output decreases*.
- The increased blood volume in the LA raises the pressure from a normal LAP of 10mmHg to up to 25mmHg.
- ↑preload leads to eccentric hypertrophy and *LV dilatation*, increasing total stroke volume, as well as forward stroke volume which returns to near normal levels: *chronic compensated MR*.
- *LA enlargement* accommodates volume overload there at lower filling pressures (15mmHg), but predisposes to *AF* and *mural thrombi*.
- *Chronic decompensated MR* exists when systolic dysfunction prevents effective ventricular contraction: stroke volume and cardiac output are reduced as blood flows into the low-resistance regurgitant pathway, and left atrial and *pulmonary pressures rise* as a result.
- Untreated decompensated MR rapidly progresses to pulmonary edema and congestive cardiac failure.
- Symptoms, LV dysfunction, LA dilatation, AF, and pulmonary hypertension are all associated with decreased long-term survival.

Symptoms and signs in chronic MR

The interval from diagnosis of MR to the onset of symptoms varies by aetiology (FED months to years, Barlow's decades). LV EF remains normal despite even severe LV dysfunction because 50% of stroke volume ejects into low-pressure LA. While most deaths are related to heart failure, the incidence of sudden death suggests ventricular arrhythmias are an important feature of the disease process. Signs include AF, prominent sustained apex beat, systolic thrill, right parasternal heave reflecting RVH due to PAH, quiet first heart sound, third heart sound audible, loud pansystolic murmur loudest at apex radiating to axilla.

Acute MR

Acute severe MR may be caused by chordal rupture, ischemic heart disease, or infective endocarditis, and it is an indication for urgent surgery. A sudden volume overload is imposed on the LV, increasing preload and resulting in a small increase in total stroke volume. Without the compensatory LA and LV dilatation seen in chronic severe MR, however, forward stroke volume is reduced, and CHF and cardiogenic shock may result. The patient with acute severe MR is always symptomatic.

Timing of mitral valve surgery

Key facts

- Severe MR reduces normal life expectancy: repair is the only treatment that can restore this to normal. Mitral replacement is associated with worse early and late mortality and morbidity than repair (Fig. 8.11).
- Symptoms, AF, PAH, and LV dysfunction or dilatation are each associated with worse survival: so they are all indications for surgery in MR.
- Early surgery may be indicated in asymptomatic patients with MR and none of the listed risk factors *if repair is very likely (>90%)*.
- MS is better tolerated than MR, is rarely amenable to repair, and may respond to balloon valvuloplasty so the threshold for surgery is higher.

Mitral regurgitation

The prognosis of chronic MR depends on both the etiology and severity of the lesion. In patients with severe symptomatic chronic MR of any etiology the prognosis is poor. The average mortality rate is ~5% per year, and may be as high as 70% at 8 years.

Patients with isolated chronic mild to moderate MR are unlikely to require surgery, and therapy is aimed at treating the symptoms and preventing complications. AHA guidelines recommend that these patients are followed up on a yearly basis, with TTE if there are clinical grounds for suspecting a deterioration in LV or mitral valve function.

In chronic ischemic MR (📖 p356) the valve itself is usually anatomically normal and the regurgitation is secondary to papillary muscle and LV dysfunction following infarction. The prognosis is poorer than in MR caused by non-ischemic pathology. CABG may improve LV function and reduce MR. If LV function is very severe (LVESD >55mm or LVEF <30%), and repair/chordal preservation unlikely, surgery may not be beneficial (📖 p357).

Acute mitral regurgitation

Acute severe MR is an indication for urgent surgery. There is no scope for compensatory changes: CO falls, LAPs increase, and pulmonary edema and cardiogenic shock ensue (📖 p401).

Mitral stenosis

It may be as long as 20–40 years between the occurrence of rheumatic fever and the onset of symptomatic MS. Once symptoms develop it may be up to 10 years before these become disabling. In the minimally symptomatic patient, 10-year survival is 80%, which drops to 10–15% once symptoms become limiting. Once there is severe pulmonary hypertension, mean survival drops to <3 years. The mortality of untreated MS is due to heart failure in 60–70%, systemic embolism in 20–30%, PE in 10%, and infection in 1–5%. Patients with a mitral valve area of <1.5cm² and NYHA functional class III–IV symptoms should be referred for surgery. There is good evidence that patients with NYHA functional class I–II symptoms and a mitral valve area <1.0cm², and severe PAH (systolic PAP >60–80mmHg) benefit from surgery.

Indications for mitral valve surgery

- Class 1: acute severe symptomatic MR, chronic severe MR *and* NYHA class II–IV *or* mild-moderate LV dysfunction. Also NYHA class III–IV moderate to severe MS if balloon valvotomy not possible.
- Class IIa: asymptomatic chronic severe MR with normal LV *if* repair >90% likely, *or* new AF, *or* PA systolic>50mmHg at rest (60mmHg exercise). Also NYHA III–IV+ severe LV dysfunction *if* primary leaflet dysfunction *and* repair likely. Also severe MS *if* PAP >60mmHg.
- Class IIb: chronic severe MR due to severe LV dysfunction despite optical medical therapy + biventricular pacing.

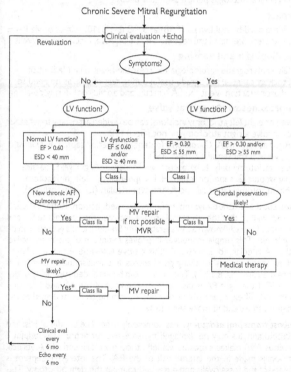

Fig. 8.11 American Heart Association/American College of Cardiologists indications for surgery in chronic severe MR. *Greater than 90% chance of repair. Reproduced from 2008 Focused Update Incorporated Into the ACC/AHA 2006 Guidelines for the Management of Patients With Valvular Heart Disease: A Report of the American College of Cardiology/American Heart Association Task Force on Practice Guidelines. *Circulation*, 2008; **118**: e523–e661. Copyright © 2008, Wolters Kluwer Health.

Mitral valve exposure

Set-up

The commonest approach is via a median sternotomy. A right minithoracotomy via the 4th ICS is used for cosmetic reasons with more proximal cannulation of the ascending aorta and administration of cardioplegia or peripheral cannulation with endoclamping or fibrillatory arrest. Left thoracotomy is used occasionally. Only the right side of the pericardium should be suspended as this rotates the heart anticlockwise, lifting the LA up towards the surgeon. Incising the caval pericardial reflections inferiorly and superiorly further improves access. Rheumatic and endocarditic repair may require autologus pericardium (🕮 p408).

Bypass

Standard aorti-bicaval bypass (CPB) at 32°C (🕮 p110) (direct or via RA ± caval snares). Sternal mitral retractor, e.g., Cosgrove, McCarthy, or Wells.

Cardioplegia and venting

* Give anterograde cardioplegia to arrest the heart via a Medicut or Stockert cannula, retrograde useful during rest of case as no need to adjust retraction. Vent the LA directly, and aortic root during de-airing.

Approaches to the mitral valve

Seven or eight left atriotomy incisions: can be divided according to whether they involve a right atriotomy or not (Fig. 8.12):
* Right atriotomy: A, *Guiraudon's* (extended superior septal), B, *Dubost*, C, vertical transeptal, D, trans ASD.
* Left atriotomy only: E, paraseptal via *Sondegaard's groove*; F, classical paraseptal; G, superior septal; H, LA appendage; I, left thoracotomy.
* No atriotomy: J, transaortic; K, transventricular; (L, autotransplant).

Paraseptal left atriotomy: most commonly used incision. Retract the lateral RA wall so that the interatrial groove between the back of the RA and the roof of the LA known as Waterston's or Sondergaard's groove, can be developed. This simple maneuver improves exposure of the mitral valve. If the LA is enlarged dissection in this groove is less necessary as a larger left atriotomy is possible giving good access. In this case the incision starts more medially (Fig. 8.12, F). This incision can be extended superiorly under the SVC if the right PA is dissected off the roof of the LA, and inferiorly to the IVC. If exposure still poor the SVC can be transected so that the incision can extended more superiorly.

Dubost transeptal atriotomy: less commonly used. The bundle of His, and tricuspid annulus may be damaged by excessive retraction. It is helpful if previous AVR makes exposure via left atriotomy more difficult. A vertical incision is made in the lateral wall of the RA. The interatrial septum is opened at the fossa ovalis and extended to meet the right atriotomy. This is continued across the lateral aspect of the LA into the right SPV. Thin SPV may tear with retraction and are difficult to repair.

Guiraudon's (superior) vertical transeptal approach: RA opened longitudinally (appendage to IVC), fossa ovalis incised longitudinally, right atriotomy extended between AV groove and appendage to meet septal incision, and dome of LA incised from the junction of these incision, away from the aortic root for 2–3cm. Gives good exposure of the anterior mitral annulus without excess retraction: tears in the LA dome may require patch closure and reinstutution of bypass to repair.

Closing the atriotomy

Use a continuous 3/0 Prolene in a single or double layer, starting at either end and tying in middle. *Pitfalls:* (1) closing off the RSPV orifice, (2) incomplete repair of the roof of the LA, (3) failure to evert the suture line predisposing to thrombus, (4) narrowing SVC, (5) sewing PA catheter into suture line. De-airing is described on 📖 p114.

Difficulty exposing the mitral valve

- Exposure is more difficult if there is a previous AVR, or LA is not dilated, e.g., acute MR from endocarditis; so think ahead.
- Exposure starts with set-up: hitch only right side of pericardium, incise caval pericardial reflections, in reop may need to free apex.
- Exposure helped by direct caval cannulation, lift up on caval snares.
- Place one retractor above the anterior annulus (not too deep or valve pushed posteriorly) and one at the posteromedial commissure, and tilt the table away from you slightly.
- Steadily increase retraction on each over several minutes.
- Make sure right heart and aortic root are fully decompressed.
- Assistant pressing down gently on aortic root with forceps handle can bring anterior annulus better into view.
- Extend incision superiorly onto dome LA ± inferiorly behind IVC ± towards fossa ovalis via intra-atrial septum (modified Dubost).
- Placing the commissural traction ± annular sutures where possible and pulling up usually brings all of the valve into view.

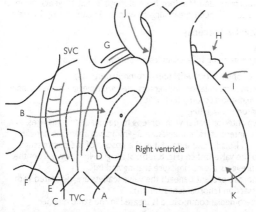

Fig. 8.12 Approaches to the mitral valve (for label key see text). Original drawing by Prasanna Simha MD. (See text for explanation of letters.)

Mitral valvotomy

Key facts

- Indicated for MS (usually rheumatic).
- Options are surgical or percutaneous (balloon mitral valvotomy BMV).
- Surgical approach either closed (without CPB) or open (requires CPB).
- Closed mitral valvotomy largely replaced by BMV in developed world.

Closed mitral valvotomy

First performed by Sir Henry Souttar in the UK in 1925. The basic principles of the operation remained unchanged for three decades until the advent of cardiopulmonary bypass enabled the surgeon to work on the mitral valve under direct vision, in a still, bloodless field.

Indications for closed mitral valvotomy

- Severe symptomatic MS
- Patients should not have MR, and not have heavily calcified valves.

This technique has mostly been superseded by BMV for suitable patients in the West (and mitral replacement where BMV is contraindicated—see 📖 p407). Closed mitral valvotomy is only really still used in countries where rheumatic disease is prevalent and cost or lack of access to technology precludes BMV.

Technique of closed mitral valvotomy

Bypass is not required for closed valvotomy, which is performed via a left thoracotomy, with a finger inserted onto the valve via the LA appendage using a purse-string to prevent blood loss or air embolism, while a Tubbs dilator is passed into the LV via the apex and then opened within the orifice of the valve (Fig. 8.13a).

Results of closed mitral valvotomy

These are comparable to BMV with good improvement in valve area, low operative mortality, and freedom from stenosis for 5–10 years for most patients. 1/3 to 1/2 need repeat surgery within 15 years, 3/4 by 20 years.

Open mitral valvotomy

Indications

- Severe symptomatic MS—main lesion commissural fusion.

Technique of open mitral valvotomy (commissurotomy)

- Aorto-bicaval cannulation with antegrade cardioplegia via sternotomy or right mini-thoracotomy (📖 p110).
- Left atriotomy (📖 p404).
- Pull down anterior leaflet with forceps to delineate commissures.
- Incise the anterolateral commissure 3–4mm away from the annulus with a no. 11 blade, and extend it in the groove of the commissural fusion to the valve orifice (Fig. 8.13b). Staying 3–4mm away from the annulus prevents the commissure tearing and MR.
- Fused chordae present beneath the valve leaflets are separated with sharp dissection (chordal fenestration).
- The posteromedial commissure is treated in the same manner.

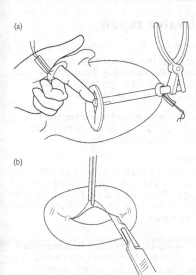

Fig. 8.13 (a) Closed mitral valvotomy. (b) Open mitral commissurotomy.

- Bulky calcium deposits may be removed from the leaflets and annulus with a bone nibbler, taking extreme care to avoid embolism.
- Satisfactory results can be obtained in the absence of calcification using either a finger or a Tubbs dilator to open up the valve.

Results of open mitral valvotomy
Comparable to BMV and open valvotomy in terms of valve area, operative mortality, and freedom from stenosis and reoperation in selected patients.

Balloon mitral valvotomy
Usually performed using transvenous approach with transseptal puncture. The initial results of percutaneous Inoue BMV versus surgical valvotomy are comparable, and both interventions have low rates of restenosis providing good functional outcomes at up to 3 years. At 3 years, however, valve areas in the BMV group are greater than in the surgery. In view of this, as well as the lower cost and morbidity of the percutaneous approach, percutaneous approach is recommended in patients without any contraindications,

Relative contraindications to BMV
- >2+ MR.
- LA thrombus.
- Wilkins score ≥ 8 (range 4–16), or Cormier group 3.
  - ↓leaflet mobility.
  - ↑leaflet/subvalvar thickening, calcification especially commissures.
- Severe concomitant CAD or AS requiring surgery.

Planning mitral valve repair

Key facts

- Match surgeon expertise to repair complexity to avoid replacements.
- Repair complexity depends on valve morphology: looking at the report is not enough—you *must* understand the images, before you start.
- History provides clues about etiology which helps predict morphology.
- MR is dynamic—3+MR on TTE in awake patient, may become trace MR on TEE in fasted patient under GA—always look at the pre-op films and do not rely on the pre-bypass TEE to plan repair.

Carpentier's classification

Carpentier classified MR as type I, normal leaflet motion; type II, excessive leaflet motion; type IIIa, restricted leaflet opening; type IIIb, restricted leaflet closure (see Table 8.3, p400). This is used with the anatomical division of each leaflet into three zones shown in Fig. 2.5. A reproducible system of repair is based on this nomenclature.

Planning the repair

- Review history for etiology—endocarditis, rheumatic fever, long patient long history murmur = Barlow's older patient, short history = FED.
- Review TTE and TEE in detail for leaflet dysfunction and lesions.
- Intraoperative inspection to confirm lesions.

> ### Predicting repair complexity
>
> - Valve analysis: clues from history, preoperative echo.
> *Lesions associated with more straightforward repair*
> - Type II *isolated* P2 from degenerative disease.
> - Type IIIb from ischemic disease.
> *Lesions associated with more complex repair*
> - Multisegment or bileaflet prolapse, in Barlow's disease.
> - Type IIIa lesion from rheumatic disease.
> - Lesions related to infective endocarditis, e.g., leaflet perforation.
> - Cleft mitral valve, primary SAM, previous failed mitral repair.

Set-up

Sternotomy or MICS (p466) MICS less appropriate for endocarditis. Aorto-bicaval CPB, cardioplegia antegradely ± retrograde. The LV is vented directly through the mitral valve. TEE. Harvest pericardium if type IIIa rheumatic or endocarditis with perforation, fix in 0.08% glutaraldehyde for 20min, then rinse in 3 × 2min washes in saline.

Atriotomy

Usually paraseptal left atriotomy in Sondergaard's groove (p404).

Assessment of the valve

This is the point at which a final decision can be made as to whether and what kind of repair is possible, or whether the valve must be replaced.

- Look for jet lesions on atrial wall to confirm direction regurgitant jet: anterior jet lesion = posterior leaflet prolapse or anterior restriction.
- Pressurize LV by injecting saline through the mitral valve using a bladder syringe with a flexible extension to see where the leaks are.
- Using two calibrated Carpentier hooks or nerve hooks of equal length examine each element of the valvular apparatus.
- First assess the annulus for dilatation (should be roughly same surface area as normal anterior leaflet).
- Next examine the chordae, distinguishing between normal primary chordae and abnormal stretched, ruptured, and fused chordae.
- Then, using the commissures as a fixed reference point, work systematically along each leaflet with the nerve hooks, assessing the location and degree of prolapse by gently lifting the edge of the leaflet with one hook and comparing the excursion with the fixed point of the nerve hook at the commissure.

Types of repair

These are outlined on 📖 p410. Common techniques illustrated in Fig. 8.14.

Testing the repair

This is done in several ways:
- Firstly by pressurizing LV with saline: there should be no residual leak.
- The line of leaflet coaptation should be symmetrical, parallel to and closest to the posterior annulus. It can be marked with ink, saline aspirated, and the area of coaptation beneath the ink checked—ideally >10mm for durability but <14mm to avoid SAM (📖 p190).
- Formal and definitive assessment can only be carried out by TEE once the heart is off bypass: up to 10% of patients will have more than mild MR and it is vital to go back on bypass to carry out further repair of valve replacement at this stage.

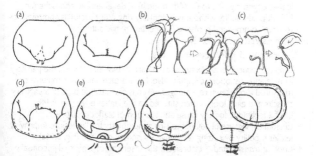

Fig. 8.14 Top row. Techniques for single-segment prolapse in small valve. (a) Triangular resection A2. (b) Gore-Tex loop. (c) Chordal transfer. Bottom row. Quadrangular resection of P2 prolapse and slidiing plasty. (d) Resection lines. (e) Vertical compression sutures. (f) Sliding plasty of P1 and P3. (g) Final appearance of repair with remodelling annuloplasty ring superimposed, symmetrical closure line closer and parallel to posterior annulus.

Principles of mitral valve repair

Key facts

- Severe MR reduces normal life expectancy: repair is the only treatment that can restore this to normal: indications are listed on 📖 p402.
- Replacement has worse mortality and morbidity than repair in degenerative MR, but the data for ischemic MR is less clear.
- Mitral valve repair provides excellent hemodynamic and long-term results, without the need for anticoagulation.
- Carpentier's three principles of repair: (1) restore or preserve normal leaflet motion, (2) improve coaptation, (3) remodel the annulus.
- Techniques can be categorized by which part of the valvular apparatus they correct (Table 8.4).

Leaflets

- *Quadrangular resection + sliding plasty:* this is used for posterior leaflet prolapse. A rectangular section of leaflet is excised from the area of maximal prolapse (Fig. 8.14). Several techniques allow the resected edges to be sutured together without tension: (1) sliding plasty, where the bases of the leaflet are divided from the annulus and reattached more centrally (Fig. 8.14g), (2) compression sutures (horizontal along most of the posterior annulus, and/or vertical just where the leaflet gap is (Fig. 8.14e).
- *Triangular resection:* this can be used for prolapse of the posterior or anterior leaflet (Fig. 8.14a). It is used where quadrangular resection would leave insufficient leaflet tissue for a competent repair. Historically anterior leaflet repairs have poorer durability than posterior.
- *Pericardial patch augmentation:* glutaraldehyde-fixed autologous pericardium (📖 p408) or bovine pericardium is used to extend posterior or anterior leaflet in rheumatic disease, and patch defects such as perforations in endocarditis or failed repairs.
- *Edge-to-edge:* Simple 4/0 proline suture used to approximate opposing leaflet edges, e.g., A2 to P2 (*Alfieri stitch*) in degenerative and ischemic MR. Poor durability without annuloplasty ring. Very useful at commissures to treat commissural prolapse (*Carpentier 'magic' suture*).
- *Commisurotomy:* (Fig. 8.13)

Chordae and papillary muscles

- *Loop technique:* Gore-Tex neochordae are fashioned between the papillary muscle and unsupported leaflet edge. Mohr's technique uses multiple pre-measured loops sewn to a pledget which is sewn to the base of a papillary muscle, and each loop is then sutured to the leaflet edge (Fig. 8.14b). Useful technique for any cause and location of leaflet prolapse.
- *Chordal cutting:* useful adjunct to ring annuloplasty for IIIb lesions improving leaflet mobility by cutting restrictive secondary chordae (Fig. 8.14c).
- *Chordal transfer and transposition:* the insertion of a normal secondary chord is excised, and re-attached to the flail segment leaflet (Fig. 8.14c). Transposition includes a segment of the leaflet.
- *Chordal shortening and reconstruction:* a variety of chordal shortening techniques have been described by Carpentier.
- *Papillary muscle reimplantation:* not ideal for ischemic papillary muscle rupture as the repair will not hold in necrotic muscle. The fibrous

tip of the ruptured head of papillary muscle is reattached to adjacent viable papillary muscle with mattress sutures.

Anulus

- *Reduction annuloplasty*: sutures or flexible band/ring used to reduce annular size to improve coaptation: thought to avoid SAM (📖 p191).
- *Remodeling annuloplasty*: usually complete, rigid or semirigid ring to reduce and remodel the annulus restoring systolic proportions (Fig. 8.15). Correct ring selection and sizing is critical to avoid MR and SAM, e.g.:
  - Type IIIb (ischemic)—use asymmetric down-sized rigid ischemic ring to address tethering predominantly in P2/P3 area, usually size 26–28.
  - Type II (degenerative)—use true-sized remodeling ring, pronounced saddle reduces risk of SAM post repair (📖 p191), usually size 34–40.

The ring is sized by extending the anterior leaflet with a valve hook, and comparing a valve sizer to the intercommissural distance, surface area, and height of the anterior leaflet. The ring is inserted with interrupted 2/0 or 3/0 non-absorbable braided sutures, using overlapping sutures on the posterior annulus if this is very dilated, and 1mm apart on the anterior annulus. The posterior annulus is reduced by making smaller bites in the valve-sewing ring than on the annulus, but the anterior annulus is not reduced to maintain the fixed intertrigonal distance.

Table 8.4 Common repair techniques by etiology and lesion

Etiology	Lesions	Repair techniques
Ischemic cardiomyopathy	Papillary muscle displacement, LV dilatation	Rigid down-sized ischemic ring (Fig. 8.15), ± chordal cutting
Degenerative disease	Annular dilatation	True-sized remodeling ring (Fig. 8.15)
(FED or Barlow's)	Chordal rupture or elongation	Chordal transfer, loops or Gore-Tex neo-chordae (Fig. 8.14b,c)
	Prolapse	Quadrangular resection ± sliding plasty (Fig. 8.14g) Triangular resection (Fig. 8.14a), Multiple loops, edge-to-edge
Rheumatic disease	Commissural fusion, leaflet calcification, chordal fusion	Pericardial patch augmentation, commisurotomy, chordal fenestration, ring

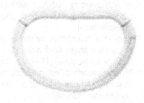

Fig. 8.15 Remodelling rings. (a) Carpentier–Edwards Physio. (b) IMR ETlogix Ring.

Mitral valve replacement

Indications for mitral valve replacement

- Repair is preferable to replacement in most cases of MR (🕮 p402).
- Class 1: acute severe symptomatic MR, chronic severe MR *and* NYHA class II–IV or mild-moderate LV dysfunction. Also NYHA class III–IV moderate to severe MS if balloon valvotomy not possible.
- Class IIa: asymptomatic chronic severe MR with normal LV *if* new AF, *or* PA systolic >50mmHg at rest (60mmHg exercise). Also severe MS *if* PAP >60mmHg.
- Class IIb: chronic severe MR due to severe LV dysfunction despite optical medical therapy + biventricular pacing.

Set-up, bypass, and exposure are as described for MV repair (🕮 p408).

Mitral valve replacement

The posterior leaflet and related subvalvular apparatus are preserved, where they will not interfere with prosthesis function. Chordal excision during MVR is associated with increases in postoperative LV end-systolic volume and wall stress, as well as a decrease in EF. Preserving the subvalvular apparatus optimizes ventricular function. Stenotic lesions are less amenable to this approach.

- To excise the valve begin with a 15 blade 2mm away from the annulus of the anterior leaflet at 12 o' clock where the leaflet tissue is usually most disease free (Fig. 8.16b).
- Continue the incision using either a McIndoe scissors or the 15 blade round to the commissural leaflet tissue at anterolateral and posteromedial commissures.
- Cut the very tips of the underlying papillary muscles. Cutting the chordae to the anterior leaflet risks scattering chordal fragments into the heart. The anterior leaflet can now be removed.
- In very elderly patients do not make overly aggressive efforts to remove subannular calcification: it may result in damage to the circumflex coronary artery, atrioventricular dehiscence or ventricular rupture and it is often possible to sew through the calcium and place a reasonable size prosthesis without undue difficulty.
- The valve is sized according to which sizer easily drops through the annulus into the ventricle taking care not to over-size or under-size the valve: a size 27 is almost always appropriate.
- The valve can be sewn using interrupted pledgetted everting or non-everting mattress sutures with a 2/0 braided non-absorbable suture, or using a semicontinuous technique with a 2/0 non-absorbable monofilament.
- Bites should incorporate the annulus, but deep bites may damage the circumflex artery (7–8 o'clock), coronary sinus (6–8 o'clock), NCC or LCC of aortic valve (11–1 o'clock), or AV node (2 o'clock) (Fig. 8.16a).
- Most surgeons orient bileaflet mechanical valves in the antianatomic position, and use everting mattress sutures to ensure that the valve leaflets move freely.

Chordal-sparing mitral valve replacement

To retain the anterior leaflet as well as the posterior leaflet, the anterior leaflet must be split centrally and folded laterally, or folded towards its base and incorporated in the suture line.

De-airing

This is described on 🕮 p114. Frustrate the valve by inserting a 16 gauge Foley catheter. Do not lift the heart once off bypass: there is a risk of atrioventricular dehiscence (bright red blood pooling in pericardial well once bypass discontinued: requires resumption of bypass, removal of the prosthesis, and challenging patch repair of the rupture. Associated mortality is high.

Pitfalls in mitral valve insertion

- Over-sizing the valve leading to atrioventricular dehiscence, or subsequent difficulty inserting appropriate size AVR.
- Damaging the circumflex artery at 6–8 o'clock (Fig. 8.16a).
- Damaging the coronary sinus at 4–6 o'clock (Fig. 8.16a).
- Distorting the NCC or LCC sinus at 10–12 o'clock (Fig. 8.16a).
- Damaging the AV node at 1–2 o'clock (Fig. 8.16a).
- Failure to keep tension on the valve sutures while parachuting down leading to loops entrapping valve mechanism.
- AV dehiscence on lifting the heart to de-air or massage after MVR.
- Posts of bioprosthetic valve may cause LVOT obstruction, or rupture through LV wall (use low profile valve in small LV/elderly).

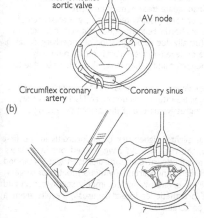

Fig. 8.16 (a) Structures at risk during MVR. (b) Excising the native valve.

Results of mitral surgery

Early mortality

- The mortality of isolated mitral ± tricuspid repair for degenerative disease in patients without pulmonary hypertension is ~1%.
- Higher operative mortality (2–5%) in patients with pulmonary hypertension, LV dysfunction, >80 years, ischemic MR, mitral replacement.

Late mortality

- Successful repair for degenerative MR restores life expectancy to that of an age-matched normal population.
- Ischemic MR is associated with much poorer survival: 1/3 of patients are dead within 5 years despite successful repair. LVEDD >65mm is associated with worse survival: <50% of patients alive at 5 years.
- Rheumatic patients are usually younger, and have good long term survival with ~80–90% still alive 10 years after surgery.

Morbidity

These include the complications of cardiac surgery in general, i.e., re-sternotomy for bleeding/tamponade (1–2%), perioperative MI (1%), stroke (1%), deep sternal wound infection(<1%), prolonged ventilation (2%), and organ dysfunction (1%) are discussed in more detail on 📖 pp253–290. Complications particularly associated with mitral valve surgery include:

Failure of repair

Patient leaving the OR with >1+MR = *residual MR*. Patient left OR with no MR but develops it later = *recurrent MR*.

- Residual MR is due to a technical issue, e.g., incorrect choice of ring, failure to close cleft, inadequate treatment of prolapse.
- Recurrent MR may occur early (usually technical, e.g., dehiscence of leaflet closure, failure of chordal reconstruction but very occasionally endocarditis) or late (usually due to progression of underlying disease).
- In the midterm, failure of degenerative repair is most commonly technical, failure of rheumatic and ischemic repair tends to be due to disease progression.
- The late failure rate for degenerative disease is ~1–2% per year, and much lower than the failure rate for rheumatic and ischemic repair, reflecting the more progressive nature of the latter two etiologies.

Prosthetic endocarditis

Mechanical valves are at slightly higher risk of endocarditis in the first 3 months after surgery, the relative risks have evened out by 5 years. The cumulative risk of prosthetic valve endocarditis is ~1% at 1 year and 3% at 5 years post-MVR. Early endocarditis (within 3 months of surgery) is usually hospital-acquired: organisms are commonly staphylococci and Gram −ve cocci. Late prosthetic endocarditis usually results from a transient streptococcal bacteraemia.

Thromboembolism

The rate of valve thromboembolism is higher than in aortic prostheses because flow velocity across the valve is slower. It is roughly 2% per year, with adequate anticoagulation of mechanical valves, and 1% per year with bioprosthetic valves. May present as stroke or systemic embolization. The management is iv heparin. *Valve thrombosis* is rare. Presents with acute onset of extreme dyspnea and orthopnea, but may be insidious. Fluoroscopy or echo to visualize if one or both leaflets not moving. Acute thrombosis can be treated with thrombolytic, but more usually this is chronic process with acute exacerbation that requires replacement (normally with a bioprosthesis to avoid repeat episode). The thrombus is usually very organized and may be superimposed on pannus. Surgical thrombectomy tempting but ineffective as unable to clear pannus and thrombus easily from ventricular aspect of prosthesis.

Paraprosthetic leak

Paraprosthetic leak is uncommon: immediate or early may be due to needle holes (tiny, and disappear after protamine), inadequate decalcification of annulus, tear, or poor suture positioning. Late new paraprosthetic leak more likely due to endocarditis. Narrow, high-velocity jets are high risk for hemolytic anemia which may be disabling (requiring multiple transfusions). Broader jets may be hemodynamically significant especially if MR was not present preoperatively. The decision whether to treat depends on balancing disadvantages of fixing paravalvular leak (e.g., reclamping diseased aorta, additional ischemic time in sick heart, severe mitral annular calcification making any improvement unlikely, high-risk resternotomy) against the disadvantages of leaving it. Prosthetic valve endocarditis is a strong indication for surgery in this context.

Prosthesis failure and reoperation

In the mitral position the lifetime risk of reoperation for bioprosthetic failure is ~45% for a 50-year-old, and this falls by just over 10% for every additional 5 years of age at the time of implantation. At 20 years after surgery ~10–15% of patients with mechanical valves will have required reop valve replacement for infective endocarditis, pannus, or valve thrombosis.

Atrial fibrillation

Around 10–20% of patients undergoing mitral surgery have a history of pre-op AF and the incidence of post-op AF is ~40%. AF is associated with thromboembolic complications including stroke, heart failure, and decreased survival so aggressive treatment of patients with a history of pre-op AF with intra-op ablation (📖 p484) is recommended. These patients are routinely anticoagulated for 3 months after surgery, may be at increased risk of thrombus formation in the early post-op period, and are often pacemaker dependent for several days after surgery.

Tricuspid valve surgery

Key facts

- Functional TR secondary to left-sided heart disease, usually MR, is the commonest cause of tricuspid valve disease.
- Isolated tricuspid valve disease is uncommon: endocarditis from IV drug abuse is one of the main causes.
- Tricuspid disease associated with congenital defects (AV septal defect, pulmonary atresia, Ebstein anomaly) is discussed on 📖 pp636–637.

Pathophysiology and morphology

Functional tricuspid regurgitation: this commonly occurs secondary to left-sided valve lesions causing pulmonary hypertension and RV dilatation. When RV dilatation develops the tricuspid annulus dilates as it is not supported by a fibrous skeleton. This is most pronounced in the posterior and anterior part of the annulus, as the septal annulus is relatively fixed. Leaflet coaptation is reduced leading to TR. Observational data suggests that in patients with >2+TR, annular dilatation, or PAH, functional TR may not resolve with correction of the left-sided lesion, and should be repaired to avoid late severe TR, which develops in a minority of patients and is associated with high morbidity and operative mortality.

Tricuspid valve endocarditis: acute tricuspid valve endocarditis is increasing in incidence. It is usually associated with sepsis from long-term ind-welling venous catheters or iv drug abuse. The causative organisms are *Pseudomonas aeruginosa* and *Staphylococcus aureus*.

Rheumatic tricuspid valve disease: most commonly this is TR predominantly due to annular dilatation secondary to severe MS. The tricuspid leaflets are often characterized by mild restriction and leaflet thickening.

Trauma: transvenous pacing wires can lead to leaflet perforation or more commonly scarring, causing TR. Traumatic TV rupture is a rare sequela of severe non-penetrating chest injury.

Carcinoid tricuspid valve disease: causes mixed tricuspid lesions (📖 p475).

Symptoms and signs

Tricuspid stenosis: the symptoms and natural history are determined by the dominant left-sided heart lesion. Tricuspid stenosis causes increased systemic venous pressure, resulting in hepatomegaly, ascites, and peripheral edema. A mid-diastolic murmur may be present.

Tricuspid regurgitation: the progression is slower than MR, and many patients are symptom-free for decades. The predominant clinical features are those of raised venous pressure. A pansystolic murmur may be present. Patients usually have moderate to severe RV failure by the time they present for surgery, as well as severe pulmonary hypertension, and moderate to severe liver dysfunction which is why isolated tricuspid valve surgery has such high mortality (~10–15%) with low cardiac output, respiratory failure, and sepsis the major problems postoperatively.

Indications for tricuspid valve surgery
- Class I: tricuspid repair for severe TR in patients having MV surgery.
- Class IIa: severe symptomatic primary TR.
- Class IIb: tricuspid repair for moderate TR *or* tricuspid annular dilatation in patients having mitral surgery.

Tricuspid valve surgery

Set-up and bypass: usually surgery is planned on the mitral valve at the same time: standard mitral set up is used. Venous drainage via bicaval cannulation is mandatory. Caval snares if no VAVD (💷 p103). If isolated TV then right thoracotomy, peripheral cannulation, beating heart, no clamp.

Right atriotomy: transverse right atriotomy, away from the AV groove, in the mid-atrium starting below the RA appendage, extending inferiorly (Fig. 8.17).

Tricuspid valve repair: the most common procedure is tricuspid annuloplasty, which may performed using a ring (rigid or flexible) or a running stitch around the annulus (DeVega) which is less durable. The tricuspid annulus tissue offers little support and sutures need to be placed and tied carefully to avoid tears, correcting TR by reducing the posterior and anterior annulus which are most prone to dilatation. The AV node is avoided by not placing sutures within the area of the triangle of Koch (Fig. 8.17). The repair can be tested by pressurizing the RV with saline instilled through the tricuspid valve while compressing the PA.

Tricuspid valve replacement: this is performed for failed repair, in endocarditis (where some surgeons advocate compete valvectomy) and carcinoid. A mechanical or bioprosthetic replacement can be used. The valve and subvalvular apparatus is excised, and the valve inserted using horizontal everting mattress sutures, with pledgets on the atrial side. It is important to avoid placing sutures at the apex of the triangle of Koch (Fig. 8.17) and sutures can be placed in the leaflet hinge instead in this area.

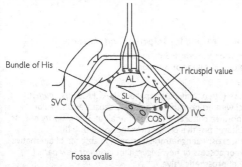

Fig. 8.17 Right atriotomy showing surgeon's view of tricuspid valve (AL, anterior; SL, septal; PL, posterior leaflet). Triangle of Koch bounded by coronary sinus (CoS), septal annulus, and tendon of Todaro inferiorly. Apex identifies conduction tissue. Dotted line represents suture placement for DeVega and partial ring annuloplasty.

Surgery for infective endocarditis

Key facts

- The pathophysiology of infective endocarditis is described in more detail on ◻ p80. This section deals with the surgical management.
- The Duke diagnostic criteria (Box 8.5) are 95% specific, with a 92% negative predictive value.
- Surgery indicated for structural valve lesions with evidence hemodynamic compromise or abscess formation.
- Optimal time to operate after embolic stroke is 7–14 days if possible.

Timing of surgery

Choosing the right time to operate can be difficult: the surgeon must define 'appropriate antibiotics', and balance need to optimize major comorbidity often including acute embolic stroke, with the fact that these patients are liable to deteriorate irreversibly. In most cases early surgical intervention is preferable to late: in case of preoperative embolic stroke delay 5–10 days if possible, if hemorrhagic stroke ideally longer.

Indications for surgery

- Class I: acute endocarditis + stenosis or regurgitation and CHF. Also acute endocarditis and AI or MR *and* PAH, ↑LAP, or ↑ LVEDP. Also fungal endocarditis. Also endocarditis complicated by heart block *or* annular *or* aortic abscess *or* fistulae between RA/RV/ LA and sinus of Valsalva *or* mitral leaflet perforation in aortic valve endocarditis. Also prosthetic valve endocarditis *and* dehiscence *or* worsening valve function *or* heart failure *or* abscess.
- Class IIa: native valve endocarditis *and* recurrent emboli and persistent vegetation *despite* appropriate antibiotics. Prosthetic valve endocarditis and bacteremia *despite* appropriate antibiotics.
- Class IIb: native valve endocarditis and mobile vegetation >10mm.

Box 8.5 Duke criteria for infective endocarditis

Definite: 2 major *or* 1 major + 3 minor *or* 5 minor.
Possible: 1 major + 1 minor *or* 3 minor.

Major criteria

- Blood culture (*Strep. viridans, Strep. bovis,* HACEK, *Staph. aureus,* enterococci with no primary focus from 2 separate cultures *or* persistent positive cultures >12h apart *or* all of 3 or majority of four separate cultures positive drawn over the space of >1h).
- Echo evidence: oscillating intracardiac mass in absence of alternative explanation *or* abscess *or* new regurgitant lesion *or* new partial dehiscence of prosthetic valve.

Minor criteria

- Predisposition/fever >38°C/emboli/blood culture or echo signs.

Technique of operation

The goals of surgery are:
- Remove infected tissue and drain abscesses.
- Reverse the hemodynamic abnormalities.
- Restore the cardiac and vascular architecture.

TEE is critical in planning surgery which may involve drainage of abscesses, debridement of necrotic tissue, closure of acquired defects such as VSD, annular abscess, fistulas, and aneurysms, in addition to valve repair and replacement.

Set-up

Median sternotomy (MICS rarely indicated because of possibility of more extensive involvement than identified pre-op), bicaval cannulation to permit access to the mitral and tricuspid valve if involved. Standard cardioplegia and venting techniques. If there are large mobile vegetations avoid handling the heart as much as possible, including placing retrograde, until the cross-clamp is on to reduce risk of emboli. Harvest pericardium for patch repair of mitral leaflet perforations (🕮 p408).

Approach

Surgery for aortic endocarditis should involve examining the anterior leaflet of the mitral valve for lesions, and if necessary, a left atriotomy. Similarly surgery for mitral endocarditis should involve inspection of the aortic valve via an aortotomy if there is any suspicion of involvement.
- Send all excised tissue and debris to microbiology.
- There is no good evidence that homograft valve replacement reduces the risk of recurrent infective endocarditis.
- Aortic valve abscesses are commonest posterior to the membranous part of the interventricular septum, and under the left coronary ostia. Mitral valve abscesses are commonest in the P2 portion of the annulus.
- For small abscesses evacuation and debridement is relatively straightforward, but in extensive root abscesses involving the AV and ventriculo-arterial junctions debridement may cause dehiscence.
- Root replacement and patch repairs of AV discontinuity are indicated.
- Abscesses around the mitral valve should also be debrided with the same regard for AV discontinuity.
- In prosthetic valve endocarditis take extra care to debride all prosthetic material: pledgets may be difficult to see (particularly if on the ventricular side of the mitral annulus) but should be removed using rongeurs, along with any calcium not debrided first time round.
- Small vegetations can be debrided and perforations in the mitral valve may be repaired with autologous pericardium.
- Some surgeons swab the local area with solutions such as povidone-iodine, and change gloves and instruments once the valve is debrided. There is no evidence that this does any harm.
- Closure, de-airing, weaning from bypass, and assessing the valve function are carried out in the standard manner.

Combined valvular procedures

Key facts

- Multivalvar disease is usually rheumatic in origin. Infective endocarditis and connective tissue disease can also cause multivalvar disease.
- There are several possible sequences: should be tailored to individual patient, e.g., need to minimize ischemic time, complex mitral repair requiring saline testing versus replacement, small aortic root, CABG.

Pathophysiology

The pathophysiology is dictated by the dominant lesion, which varies:

- **Aortic and mitral regurgitation:** this imposes a large volume overload on the LV which undergoes marked hypertrophy and eventual dilatation.
- **Aortic and mitral stenosis:** this results in a small, hypertrophied, non-compliant LV, usually with well preserved LV EF.
- **Mitral stenosis and aortic regurgitation:** the MS is usually dominant. MS restricts LV filling, blunting the effect of AR on LV volume. Even in severe AR hyperdynamic circulation and dilated LV are absent.
- **Aortic stenosis and mitral regurgitation:** the AS worsens the degree of MR. The MR causes difficulty in assessing the severity of the AS because of reduced forward flow. Patients can decompensate rapidly.
- **Mitral stenosis or regurgitation and tricuspid regurgitation:** pulmonary hypertension is usually present (see 🔖 p416 for more discussion).

Indications for surgery in moderate valve disease

Although the non-dominant lesion may be mild at the time of operation, these lesions are progressive. Rheumatic AS that was mild at the time of operation on concomitant rheumatic mitral lesion progresses to moderate to severe in 1/3 of patients within 5 years. The progression of AI is much slower and better tolerated, although distorting the aortic annulus by mitral annulolplasty ring or replacement may cause 2+AI to become severe. Regurgitant combined lesions tend to progress faster, and the prognosis in combined stenotic lesions is worse than in isolated stenotic lesions. The temptation to operate on multiple valves to avoid later surgery needs to be balanced against increased perioperative mortality and long-term morbidity of valve replacement. May need to inspect the valve in question at the time of surgery to make final decision.

Sequence of operation

Median sternotomy. If CABG is planned the LIMA and LSV are harvested before heparinization. Bicaval cannulation. The advantage of using retrograde cardioplegia is that it can be given without having to interrupt valve implantation. The patient is cooled to 32°C. There are several options for operative sequence after cross-clamping and arresting the heart:

- Sequence A: Allows saline testing of mitral repair, tricuspid and mitral exposure better before AVR in place:
  - Distal CABG anastomoses including LAD (bulldog on IMA).
  - TV repair.
  - Mitral +/– tricuspid repair then AVR.
  - Proximal anastomoses, de-air left heart, clamp off, close RA.

- Sequence B: Shortens clamp time, allows saline testing of mitral repair:
  - Distal CABG anastomoses including LAD (bulldog on IMA).
  - Mitral repair then AVR.
  - If single clamp technique perform proximals while giving hot-shot.
  - De-air left heart, clamp off.
  - Right atriotomy, TV repair beating heart, close right atriotomy.
  - Perform proximals with sidebiting clamp.
- Sequence C: No saline testing planned (mitral replacement not repair):
  - Distal CABG anastomoses, including LAD (bulldog on IMA).
  - Open aorta, excise and size aortic valve.
  - Mitral replacement.
  - Tricuspid repair.
  - Place aortic sutures and implant valve, close aortotomy, proximals.
  - Close LA, de-air left heart, clamp off, close RA.

Tips and pitfalls in combined valve surgery

- If AVR and CABG is planned, ensure aortic cannulation is as distal as possible so there is room for clamp, vent, proximals, and aortotomy: in a reop, axillary cannulation helps with this aspect (🕮 p120).
- Exposure of the mitral and tricuspid is made more difficult by an aortic prosthesis, whereas a mitral prosthesis makes it more difficult to get a large prosthesis in the aortic position.
- Cannot saline test mitral from LA if aortotomy open.
- The tricuspid valve can be operated on with the clamp off and the heart beating, which reduces ischemic time (and allows sutures affecting the conduction tissue to be removed), but increases the risk of annular tears because of friable tissue and worse exposure.
- CABG distals should be performed first and checked for bleeding:
  - This reduces the need to pick the heart up once a mitral prosthesis is *in situ*, which can cause AV dehiscence.
  - Also allows cardioplegia to be given down the grafts.
- CABG proximals can be performed with the cross-clamp on (single-clamp technique) which minimizes stroke risk from multiple clamping, and avoids need to instrument the aortotomy closure, but adds to ischemic time.
- In multivalve reop surgery tissues are less compliant and it may be very difficult to get an adequate size aortic prosthesis, and occasionally mitral prosthesis in place:
  - Ensure both valve annulus completely debrided of calcium, pannus, pledgets and any remainder of the valve sewing ring.
  - Avoid placing the largest possible prosthesis in the mitral position as this will decrease the room available for an aortic prosthesis.
  - Consider the techniques for the small aortic root (🕮 p392).
  - Occasionally aortic root enlargement with a patch extending down onto the dome of the LA roof and across the mitral annulus is required to allow implantation of appropriately-sized aortic and mitral prosthesis.

The thoracic aorta

Surgical options

A variety of operative approaches can be used in thoracic aortic disease.
See Table 9.1.

Table 9.1 Surgical options

Technique	Indication	Summary
Fenestration	Persistent organ ischemia after surgical correction of the proximal tear.	Creating holes in the dissection flap so that blood can perfuse organs being supplied by both true and false lumens. Can be done open or via percutaneous approach.
AVR and interposition graft	Abnormal aortic valve and aneurysmal or dissected ascending aorta.	AVR carried out as described on 🕮 pp378–382. Then interposition graft placed (see 🕮 p444)
Wolfe procedure	Aneurysm or dissection involving non-coronary sinus, but not the left or right	Similar to interposition graft, but with proximal scallop to recreate non-coronary sinus
Bentall technique	Abnormal aortic valve and ascending aneurysm/ dissection/endocarditis involving annulus and/or sinuses	See 🕮 p390. In the original 1968 description the coronary ostia were sutured directly to holes created in the tube graft without making buttons, and the conduit was not composite
Modified Bentall	As above	Same as the Bentall but with composite valved graft, and with the coronaries excised with a cuff to create 'buttons' and mobilized proximally (🕮 p390)
Cabrol graft	Used where coronary buttons cannot be mobilised adequately e.g., calcification, previous root replacement	Valved conduit implanted in same way as Bentall, but 8mm Dacron graft anastomosed end to end to left coronary buton, then either to aorta (hemi-Cabrol) or end to side to right coronaru buttom (full Cabrol) and then to aorta (🕮 p445)
Elephant trunk	Arch aneurysm/ dissection where descending aorta also needs replacement. 🕮 p448	Two-stage procedure where distal end of Dacron graft is left inside descending aorta after arch replacement, for later replacement of descending aorta. (🕮 pp448–451)
Homograft	Similar indications to Bentall, valuable where tissue very friable e.g., endocarditis	Described on 🕮 p386

Table 9.1 (Cont'd)

Technique	Indication	Summary
Trifurcation graft	Alternative to "island technique" (Fig. 9.7b), for arch replacement (📖 pp448–449)	
Glue aortoplasty	Obliterate false lumen in dissection, most commonly to treat extension into aortic sinuses in conjunction with interposition grafts.	Biological glues used

Endoluminal stenting is described on 📖 p431.

Pathology of aortic dissection

Definition

Blood leaves the aortic lumen via an intimal tear, separating the inner from the outer layers of the media creating a false lumen.

Classifications of aortic dissection

- Acute dissections are those presenting within 14 days.
- Chronic dissections present after 2 months.
- Subacute dissections present between 14 days and 2 months.

Stanford (Fig. 9.1)

Type A: any case in which the ascending aorta is involved.
Type B: any case not involving the ascending aorta.

DeBakey (Fig. 9.1)

Type I: tear in the ascending aorta, dissection extending to arch.
Type II: tear in ascending aorta, dissection limited to ascending aorta.
Type IIIa: tear in descending aorta, dissection limited to descending.
Type IIIb: tear in descending aorta, dissection may extend to arch and ascending aorta.

Emergency surgery is indicated for acute Stanford type A and DeBakey type I and II dissections.

Risk factors

The pathogenesis of aortic dissection is not well understood. There are several theories that might explain the etiology of the intimal tear that results in dissection. An early theory was cystic medial degeneration where the media is abnormal, but as this abnormality has been found in only a minority of patients with acute aortic dissection, this theory has lost ground. Later theories identified atherosclerotic ulceration penetrating to the media as the source of the intimal tear, but again these are uncommon at the site of the intimal tear. Finally, intramural hematoma resulting from bleeding of the vasa vasorum into the media is thought to account for sufficient stress to cause an intimal tear. Risk factors include:

- Age (up to 90% of patients are >60 years of age).
- Hypertension (chronic primary hypertension, and Sheehan and Cushing syndromes, pheochromocytoma, polycystic kidney disease).
- High cardiac output states, e.g. pregnancy.
- Connective tissue disorders (Ehlers–Danlos syndrome, Marfan syndrome, Turner syndrome, 📖 p429).
- Atherosclerosis is a risk factor only in pre-existing aneurysms.
- Bicuspid aortic valve, cystic medial degeneration, aortitis.
- Iatrogenic (catheterization, cannulation, aortic cross-clamping, AVR, proximal aorto-coronary anastomosis, IABP).
- Competitive weightlifting.
- Trauma.

Clinical features

Dissection usually results in sudden, severe, 'tearing' pain radiating from chest through to the back, and sometimes neck and arms. About 30–40% die immediately. A minority of patients present with asymptomatic, usually chronic, dissections picked as incidental findings on CT. Complications of aortic dissection include:

- Arch vessel occlusion causes stroke in 5% of type A dissections.
- Myocardial ischemia occurs in up to 20% of type A dissections.
- Hemopericardium occurs in about a 1/4 of type A dissections.
- Severe AI occurs in about 1/3 of type A dissections.
- Occlusion of vessels may lead to upper and lower limb, mesenteric, and renal ischemia: peripheral vascular examination is abnormal in 20%.
- Paraplegia develops in 2–5% of type B dissections as a result of spinal artery occlusion.
- Rarely acute aortic dissection may cause SVC syndrome, hemoptysis, airway compression, and Horner's syndrome.

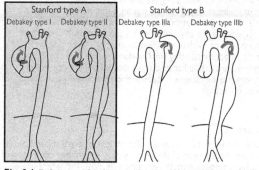

Fig. 9.1 DeBakey and Stanford classifications of aortic dissection.

Pathology of aortic aneurysms

Key facts

An aneurysm is defined as a permanent localized dilatation of an artery by at least 50% compared to normal. The dimensions of the normal aorta are (uncorrected for body mass index):

- Annulus: 2.8–3.2 cm (2.1cm/m² adjusted for BSA).
- Sinus of Valsalva: 3.4 ± 0.3 in men, 3.0 ± 0.3 in women.
- Sinotubular junction: 2.4–3.0cm (1.9cm/m², or roughly 0.9x annulus).
- Mid ascending aorta: 2.6–3.4cm.
- Mid arch 2.4–3.1 cm.
- Mid descending aorta 2.8cm in men, 2.6cm in women.
- At the celiac axis 2.3cm in men, 2.0cm in women.
- Infrarenal aorta 1.9cm in men, 1.5cm in women.

Classifications of aortic aneurysm

- A *true aneurysm* involves all layers of the arterial wall.
- A *false or pseudoaneurysm* usually has an outer wall consisting of adventia, organized thrombus, and surrounding structures.
- A *mycotic aneurysm* is any aneurysm caused as a result of infection.
- Aneurysms can be further classified by location: ascending, arch, descending, abdominal using the *Crawford classification* (Fig. 9.2).
- Aneurysms are classified according to shape (*fusiform or saccular*).
- Aneurysms may be classified according to complicating pathology: (*ruptured, dissecting*).

Risk factors

Aortic aneurysm formation is usually due to loss of elasticity and tensile strength in the medial layer of the aorta, which is normally composed of elastin, collagen, smooth muscle cells which degrade and synthesize elastin, and ground matrix. Elastin content is highest in the ascending aorta and the media becomes thinner distally. In typical aortic aneurysms there is fragmentation of elastin fibres within the media and loss of smooth muscle cells. This is called *cystic medial degeneration*. The ascending aorta expands and recoils with systole and diastole respectively, maximizing forward flow. When elasticity is lost, the aorta begins to dilate. The aorta dilates normally with age. Risk factors for aneurysm formation include:

- Age (up to 90% of patients are >60 years of age).
- Hypertension, atherosclerosis, smoking.
- Connective tissue disorders (Ehlers–Danlos syndrome, Marfan syndrome, Turner syndrome, Loeys–Dietz syndrome ⬚ p429).
- Cystic medial degeneration.
- Aortitis (Takayasu's arteritis most commonly involves the arch).
- Aortic stenosis, bicuspid aortic valve: two mechanisms—(1) post-stenotic dilatation, (2) increased medial degeneration in bicuspid AV so expansion is faster and risk of aortic aneurysm and dissection 10x that

of normal population (1:1000 vs. 1:10 000). Aortic aneurysm is still rare in patients with bicuspid valve, but they represent a high proportion of aneurysm patients.

- Syphilis (characteristically ascending aneurysms).
- Bacterial infection (most commonly *Staphylococcus aureus, Staphylococcus epidermidis, Salmonella, Streptococcus*).
- Trauma is a rare cause of true aneurysms, but iatrogenic trauma (surgery or intervention) is a common cause of pseudoaneurysms.

Connective tissue disorders

- *Marfan syndrome* is an autosomal dominant connective tissue disorder with an incidence of 1:10 000 which causes a fault in the fibrillin gene of chromosome 15: abnormal *elastin* fibres are prone to disruption and cystic medial degeneration occurs at an early age; commonest cause of death is aortic dissection.
- *Ehlers–Danlos syndrome* is an inherited disorder of connective tissue with several subtypes of which type IV is associated with cardiovascular malformations due to defect in *collagen* formation: rupture of mesenteric vessels more commonly than thoracic aneurysm formation.
- Familial aneurysms that are not due to Marfan or Ehlers–Danlos syndromes are aneurysms occurring in families with a strong history of aortic aneurysm and dissection, and may be linked to the 5q locus.

Clinical features

- About 1/3 of patients are asymptomatic: the aneurysm is an incidental finding on CXR, or TTE or cardiac catheterization.
- About half of patients present with anterior chest pain.
- Acute onset pain suggests dissection or impending rupture.
- Hoarseness from arch aneurysms stretching recurrent laryngeal nerve.
- Examination is frequently unremarkable but 10–20% of patients have associated abdominal aneurysms.

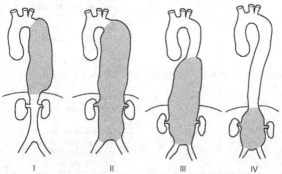

Fig. 9.2 Crawford classification of thoracoabdominal aortic aneurysms.

Diagnosis of type A dissection

Imaging

- The primary role of the diagnostic modalities is to differentiate between a type A dissection (an indication for emergency surgery) and a type B dissection. A secondary role is assessing the extent of dissection which dictates surgical approach.
- As a broad rule, centers planning to refer suspected acute type A dissections should use the imaging modality in which they have most expertise that can be done with minimum delay: an expertly performed TEE is more sensitive and specific, for example, than an inexpertly performed and interpreted CT angiogram (CTA); neither should delay referral.

Table 9.2 Imaging modalities used in diagnosis of type A dissection

Imaging modality	Sensitivity	Specificity	Comments
TEE + Doppler	96–100%	86–100%	Widely available, familiar. Dynamic images generated. Shows coronary ostia, LV function, AI, pericardium, pleura
CT angiography	90–100%	90–100%	Quick, readily available, familiar Shows pleural + pericardial space Shows head and neck vessels IV contrast may cause renal failure
MRI	98–100%	98–100%	Gold standard Detailed dynamic images of aorta, pericardium, pleura, LV, AV, flow in branch vessels and false lumen Not easily available or accessible Contraindications (🔲 p440)
Aortography	80–90%	88–95%	Until recently gold standard Facilities and expertise not as widely available Arterial access often difficult Can precipitate rupture Shows perfusion of true and false lumens, flap, coronary arteries, AI

Investigations

- In the hemodynamically unstable patient where there is a high index of suspicion (e.g., in the patient with crushing chest pain already known to have an aneurysm) it is reasonable to transfer directly to the operating room, anaesthetize and perform a TEE. If the TEE is positive, lines are placed so that it is possible to proceed directly to surgery: if the TEE is negative, invasive monitoring will allow the patient to undergo additional investigation.
- In more stable patients a CTA can be obtained quickly, with a plan to transfer the patient directly to the operating room, without delaying to insert monitoring lines or treat pressure if the CTA is positive.
- Blood tests are usually normal: raised creatinine and LFTs sometimes indicate chronic hypoperfusion states, and raised troponin suggests involvement of coronary ostia.
- EKG should be inspected for signs of ischemia, but in 30% of patients in whom the coronary ostia are involved EKG changes are non-specific.
- CXR may show a widened mediastinum, cardiomegaly secondary to pericardial effusion, and signs of pleural effusion (usually left).
- Coronary angiography is difficult and hazardous, and the same information can be obtained by CTA: most patients with type A dissections go to surgery without cardiac catheterization.

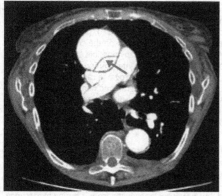

Fig. 9.3 CT scan of a type A dissection. A Type B dissection is shown on 📖 p17 (Fig. 1.4 and b).

Management of type A dissection

Natural history

- 30% of patients die immediately, 50% die within 48h, medical management has a 60% in-hospital mortality. Operative mortality is 20–30%. 1-year survival is about 66%, 5-year survival is 45–55%.
- Mode of death in acute presentation may be *rupture, cardiac tamponade, AMI, stroke, cardiogenic shock from acute severe AI*.

Indications for surgery

- The aim of surgery is to treat/prevent the causes of death.
- An acute type A dissection is an indication for emergency surgery.
- A subacute type A dissection is an indication for urgent surgery.

Contraindications to surgery

- Advanced age (> 05 years) or frailty are relative contraindications
- Incurable malignancy or other terminal illness.
- Chronic dementia or irreversible, profound brain injury.
- AMI, coma, stroke, paraplegia, renal failure, acute limb and visceral ischemia increase risks of surgery, but may improve following repair of the dissection, so are not contraindications to surgery.

Planning surgery for type A dissection

The main variables to think about are: (1) the *extent of resection* (root or arch replacement required?), (2) *cannulation* strategy, (3) need for *circulatory arrest*, (4) can the aorta be clamped (dictates *sequence* of distal vs. proximal anastomosis as well as need for DHCA), (5) *myocardial protection* strategy, (6) *venting*. The impact of each on the conduct of surgery is outlined on 📖 pp433–435. There are many possible scenarios:

- The arch and root are normal: a simple interposition graft using aortocaval cannulation, direct ostial ± retrograde cardioplegia, no DHCA.
- Distal aorta aneurysmal: interposition graft and hemiarch replacement with DHCA using axillary cannulation, ostial ± retrograde cardioplegia.
- Root aneurysmal: root replacement with or without DHCA.
- Arch involved: DHCA ± selective or retrograde cerebral perfusion.

Monitoring lines

At least two arterial lines are helpful as dissection or cannulation of arch and distal vessels may lead to misleading arterial pressure measurements.

- A right radial line is useful in right axillary cannulation to detect hyper- (or hypo-) perfusion of the right arm if a side-graft cannulation technique is used, but pressures transduced from it during bypass may bear little correlation with systemic pressures, especially in direct right axillary artery cannulation (📖 p120).
- Left axillary or femoral lines give more accurate central arterial pressure than a radial line which is usually damped by end of case.

Prepping and draping

- Drape for a full sternotomy, but include the lower neck in the field in case the incision has to be extended for arch involvement, and the whole infraclavicular area to allow axillary cannulation.

- Shave and prep both groins for possible cannulation.
- Prep and expose thighs in case saphenous vein is required.

Incision

- Type A dissections are repaired via a median sternotomy: may need to extend up into neck, so always prep and expose this area as well.

Cannulation

Very large aneurysms may make access to RA difficult, and may preclude safe aortic cannulation. The main options are:

- Central cannulation with venous return via a two-stage cannula in the RA and arterial return to the distal ascending aorta or arch (fastest option in an emergency, can use TEE to identify true lumen).
- Fem–caval cannulation, with the femoral arterial cannula placed either before or after opening the chest (if dissection extends to the femoral vessels it is important to cannulate the lumen in which blood is flowing, irrespective of whether it is the true or false lumen). Next fastest.
- Fem–fem cannulation: may be favoured if rupture suspected, as patient can be cooled in readiness for DHCA without opening pericardium, which may precipitate acute rupture.
- Axillo-caval cannulation: axillary cannulation usually before sternotomy, slowest of all options in an emergency, but less risk of stroke or cannulating false lumen, and facilitates selective cerebral perfusion (📖 p125).
- Use bicaval cannulation if retrograde cerebral perfusion is planned.

Myocardial protection

- Depending on the nature of the ascending aorta it may be preferable not to clamp it: bypass is commenced and the patient cooled, the heart fibrillates around 32°C, and retrograde cardioplegia is given at regular intervals to supplement cardioprotection from profound systemic hypothermia. If there is AI the LV must be vented to prevent distention.
- Antegrade can be given directly via coronary ostia after aortotomy.

Venting

- The LV via the right superior pulmonary vein (usually much less difficult to access once bypass commenced) or LV apex.
- Pump sucker placed in the LV via the aortic valve.

Cerebral protection

- Cool to 18°C (usually safe to assume DHCA will be needed).
- DHCA mandatory (📖 p125) if the arch is involved, or if the distal repair may only be performed with the cross-clamp off.
- Cerebral perfusion during DHCA may be none, retrograde, or from selective perfusion (📖 p125).

Overview of initial set-up

- Ensure the patient is monitored with two or more arterial lines.
- Prep and drape the patient, cannulate right axillary or femoral artery.
- Open the chest, give full-dose heparin, and then place purse-strings.
- Cannulate RA, go on bypass, start cooling, separate aorta from the PA.
- Either cross-clamp the distal ascending aorta or open the ascending aorta once the required systemic temperature is reached.
- Give cardioplegia directly into the coronary ostia or retrograde.

Repair of type A dissection

Key facts

- In the acute setting it is usually safest to focus on treating the immediately life-threatening complication of ascending aortic rupture: aortic arch resection is limited to the proximal arch, and valve involvement addressed by resuspension of the commissures rather than attempting root replacement. If the dissection extends into the coronary sinuses bioglue and a careful proximal suture line on the interposition graft should prevent progression, as the coronary ostia are usually spared.
- If it is safe to clamp the ascending aorta (avoid in large aneurysms where rupture is a risk); the proximal anastomosis can be completed while the patient is cooled.
- The distal anastomoses can be performed with the cross-clamp on (no need for circulatory arrest) or off (deep hypothermic circulatory arrest (DHCA) required), depending on how far distally the dissection extends, and whether the aorta can be safely clamped.
- Cannulation options are discussed on 🕮 p433: aorto-caval is fastest in emergencies but may be contraindicated: femoral-caval is next fastest, followed by axillary cannulation which takes more time, but minimizes risk of cannulating false lumen and stroke, and permits selective cerebral perfusion during arch replacement without moving cannula.

Interposition graft

This technique is preferred for DeBakey type II dissections, not involving the aortic root. It supersedes the older graft inclusion technique, where aortic tissue was preserved and wrapped around the interposition graft.

- Set-up is described on 🕮 pp432–433.
- Bypass is established via aorto-caval cannulation.
- The perfusionist begins to cool the patient to 28°C.
- The aortic clamp is placed just proximal to the innominate artery.
- Give cardioplegia anterogradely via a Medicut cannula into the root, or retrogradely via a coronary sinus cannula, to arrest the heart.
- Open the aorta transversely and use a pump sucker to vent the heart.
- Inspect the aortic lumen and the aortic valve: if the dissection extends past the sinotubular junction this will need reconstruction, if intimal tear extends distal to the cross-clamp circulatory arrest is required to inspect and repair the distal ascending aorta, in which case continue cooling to 18°C.
- Give cardioplegia directly into the coronary ostia and/or retrograde.
- Transect the aorta 5–10mm distal to the sinotubular junction (Fig. 9.4).
- If the dissection extends to the sinotubular junction reconstruct the aorta using bioglue to reapproximate the intima and media, and secure the whole thing with 4/0 Prolene running stitches anchoring a strip of PTFE felt all the way around the proximal aorta.
- Size the proximal aorta: size 26–28 usually appropriate.
- Suture the proximal aorta and felt to a Dacron graft with double-ended 4/0 Prolene RB needle running suture, starting forehand inside

to out, aorta to graft, a few bites further away from 6 o'clock (Fig. 9.4), running towards you until you need to take bites in two, then taking other arm and run it up the wall furthest away from you in two bites, then across the top towards you forehand in single bites. It's usually worth tightening the whole anastomosis with nerve hooks before tying.

- Transect the distal aorta and bevel the Dacron tube to match size.
- If the distal anastomosis is to be carried out without the cross-clamp, stop bypass when the temperature is 18°C, clamp lines, stop vents, and remove the cross-clamp: this anastomosis should take <20min.
- Suture the distal cuff of ascending aorta to the distal graft, with felt strip, in the same way as the proximal aorta (starting forehand inside to out, graft to felt to aorta, a few bites further away from 6 o'clock (Fig. 9.4), running towards you until you need to take bites in two, then take other arm of suture and run it up the wall furthest away from you in two bites, then forehand across the top. If size mismatch cheat on the top, never the bottom where leaks are awkward to fix.
- As the distal anastomosis is completed the graft is allowed to fill retrograde, remove the arterial line clamp and ask the perfusionist to come on at 500mL of flow, shake the graft so it de-airs fully and suction debris, come up further on flows and tie, then come fully up, unclamp venous line and vents, and resume bypass.
- Place a vent in the graft, and carry out standard de-airing (📖 p114).

Hemostasis

- Look for any 'spurters' and fix with 4/0 pledgetted Prolene with the flows down. For everything else pack and reassess **after** protamine has been given *and* any coagulopathy (usually platelet dysfunction) **completely** corrected: using Prolene to treat non-surgical bleeding begets more bleeding and coagulopathy. **Cabrol patch** is described on 📖 p445.

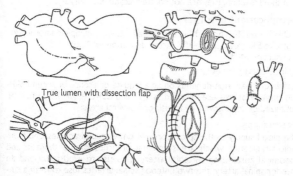

Fig. 9.4 Technique of performing an interposition graft for a type A dissection. Although a longitudinal aortotomy is shown, a transverse aortotomy is more commonly performed.

Management of type B dissection

Natural history

- Type B dissections have an initial hospital mortality of about 10%. About 2/3 of remaining patients have no complications requiring operation. 50% of unoperated patients, however, die within 3–5 years, of rupture or complications related to end-organ ischemia.
- Operative mortality is 5–15%, with a 5–30% risk of paraplegia depending on the presentation. After operation 1-year survival is about 65%, 5-year survival is 50%, 10-year survival 30%.

Indications for surgery

Medical treatment is primarily aimed at maintaining low arterial BP and reducing force of ventricular ejection. Labetolol (250mg in 250mL 5% dextrose at a rate of 2–8mg/min) is the best agent for this in hospital. Complications requiring emergency surgery include.

- Aortic rupture, periaortic or mediastinal hematoma, hemothorax.
- Dissection in pre-existing aneurysm.
- Rapid increase in aortic diameter.
- Ischemia of limbs and viscera.
- Intractable pain despite optimal medical management, progression.
- Marfan syndrome.

Contraindications to surgery

- Advanced age (>80 years) or frailty are relative contraindications.
- Incurable malignancy or other terminal illness.
- Chronic dementia.
- Severe pulmonary disease favours stenting over surgery.
- Irreversible, profound brain injury.
- New stroke, paraplegia, renal failure, acute limb and visceral ischemia increase the risks of surgery, but as they may improve following repair of the dissection, they are not contraindications to surgery.

Complications of surgery

- Death 10–15% (up to 50% in elderly patients with multiple comorbidity).
- Stroke 5%, paraplegia 5–10% (acute dissection ~30%, chronic dissection ~10%).

Spinal cord protection

Spinal cord perfusion depends on an adequate difference between MAPs and intracranial pressure (dictated by CVP and CSF pressure). This may be optimized perioperatively by focusing on several areas:

Arterial supply

The blood supply to the spinal cord is from vertebral arteries, and from radicular arteries which are segmental branches of the thoracic and abdominal aorta. Each vertebral artery gives rise to a posterior and an anterior spinal artery: the two anterior spinal arteries fuse to form a single midline vessel which travels along the median fissure of the spinal cord. Below the neck all three spinal arteries unite to form a continuous series of anastomoses with posterior intercostal (radicular) arteries. In its lower segments the spinal cord depends more on radicular arteries. Some surgeons believe a consistent and large radicular artery (artery of Adamkiewicz) present at T12–L2 provides the arterial supply for the lower 2/3 of the cord, but it has not been demonstrated consistently.

Surgical technique

There are several approaches. *Preventing hypotension* is key to all.

- *Reimplant large radicular arteries* below particularly below T10 (disadvantages include longer ischemic time and risk of bleeding).
- *Monitor somatosensory evoked potentials (SSEPs) and motor evoked potentials (MEPs)* which give a better indication of anterior cord function, clamping intercostals vessels sequentially but only dividing them if no change in SSEP is seen after 10min of clamping.
- *Minimize ischemic time by perfusion of vessels downstream* of the distal graft anastomosis rather than 'clamp and go' technique.

Cooling and hypothermia

Systemic hypothermia offers some protection to cord ischemia primarily by reducing cord temperature during the ischemic period: systemic hypothermia is more widely used than surface and intrathecal cooling.

Cerebrospinal fluid withdrawal

Intra- and postoperative withdrawal of cerebrospinal fluid to maintain CSF pressure 10–20mmHg is aims to increase cord perfusion by increasing the difference between intracranial and arterial pressure.

Pharmacological methods

The most important pharmacological adjuncts are vasopressors, given to *maintain MAPs 90–100mmHg* postoperatively: late onset paraplegia is associated with ↓BP. Corticosteroids, sodium thiopental, prostaglandin E, and O_2 free radical scavengers are adjuncts of unproven importance.

Endoluminal stenting

A proportion of patients with acute or chronic type B dissections are candidates for endoluminal stenting.

Indications

For the stent to remain *in situ* there needs to be a neck of 2cm of normal aorta both proximally and distally. The precise indications for endoluminal stenting still a matter of debate, but most patients, particularly older patients with multiple comorbidity, should be considered for stenting for the following purposes:

- Stenting of true lumen to seal entry tear.
- Stenting of static obstruction of a branch artery.
- Balloon fenestration of dissection flap and stenting of true lumen for visceral or lower limb hypoperfusion.
- Stenting of true lumen to enlarge compressed true lumen.

Complications of endoluminal stenting

- Hospital mortality (MI, aneurysm rupture) 5–10%.
- Paraplegia 5–10% (depends on morphology), stroke 2–5%.
- Stent migration 2–5%, organ ischemia 2–5%.

Repair of type B dissection

Key facts

- The aim of repair is to resect as much of the involved aorta as possible while minimizing risk of spinal cord and end organ ischemia.
- The tear is usually at the origin of the left subclavian artery. The aorta containing the intimal tear must be resected, but it is frequently not possible to obliterate the entire false lumen.
- Repair can be done off bypass, on bypass, with or without deep hypothermic circulatory arrest, or partial left heart bypass depending on the extent of the dissection, with or without renal artery perfusion:
  - **Full bypass** allows control of BP, and option of **DHCA** which improves ability to control proximal portion (especially if arch involved), eliminates bleeding collaterals, as well as allowing BP control and lower body to be perfused.
  - **Partial left heart bypass** (📖 p125) also allows BP control and distal perfusion, but without coagulopathy associated with full heparinization and use of oxygenator. Arterial return is to the femoral artery, with venous drainage from the left inferior pulmonary vein, or left atrial appendage.
  - **'Clamp and go'** avoids the coagulopathy and inflammatory picture associated with bypass, but relies on a fast anastomosis as the lower body warm ischemic time is longest with this technique, and risks upper body hypertension once the descending aorta is clamped.
- Spinal cord protection strategies aim to minimize paraplegia risk (📖 p437).

Set-up

- Ensure that the patient has external defibrillator paddles, right and left radial arterial lines (the left subclavian may be snared or clamped), and that the groins are shaved.
- A double-lumen ET tube facilitates left lung decompression.
- Prep and drape the patient in the right lateral position, with the pelvis as horizontal as possible to allow access to both groins.
- Make a left posterolateral thoracotomy incision in the 5th intercostal space, and divide the costotransverse ligaments of the 5th and 6th rib to permit maximum exposure without requiring rib fracture (📖 p39).
- A thoracoabdominal incision (Fig. 9.5) is required if the abdominal aorta is involved: the abdominal exposure is normally retroperitoneal but peritoneum can be opened if there is a need to view viscera, e.g., concern about ischemia.
- Once the thoracic aorta is exposed secure the left subclavian artery, and preserve the **left vagus and recurrent laryngeal nerves**.
- The thoracic aorta is freed from the left common carotid artery as far as the distal extent of the resection, clipping and dividing the spinal arteries in the segment to be resected.
- If left heart bypass is to be used, open the pericardium and place a 4/0 Prolene purse-string in the left inferior pulmonary vein and cannulate with a 14F cannula, with arterial return to either the distal descending aorta, or the femoral artery providing flow rates of 1–2L/min.
- If total cardiopulmonary bypass is required, use fem–fem cannulation.

Repair

- Once fully heparinized go on bypass and place vascular clamps on the aorta proximal and distal to the area of resection.
- Maintain right radial artery pressures at 100–130mmHg and femoral artery pressures at 60–70mmHg.
- Open the aorta longitudinally and ligate bleeding intercostals arteries: this can be done sequentially while monitoring SSEPs and MEPs (📖 p437).
- Transect the aorta at least 1cm distal to the origin of the left subclavian artery.
- For proximal anastomosis use pledgetted 4/0 Prolene (Fig. 9.5): in a stage II elephant trunk (see 📖 p449 for stage I), the proximal anastomosis is to the distal end of the Dacron graft left at the previous operation, which is located and orientated under a brief period of circulatory arrest with clamp off.
- When this anastomosis is complete, reposition the proximal clamp on the graft which is allowed to fill with blood, so that the anastomosis can be inspected (Fig. 9.5).
- If the proximal anastomosis is satisfactory, transect the distal aorta, cut the graft to fit and perform the anastomosis with 3/0 Prolene, Teflon strips, and biological glue as indicated.
- Depending on the level and extent of resection, renal and celiac arteries may be reimplanted into the Dacron graft at this stage.
- Wean bypass, reverse heparin, and secure hemostasis.

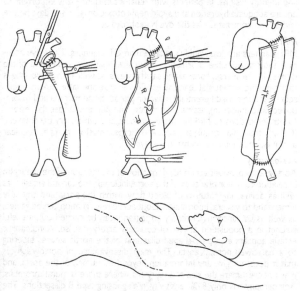

Fig. 9.5 Technique of repair of descending aorta.

Diagnosis of aortic aneurysm

Key facts

- The role of imaging in chronic aneurysms is to establish and monitor the size of the aneurysm, and define the anatomy and comorbidity.
- CT is the most widely used modality, but MRI is a useful adjunct.
- Additional assessment includes echocardiography and coronary angiography.

Imaging

CT

CT scanners are widely available and the images familiar to all clinicians. CT provides accurate and reproducible information about size, anatomy, and extent of the disease, so it is used for 6-monthly assessment of chronic aneurysms: these must be *standardized assessments* as estimates of aneurysm size can vary widely between scans, and within a single test depending on where the measurement was taken and how perpendicular the measure was to the wall of the aorta. CT angiography (i.e., with iv contrast) provides additional information about intramural hematoma, thrombosis, and dissection. Detailed 3D reconstructions can be used to help operative planning. The abdominal aorta is always imaged as 25% of patients with thoracic aneurysms also have abdominal aneurysms. CT angiography can be performed to image coronary and carotid anatomy and identify lesions. In patients with renal insufficiency it is important to ensure adequate hydration and avoid nephrotoxic drugs in the days before and after a contrast CT as the dye is nephrotoxic.

MRI

MRI scanners are less widely available than CT scanners. They give accurate and reproducible information about size, anatomy, and extent of the disease in transverse, coronal and sagittal views, as well as dynamic images that can pinpoint intimal tears, assess flow in true and false lumens of dissected aneurysms, differentiate between periaortic hematoma and thrombosed false aneurysm, assess LV function, and peripheral vascular lesions. Contraindications to MRI include permanent and temporary pacemakers, ICDs, intracranial aneurysm and AVM clips, infusion pumps, cochlear implants, and metal fragments in the eye.

Aortography

Aortography provides accurate information of the location of the aneurysm in relation to major branches of the aorta, including the carotid arteries, as well as delineating patterns of blood flow within the aorta and any false lumen, and to viscera. Information about aortic regurgitation can be gained, as well as LV function. Coronary angiograms can be carried out, a useful adjunct in a population at risk of coronary artery disease. Annuloaortic ectasia appears as a pear-shaped dilatation of the aortic sinuses tapering to a narrower normal aorta. The main disadvantage of aortography is that it does not give any information beyond the lumen of the aorta, and may underestimate the size of aneurysms where there is mural thrombus. Aortography has only 84% sensitivity in diagnosing type B dissections. The contrast used is nephrotoxic. Aortography is an invasive procedure that may be difficult to carry out in patients with severe peripheral vascular disease.

Other investigations

Cardiovascular system
- EKG with stress testing if indicated.
- TTE: mitral valve disease frequently accompanies aortic aneurysms, and in Marfan disease the incidence is as high as 30%.
- Coronary angiography for male patients >35 years and females >45 years, or with a history suggestive of ischemic heart disease: 25% of patients undergoing repair of ascending aneurysms have concomitant coronary artery disease.

Respiratory system
- CXR.
- Lung function tests in patients with COPD or long history of smoking.
- Spirometry and ABGs will assist the anesthesiology assessment of whether these patients will tolerate single lung ventilation, and establish a baseline function.
- Early admission for antibiotics, nebulized bronchodilators, and physiotherapy improves outcome in patients with significant COPD.

Renal function
- Urea and creatinine, GFR.
- Preoperative hydration, fluid balance monitoring, and occasionally admission to ICU for invasive monitoring and inotropic support in an attempt to optimize function may be indicated.

CNS function
Consider duplex of the carotid arteries in patients with severe atherosclerotic disease, or a history of TIA or stroke.

Management of aortic aneurysm

Natural history

Thoracic aortic aneurysms have a 5-year survival of about 40%, compared to 20% for thoraco-abdominal and abdominal aneurysms. The 5-year survival of chronic dissecting aneurysms may be as low as 13%. Thoracic aneurysms increase in size by about 0.4cm per year, with arch aneurysms increasing fastest. Larger aneurysms (>6cm) expand faster than smaller aneurysms, predicted by Laplace's law: aneurysms >8.0cm in diameter increase in size by up to 0.16cm per year. *The size of aneurysm at presentation is the most important predictor of risk of rupture*. The annual risk of rupture of aneurysms between 6.0–6.9cm is fourfold that of aneurysms of 4.0–4.9cm. Median size of rupture or dissection of ascending aneurysms is 5.9cm, and 6.9cm for descending aneurysms. Once symptoms develop the mean time to rupture is about 2 years. *The annual risk of rupture, dissection, or death is 5–6% for aneurysms 5.0–5.9cm, and 10–15% for aneurysms >6.0cm. Elective operative mortality is:*

- 1–5% for elective repair of ascending aneurysms, with 85% 5-year survival (operative mortality of aortic root replacement is as low as 1% in experienced centres, but nationally mortality is closer to 7%).
- 5–10% for repair of arch aneurysms, with 75% 5-year survival.
- 5–10% for repair of descending aneurysms, with 60% 5-year survival.
- 5–10% for repair of thoracoabdominal aneurysms, with 60% 5-year survival.

Mode of death in unoperated thoracic aneurysms

- Rupture (40–70%).
- Dissection.
- Cerebral embolism.
- Visceral embolism.

Indications for surgery

Ascending aorta

- Acute dissection (emergency).
- Symptomatic aneurysms.
- Asymptomatic aneurysms >5.5cm.
- Aneurysms >5.0cm and known connective tissue disorder.
- Aneurysms >5.0cm and bicuspid aortic valve requiring replacement.
- Moderate to severe aortic regurgitation.

Aortic arch

- Symptomatic aneurysms.
- Aneurysms >5.5cm.
- Documented progressive enlargement.
- Potential source of emboli in patient with embolic cerebral events.

Descending aorta

- Symptomatic aneurysms.
- Asymptomatic aneurysms >6.5cm.

- Documented progressive enlargement.
- Aneurysms associated with chronic type B dissection.

Contraindications to surgery

- Advanced age (>85 years).
- Incurable malignancy or other terminal illness.
- Irreversible, profound brain injury, chronic dementia.

Controversies

Borderline aorta (4.5–4.9cm)

In light of newer data on rates of dissections in aorta <5.0cm, and low mortality in experienced centers with elective intervention, the 2008 AHA/ACC and 2007 ESC guidelines say essentially the same thing: repair/replacement of the ascending aorta and/or root is indicated for:

- Any patient if the diameter of the ascending aorta >5.0cm, or the rate of increase is >0.5cm/year.
- Patients undergoing aortic valve replacement if the ascending aorta >4.5cm.
- Lower thresholds may be considered in young patients of small stature.
- 2010 AHA/ACC thoracic aorta guidelines recommend cut-offs of 4.5cm for patients with Loeys–Dietz syndrome, or the TGFBR1 and 2 mutations.

Root replacement or interposition graft with aortic valve replacement

The decision whether to replace the coronary sinuses boils down to a balance between the incremental operative mortality of a complete root replacement compared to AVR + interposition graft (3–5%), and the long-term risk of dissection or aneurysm formation of the residual native tissue. In older patients without an obvious connective tissue disorder, an interposition graft is probably most reasonable as the risk of late complications from the native aortic sinuses is low and root replacement is associated with higher mortality. In younger patients with Marfan or other connective tissue disease, complete root replacement or valve-sparing root replacement is more frequently indicated as it can be performed with low operative mortality and they are otherwise at higher risk of late complications from the native aortic sinuses.

Indexing aortic size to body surface area

There are several methods of adjusting these cut-offs for patient size:

- Svensson et al.[1] reported that if aortas were replaced when πr^2 (cm)/(height (m) >10 that 95% of dissections in their retrospective series would have been avoided.
- Ergin et al.[2] recommended intervention based on multiples of the normal diameter for a 40-year-old patient with a BSA of 2m², ranging from 1.3 in Marfan disease to 1.5 in asymptomatic patients with no history of connective tissue disorder.

References

1. Svensson LG et al. Relationship of aortic cross-sectional area to height ratio and the risk of aortic dissection in patients with bicuspid aortic valve J Thorac Cardiovasc Surg 2003; 126:892–3.
2. Ergin MA et al. Surgical treatment of the dilated ascending aorta: when and how? Ann Thorac Surg 1999; 67:1834–9.

Surgery for ascending aneurysms

Key facts

- The aim of surgery is to resect all aneurysmal aorta, anastomosing tube graft to relatively normal aorta. Depending on which segments of the proximal ascending aorta are affected this may involve a simple interpositional graft, replacement of the aortic valve, replacement or remodelling of the aortic root.
- If the aneurysm is quite proximal it may be possible to perform the distal anastomosis with the cross-clamp on. More distal involvement requires removal of the cross-clamp, to do a hemiarch replacement under 15–20min of hypothermic circulatory arrest (🕮 p435).

Set-up

Sternotomy. Axillary or femoral (🕮 p120) or low aortic cannulation (the cannulation site will be excised with the aneurysmal segment under DHCA). High aortic cannulation only if intention is to leave the distal ascending aorta in place, and perform anastomosis with clamp on.

Operative techniques

Interposition graft

This involves replacing the aneurysmal aorta with a tube graft. The aortic valve may or may not be replaced. The sinuses are preserved and so there is no need to reimplant the coronaries. It is usually possible to perform without circulatory arrest. The technique is described on 🕮 p434.

- It is suitable for aneurysms limited to the ascending aorta and not involving the aortic root (proximal to the sinotubular junction).
- In young patients with dilated sinuses, or in patients where there is evidence of chronic dissection or other pathology (e.g., abscess formation) involving the sinuses or annulus root replacement is required.
- In elderly patients with moderate sinus dilatation an interposition graft is usually a better option than a root replacement as the risk of complications from leaving the sinuses intact is probably lower.
- In acute type A dissection it is preferable to perform an interpositon graft, even if there is some evidence of dissection into the sinuses, as root replacement in this setting is much more difficult (tissues are friable, bleeding may be insurmountable). Dissected sinuses can be reapproximated with bioglue, a Teflon strip, and a running 4/0 Prolene prior to performing the proximal interposition graft anastomosis.

Root replacement

This is indicated when ascending aortic aneurysms involve the aortic root, and severe valvular disease means that it is not possible to preserve the aortic valve. The aortic root and aneurysmal aorta is replaced with a composite conduit with a mechanical (Bentall) or bioprosthetic valve (bio-Bentall) or a homograft aortic root and aorta harvested *en bloc* from a cadaveric human heart. This requires mobilization and reimplantation of the coronary ostia. The technique is described on 🕮 pp386–391.

Ross procedure

This technique involves aortic root replacement with the patient's own pulmonary trunk, which is in turn replaced with a pulmonary homograft, and more limited indications. The technique is discussed on 📖 pp388–389.

Aortic valve-sparing procedures

Several techniques reduce the size of the aortic root without replacing the aortic valve, although it is usually resuspended within the tube graft, which replaces the resected segment of aorta. These techniques are described on 📖 p446. External wrapping of the aorta is very occasionally used in patients too frail to undergo a more extensive procedure.

Tips and pitfalls in aortic root surgery

Cabrol graft

This is useful in aortic root replacement where the coronary buttons are too friable, adhesed, calcified, or fibrosed to permit mobilization enough for them to be anastomosed to aortic conduit without tension. It is a particularly useful adjunct in reoperative root replacement, if the original aortic conduit has to be excised. A length of SVG, or more commonly an 8mm Dacron graft, is sewn end-to-end to the left coronary button with continuous 6/0 Prolene (buttressed if necessary with a 2mm Teflon felt strip) wrapped round the graft so that it can be sewn end-to-side to the right coronary button, and then end-to-side to the aortic conduit. In *hemi-Cabrol* just one coronary button is anastomosed in this way.

Cabrol patch or shunt

This is a bail-out technique for uncontrollable hemorrhage at the end of the case, usually from the proximal anastomotic or coronary button suture lines. In the original description the RA appendage was sewn to the aneurysmal sac, decompressing the perigraft space and allowing autotransfusion to the patient. Numerous modifications exist. Sewing a 10 x 8cm bovine pericardial patch to all the anterior surface of the heart and great vessels (usually the SVC, RA, RVOT, PA, ascending aorta), and just prior to closure creating a 1–2cm incision in the RA underneath the patch, works well to autotransfuse all blood loss into the RA, if there is no connection between the aortic root and the posterior pericardial sac. If the root communicates with the posterior pericardium, packing the posterior pericardial well and waiting before chest closure usually works surprisingly well. If the patch appears tense, you need to enlarge the right atrial hole (can be done via the suture line or a purse-string). These patches can be left in place (the shunt eventually disappears) or taken down a day or so later—remarkably little bleeding from the right atriotomy is seen at takedown in most patients.

Right coronary ischemia

The right coronary button is more frequently the source of problems that can compromise separation from bypass, than the left button—possibly because it is more prone to distortion and kinking as the heart fills. Even a tiny non-dominant RCA can result in severe RV dysfunction if it is not accurately reimplanted: have a low threshold for performing a hemi-Cabrol or a bypass graft.

Valve-sparing surgery

Key facts

- Important aortic root pathology necessitating surgical correction frequently coexists with *structurally normal aortic valve leaflets*.
- Any technique that allows root reconstruction without valve replacement avoids some of the disadvantages of aortic valve replacement (📖 pp370–371). A large number of valve sparing root techniques have evolved, which can be divided into two main groups:
  - *Remodeling* techniques, e.g., the *Yacoub* in which a tailored graft is sewn to the remnants of the individual aortic sinuses, preserving dispensability and creating neosinuses, but not reinforcing the annulus, in a technically slightly easier procedure (Fig. 9.6).
  - *Reimplantation* techniques, e.g., the *David* in which the whole aortic root is replaced by a Dacron tube, secured to the annulus, in a technically more demanding procedure (Fig. 9.6).

Valve-sparing techniques

Remodeling: 1979 Yacoub

A Dacron graft, sized to the internal aortic diameter, is tailored to individually replace the resected sinuses (Fig. 9.6). The commissural pillars are resuspended within the Dacron graft so that the leaves of the graft replace each coronary sinus, and so that they are stretched upwards slightly maintaining tension on the valve leaflets. The coronaries are reimplanted as buttons.

- The technique is supposed to be technically easier than the David.
- Disadvantages are that the annulus is not stabilized (potentially a problem in patients with connective tissue disorders), and the sinotubular junction is not narrowed, so connective tissue disorders are a relative contraindication (long-term risk of annular dilatation and recurrent AI).
- Most useful in smaller roots because of the more physiologic dynamics.

Reimplantation: 1992 Tirone David I (TDI), 1995 TDII, Seattle, 1996 TD III, 1997 TD IV, 2002 TD V

This technique was designed for patients with dilatation of the sinotubular junction, dilation of the sinuses of Valsalva and annulo-aortic ectasia. The aortic valve is reimplanted within a Dacron tube-graft (Fig. 9.6) sized to the external aortic diameter. The root is excised leaving the ostia on 10mm buttons of sinus aorta, and the proximal coronary arteries mobilized. The Dacron graft is parachuted down onto the base of the aortic root, via pledgetted sutures placed through the base of the aortic outflow tract. The valve commissures are resuspended within the Dacron graft, the coronary buttons sewn into holes created within the tube graft, and the distal anastomosis performed. The annulus is stabilized by the Dacron graft. The TD III added a Teflon felt strip to buttress the annulus. The 1995 Seattle and the TD IV and V scalloped and plicated larger grafts to create more bulbous neosinuses.

- The technique has a longer learning curve than the Yacoub.
- The advantage is that the annulus is stabilized, so patients with annuloaortic ectasia and connective tissue disorders may be less prone to late annular dilatation and recurrent AI.
- Early iterations did not recreate sinuses, changing the root dynamics, contributing to abnormal leaflet stresses and late recurrence of AI.

Choice of technique

Lesion	Causes	Technique
Annulus normal, STJ enlarged	Aortic ectasia Aneurysm	Yacoub
Annulus and STJ normal	Aortic dissection	Interposition graft and glue sinuses, or replace non-coronary, or Yacoub
Annulus and STJ enlarged	Annuloaortic ectasia Marfan	David, or interposition graft

Patient outcomes

Perioperative elective mortality is approximately 1–2% (young patients):
- 10-year survival is 80–90% (close to normal population).
- Freedom from reoperation at 10 years is highly variable—while Tirone David reports 90–98%, this is lower elsewhere (75% where the Yacoub was used in Marfan syndrome), and not a direct reflection of freedom from mod-severe AI which was 85% at 10 years in the David series, i.e., not dissimilar to bioprosthetic AVR.

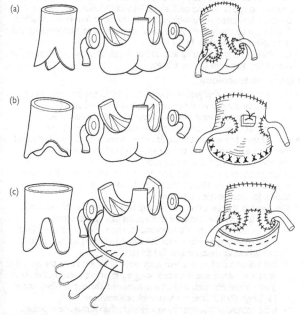

Fig. 9.6 Examples of valve sparing aortic surgery. (a) Yacoub repair. (b) Seattle repair. (c) Tirone III repair.

Arch replacement

Key facts

- Aneurysms and type A dissections may involve the distal ascending aorta and arch: the main options for arch replacement are:
  - **Island** technique (Fig. 9.7b).
  - **Trifurcated graft** (Fig. 9.7d) which has largely superseded the Island technique as it is easier to selectively perfuse the brain reducing DHCA, replaces the entire arch, and anastomosis is limited to the usually less diseased head and neck vessels.
  - **Stage I elephant trunk** (Fig. 9.7a) is an adjunct to either of the above techniques where the aneurysmal descending aorta will need later replacement (usually >3 months after the stage I).
- Aortic arch surgery mandates cerebral protection in addition to myocardial protection (🕮 p124). DHCA is almost invariably required as the distal anastomosis must be performed with the cross-clamp off and the head and neck vessels must be reimplanted if the arch is replaced.
- DHCA may be supplemented by direct antegrade perfusion, selective cerebral perfusion, or retrograde cerebral perfusion (🕮 p124).

Set-up

- Set-up is described on 🕮 p444: an extended sternotomy may be used so prep and drape to expose neck and axillary cannulation sites.
- Bypass is instituted via fem-bicaval, axillo-caval, or fem-fem cannulation (which can be changed to aorto-caval cannulation at a later point) and the patient is cooled to 15°C.
- Cardioplegia is given retrograde and/or antegrade, and a right superior pulmonary vein vent usually placed.

Operative technique

- When the nasopharyngeal temperature is 15°C, the patient is placed in Trendelenburg, caval tapes secured, and the SVC pipe clamped temporarily to eliminate negative pressure in the cerebral venous system that might entrain air emboli when the aorta is opened.
- Dissect the phrenic and the vagus nerves from the anterior surface of the aorta, and dissect out the proximal 1cm of the innominate artery, left common carotid, and subclavian.
- Select and trim a trifurcation graft to fit: sizes of the two distal arms are usually 8mm or 10mm, and the graft may have an additional side branch for later aortic cannulation.
- The pump is stopped, the cross-clamp is removed, and blood vented from the arch so that the arch and vessels can be inspected.
  - If the dissection flap or aneurysmal portion does not extend into the arch an anastomosis with the distal ascending aorta can be carried out as described on 🕮 p435.
  - If the dissection flap or aneurysmal portion extends into the arch, but does not extend into the descending aorta or arch vessels, the aorta is transected obliquely and an anastomosis fashioned similarly under 15–20min DHCA: this is a **hemiarch replacement**.
  - If the pathology involves the whole arch, then it must be replaced, and the arch vessels reimplanted: the *trifurcated graft technique* is described next.

- Transect the aorta distal to the origin of the left subclavian, and the head and neck vessels close to their origin (Fig. 9.7).
- Using continuous 4/0 Prolene on an SH needle starting forehand well to the left of the heel, inside to out on the Dacron and outside to in on the native vessel, running the suture round to the heel and then up side nearest you, then taking the other arm and running it forehand towards you across the top: complete the left subclavian, then left common carotid and then innominate artery anastomosis. The Dacron can be bevelled to fit.
- If axillary cannulation was used, the pump is then resumed at 50mL/min to de-air the graft, the proximal end of which is then clamped and selective cerebral perfusion commenced (□ p125).
- A Dacron graft is selected to fit the distal anastomosis (24–30mm) and using a strip of Teflon felt to buttress either sewn end-to end or as an elephant trunk (where the graft is invaginated with the inner portion then pulled out to complete the proximal anastomosis (Fig 9.7a), while the outer portion marked with three metal clips remains in the descending aorta for the Stage II descending repair). This can be de-aired and clamped and perfusion begun to the lower body.
- The proximal ascending aorta anastomosis, which may involve a root replacement (□ p444) or simple interposition graft (□ p434) is completed, and a graft-to-graft anastomosis using 4/0 Prolene between the proximal and distal grafts is performed (taking care to leave a landing zone for the trifurcated graft), and normal cardiopulmonary bypass resumed.
- The trifurcated graft is anastomosed finally, selective cerebral perfusion is over and the patient is rewarmed.

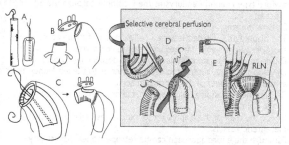

Fig. 9.7 Arch replacement. (a) Invaginating Dacron graft for elephant trunk. (b) Set-up for Island technique. (c) Stage I elephant trunk using island technique for arch. Gray box shows trifurcated graft technique. (d) Stage I elephant trunk with selective cerebral perfusion. (e) Completed arch replacement with trifurcated graft.

Repair of descending aneurysms

Overview

The natural history and pathology, are discussed on 🕮 p48. The aim of surgery is to resect all aneurysmal aorta, reimplanting the larger radicular arteries and all involved visceral arteries. If the arch is not involved circulatory arrest is not required, and it may be possible to use partial left heart bypass instead of full cardiopulmonary bypass (🕮 p125). The variable extent of thoracoabdominal aneurysms makes accurate preoperative imaging vital. Spinal protection is an important part of surgery on the descending aorta as the blood supply to the spinal cord is usually compromised (🕮 p436) resulting in paraplegia rates as high as 20%. Techniques of spinal protection are described on 🕮 p437, including:

- Surgical technique.
- Spinal fluid withdrawal.
- Hypothermia and topical cooling.
- Pharmacological adjuncts.

Set-up

This is as described on 🕮 p438. Double-lumen ET tube for single-lung ventilation. The patient must be positioned in the right lateral position with the hips rotated so that the left groin is accessible.

Incision

Crawford type I and II aneurysms are approached via the 6th rib space through a lateral thoracotomy extended via a gentle curve into a midline laparotomy incision extending to the umbilicus if required (Fig. 9.5). For Crawford type III and IV aneurysms the incision is through the 8th or 9th rib spaces.

- Deflate the lung.
- The diaphragm is divided leaving a 1–1.5cm rim of tissue at the thoracic wall, to avoid damage to the phrenic nerves.
- Divide the retroperitoneum lateral to the descending colon.
- Develop the plane anterior to psoas, posterior to the left kidney as far as the lateral aspect of the abdominal aorta.
- Retract the descending colon, spleen, tail of pancreas, and left kidney to the right.
- Divide the crux of the diaphragm to expose the celiac axis, renal and mesenteric vessels.
- Although the entire approach can be retroperitoneal particularly where extensive adhesions from previous laparotomies make an open approach difficult, an open approach makes it possible to asses the viscera after reperfusion.

Venting

The heart can be vented through the left inferior pulmonary vein, or the apex.

Options for cardiopulmonary bypass

'Clamp and go'

Cardiopulmonary bypass is not used, the patient is not cooled. There is no control of upper body hypertension on clamping the descending aorta, and no perfusion to the lower body during this time. It is used in emergencies if cardiopulmonary bypass is not available, and in elective situations may be preferred by some surgeons.

Full cardiopulmonary bypass with deep hypothermic circulatory arrest

The technique of deep hypothermic circulatory arrest is described on 📖 p124. In repair of descending aortic aneurysms the following options for cannulation are available:

- Fem-fem cannulation.
- Fem-fem bypass augmented with flow from the PA.
- Axillo-femoral bypass.
- Arterial drainage from left subclavian or distal aorta.

CPB is instituted as soon as possible and cooling started. Various methods of spinal cord protection may be used (📖 p437). The heart is vented as soon as it starts to fibrillate. Once the nasopharyngeal temperature is 15°C venting is stopped (to prevent entraining air into the heart) and bypass is discontinued. The aorta distal to the aneurysm is either clamped or, if this is not possible due to heavily calcified atheroma or poor access, a Foley catheter balloon is inflated with saline to occlude the lumen.

Partial left heart bypass

Left heart bypass consists of drainage of oxygenated blood via a cannula placed in the LA or one of the left pulmonary veins, which is then pumped using an in line centrifugal pump into either the left common femoral artery or the distal aorta. Bypass flows of up to 1.5L/min are adjusted to maintain a distal arterial pressure of 60–70mmHg. The upper body circulation proximal to the cross-clamp maintains near normal perfusion pressures. The aorta is clamped either side of the aneurysmal segment. Depending on the extent of the aneurysmal segment this allows constant perfusion of abdominal visceral, lower limbs, and spinal cord. As each arterial branch is reanastomosed to the graft the clamp can be moved distally. The advantages of left heart bypass are:

- Reduced risk of stroke from aortic cannulation.
- Reduced risk of aortic dissection.
- Reduced pulmonary dysfunction postoperatively.
- Some surgeons use a reduced dose of heparin (1000U/kg).

Traumatic aortic transection

Key facts

Traumatic aortic transection is caused by massive deceleration injuries. The force needed to rupture the aorta is equivalent to an intraluminal pressure of >2000mmHg. High-speed impacts result in continued forward movement of the distal end of the aortic arch, against the upper descending aorta which is held stationary relative to the thorax by the ligamentum arteriosum, intercostal arteries, and origins of the head and neck vessels. As a result almost 50% of acute aortic transactions occur in the very proximal descending aorta near the aortic isthmus, 1cm distal to the origin of the left subclavian. <10% occur in the ascending aorta. The remainder occur in the distal thoracic aorta, often in combination with vertebral fractures.

- Transection may be complete, including adventitia and pleura.
- Adventitia and/or pleura may be spared.
- The aortic intima may be spared.
- False aneurysms result from partial transactions: they calcify, enlarge, and eventually often rupture.

Natural history

When transection is complete death is almost instantaneous as there are no tissues to tamponade hemorrhage. Tears that spare the adventitia or pleura result in proportionately smaller hemorrhages into the retroperitoneal tissues that result in severe chest pain radiating through to the back, hemorrhagic shock, and left hemothoraces. Risk of death is greatest immediately after the transection, and although the instantaneous risk of death decreases with time it levels off after 7 days leaving a low constant risk of death from hemorrhage.

- 48% of untreated patients are dead within 48h.
- At 10 years the predicted 5-year mortality from rupture is 20%.

Diagnosis

The classical features of a widened mediastinum on CXR may not be apparent: features to look for include rightward shift of the trachea, blurring of the sharp outline of the proximal descending aorta, and opacification of the aorto-pulmonary window. Aortography is being replaced by MRI as the gold standard for imaging, although the usual caveats about availability of MRI apply. Spiral CT has a lower specificity, but may be vital in the diagnosis and management of associated injuries.

Indications for surgery

Urgent surgical repair is indicated for stable patients with contained aortic injury who do not require laparotomy, craniotomy, pelvic stabilization, or thoracotomy for bleeding. Emergency repair is indicated for:

- Signs of impending rupture.
- Hemothorax.
- Contained hematoma.

After 10–14 days aortic transactions may be treated as chronic aortic aneurysms (☐ p450). Hypertension should be avoided.

Outcome

Variability in outcome reflects the range in severity of transection ranging from moribund patients exsanguinating from complete tears, to stable patients with contained hematomas.
- The operative mortality in the former group is >40%.
- This compares to <5% in the latter group.
- Overall hospital mortality is 30%.

Technique

The techniques are similar to those described on ☐ pp438–439. The same adjuncts for spinal cord protection are often not feasible in the critically ill trauma patient. The main differences between the technique described on ☐ pp438–439 for repair of a type B dissection, and repair of a traumatic transection are:
- Dissection around the isthmus (the usual location of a tear) is only started once proximal and distal aortic control has been established.
- 'Clamp and go', where the aorta is simply cross-clamped just distal to the left subclavian artery, and the section including the tear is replaced with a Dacron graft, is useful in trauma centers where extracorporeal bypass may not be an option, and for rapid control of continued hemorrhage: cross-clamp times of <30min result in low paraplegia rates, but most cross-clamp times are significantly longer.
- Lower body perfusion systems, e.g., left heart partial bypass (☐ p451) (if available) should be chosen with the aim of using the least amount of heparin possible, because of the risk of concomitant intracranial hemorrhage.

Endoluminal stenting
- Endoluminal stenting is increasingly used instead of surgery for traumatic aortic rupture, as it appears to offer similar short-term survival, without the need for thoracotomy, single lung ventilation, or cardiopulmonary bypass.
- Gore Tag® grafts are used to cover relatively short segments (5–10cm).
- There is little long-term outcome data available.

Less invasive options

Smaller incisions

Anterior MIDCAB

There are two main options: (1) 6–10cm incision from the left border of the sternum over the 4th rib which may be resected (Fig. 10.1a), or (2) a 5–7cm muscle splitting incision over the 4th rib space extending towards the nipple, from 2cm lateral to the left sternal edge. A Finochietto, West self-retaining or soft-tissue retractor is used. The pericardium is hitched to the chest wall with 1/0 silk sutures. Suitable for:

• MIDCAB (minimally invasive direct coronary artery bypass grafting).
• Endo ACAB (endoscopic atraumatic coronary artery bypass grafting).

Right minithoracotomy

A 6–10cm incision is made along the 4th rib space extending from the level of the nipple to the anterior axillary line, or following the breast crease (Fig. 10.1d). Pectoralis major is divided or split, and the intercostal muscle raised off the inferior rib anteriorly to 1cm lateral to the sternum (avoiding the RIMA) and laterally round to the costal angles to mobilize the rib space. A mini Cosgrove, McCarthy, or similar mitral retractor with narrow blades is placed between the ribs and the pericardium opened well above the right phrenic nerve. It is possible to cannulate the aorta, SVC, IVC, and coronary sinus directly through this, or peripherally in order to create more space (📖 p120). This incision is useful for:

• Mitral and tricuspid repair.
• ASD repair.

Hemisternotomy

A full sternotomy can be performed through a very low 6–10cm skin incision in most patients and gives excellent access for mitral and aortic surgery. A *hemisternotomy* is an alternative where only the upper or lower 2/3 of the sternum is divided. Its main disadvantage is the risk of tearing the IMA or intercostals when opening the retractor. A 6–10cm incision is made in the midline from an inch or so above the xiphisternum to an inch or so below the angle of Louis. The sternum is divided from xiphisternum to the 3rd or 4th intercostal space where it is 't'd' to the right (*lower hemisternotomy*) or from the sternal notch down to the 3rd or 4th intercostal space (*upper hemisternotomy*) (Fig. 10.1b). The tissue over the 4th rib space is divided as far as pectoralis major which may be entered in a muscle splitting fashion, or divided with cautery. Occasionally it may be necessary to divide or resect part of a rib to obtain better access. This incision is used for:

• Upper hemisternotomy: aortic valve surgery, thymectomy.
• Lower hemisternotomy: mitral and tricuspid valve surgery, ASD.

Subxiphoid incision

This approach is described on 📖 p490, and involves a 4–6cm incision extending from the xiphoid process which is divided, caudally (Fig. 10.1c). The pericardium is entered above the diaphragm. This approach allows access to:

• The PDA and distal OM vessels if extended caudally.
• Pericardial window.
• Access in reoperative cases for epicardial ablation.

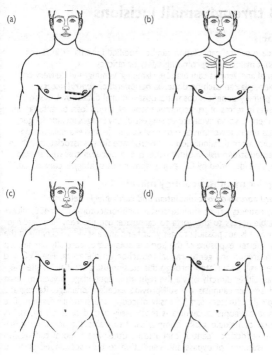

Fig. 10.1 (a) Left anterior minithoracotomy (MIDCAB), (b) hemisternotomy (AVR), (c) subxiphoid approach (pericardial window), (d) Right anterolateral minithoracotomy (mitral, tricuspid, ASD closure).

Thorascopic approaches

A modification of the left VATS approach described for thoracic procedures, requiring double lumen intubation and single lung ventilation (📖 pp686–687) can be used to harvest the LIMA and RIMA, and perform distal coronary anastomoses (usually directly via a MIDCAB incision). The main differences in set up are:

- External defibrillator paddles are placed.
- The radial arterial line should be sited on the right side.
- The patient is placed at a 30° angle (Fig. 10.3) with the hips horizontal and the left arm above the head.
- The patient is prepped so that the groin and the midline are accessible.
- The port sites are positioned as described on 📖 pp460–461.
- CO_2 is infused at 6–8mmHg by a pressure-regulated insufflator.
- A Harmonic scalpel is used by most surgeons to harvest the LIMA as there is less smoke, and local heat injury is less.

CPB through small incisions

Key facts

- Standard central cannulation can be modified for smaller incisions without majorly compromising safety or efficacy.
- Arterial and venous cannulation, clamping, venting, and delivery of cardioplegia can each be done via **peripheral or central access**.
- The primary benefit is cosmetic: observational data shows mixed benefits in terms of pain control, recovery, blood loss, or extubation, and there is some evidence to suggest disadvantages include longer bypass times, lower mitral repair rates, and under-revascularization.
- Femoral arterial cannulation and retrograde flow is associated with an **increased stroke risk** in older patients and vasculopaths, who should always be identified by CT angiography if this strategy is considered.

Set-up for minithoracotomy mitral

Standard aorto-bicaval cannulation and cardioplegia delivery

In many patients a right 4th intercostal minithoracotomy (🕮 p456) allows reasonable access to the aorta to cannulate: use the Fem-Flex Seldinger cannula as it is not possible to get your hand and a standard cannula in the incision. Better exposure of the aorta is obtained by carefully hitching up the pericardium and gentle caudal retraction on the aorta. The SVC and IVC are easily cannulated through this incision using standard single-stage cannulas, either directly or via the right atrial appendage. If vacuum assist is used, smaller cannulas will still provide excellent drainage. Retrograde cardioplegia catheters can be easily placed in the standard fashion. The antegrade cardioplegia cannula is most easily placed once on bypass. A Chitwood or flexible snake clamp is used to clamp the aorta. Lung isolation is needed for central cannulation: otherwise femoral cannulation allows institution of bypass and ventilation to be discontinued prior to thoracotomy.

Peripheral alternatives

Any of these can be used to improve access or reduce incision size:

- Femoral arterial cannulation (avoid in elderly or arteriopathic patients).
- Femoral venous cannulation (percutaneous or open) usually with vacuum assist to enhance venous drainage.
- Percutaneous internal jugular vein cannulation (anesthesiology).
- Percutaneous internal jugular retrograde cardioplegia cannulation.
- Fibrillatory rather than cardioplegic arrest (if no more than trace AI).

Port-access bypass

This involves fem-fem bypass, but also occludes the ascending aorta with a balloon (the **endoclamp**) inserted via the femoral artery allowing delivery of antegrade root cardioplegia. The heart can be arrested on bypass, enabling mitral valve surgery, as well as CABG, to be carried out through smaller, usually thoracotomy or thorascopic (port), incisions. Aortic surgery is not possible because of difficulty maintaining the balloon occlusion distal to the aortotomy without occluding the head and neck vessels. Aortic dissection complicates around 1% of port access CPB.

Technique

As the surgeon is not able to visualize the cannulas or cardioplegia delivery system additional monitoring is mandatory. Radial arterial lines are sited bilaterally, and TEE routinely used so that migration of the arterial cannula or cardioplegia delivery system can be detected.

- Make a 2–3cm groin crease incision overlying the femoral vessels.
- Obtain proximal and distal control of the vessels with slings.
- After heparinization pass a 22F venous cannula into the RA via the femoral vein under TEE control, so the tip is in the SVC.
- Using vacuum assist enhances venous drainage.
- Cannulate the femoral artery with a dual port arterial return catheter and position the tip of the cannula in the aortic arch using TEE.
- Again under TEE pass the endoclamp down the second limb of the femoral cannula so that the tip sits just above the sinotubular junction.
- The endoclamp consists of a triple lumen catheter with an inflatable balloon at the tip: the balloon is inflated to occlude the aorta via the first lumen, the second allows aortic root pressure to be transduced and is used as a root vent, and the third delivers cardioplegia (Fig. 10.2).
- After institution of CPB inflate the endoclamp with 20–30mL of saline, aiming for a balloon pressure of 250–350mmHg. De-airing is critical.
- If there is any forward ejection of the heart the balloon will migrate distally, so it is important to ensure complete emptying of the heart.
- It is possible to puncture the balloon (e.g., while placing anterior mitral annuloplasty sutures): completing the procedure under fibrillatory arrest or replacing the balloon are both options.

Contraindications to port-access bypass

- Severe peripheral vascular disease.
- Intraluminal atherosclerosis of the aortic arch.
- Aortic valve or ascending aorta procedures.

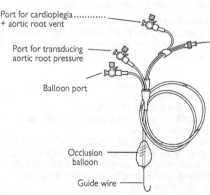

Port for cardioplegia ....
+ aortic root vent

Port for transducing — aortic root pressure

Balloon port

Occlusion — balloon

Guide wire —

Fig. 10.2 Port-access endoclamp.

LIMA harvest via small incisions

Key facts

The LIMA can be harvested to a variable extent through several incisions. It is important to obtain a long length (preferably the entire length) of LIMA because:

- If the LIMA is tethered to the chest wall it will tend to kink.
- If the LIMA is short it will place the anastomosis under tension.
- A short length of LIMA will not reach the LAD in patients with distal disease or COPD.
- A long length facilitates sequential grafting.
- The risk of coronary steal from patent IMA branches is avoided.

Anterior, lateral, and mid-lateral MIDCAB incisions

There are a number of specialized retractors which enable the LIMA to be harvested from 1st to 5th rib space from the right of the patient in a manner similar to that used in a median sternotomy approach (Fig. 10.3).

Thorascopic IMA takedown

This is an alternative method of harvesting the IMA which has several advantages. Firstly, rib resection and retraction are avoided. Secondly, the entire length of the IMA can be mobilized, avoiding kinking, tension on the anastomosis, and IMA steal. Harvest takes longer, with a longer learning curve. Double lumen intubation and single lung ventilation is required, which not all patients tolerate well. Insufflation of CO_2 may result in hemodynamic compromise. Uncontrollable hemorrhage may mandate median sternotomy.

Patient selection

The following are relative contraindications to thorascopic LIMA harvest:
- Lung disease making single lung ventilation impossible.
- Previous thoracic surgery resulting in pleural adhesions.

Anesthesia and positioning the patient

This is described on 🕮 p686. The patient's left armpit should be shaved. It may be helpful to mark the anterior and midaxillary lines as well as the 4th rib space and midline with indelible pen prior to prepping.

Positioning the ports

- Triangulate the port sites, which prevents the instruments from interfering with each other during use.
- Make three incisions of 1.5mm with a 15 blade.
- Use a mosquito or Dunhill to dissect down to the intercostal space.
- Ask the anesthetist to deflate the lung.
- Place the camera port at the 5th intercostal space along the anterior axillary line, which gives the best view of the length of the LIMA.
- The two instrument ports are placed using the camera internally to obtain optimal positioning, usually along the midaxillary line, one or two rib spaces either side of the camera port.
- Placing the instrument ports below and away from the LIMA gives better access for harvesting than placing them too close or directly opposite.

Harvesting the LIMA thoracoscopically

Filmy adhesions can usually be divided without wasting too much time, but dense adhesions make introduction of ports and instruments hazardous, and the thorascopic approach should be abandoned. If the LIMA is not obvious, it is easiest to identify it just distal to its origin from the subclavian artery where it is covered by a thin layer of parietal pleura. The middle 1/3 is frequently covered by fat, and the distal 1/3 by the innermost intercostals and pericardial fat. The camera can be held either by an assistant or by a voice-activated arm.

- Incise the parietal pleura lateral to the LIMA with cautery.
- Retract the pleura with forceps and use a combination of cautery and blunt dissection with the blade of the diathermy to separate the LIMA pedicle from the thoracic wall.
- LIMA branches are best divided by direct coagulation as clipping individual branches means frequent instrument changes, increasing operative time and the risk to adjacent structures.
- Some surgeons advocate skeletonizing the LIMA as a more precise dissection and longer length is allowed: this is at the risk of increased trauma to the LIMA.
- Insufflation of CO_2 to a pressure of 5–15mmHg, if tolerated by the patient, enlarges the operative field facilitating the distal dissection.
- Once an adequate length is secured heparin is given (150U/kg).
- The LIMA is ligated with two large clips and all but a few muscle strands divided, so that it is held in the anatomical orientation while the thoracotomy incision is made, through which it can be brought under direct vision.

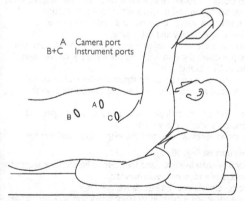

A   Camera port
B+C Instrument ports

Fig. 10.3 Positioning the patient and port sites.

SVG harvest via small incisions

Key facts

- In addition to significant postoperative pain and decreased mobility, the standard method of harvesting the saphenous vein through a long, continuous incision results in delayed wound healing due to cellulitis, lymphoceles, edema, large skin flaps, fat necrosis, hematoma, sympathetic dystrophy.
- Much of this can be avoided by using either endoscopic or hybrid approaches which maintain skin bridges.
- The advantage of the standard open approach is that the 'no touch' technique preserves endothelial integrity: minimally invasive approaches result in much more direct handling of the vein and there is some observational data suggesting this may be associated with reduced long-term patency rates.

Methods of minimally invasive SVG harvest

There are several systems for minimal access harvest. In skilled hands all of them result in comparable quality conduit. Endoscopic techniques have a much longer learning curve: they are therefore better suited to surgical assistants on long-term contracts than surgeons on short training rotations. An alternative is using a stripper, which allows vein to be harvested through multiple small stab incisions without a camera.

Using a stripper (Fig. 10.4a)

A stripper is simply a 1cm metal ring, mounted at an angle on a long handle. This method is quicker than conventional harvest as there is no long incision to close, but real care should be taken to avoid avulsing small branches and damaging the endothelium with too much traction.

- Expose the saphenous vein at the groin and ligate it proximally.
- Place a 0/0 silk suture distally and cut it long.
- Pass the suture and the vein through the ring end of the stripper and pass the stripper down the vein until you meet resistance with skin tethering causes by a branch.
- Make a 1.5cm incision down onto the stripper where it has come up against a branch, and pass the stripper and vein up through the incision.
- Remove the vein from the stripper and the incision, and ligate and divide the branch is usually easily visible.
- Continue as far as necessary and test the vein in the usual manner.

Endoscopic vein harvest (Fig. 10.4b)

There are several systems available, and they offer different approaches to the various aspects of endoscopic vein harvest:

- The saphenous vein is identified just above the knee.
- The subcutaneous space is created by blunt dissection anterior to the vein either by a transparent blunt-tipped dissector under endoscopic vision, with an airtight space maintained by a balloon inflated at the incision and CO_2 insufflation: excellent vision is provided by the scope.

- Dissection is carried out with long-handled, blunt 'U' tipped instruments: side branches are clipped and divided with diathermy.
- Similar techniques have been used for radial artery harvest.
- Experienced surgical assistants take no longer to extract the length of vein in this way than by the open technique: the main issue is not one of time but one of quality, and the learning curve is around 200 cases.

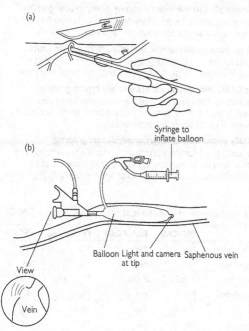

Fig. 10.4 (a) Using a vein stripper. (b) Endoscopic vein harvest.

CABG via small incisions

There are several methods of carrying out minimally invasive CABG. Four representative methods are described briefly in Box 10.1, and the techniques, their advantages and disadvantages listed in Table 10.1.

Box 10.1 Techniques of minimally invasive CABG

MIDCAB (minimally invasive direct coronary artery bypass grafting)
- LIMA harvesting and coronary artery anastomosis are performed, without bypass, through a small anterior thoracotomy incision.

EndoACAB (endoscopic atraumatic coronary artery bypass grafts)
- LIMA is harvested thoracoscopically, then coronary anastomosis is performed, off-pump, through a small anterior thoracotomy incision.

Port-access CABG (port-access coronary artery bypass grafting)
- LIMA harvesting, and coronary artery anastomosis on bypass, are performed through a small anterior thoracotomy, aortic occlusion and delivery of cardioplegia are endovascular.

TECAB (totally endoscopic coronary artery bypass grafting)
- LIMA harvesting and coronary artery anastomosis are performed, off bypass, thoracoscopically: the coronary artery anastomosis is usually performed with robotic assistance, and/or anastomotic aids (Fig. 10.5).

Table 10.1 Comparison of four methods of minimally invasive CABG

	MIDCAB	EndoACAB	Port-access	TECAB
Single lung ventilation	No	Yes	No	Yes
TEE/X-ray guidance	No	No	Yes	No
Arterial monitoring	R radial	R radial	R+ L radial	R radial
Femoral cannulation	No	No	Yes	No
Beating heart	Yes	Yes	No	Yes
Cardioplegia	No	No	Yes	No
Heparinization	Partial	Partial	Full	Partial
Endoscope required	No	Yes	No	No
Robot required	No	No	No	Yes
Thoractotomy incision	8–10cm	6–8cm	8–10cm	No
Ribs divided/excised	Yes	No	Yes	No
LIMA to LAD possible	Yes	Yes	Yes	Yes
Grafts to PDA, OM	No	Yes	No	Yes
Top-ends possible	No	Yes	No	Yes
Anastomotic devices	Not routinely used but helpful in TECAB (Fig. 10.5)			
Stenting some lesions	Inaccessible lesions stented in 'hybrid' procedures			

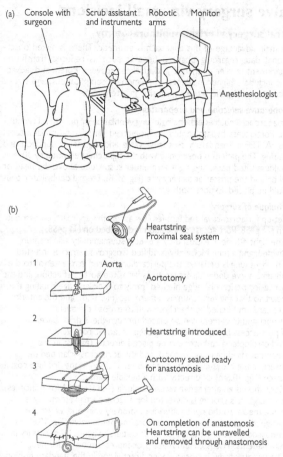

(a)
Console with surgeon
Scrub assistant and instruments
Robotic arms
Monitor
Anesthesiologist

(b)
Heartstring
Proximal seal system

1   Aorta
Aortotomy

2
Heartstring introduced

3
Aortotomy sealed ready for anastomosis

4
On completion of anastomosis Heartstring can be unravelled and removed through anastomosis

Fig. 10.5 (a) Set up for robotic surgery. (b) Device for performing proximal coronary anastomosis without using a clamp on the aorta.

Valve surgery via small incisions

Mitral surgery via right minithoracotomy

The main advantage of this approach is cosmetic. There is mixed observational data regarding possible benefits such as reduced transfusion requirement, earlier discharge, and quicker recovery. Potential disadvantages include a higher incidence of pulmonary complications, and stroke related to retrograde arterial perfusion in arteriopaths.

Preoperative selection and preparation

This approach requires either single lung ventilation or peripheral cannulation. Port-access bypass should be monitored via bilateral radial arterial lines. A TEE is mandatory to assess valve and ventricular function and de-airing. The patient is positioned with the right chest elevated by 30–45°, shoulders tilted back, and right arm either suspended above the head or well behind the posterior axillary line (Fig 10.6). Eternal defibrillator pads should be placed. Expose both groins.

Technique of surgery

- Set-up for aorto-caval and fem-fem bypass via this approach is described on 🔲 p458. Port-access cannulation is described on 🔲 p458.
- The right 4th rib is exposed by a 6–8cm submammary skin incision, divided, and a mini-McCarthy/modified Cosgrove retractor inserted.
- The right lung is deflated, the pericardium incised 2cm anterior to the phrenic nerve under direct vision as far as the aortic reflection, and the posterior pericardial edge hitched firmly to the skin edge rotating the heart so that the left atrium is uppermost (Fig. 10.6), and the anterior pericardium hitched to the chest wall to expose the aorta.
- A port and 0° camera can be placed through the 3rd rib space.
- If port-access bypass is not being used, an aortic root vent and cardioplegia catheter can be placed directly (easiest in the decompressed heart on bypass), and the aorta cross-clamped by inserting the cross-clamp through a 5mm incision in the 3rd intercostal space (Fig. 10.6m) or directly with a flexible clamp.
- Fibrillation is an alternative to cardioplegia (see 🔲 p121 for principles).
- Sondergaard's groove is dissected for 1–2cm, a small atriotomy is made medial to the right superior pulmonary vein, and a purpose designed retractor inserted to expose the mitral valve (Fig. 10.6).
- Endoscopic instruments are used. Knot-tiers may not be necessary in slim patients. Tricuspid and maze procedures can be performed.
- The left atriotomy is closed under direct vision in the standard fashion.

Aortic valve surgery

The aortic valve can be accessed via an upper sternotomy incision (🔲 p456) or a small right anterior thoracotomy. The technique is a modified version of the standard open technique, although port-access bypass can be used instead of aorto-caval bypass. Retrograde cardioplegia is used if desired, and the heart is vented via the right superior pulmonary vein, or LV via the dome of the LA. De-airing is carried out under TEE guidance in the standard fashion (🔲 p114), but lifting the heart is done using internal defibrillator paddles.

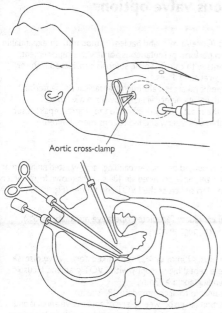

Aortic cross-clamp

Fig. 10.6 Minimal access mitral valve surgery.

Percutaneous valve options

Key facts

- Pericardial valves (CoreValve™ and Sapien™) mounted on expandable
  stents are used to perform percutaneous aortic valve replacement,
  currently in patients with calcific aortic stenosis considered high- or
  very high-risk surgical candidates.
- Access is via the femoral artery, although transapical (left anterior
  thoracotomy) and axillary artery via cut-down are also used.
- The MitraClip is the most widely used option for mitral repair: results
  are less comparable to surgery, and indications more limited.

Corevalve™

Device

Porcine pericardium mounted on a self-expanding, large waisted nitinol stent
in 22mm and 26mm sizes, now delivered via 18F sheaths (down from earlier
25F and 21F), designed to sit across the LVOT and sinuses (Fig. 10.7a).

Indications

- High-risk surgical candidate (predicted operative mortality ≥15%).
- Symptomatic, severe, degenerative AS.

Contraindications

- Native aortic annulus <20mm or >27mm, mixed aortic valve disease
  (AI >3–4+), severe septal hypertrophy with LVOT gradient, bicuspid
  aortic valve, ascending aorta >43mm.
- Femoral arteries unable to accommodate 18F sheath.
- Aortic root angulation (angle between plane of aortic valve annulus and
  horizontal plane/vertebrae) >70° (femoral access) or >30° (axillary access).

Results

- Procedural success rate close to >90% in most recent series.
- 30-day mortality 0–25%, stroke (0–10%), conversion to surgery (0–8%).
- Need for PPM insertion (0–36%).
- Complications include paravalvular leak >2+ (4–35%), tamponade
  2–10%), malpositioning, aortic dissection (0–4%), blood transfusion 2U
  (3–24%), vascular complications (10%), 30-day MACCE 3–30%.
- Procedure duration 2–3h, length of stay 7–17 days.

Sapien valve

Device

Bovine pericardium mounted in a balloon expandable 16mm long tubular
stent in 26mm sizes, now delivered via 22F sheaths designed to sit across
the annulus (Fig. 10.7b).

Indications

- High-risk surgical candidate (predicted operative mortality ≥15%).
- Symptomatic, severe, degenerative AS.

Contraindications

- Native aortic annulus <18mm or >25mm on echo.
- Mixed aortic valve disease (AI >3+) or severe MR.

- Severe septal hypertrophy with LVOT gradient.
- Bicuspid or non-calcified aortic valve, active endocarditis, bulky calcified aortic valve leaflets in close proximity to coronary ostia.
- Significant abdominal or thoracic aortic disease, e.g., aneurysm (>5cm), marked tortuosity, aortic arch atheroma, narrowing of abdominal aorta with calcification or irregularities, ileofemoral calcification, or vessels <7mm for 22F catheter.
- Femoral arteries unable to accommodate 18F sheath.
- Aortic root angulation (angle between plane of aortic valve annulus and horizontal plane/vertebrae) >70° (femoral access) or >30° (axillary access).

Results

- PARTNERS trial[1] randomized to transcatheter (n=348) or surgical replacement (n=351).
- Procedural success rate 95%.
- 30-day mortality 3.4% Sapien vs. 6.5% surgery (p=0.07), 1-year mortality 24 vs. 27% (p=0.44).
- Strokes: Sapien 5.5% vs. surgery 2.4% (p=0.02) and at 1 year 8.4 vs. 4.3%.
- 12% moderate AI in Sapien (vs. 0.9% after surgery).
- Major vascular complications 11% in Sapien vs. 3% in surgical group (p < 0.001), major bleeding 9 vs. 19.5% (p=0.006).
- Shorter hospitalization with Sapien (6 vs. 12 days) no functional difference at 1 year.

MitraClip

Device

4mm wide, cobalt-chromium implant with two arms designed to clip the anterior and posterior mitral leaflet together (edge-to-edge repair, 📖 p410) delivered by atrial transseptal puncture (Fig. 10.7c).

Indications

- MR 3–4+, primary jet originating from malcoaptation of P2 and A2 (📖 p408).

Contraindications

- Mitral valve orifice <4.0cm², flail segment ≥15mm wide, flail gap ≥10mm, or coaptation depth >11mm/vertical coaptation depth <2mm if leaflet tethering, significant adjacent cleft, bileaflet flail.
- Severe mitral annular calcification, lack of chordal support, prior mitral surgery, endocarditis, rheumatic heart disease, ASD, or PFO.

Results

- At 1 year freedom from death, surgery, and grade 3 or 4+ MR was 55% in the MitraClip goup and 73% in the surgery group (p <0.001).
- Major adverse events at 30 days were the same for death (1%), stroke (2%), emergency cardiac surgery 2–4%, and the difference in adverse events reported was due to increased blood transfusion in the surgery arm.

Reference

1. Smith CR et al. Transcatheter vethus surgical aortic-valve replacement in high-risk patients. New Engl J Med 2011; 364:2187–98.

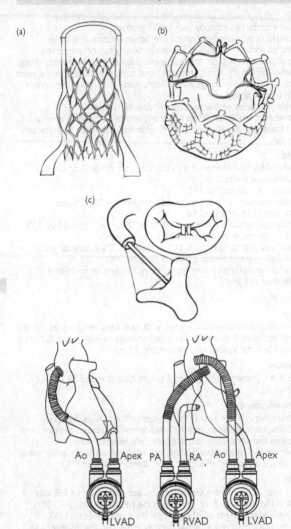

Fig. 10.7 (a) Corevalve aortic prosthesis. (b) Sapiens aortic prosthesis. (c) Mitraclip. Various assist devices: (Top right) Thoratec Heartmate VE. (Top left) Jarvik 2000 implanted with outflow in descending aorta. (Middle) Tandem and Impella devices. (Bottom left) schematic of implantation of Thoratec LVAD. (Bottom right) schematic of Thoratec biventricular device.

Other conditions

Myxoma

Key facts

- Myxomas are composed of pluripotential **subendocardial mesenchymal** cells (📖 p84) and are the commonest type of primary cardiac tumor, compromising 40–50% of all benign cardiac tumors.
- They are 2–3× commoner in women, occurring in the 3–6th decade. 5% show autosomal dominant inheritance.
- 70% of sporadic myxomas occur in the LA.
- They are an indication for urgent removal, to reduce the risk of systemic embolism

Presentation

Symptoms and signs depend on the location of the myxoma and the degree to which RV and LV filling is compromised. Often incidental finding in asymptomatic patient. Embolic and constitutional features coexist

- LA myxoma (75%): episodic dyspnea, hemoptysis, syncope.
- RA myxoma (20%): episodic dyspnea, signs of right heart failure, ascites and hepatic congestion, ↑JVP, edema.
- **Embolic features** (30–40%): mostly systemic, **stroke**, retinal, visceral, coronary, aortic saddle embolus, PE rare.
- Very large mobile tumors may transiently occlude AV valve leading to loss of cardiac output (which can occasionally be restored by placing patient in steep Trendelenburg to dislodge tumor) and **sudden death**.
- Systolic murmurs (impeded AV closure/narrowing outflow tracts).
- Diastolic murmurs (obstructed filling of RV or LV).
- Widely split S2 (delayed closure of mitral valve), 'tumor plop'.
- Constitutional features: fatigue, fever, rash, pyrexia, athralgia, myalgia, ↓weight, ↓Hb, ↓Plts, ↑CRP, ↑ESR.

Investigation

- EKG changes are non-specific and include AF and bundle branch block.
- CXR changes are non-specific: calcification is unusual, signs of LA enlargement and pulmonary edema may feature.
- Echocardiography is diagnostic: TEE can detect masses as small as 1–3mm and a **pedunculated, smooth mobile mass sitting in the LA** almost pathognomonic of LA myxoma.

Natural history

Myxomas are usually benign, but the tumor occasionally metastasizes to brain, sternum, vertebra, pelvis, or scapula. Once myxomas become symptomatic death usually occurs within 1–2 years. There is a significant risk of sudden death: 10% of pre-op patients die of embolic phenomena.

- Hospital mortality after resection of atrial myxomas is about 1–5%.
- Hospital mortality after resection of ventricular myxomas is about 10%.
- 1–2% of sporadic myxomas recur, compared to up to 75% of familial.

Indications for operation

Myxomas have been traditionally considered as an indication for urgent surgery (within 24h of diagnosis).

Surgical technique for left atrial myxoma

Minimize handling the heart to avoid fragmentation of the tumor. In the rare event of sudden loss of cardiac output before bypass is instituted as a result of a large tumor occluding flow into the LV, place the patient in steep Trendelenburg to allow the tumor to roll back into the LA restoring output, start chest compressions if needed, and open emergently.

Set-up

- Standard invasive monitoring including TEE.
- Median sternotomy (right anterolateral thoracotomy an option).
- Incise the pericardium away from the midline so that you can harvest a patch for repair of large defects.
- Insert a mitral retractor hitching up the right pericardium only.
- Standard aorto-bicaval cannulation with snares and/or vacuum assist, CO_2 insufflation, and an aortic root vent.
- Surgery is performed with the heart fibrillating, or clamped with antegrade cardioplegic arrest at 32°C.
- Pump suckers, vents, and cell salvage may be used as they add little to the risk of embolizing tumor cells arising from bypass.

Atriotomy and tumor excision

- Atriotomy is dictated by the location of the tumor which is usually attached to the left side of the interatrial septum: this is best approached via an *oblique right atriotomy*, then incising the floor of the right atrium in a *transseptal approach*
- Exposure is gained as in a tricuspid repair, with retractors and by extending the incision if appropriate (📖 p404).
- The tumor is most commonly attached by a stalk, which may be broad based, to the atrial septum: this base should be excised with a *5mm margin* of full thickness septum.
- A sterile *dessert spoon* is useful to help evacuate the friable, gelatinous tumor without fragmenting it.
- Once the tumor is removed inspect the whole of the LA, the LV, and what can be seem of the RA through the septal defect, and RV through the tricuspid valve, for any other myxomas, which should be excised.
- Ventricular myxomas are excised with a partial thickness of ventricular wall: the approach is usually via the LA and RA for LV and RV tumors respectively.
- Occasionally myxomas arise from valves, or damage valves by a 'wrecking ball' effect which requires reconstruction or replacement.
- Thoroughly irrigate with water (may lyse residual tumor cells) and a waste sucker (not cell salvage).

Closure

- Repair small septal defects (<1–2cm) with double layered 4/0 running Prolene, and larger defects with the pericardial or Dacron patch, de-airing the LA by asking the anesthesiologist to ventilate, displacing air from the LA as the suture line is completed (📖 p120).
- Place RV pacing wires as tumor excision can compromise SA node artery which crosses the interatrial septum, leading to sick sinus syndrome.

Other cardiac neoplasms

Key facts

Pathology and indications for operation of primary cardiac neoplasms, including lipomas, papillary fibroelastomas, rhabdomyomas, angiosarcomas, and rhabdomyosarcomas, are outlined on 📖 p84. These tumors are removed by open heart surgery where possible.

Right atrial spread of infradiaphragmatic tumors

Pathology

Infradiaphragmatic tumors that extend up the IVC into the RA normally involve both the endothelium of the IVC and the endocardium of the RA. Tumors include:
- *Renal cell carcinoma* (by far the commonest).
- Renal adenocarcinoma.
- Wilms tumor.
- Uterine leiomyosarcoma.

Diagnosis

- Cardiac symptoms do not occur until quite late. Extension into the right atrium may be suspected from CT imaging performed in order to stage tumors, and can be further assessed by TEE or MRI.

Indications for surgery

Renal cell carcinoma extension without distant metastasis is one indication, although indications in less common tumors are less well established. After combined nephrectomy and resection of atrial renal cell carcinoma:
- 5-year survival is ~65%.
- 10-year survival is ~60%.

Surgical technique

The nephrectomy and resection of atrial extension are most commonly performed as a combined procedure. It is often possible for the vascular surgeons to complete the entire procedure without cardiopulmonary bypass from the abdomen. Occasionally this is not possible, and *cardiopulmonary bypass* is required for an approach via the RA. As no venous return can be obtained from the IVC while the tumor is being excised *deep hypothermic circulatory arrest or low flows* at deep hypothermia are required.
- A TEE probe is placed in addition to routine invasive monitoring.
- The patient is prepped and draped as for CABG, but exposed from clavicle to groin, with no drapes over the umbilicus.
- A median sternotomy incision is extended to a midline laparotomy as far as the pubis.
- The SVC and RA are cannulated (do not use a two-stage cannula), aortocaval bypass commenced using vacuum assist, and the patient cooled to 18°C, venting either the LV or the right superior pulmonary vein.
- Pump suckers, vents, and cell salvage may be used as they add little to the risk of embolizing tumor cells arising from bypass.
- The abdominal tumor and involved kidney is mobilized ready for excision during cooling.

- At 20°C the aorta is cross-clamped, cold blood cardioplegia given into the root, the SVC snared, and the RA opened.
- Flows can be reduced or stopped for up to 35min at this temperature, usually 5–10min of low flow or DHCA are necessary to clearly visualize the tumor in the IVC orifice.
- A rough sucker is used to remove blood from the vicinity of the tumor in the RA as it is dissected free of the endocardium.
- Blunt dissection to free the tumor from the endothelium of the IVC.
- Once the tumor has been removed from the RA and IVC, the renal pedicle is ligated and divided, and the kidney removed.
- The RA is closed and the IVC cannulated in the normal manner so that full flow bypass can be established and the patient rewarmed.

Carcinoid heart disease

Pathology

Carcinoid tumors arise from the *argentaffin cells of the GI tract*. They occur in the ileum, pancreas, ovaries, and testes, and they secrete large amounts of serotonin (5HT). 10% metastasize, usually to the liver. 10% result in *carcinoid syndrome* which is characterized by flushing, bronchospasm, diarrhea, and telangiectasia. In 50% of cases of carcinoid syndrome fibrosis involves the right heart valves. Severity of cardiac involvement correlates with serum levels of 5HT. Cardiac involvement results in *tricuspid and/or pulmonary valve regurgitation* due to thickening and restriction of the valve leaflets, and is usually limited to the right-sided valves. Metastasis to the heart is rare.

Diagnosis

The described symptoms may be accompanied by signs including the systolic murmur of TR. While carcinoid syndrome is diagnosed from symptoms, imaging identifying the tumor, serum 5HT and urinary 5-hydroxy-indoleacetic acid, cardiac lesions are best assessed by echocardiography. Valve leaflets appear short and thick with a characteristic 'dagger' appearance in color modes.

Indications for surgery

Valve lesions progress rapidly and cause CHF in untreated patients, who have a poorer prognosis than carcinoid patients without cardiac involvement. Operative mortality 10–20%. Liver metastases are not a contraindication to surgery as they are indolent and treatable, but predispose the patients to *carcinoid crises* (profound hypotension), triggered by catecholamine use, and prevented and treated by octreotide infusion which should be maintained throughout the perioperative period.

Techniques of surgery

Valve repair is not usually possible. Pulmonary and tricuspid replacement (📖 p417) is performed, usually with bovine pericardial patch augmentation of the RVOT. Bioprostheses are preferred despite accelerated degeneration if 5HT levels are high, as mechanical valves and anticoagulation make postoperative care and future resection of liver metastases challenging.

Massive pulmonary embolism

Key facts

- *Acute PE* is common in patients with multiple risk factors, particularly if not on thromboembolic prophylaxis.
- The majority of cases are managed medically with *heparinization or thrombolysis:* indications for emergency surgery are unusual but include near complete occlusion of both pulmonary arteries with either evidence of hemodynamic compromise (hypotension, shock, cardiac arrest) or RV dysfunction, or large intracardiac thrombus.

Pathology

Risk factors for venous thromboembolism

In 1856 Rudolf Virchow linked DVT and PE to *a triad of venous stasis, vein wall injury, and hypercoagulability.* Known risk factors for DVT include:

Venous stasis
- Immobility (surgery, trauma, paralysis, medium- and long-haul flights).
- Failure of deep venous valves, venous dilatation.
- Compression of veins (pregnancy, bulky intra-abdominal tumors and cysts, deck chairs, poor padding on operating table, tourniquets).
- Low cardiac output, right heart failure.

Endothelial injury
- Previous DVT, traction on vein branches during surgery.

Hypercoagulability
- Dehydration, age, malignancy, smoking, pregnancy.
- Oral contraceptive pill, factor V Leiden, C and S deficiency.

Venous thrombus most commonly forms in the deep veins of the leg: 90% of clinically detected PEs are associated with leg DVT. Thrombus may propagate into the iliac veins or spontaneously detach travelling through the right side of the heart into the PA, either as a single large clot which may lodge straddling the pulmonary trunk (saddle embolus) or as smaller fragments which tend to migrate to the lower lobes, right more than the left. Old-established DVT is usually firmly attached to the vessel walls and less likely to embolize than a new clot which is usually only attached to the vein wall at its site of origin. The thrombus rapidly becomes covered in a layer of platelets and thrombin. As a result of acute PE several pathological changes occur:
- RV pressure rises causing RV dilatation.
- RV stroke volume and consequently LV preload fall.
- Systemic hypotension results in reduced coronary blood flow.
- Alveolar dead space increases causing $\downarrow\downarrow PaO_2$.
- Except in massive PE, hyperventilation often causes $\downarrow PaCO_2$.
- Pulmonary vasoconstriction is caused by release of serotonin, ADP, thromboxane, platelet activating factor and platelet derived growth factor, anoxia, and ischemia further compromising RV function.

Diagnosis of pulmonary embolism

PE is incorrectly diagnosed in almost 75% of patients. The differential includes acute MI, aortic dissection, septic shock, chest infection, hemothorax, and pneumothorax. *Massive PE* is PE resulting in hemodynamic compromise, or >30% of the pulmonary vasculature is compromised.

Clinical features of pulmonary embolism
- Symptoms: dyspnea, pleuritic or dull chest pain.
- Signs: tachypnea, tachycardia, hypotension, elevated JVP, pallor.
- Risk factors for or clinical evidence of DVT.
- Bedside tests: EKG shows RV strain pattern (S1, Q3, T3) but this is neither a specific nor a sensitive test.
- $\downarrow PaO_2$, $PaCO_2$ may be low.
- CXR may show consolidation and effusion early on.
- TTE or TEE shows RV dilatation, TR, and RA or RV thrombus.
- Pulmonary angiography, spiral CT, and VQ scanning are diagnostic.

CT

This is the most readily available modality in most centres. CT angiography has a sensitivity of 90% and a specificity of 95% for large PEs. Subsegmental PEs are frequently not picked up.

Ventilation-perfusion scans

A gamma camera images uptake of inhaled krypton-81m and emission of injected technetium 99m. PE shows up as a perfusion cold spot (emission of ^{81}Kr but no ^{99}Tc). Pneumonia, atelectasis and previous PE also cause VQ mismatches so are relative contraindications to a VQ scan. VQ scans have a 98% sensitivity and low specificity in the diagnosis of acute major PE. Results are given as high, intermediate, or low probability of PE.

Pulmonary angiography

Pulmonary angiography is the gold standard investigation for acute PE. The associated mortality is 0.2%, and it should not be carried out in hemodynamically unstable patients.

MRI

This has a specificity of 80% and a sensitivity of 77%. It is better at identifying subsegmental PEs than CT scans, but limited availability and high cost mean that MRI is not a routinely used modality.

Outcome

- The 30-day mortality of acute massive PE is about 50%.
- About 10% of mortality occurs within the first hour.
- Up to 80% of mortality occurs within the first 2h.
- The mortality of surgical intervention is up to 70% for patients requiring CPR or mechanical circulatory support preoperatively.
- The operative mortality of stable patients is about 10–20%.

Pulmonary embolectomy

Key facts

- This a surgical emergency: patients may be in extremis.
- The embolus is removed on CPB via two arteriotomies in the MPA and RPA, periods of low flow or circulatory arrest may be needed.
- An IVC filter should be placed intraoperatively or immediately after.
- There is often severe RV dysfunction postoperatively.

Management

CPR may be indicated. Otherwise:

- Sit up and give 100% O_2.
- Patient may require intubation before arrival in the OR.
- Get iv access and give heparin 5000U bolus iv.
- Start a heparin infusion (50,000U heparin in 50mL of normal saline) at 1000–2000U/h

Indications for surgery

- Patients with a definite diagnosis of acute massive PE and life-threatening circulatory insufficiency or moderate to severe RV dysfunction, in whom thrombolysis is contraindicated or unsuccessful.
- Large right atrial or ventricular thrombus.

Contraindications

Advanced age, frailty, or comorbidity, prolonged CPR.

Technique of pulmonary embolectomy

- Contact interventional radiology or cardiology to arrange placement of IVC filter either in OR or in catheter lab after surgery.
- Ask for gallstone forceps: it may take cardiac team a while to locate these from general surgery.

Set-up

- Standard invasive monitoring with TEE.
- Midline sternotomy, full heparinization.
- Aorto-bicaval cannulation with caval tapes or vacuum assist (exercise caution when placing the IVC cannula if there is RA thrombus—simply placing it carefully into the RA is sufficient for institution of CPB), and aortic root vent.
- Cardioplegic or fibrillatory arrest.
- Moderate hypothermia (32°C).

Procedure

- Evacuate any clot from the RA and RV via a right atriotomy first: snare the cavae if not using vacuum assist and make an oblique right atriotomy, which can be retracted open using a Cosgrove retractor.
- Close the atriotomy using 4/0 Prolene double layer suture.
- The PA is opened longitudinally 1–2cm distal to the pulmonary valve and the incision extended to the left PA (Fig. 11.1).
- Thrombus is removed ideally using gallstone forceps which are a perfect size and shape for this, and come in a range of curvatures

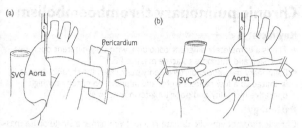

Fig. 11.1 Pulmonary embolectomy. (a) Left pulmonary arteriotomy (which does not extend past the pericardial reflection). (b) Right pulmonary arteriotomy (which may be even more readily accessed *lateral* to the SVC immediately medial to the pericardial reflection).

which are great for getting around the pulmonary branch arteries. Sponge holders are too straight and large for more distal clots.

- The right PA is opened either between the aorta and the SVC (mobilizing the SVC as far as the innominate and retracting improves exposure) or more easily lateral to the SVC which improves access to more distal branches and is easier to repair.
- Use a nerve root or vein retractor to hold the arteriotomies open.
- A sterile fiberoptic bronchoscope may be used to visualize thrombus in lower level pulmonary vessels, and gently compressing the lung and hilum can help to propel thrombus into the larger pulmonary vessels where it can be suctioned out.
- Take care not to inadvertently grab the PA branch bifurcations instead of clot when extracting blindly as this will cause hemoptysis from localized ruptures postoperatively.
- Aim to extract clot that tapers down to fine point, indicating that it has not broken off in the distal arteries.
- Flush copiously with saline and suction, which improves visualization of remnants of thrombus, and flushes out debris.

Closure

- Close the arteriotomies with 4/0 Prolene SH needle, double layer.
- De-air and wean from bypass in the standard fashion: moderate inotopic support for RV dysfunction usually required.
- An IVC filter can be placed percutaneously at this point, or after transfer back to cardiac catheterization labs: some surgeons place it directly under vision while on bypass.
- CVP, RVEDP, and PAP should be much lower than preoperatively.

Postoperative management

- Heparinization once bleeding stopped (within 6–12h): this is because the pulmonary endothelium may be thrombogenic.
- Start warfarin, and run thrombophilia screen if not already done.

Chronic pulmonary thromboembolism

Key facts
- This is a completely different condition, with very different operative approach and outcome to acute massive PE.
- Pulmonary thromboendarterectomy performed for chronic disease is limited to a few centers to try and improve on historically high operative mortality and poor long-term outcomes.

Pathology
Chronic thromboembolic disease results from either a single acute massive PE that does not resolve, or repeated smaller PEs. There are several reasons why emboli fail to resolve:
- Large volume of clot may overwhelm the thrombolytic cascade.
- If the clot obstructs the vessel lumen, thrombolytics cannot reach it all.
- PEs tend to occur in people with abnormalities of thrombolysis
- The clot may be made of material other than thrombus that will not resolve, e.g., tumor fragments particularly myxoma, fat, already organized thrombus; or be associated with indwelling lines.

Clot that does not resolve either becomes canalized and endothelialized, or becomes a solid mass of dense fibrous material, with its own capillary blood supply, that completely obstructs the vessel lumen. Pulmonary hypertension results. This is not because of simple obstruction to flow: patients do not develop pulmonary hypertension after pneumonectomy. Sympathetic stimulation and humoral changes contribute. The proximal vasculature becomes dilated and the distal vasculature shows intimal proliferation and medial hypertrophy.

Presentation
Symptoms and signs are non-specific, and generally do not develop for months to years. Symptoms and signs reflect pulmonary hypertension and RV failure and include exertional dyspnea, fatigue, exertional presyncope, angina, hemoptysis, hypoxia, cyanosis, peripheral edema, ↑JVP, cannon v wave, sternal heave, pansystolic murmur of TR, mid-diastolic murmur of PR.

Investigation
- EKG shows right heart strain pattern (right axis deviation and dominant R wave in V1).
- CXR may show oligemia or abrupt cut-offs of the hilar vessels.
- Pulmonary function tests show non-specific changes such as mild restrictive disease and reduced DLCO, but are important in excluding COPD or restrictive disease as a cause of pulmonary hypertension.
- PA pressures are raised on right heart catheterization, and may be suprasystemic. Pulmonary artery O_2 sats are low.
- VQ scans are the single best screening test, but underestimate defects.
- CT and MRI scans are increasingly used.
- Pulmonary angiography is useful but needs expert interpretation.
- Coronary angiography is performed in patients over 45, or with risk factors for coronary artery disease.

Outcome

Patients remain asymptomatic for months to years. Untreated survival is low and correlates with the degree of pulmonary hypertension:
- 5-year survival for patients with PAP 40mmHg is 30%.
- 5-year survival for patients with PAP >50mmHg is 10%.
- Operative mortality is 5–25%.
- 6-year postoperative survival is ~75%.

Pulmonary thromboendarterectomy

Indications for surgery

The goals of surgery are prognostic and symptomatic: prevention of RV, prevention of extension of thrombus.
- Symptomatic patients with hemodynamic or ventilatory impairment.
- Marked pulmonary hypertension on exercise.

Contraindications to surgery
- Subsegmental thrombi.
- Severe underlying COPD or restrictive lung disease.
- Advanced age, frailty, comorbidity.

Technique of surgery

The set-up is as described for pulmonary embolectomy (📖 p478), but DHCA is required for complete endarterectomy because of copious flow from bronchial collaterals which develop in chronic pulmonary hypertension. Any lung dissection is technically challenging because of the collaterals from bronchial, diaphragmatic, intercostal, and pleural vessels. A median sternotomy gives access to both sides. Bronchial collateral flow means that venting the left heart is mandatory during cooling.
- During cooling the SVC and right PA are mobilized, and slings placed around the SVC, PA, and aorta.
- The right PA is opened longitudinally, medial to the SVC and any loose thrombus removed, but there is frequently no loose thrombus.
- It is possible to begin the thromboendarterectomy while still cooling, if the bronchial circulation is not copious.
- A microtome knife is used to develop the plane of the endarterectomy, which should be easy if the correct plane is entered, and reveal a pearly white vessel media with no residual plaque.
- If the plane is too deep the reddish adventitia becomes visible, and there is a real risk of perforating the pulmonary artery.
- Each endarterectomy is followed to a segmental branch and should taper off gradually, becoming free spontaneously without breaking off.
- It is possible to resume bypass while repairing the right PA and beginning the dissection on the left.
- ASDs are repaired and other concomitant procedures, including insertion of a Greenfield IVC filter, are carried out during rewarming.

Postoperative management

Moderate to severe RV dysfunction is managed with inotropes and inhaled pulmonary inodilators, e.g., nitric oxide. See also 📖 p191.

Permanent pacemaker

Key facts

- Indications for permanent pacemaker insertion (📖 p263) include complete heart block, Mobitz type II and symptomatic Mobitz type I second-degree heart block, as well as trifascicular block.
- Permanent pacemaker insertion may be carried out using a combination of percutaneous Seldinger technique to place endocardial leads via the subclavian veins, as well as open dissection of a pocket usually in the infraclavicular fossa to place the pacing box.
- Occasionally lack of access due to SVC obstruction or occlusion means that placement of endocardial wires is impossible and permanent epicardial leads are placed via a VATs or minithoracotomy approach.

Placing a permanent epicardial system

Set-up

- Ensure that you have the correct pacing system in the OR, and that a cardiac technician is present to test the system as soon as it is in place.
- General anesthesia, with arterial and central line.
- Ensure the patient's chest and abdomen are shaved.
- Prep and drape the patient so that they are exposed from above the umbilicus to the suprasternal notch, as the incision may rarely have to be extended into a median sternotomy to control bleeding.

Procedure

- Make a 5–6 cm longitudinal incision running from 1cm above the xiphoid process towards the umbilicus (Fig. 10.1c).
- Cautery down to the xiphisternum, controlling the vein that runs across the sternum at the level of the sterno-xiphisternal junction.
- Continue down the length of the incision as far as the rectus muscle.
- Using a finger, develop a pocket in the plane between rectus and the rectus sheath lying below it, large enough for the pacing box.
- Place a self-retainer in the incision and divide the xiphisternum with Mayo scissors.
- Staying close to the underside of the xiphisternum, use a finger to develop the plane between the sternum and the pericardium: it should be possible to easily feel a ventricular impulse.
- Open the pericardium with a Mackindo scissors, extending the opening as far as required to visualize the RA and the RV, and place stay sutures which can be locked around the retractor.
- If atrial wires are required place these first by retracing the RV leftwards gently using the handles of the Mackindo scissors to expose the base of the RA.
- The easiest pacing system to insert comes with a long-handled applicator and is inserted with a simple punch and twist action.
- Ventricular wires are placed in the same manner, taking care to avoid the PDA and great cardiac vein.

- Take care to identify which wire is atrial and which is ventricular before letting the cardiac technician test them, and then connecting them to the pacing box.
- Place the pacing box in the pocket beneath rectus, tucking redundant lengths of wire into the pericardium.
- Place a redivac drain the pericardium if there is any bleeding and close the soft tissues in layers with 1/0 Vicryl continuous sutures.

Surgery for atrial fibrillation

Key facts

- AF increases morbidity and mortality from thromboembolic events (TEs), particularly stroke (📖 p219) despite optimal anticoagulation and rate control.
- Ablation procedures, performed with a variety of energy sources, at the time of cardiac surgery (usually mitral) can restore sinus rhythm in up to 70% of patients at 1 year.
- The Cox–maze cut-and-sew procedure has freedom from AF at 1 year reported to be as high as 98%, and in a few centers is performed as a stand alone procedure for refractory AF.
- LA appendage ligation is a useful adjunct to reduce risk of TEs.

Pathology

AF is characterized by irregular, disorganized atrial impulses at a rate of 350–500/min, and ineffective atrial contraction. P waves are absent from the EKG. The resulting arterial waveform is irregular in rate and amplitude. Atrial flutter is characterized by regular atrial impulses at a rate of 250–350/min, variable AV block. P waves often have a saw-toothed appearance and the arterial waveform is regular in rate and amplitude. AF has a prevalence of 6% in the over 65s.

- AF is *induced* by focal areas of enhanced automaticity in the atria, mostly in and around the *pulmonary veins*, and much less frequently around the SVC and coronary sinus.
- AF is *maintained by macro re-entry circuits* throughout the atria which become more persistent the longer AF lasts.
- Treating paroxysmal AF must stop induction pathways, whereas treating permanent AF must address maintenance pathways.
- Ineffective atrial contraction not only reduces cardiac output by up to 30%, but also results in blood stasis which predisposes to mural thrombus, particularly in the *LA appendage* (which has a narrower neck compared to the RA appendage).
- Risk factors for AF are age, dilated LA, recent cardiac surgery, recent pneumonectomy, sepsis particularly pneumonia, hypokalemia, hyopomagnesemia, withdrawal of antiarrhythmics.

AHA classification of atrial fibrillation

- *Recurrent*: two or more episodes.
- *Paroxysmal*: recurrent AF >7 days, terminating spontaneously.
- *Persistent*: recurrent AF >7 days terminated medically.
- *Permanent*: AF that cannot be permanently terminated medically.

Surgical options

Maze procedure

This is the definitive surgical treatment for chronic AF: it is indicated as a stand-alone procedure in patients that have failed maximal medical therapy and are either symptomatically compromised by AF or have had embolic events. The

Cox–maze III interrupts conduction routes of the most common re-entrant circuits, providing a single pathway from the sinus node to the AV node.

- The name 'maze' arises because conduction to the rest of the atria is maintained by providing multiple blind pathways off the main route, preserving atrial contraction, but preventing re-entrant circuits.
- Conduction is interrupted by creating *full thickness lesions* in the atrial wall: this can be done using incisions which are then resutured, or energy sources including *cryoablation* (employing nitrogen-cooled probes to a temperature of −150°C), unipolar or bipolar *radiofrequency*, or *microwave ablation*.
- The advantage of using *cut-and-sew* is that large atria can be reduced in size, minimizing the risk of macro re-entry circuits. This takes longer than using ablation energy sources (40min to 1h, compared to 10–20min), and the risk of bleeding is greater.
- The advantage of ablation is smaller surgical incisions: unipolar is used in small, delicate areas; bipolar is used over long tracts.
- Set-up requires bicaval cannulation: electrophysiological mapping is not routinely performed preoperatively, as macro re-entry circuits change constantly, and the incisions in the maze procedure (Fig. 11.2) are fixed.

Modified maze and pulmonary vein isolation

These more limited lesion sets take less time than performing the classic Maze, and in selected cases can be done without bypass with concomitant OPCAB. Patients have a 60–75% freedom from AF postoperatively, compared to >90% with the cut-and-sew Maze. The disadvantage of pulmonary vein isolation is the risk of refractory atrial flutter in some patients, which may be more symptomatic than AF.

Biatrial cryomaze at the time of mitral surgery

This is indicated for patients undergoing mitral surgery, with any previous history of AF. The LA lesion set is performed under cardioplegic arrest, before oversewing the LA appendage (4/0 running Prolene double layer) and placing annuloplasty sutures. The right atrial lesion set can be performed with the clamp on or off. Patients should be started on amiodarone and anticoagulated for 3 months as atrial transport remains abnormal, and the endocardial lesions are thrombogenic.

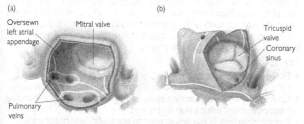

(a)
Oversewn left atrial appendage
Mitral valve
Pulmonary veins

(b)
Tricuspid valve
Coronary sinus

Fig. 11.2 Pattern of incisions in the Cox–maze III procedure. (a) Left atrium. (b) Right atrium. Reproduced from Chikwe J et al. Current concepts in ablation of atrial fibrillation. *Semin Cardiothoracic Vasc Anesth* 2009; **13**: 215–24. © SAGE Publications Ltd./SAGE Publications, Inc., All rights reserved. 2009.

Surgery for HOCM

Key facts

- *Hypertrophic obstructive cardiomyopathy (HOCM)* is a subtype of hypertrophic cardiomyopathy causing LVOT obstruction, which may be complicated by SAM and mitral regurgitation (📖 p190).
- This can be treated by septal myomectomy ± mitral repair.

Pathology

Hypertrophic cardiomyopathy (HCM) is a group of heterogenous sarcomere disorders caused by mutations in the β-myosin heavy chain gene on chromosome 14 (q11–q12), in cardiac troponin-T on chromosome 1, and in α-tropomyosin on chromosome 15, transmitted in an autosomal dominant fashion or occurring spontaneously.

- HOCM is characterized by hypertrophy of the LV and the septum, usually maximal in the outflow portion of the ventricular septum, with maximal thickening lying below the free edge of the anterior mitral leaflet (*basal*) or it may be more **diffuse**.
- Mitral valve leaflets are disproportionately long and thick, and 20% of HOCM patients have MR, usually as a result of systolic anterior motion (*SAM*) of the anterior mitral leaflet, which exacerbates the LVOT gradient which may be as much as 120mmHg.
- The left ventricular cavity is small, with an S shape in young patients.
- Although coronary arteries are usually larger than normal, inadequate capillary flow occurs during diastole because of abnormal relaxation, and septals may be obliterated during systole: myocardial infarction can occur in HOCM in the absence of atherosclerotic disease.
- Although cardiac output is often supranormal in the early stages of disease, progressive fibrosis leads systolic and diastolic dysfunction, compounded by arrhythmias and ischemia.

Presentation and natural history

Onset of symptoms occurs in any decade and includes angina, effort dyspnea, syncope, and exertional presyncope. LVF results in orthopnea and paroxysmal nocturnal dyspnea. The triad of signs is: (1) bifid arterial pulse, (2) palpable left atrial contraction, and (3) late ejection systolic murmur at the left sternal edge. Although the clinical course may be stable over long periods, sudden death, heart failure, and peripheral embolization may occur. Annual mortality of symptomatic HOCM is about 3%. Risk factors for sudden death include young age, syncope, myocardial ischemia, and sustained VT on ambulatory monitoring.

Investigation

- EKG shows an LV strain pattern: Q waves, signs of LV hypertrophy, right and left bundle branch block, and atrial hypertrophy also feature.
- CXR shows moderate cardiomegaly, and signs of heart failure including frank pulmonary edema may be present.
- Echocardiography is diagnostic: asymmetric septal hypertrophy and SAM give the diagnosis; and the exact morphology, degree of LV dysfunction, LVOT obstruction and amount of MR can be quantified.
- Coronary angiography is performed to diagnose CAD, and ventricular pressure gradients may be measured directly if TEE equivocal.

Septal myectomy

Indications

Septal myectomy should be considered in any patient symptomatic despite maximal medical therapy, and whose LV gradient at rest, on exertion, or after an ectopic beat is >50mmHg.

Technique of surgery

Standard bicaval CPB (in case the mitral valve requires repair) under cardioplegic arrest, via a median sternotomy, with monitoring and TEE. The LV is approached via a transverse or oblique aortotomy (Fig. 11.3)

- If the right aortic cusp is carefully retracted, the bulge of hypertrophied septum can be seen and incised in a longitudinal direction exactly below the lowest point of the right aortic cusp. (Fig. 11.3).
- A second incision is made parallel to this as far leftwards as possible, and both incisions are continued down to the apex as far as possible
- A transverse incision is made between the 2 vertical incisions and continued downwards so that a long, 1–1.5cm thick rectangular strip of septum is excised (Fig. 11.3). Angle the blade towards the horizontal not vertical plane to excise maximal muscle. Residual hypertrophy can be digitally palpated and resected using rongeurs.
- *Anomalous papillary muscles* and thickened chordae which insert into the anterior mitral leaflet should be resected, taking care to preserve primary chordae to avoid causing mitral prolapse and MR.
- Avoid creating a **VSD** by not resecting too far towards the RCC/NCC junction where the septum is thinnest, or close to the annulus.
- Once the aortotomy is closed and the heart is de-aired, the gradient across the LVOT can be assessed by TEE: significant gradient warrants further resection, and moderate or worse MR should be corrected.

Results of surgery

Myectomy has a hospital mortality of 2–5%, a 5-year survival of 80–90%, and 10-year survival of 70–85%. Symptom relief depends on relief of LVOTO: 90% of patients are NYHA class I/II postoperatively.

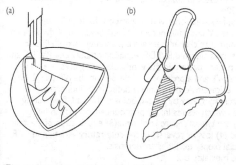

(a)   (b)

Fig. 11.3 Technique of myectomy. (a) View through the aortic valve. (b) Cross-section of the LVOT showing the position of the myocardium that is removed.

Chronic constrictive pericarditis

Key facts

- Constrictive pericarditis may be idiopathic (the most common) or associated with other conditions including prior cardiotomy (📖 p82).
- Cardiac catheterization shows equalization of LVEDP and RVEDP, a dip plateau pattern in the ventricular filling pressure curve, and a prominent 'y' descent in the JVP, and is needed to differentiate between this and restrictive cardiomyopathy (Table 2.4).

Pathology

Constrictive pericarditis may be idiopathic or associated with inflammatory or infective processes, or due to connective tissue disorders, systemic diseases including uremia and hypothyroidism, neoplastic, traumatic (including surgery), and physical agents such as radiotherapy. The visceral pericardium becomes a thick rind-like layer, densely adherent to the heart, and preventing normal function resulting in a tamponade-like picture. Occasionally calcifies.

Presentation and natural history

Constrictive pericarditis may be asymptomatic for years. Fatigue progresses to effort dyspnea, hepatomegaly and ascites with peripheral edema. Orthopnea and paroxysmal nocturnal dyspnea is uncommon. Signs include ↑JVP, *Kussmaul's sign* (failure of JVP to fall during inspiration), pulsus paradoxus, systolic retraction in the left parasternal region, and 'pericardial knock'. Salt and water retention is a key feature. The average life expectancy once symptoms appear is 5–15 years.

Investigation

- Biochemical abnormalities include hypoproteinemia secondary to protein-losing enteropathy, with ↓albumin and gamma globulin.
- EKG shows non-specific ST-segment and T wave changes, and the QRS complexes are low voltage.
- Calcification is present in 40% on the CXR, with enlarged cardiac silhouette in 30%.
- Echocardiography reveals that with inspiration the RV fills supranormally but the LV underfills because of left deviation of the septum, and will also detect thickened pericardium and pericardial effusion.
- Cardiac cath shows elevated RVEDP, equalization between RVEDP and LVEDP, a dip plateau pattern in the ventricular filling pressure curve ('square root sign'), and a prominent 'y' descent in the JVP (Fig. 2.16).
- Constrictive pericarditis can be differentiated from inoperable restrictive cardiomyopathy by a rapid bolus of 1000mL fluid during catheterization which results in: (1) pronounced increase in filling pressures, (2) the typical square root sign, (3) equalization of diastolic pressures, and (4) loss or reversal of the respiratory variation in RAP.
- Endomyocardial biopsy excludes amyloidosis.
- The operative mortality is 2–3%.
- 5-year operated survival is about 65%.
- 5% of patients continue in heart failure after surgery.

Indications for surgery

The diagnosis of symptomatic constrictive pericarditis is indication for operation. The operative mortality and failure to achieve symptomatic improvement is high in patients with a history of chest irradiation and NYHA status III–IV.

Technique of surgery

Pericardiectomy can be carried out via a left anterolateral thoractomy, which gives the best access to the LV allowing all the pericardium covering to be removed. Or via a median sternotomy which facilitates access to the RV and CPB. It is possible to carry out pericardiectomy without CPB, although not all hearts tolerate the manipulation necessary to clear the LV without CPB. Pericardiectomy via a median sternotomy is described.

- External defibrillator paddles should be placed.
- The groin should be prepped and draped.
- The pericardium is incised vertically with a 15 blade starting over the RV near the diaphragm where it is easier to find a plane.
- Dissection continues over the ventricular surface, taking care not enter myocardium.
- The right and left phrenic nerve are preserved by dissecting them from the pericardium with a pedicle of fat and soft tissue (Fig. 11.4)
- The plane is extended across the lateral walls of the RA, across entire LV until that is freed as far as the AV groove and diaphragm.
- The cavae do not need to be freed, but the pulmonary trunk does.
- Islands of plaque may be left where pericardium is densely adherent and coronary vessels are likely to be present, such as the AV groove.
- Where it is impossible to separate pericardium from the epicardium, without revealing the dark red, raw bulging myocardium, the pericardium can be cross-hatched to reduce constriction (Fig. 11.4).

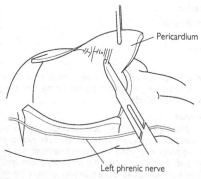

Peri cardium

Left phrenic nerve

Fig. 11.4 Technique of pericardiectomy.

Chronic pericardial effusion

Key facts

- Pericardial effusions are most commonly due to malignancy, or post-cardiotomy Dresslers' syndrome (📖 p264).
- They can be managed by needle pericardiocentesis: surgical pericardial window is useful for recurrent effusions and for obtaining histology.

Pathology

The causes of chronic pericardial effusion include:

- Malignancy involving the pericardium (most commonly from breast and bronchial carcinoma), and malignant syndromes.
- End-stage renal failure, dialysis.
- Collagen vascular diseases.
- Dresslers' post-cardiotomy syndrome.

Presentation

Symptoms may include pericarditic chest pain, angina pectoris, dyspnea, fever, palpitations. Chronic pericardial effusions may be asymptomatic. Signs may include those of cardiac tamponade i.e. ↑JVP, ↓BP, tachycardia, pulsus paradoxus and Kussmaul's sign, as well as a pericardial rub and pedal edema. Chronic pericardial effusion may cause death from tamponade, resolve after pericardiocentesis, or evolve into restrictive chronic pericarditis. Prognosis depends upon the etiology.

Investigation

- EKG shows widespread concave upwards ST segment elevation if acute pericarditis is present, but in chronic pericardial effusion the EKG is often normal or shows low voltages.
- CXR may show an enlarged, 'globular' cardiac silhouette.
- Echocardiography is diagnostic.

Indications for operation

- Relief or prevention of tamponade.
- Symptomatic relief.

Techniques of surgery

Pericardiocentesis

This percutaneous approach to aspiration of a pericardial effusion is described on 📖 p246. It is most commonly carried out by the cardiologists. TTE or TEE guidance is a useful adjunct.

Subxiphoid pericardial window

3–5cm incision in midline starting over xiphoid and extending inferiorly. Divide upper 1–2cm of linea alba and resect xiphoid with bone nibblers. Smooth any sharp bony fragments with bone file. Retract sternum anteriorly, divide pericardial fat, and identify pericardium superior to diaphragm. Carefully grasp pericardium and nick it, and make a 3×3cm window either laterally so that fluid drains into the pleura, or inferiorly so that fluid drains into the pericardium. A Redivac drain should be placed: this can bed removed after 2–3 days if 24 drainage is <25mL.

Video-assisted thorascopic pericardial window

This can be done via a left- or right-sided approach: the advantage of a left-sided approach is that less respiratory compromise is created by dropping the smaller left lung, and the pericardium is closer to the chest wall (helpful if adhesions mean this has to be converted to a minithoracotomy). TEE assessment of where the effusion is largest can decide approach. The approach for left VATS is as described on 📖 p686. The 3x3cm window is created in the pericardium several centimeters anterior to the phrenic nerve, using cautery scissors. If the pericardium does not 'tent' when you grasp it, pick another site to incise as it may be adhesed to the heart. Two intercostal drains are placed via the port sites, and this is placed on suction, and removed when drainage is <50mL/24h.

Advantages and disadvantages of VATs vs. subxiphoid approach

- If patient has evidence of **tamponade**, subxiphoid approach allows quickest relief: if tamponade is marked (hypotension, tachycardia, or RV diastolic collapse on echo) then *surgeon should scrub, prep and drape patient, before induction*, as this can cause loss of cardiac output which will only be relieved by evacuation of effusion.
- Both approaches can result in injury to heart if the pericardium is adhesed at the site of resection: this is easier to control via a subxiphoid approach.
- VATs approach allows aspiration of any pleural effusion, cytology and histology—potentially helpful in malignant disease.
- VATs approach requires set-up for single lung ventilation: in patients with hemodynamic compromise this may not be tolerated.

Outcomes

- Usually possible to remove drains and discharge patients within 48–72h.
- Perhaps 5–10% recurrence rate depending on technique, size of window and etiology: pleural effusion is usually not problematic.

(a)

(b)

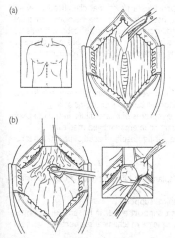

Fig. 11.5 Technique of subxiphoid pericardial window.

Heart failure

Key facts

• Heart failure affects 1–3% of the population, affecting 6 million in the US alone, and accounts for up to 2% of health expenditure.
• The 1-year mortality of NYHA grade IV heart failure is about 60%.
• Ischemic heart disease accounts for around 60% of heart failure.
• Heart failure may be predominantly due to **systolic** and/or **diastolic** dysfunction, and classed clinically as **acute or chronic**, **left and/or right**, and graded by one of three main classification systems (see Box 11.1)

Etiology and pathophysiology

Pathophysiology is described on ☐ p76. Etiology is detailed on ☐ p76, and varies widely between patient populations, e.g., coronary artery disease accounts for 75% of cases of chronic heart failure in white male patients, but only 30% of cases in females. Dilated cardiomyopathy accounts for around 30% of patients on transplant waiting list, and end-stage valvular heart disease a further 5–10%.

Box 11.1 Definition of heart failure

The AHA describes heart failure as 'a clinical syndrome that is characterized by specific symptoms (dyspnea and fatigue) and signs (fluid retention. There is no diagnostic test…because it is largely a clinical diagnosis that is based on a careful history and physical examination)'. Many surgical studies use a definition of LV ejection fraction <30%. Diastolic heart failure is defined as symptoms or signs of heart failure, and abnormal LV relaxation, filling or diastolic distensibility.

Classification of heart failure

The NYHA grading (☐ p2) provides a functional classification which describes symptom severity, is useful for assessing response to treatment, and is widely used in cardiac surgery risk stratification. It was not designed specifically with heart failure in mind and does not correlate well with formal exercise testing, so the ACC/AHA introduced an alternative staging:

ACC/AHA staging system

• Stage A: patient at high risk for developing heart failure in the future.
• Stage B: a structural heart disorder but no symptoms at any stage.
• Stage C: previous or current symptoms of heart failure in the context of an underlying structural heart problem managed medically.
• Stage D: advanced disease requiring hospital-based support, a heart transplant, or palliative care.

UNOS waiting list priority

In patients listed for heart transplant the UNOS status is used to prioritize management (☐ p507):
• Status 1A: patient on mechanical support.
• Status 1B: patient on inotropic support either in hospital or at home.
• Status 2: patient not on inotropic or mechanical support.

Presentation

- **Left heart failure** is characterized by orthopnea, paroxysmal nocturnal dyspnea, and dyspnea at rest, because of pulmonary edema.
- **Right heart failure** presents with hepatic congestion (abdominal discomfort), ascites, and peripheral edema. Congestive heart failure presents with both sets of symptoms.
- Many patients may present immediately or months to years following an MI, with exertional fatigue, dyspnea, and fluid retention.

Investigation

- EKG may show Q waves from old infarctions, AF, wide QRS.
- CXR may show cardiomegaly, pulmonary edema, pleural effusions.
- Echo is diagnostic and quantifies LV and RV function and dimensions, regional wall motion abnormalities, dilatation, hypertrophy, and valvular disease. Exercise or dobutamine stress echo can further identify contractile reserve and hibernating myocardium.
- Viability can be assessed using thallium or technetium (p28).
- MRI is useful to quantify ventricular and valve function and dimensions, ischemia and infarcts (using gadolinium) and viability (dobutamine).
- Deranged LFTs, electrolyte ($\downarrow Na^+$, K^+) and hematological ($\downarrow Hb$) abnormalities are not unusual.
- Right heart catheterization is indicated to assess PVR, PAP, and cardiac output, and coronary angiography is performed in at-risk patients to identify coronary disease.

Medical management

Treatment is directed at treating risk factors and underlying causes, symptom relief, and improving prognosis.

- **Loop diuretics** (furosemide 40–120mg daily, or bumetanide 1–4mg daily) are titrated to response to relieve symptoms of fluid retention, together with potassium-sparing diuretics (spironolactone 50–200mg daily, or amiloride 5–10mg daily) to prevent hypokalemia, and thiazide diuretics (metolazone 2.5–5mg once or twice weekly) in resistant cases.
- **Nitrates** (ISMN 30–120mg daily) improve symptoms by a minor reduction on systemic and pulmonary vascular resistance, and improved coronary perfusion.
- **ACE inhibitors** (captopril 12.5–50mg three times daily, enalapril 10–20mg twice daily) improve symptoms and prognosis through afterload reduction, but patients with renal dysfunction or on potassium-sparing diuretics must be monitored closely for hyperkalemia.
- Careful use of β-**blockers** (bisoprolol 1.25–5mg twice daily, carvedilol 3.125–10mg twice daily) improves symptoms and long-term prognosis through a favourable effect on diastolic function.
- **Digoxin** (62.5–375 micrograms daily) has a mild positive inotropic effect in addition to its antiarrhythmic effect.
- **Atrio-biventricular pacing**, which restores synchronous ventricular contraction, may improve symptoms in patients with widened QRS, and CHF patients should be considered for prophylactic AICD.

Surgery for heart failure

Key facts

Surgical options for heart failure include revascularization, valve surgery, LV remodeling, VADs (📖 pp498–501), and transplantation (📖 pp506–519).

Coronary artery bypass grafting

Coronary artery disease (CAD) is the commonest cause of heart failure. Operative mortality for isolated CABG in selected patients with chronic severe LV dysfunction is around 5%, compared to patients with preserved LV function where it is 1–2%, and long-term survival is poorer. However, selected patients with severe LV dysfunction and CAD still derive significantly more benefit from surgical revascularization than they do from PCI or medical management, in terms of symptoms, freedom from revascularization and survival. Patients with poor LV being considered for CABG should have: (1) **severe, obstructive CAD** with (2) **adequate targets, and** documented evidence of (3) **ischemia** and (4) **substantial viability**. If dyspnea and other failure symptoms predominate over angina then the benefits of CABG are less clear. Patients with severely dilated LV have low likelihood of showing improvement in LVEF, even if they have large areas of viability: concomitant ventricular restoration (📖 p495) may have a role in ameliorating symptoms of heart failure.

Adjuncts to standard management in CABG patients with poor LV
- Preoperative assessment of myocardial viability:
  - Technetium and thallium SPECT, or PET (📖 p28).
  - Dobutamine stress echocardiography (📖 p25).
  - MRI (📖 p29) dobutamine or gadolinium.
- Preoperative nesiritide or NTG infusion to reduce RV afterload, improve myocardial perfusion, and treat pulmonary edema.
- Prophylactic IABP may decrease mortality but carries substantial morbidity in arteriopaths.
- Aggressive myocardial protection with blood cardioplegia given antegradely, retrogradely and down grafts at frequent intervals.

Mitral valve surgery

MR may be the cause or the consequence of heart failure. Organic leaflet disease, e.g., leaflet prolapse causing type II MR (📖 p400) can eventually result in severe LV dysfunction as a result of chronic volume overload. Type IIIb MR (📖 p356) results from LV dilatation which causes posterior displacement of the posteromedial papillary muscle and restricted closure of normal leaflets, as a result of ischemic cardiomyopathy. Dilated cardiomyopathy causes annular dilatation resulting in failure of normal leaflets to coapt causing type I MR. Deciding whether a patient presenting with severe MR and severe LV dysfunction will benefit from surgery or has 'missed the boat' is a common dilemma, particularly as LV function is overestimated in the presence of severe MR:
- Although the operative mortality is 5–15% and patients will still have severe LV dysfunction, surgery is likely to improve symptoms, and may improve survival in patients with LV dysfunction due to MR, if the valve can be repaired. In valves that must be replaced chordal preservation is necessary to achieve prognostic and symptomatic benefit.

- Where MR is secondary to severe LV dysfunction the advantages of mitral surgery over optimal medical management (e.g., β-blockers, ACE inhibitors) and ventricular resynchronization have not been demonstrated. Certain subsets of patients, e.g., those with ischemic cardiomyopathy, suitable targets and evidence of viability; gain symptomatic and prognostic benefit from repair (with a rigid, downsized, remodeling ring).

Left ventricular remodeling

This includes a number of procedures, all of which are based on **Laplace's law** (reduction in LV radial dimensions lead to a reduction in wall tension, and hence improvement in ventricular function).

The Batista procedure (partial left ventriculectomy)

Designed for DCM. Largely been abandoned because of high mortality and morbidity. It involves resection of the posterolateral LV wall, between or including papillary muscles. Mitral repair is sometimes performed from the ventricular aspect. DCM does not affect the LV homogeneously: improved outcomes have been reported when this procedure is limited to patients in whom the lateral LV wall is worst affected.

Dor procedure (left ventricular restoration)

Designed for ischemic cardiomyopathy, the *Dor procedure* excludes scarred dyskinetic and akinetic segments, reshaping the ventricle from its pathological spherical shape and restoring its more physiological elliptical shape. It is usually performed with full revascularization ± mitral repair.

- The LV is opened through scar tissue, subtotal endocardiectomy is performed, the scar tissue is excluded using a circumferential endoventricular purse-string, leaving a smaller LV cavity (often sized using shaped balloon inflated with saline to a volume 50–60 × BSA), and the residual apical defect closed with a Dacron patch (📖 p351).
- Operative mortality has been reported at <2%, with 3-year survival of over 75%, and sustained improvement in NYHA class.
- The STICH trial[1] found that adding SVR to CABG did not improve mortality, symptoms or hospitalization for CHF compared to CABG alone in these patients, but there are several problems with the data (📖 p349).

Cellular cardiomyoplasty (cell transplantation)

These techniques, which are in the early clinical trials, involve implanting cultured suspensions of cardiac, skeletal, or smooth muscle cells; or progenitor cells harvested from bone marrow into injured myocardium.

- Can be done percutaneously with cells infused into coronary arteries in infarcted territory; or directly during surgical revascularization.
- Initial experience suggests that implanted cells engraft within the infarcted region but evidence of clinical benefit from improved regional perfusion, wall thickening and motion, and global motion is lacking.
- Skeletal myocytes implanted into an infarct region adopt a similar morphology to cardiac myocytes but do not have synchronous contractility, and may contribute to arrhythmias.

Reference

1. Jones RH et al. Coronary bypass surgery with or without surgical ventricular reconstruction. *NEJM* 2009; **360**:1705–17.

Ventricular assist devices

Key facts

These are devices that unlike IABP (📖 p192), cardiopulmonary bypass (📖 p102), and ECMO (📖 p500), are anastomosed to the appropriate atrium and outflow vessels to provide augmentation of ventricular outflow.

Types of ventricular assist devices

Side of heart assisted: left, right and biventricular

- The left ventricular assist device (*LVAD*) receives inflow from the LA or LV, and outflows into the aorta.
- The right ventricular assist device (*RVAD*) receives inflow from the RA or RV and outflows into the pulmonary artery.
- The biventricular assist device (*BiVAD*) consists of an RVAD and an LVAD attached in parallel, or a dual chamber device known as a total artificial heart (*TAH*), e.g., Abiomed.

Pulsatile versus non-pulsatile

- Pulsatile: most devices employ pneumatic pumps to drive pusher plates or compress polyurethane sacs giving stroke volumes of up to 85mL (e.g. *Thoratec PVAD, IVAD, AB5000, Berlin heart*), but some electric devices, e.g., *Novacor, Heartmate XVE* are also pulsatile.
- Non-pulsatile devices may be axial, centrifugal, or bearingless magnetic levitators and are generally smaller with fewer moving parts and less surface area in contact with blood, and therefore less thrombogenic, less prone to driveline infections, quieter, and more durable than pulsatile devices.
  - Axial flow pumps include *Heartmate II, MicroMed DeBakey, Jarvik 2000, Impella* (small enough to be inserted percutaneously).
  - Centrifugal devices: *Levotronics, Ventrassist, Tandem Heart.*
  - The *Duraheart* is a bearingless magnetic device.

Intracorporeal (implantable) vs. extracorporeal (external devices)

- Most devices can be implanted, usually intra- or extraperitoneally.
- VADs using axial flow technology (Jarvik 2000, Thoratec HeartMate II, and the DeBakey VAD) can be implanted into small patients.
- VADs used for short-term support, e.g., Centrimag are usually left externally. Pediatric devices, e.g., Berlin Heart, are usually external.
- Electromagnetic flow coupling removes the need to have a power line passing externally, reducing the risk of infection which is the main cause of complications leading to VAD failure or removal.

Indications

These devices are currently indicated for:

- *Bridge to recovery, bridge to decision* (for temporary support in patient with cardiogenic shock with questionable neurologic or end-organ status), **bridge to bridge**:
  - Ultra-short-term, e.g. post AMI cardiogenic shock: Impella, Tandem Heart (both percutaneous, deliver 2–3L cardiac output).
  - Short term, e.g. post cardiotomy cardiogenic shock, myocarditis: Levitontrix Centrimag).

• Short- to long-term, e.g., acute fulminant myocarditis: Thoratec PVAD, AB 5000.
• *Bridge to transplantation*: Heartmate, Heartware, Duraheart, Ventrassist, Debakey.
• *Destinational* (permanent) therapy for patients with refractory heart failure who are not eligible for transplant: Heartmate, Duraheart, Ventrassist, Debakey.

Management of cardiac disease in VAD candidates

Coronary artery disease

Management of CAD depends on the indication for VAD insertion: in high-risk patients undergoing VAD insertion to support revascularization CABG is carried out siting top-ends on the lesser curve of the aorta, leaving plenty of space for LVAD insertion. For implantable long-term LVADs, left-sided grafting is usually not performed, but RCA grafting may be indicated to avoid RV failure post LVAD insertion (📖 p499).

Valvular heart disease

• *Aortic incompetence* >2+ must be treated to prevent blood regurgitating back to the device: leaflets are partially oversewn or bioprosthetic valve replacement is performed.
• *Aortic stenosis* does not need treatment in bridge to transplant patients, but in bridge to recovery patients using a bioprosthetic rather than mechanical valve prosthesis reduces risk of thromboembolism.
• *Mitral regurgitation* generally does not need correction.
• *Mitral stenosis* is addressed to avoid a low output syndrome resulting in the reduction in LV inflow: a bioprosthetic replacement.
• *Tricuspid regurgitation* may improve with improvements in right heart failure, but severe TR should be addressed with annuloplasty (📖 p417).
• *PFO* closed if present.
• A *mechanical AVR* is replaced with a bioprosthesis to reduce risk of thromboembolism associated with stasis across the AVR; if there is a *mechanical MVR* this is left *in situ* and the patient anticoagulated.

Principles of LVAD implantation

• Median sternotomy or sternum-sparing incisions are used: VADs can be implanted on- or off-pump. The pocket for implantable VADs is intra-or extraperitoneal, driveline tunnelled across abdominal wall.
• LV apex is used for inflow: any thrombus is removed and interrupted pledgetted 2/0 Ethibond mattress sutures are placed circumferentially around the ventriculotomy, then through the sewing cuff of the inflow cannula, and tied down.
• The outflow cannula is anastomosed to the greater curvature of the ascending aorta after longitudinal aortotomy with a side-biting cross-clamp. This is done proximally to leave adequate distal aorta for transplantation. The outflow graft is curved gently to the right to avoid kinking and proximity to the midline (facilitating future resternotomy).
• During and after connection of the graft to the device, de-airing is performed though the graft and ascending aorta.
• The VAD is initiated at low speed on partial CPB and full speed is achieved when off CPB (to avoid entraining air).

The VAD patient

Basic principles

- In *LVADs* the LV is connected to the ascending aorta via a pump (□ p496) unloading the LV, optimizing myocardial O_2 supply:demand.
- The aortic valve should open only intermittently: pump output equals cardiac output and the arterial trace is flatline in a non-pulsatile device.
- LVADs deliver up to 10L/min, percutaneous devices (e.g., Impella and Tandem) deliver 2–3L/min.
- In *RVADs* the RA is connected to the PA via a pump (□ p496), which unloads the RV allowing it to recover function. Satisfactory LV function is required for adequate systemic perfusion. RVAD flow is initiated at 2.0–2.5L/min to achieve LAP and RAP 8–16mmHg.
- In *biventricular assist devices* (*BiVADs*) the RVAD and LVAD connected as described earlier, operating in series.
- Flow is determined at the console: alterations in heart rate and filling lead to a compensatory change in stroke volume. A cardiac index of 3.0–5.0L/min, LAP and RAP 10–12mmHg are usual targets.
- LVAD and RVAD rely on adequate function of the unassisted ventricle.

Anticoagulation management for VAD patients

- Postoperative anticoagulation differs between VADS and institutions.
- *Percutaneous short-term devices* (e.g., Impella, Tandem Heart) iv heparin is started immediately.
- *Implantable* VADs (e.g., Jarvik, Thoratec Heartmate II)) usually no anticoagulation is given for first 24–36h immediate postoperatively. Aspirin and warfarin is started after that if no excessive bleeding. Intravenous heparin can be used until INR 2–3.0. Platelet studies can be performed to see the effectiveness of aspirin.
- *Surgical temporary assist devices* (e.g., Centrimag) iv heparin (target APTT 70–90) is usually started 24–48h postoperatively (earlier in LVADs/BiVADs as compared to RVADs). Lower APTT (target 50–70) is required for heparin-bound circuits and cannulas.
- A higher APTT is required in low speed operation or weaning mode.

Common problems

Inability to achieve satisfactory flows

- May be due to hypovolemia, kinking of the inflow or outflow lines, failure of the unassisted ventricle, ventricular arrhythmias, and thrombosis of the device. Check that the external inflow and outflow lines are not kinked. Ensure that the patient is optimally filled and correct arrhythmias. Get a TEE to diagnose tamponade, failure of non-supported ventricle, malplacement of the inflow cannula.

Mediastinal bleeding

- 20–50% of VAD patients bleed excessively postoperatively and reoperation rates for bleeding are high. Multiple factors contribute including surgical suture lines, emergency and reoperative surgery, coagulopathy, or anticoagulation. Antifibrinolytics are given on induction, and meticulous surgical hemostasis is carried out in an attempt to reduce bleeding complications. If the surgeon is confident there is no surgical source, any coagulopathy is corrected aggressively: continued excessive bleeding requires re-exploration. Massive transfusion is described on 📖 p149.

Right ventricular failure

Occurs in 10–20% of patients with LVADs. Suggested by rising CVP, falling VAD flows. RVEDP equal to CVP. TEE diagnostic. It is associated with large volume transfusion (may be cytokine mediated). Medical management— avoiding volume overload. Phosphodiesterase inhibitors, inhaled nitric oxide or prostaglandins, inotropes to increase RB contractility and reduce after-load through lowering PVR. RVAD is required in refractory cases with low RVSWI (RV stroke work index) with higher CVP and lower PA pressures.

Thromboembolism

The incidence is about 5–15 %, higher in the setting of clinically important infections. Head CT to rule out hemorrhage before increasing APTT.

Management of sepsis in VAD patients

Nosocomial infections result in prolonged hospitalization, poor nutritional status, immune suppression from chronic illness, and multiple indwelling monitoring lines. Prevention is critical: strict asepsis during surgery and any intervention, contact precautions, driveline site care, cultures whenever clinical features of infection and appropriate antibiotics. Sepsis is aggressively treated with antibiotics according to sensitivity. For implantable devices driveline site or pump pocket debridements, explant of VAD or urgent transplantation may be required.

Other problems

- *Renal or hepatic dysfunction*: occurs in 1/3 of cases (📖 p236, p276).
- *Hypoxia*: inline oxygenator can be temporarily added to some circuits.
- *Hemolysis*: occurs in ~5 % cases. Patients have anemia, high indirect bilirubin, LDH and free plasma hemoglobin, low haptoglobulin levels. Reduction in VAD speed, and correction of anemia is usually sufficient.
- *Device failure*: usually needs device exchange. Can be explanted.

Weaning VAD support

Weaning is performed with echo assistance (watching LV, RV, septum, volume status). CVP, MAP, PAP, PCW, mixed venous sats are observed for normal/acceptable values. Adequate anticoagulation must be ensured. Small inotropic support is usually required.

Conduct of a code when a patient has a VAD

- ABC: call for help, protect the airway, give O_2—remember VAD patients may stroke, aspirate, and have respiratory causes of arrest.
- Try to feel pulse, assess BP, assess VAD function (look at console and any alarm messages, auscultate pump), assess rhythm:
  - If power failed, may be possible to switch to back-up or hand pump.
  - If no adequate BP *start chest compressions*: risk of rupturing heart is lower than immediate risk of no output.
  - Shock VF/VT: no need to disconnect device.
- Get iv access, give epinephrine and volume, get arterial access and assess PaO_2, $PaCO_2$, and pH and treat aggressively.

Extracorporeal membrane oxygenation

Key facts

- ECMO, also known as extracorporeal life support (ECLS) is based on the same principles as CPB (📖 p192), with several key modifications that allow support to continue for days rather than hours.
- Its primary role is in management of acute respiratory insufficiency in children: it is used as a salvage strategy in adults.
- ECMO is usually instituted via the groin, open or percutaneously, but can also be instituted via central cannulation.

Basic principles

- There are two main types of ECMO: *venovenous* provides respiratory support, and *venoarterial* provides both respiratory and hemodynamic support.
- A typical ECMO circuit consists of:
  - Heparin-bonded circuit usually connecting to femoral venous cannula to the pump and oxygenator, with inflow to a femoral arterial or venous cannula depending on whether it is venovenous or venoarterial ECMO.
  - A hollow-fiber oxygenator with integrated heat-exchanger.
  - Centrifugal pump (these are afterload and inflow dependent, i.e., if downstream or inflow obstruction occurs pump flows will decrease).
- An ECMO circuit differs from a CPB circuit in several regards, that means it can be used for longer periods and with lower heparin levels without the same degree of inflammatory response, coagulopathy, or thromboembolic complications.
  - Use of heparin bonding and hollow-fiber membrane oxygenators.
  - The absence of reservoirs, eliminating blood stasis.
  - The absence of cardiotomy suction and air entrainment, reducing hemolysis and activation of inflammatory and clotting cascades.

Indications for ECMO

Adults

- Severe acute potentially reversible respiratory failure: the CESAR (Conventional ventilatory support versus ECMO for Severe Acute Respiratory failure) trial randomized 180 adults to ECMO or conventional management, with better outcomes at 6 months in the ECMO group. Patients >65 years were excluded.
- No large-scale studies of ECMO for cardiac failure in adults: survivals reported around 20–40% depending on indications for venoarterial ECMO in patients post cardiac arrest, severe cardiogenic shock or failure to wean from CPB.
- It is occasionally used as a bridge to transplant in place of a VAD.

Children

- The indications for ECMO in children are outlined on 📖 pp538–539.

Technique

The technique used very much depends on the setting (e.g., bedside emergency vs. failure to wean from CPB), and whether venovenous (respiratory support only) is intended, or venoarterial for respiratory and hemodynamic support. Generally institution via peripheral percutaneous cannulation is fastest in the bedside setting, when surgical instruments and assistance is not available. In the operating room, femoral cut-down (especially when peripheral pulses are not palpable due to obesity or low output states) allows rapid, accurate placement of both cannulas.

- The CPB cannulas can be used: they are normally reinforced with additional purse-strings and snares.
- Alternatively femoral cannulation—the patient can be weaned and ECMO discontinued at a later date without reopening the chest.
- Advantages of closing the chest include reduced bleeding and infection risk, less need for sedation and repeat anesthetic, and more rapid weaning from the ventilator if that becomes an option.

Failure to wean from cardiopulmonary bypass

- A femoral cut-down is made as for peripheral cannulation (📖 p120). If the patient is stable on CPB an 8mm Dacron graft can be sewn onto the femoral artery, and cannulated with a 14 Sarns: this ensures adequate distal as well as antegrade perfusion.
- Alternatively an 18F Fem Flex II can be inserted through the skin and into the femoral artery under direct vision using a modified Seldinger technique: arterial cannulas inserted in this way should be removed under direct vision, with closure of the arteriotomy with 6/0 Prolene, as the lack of surrounding tissue precludes hemostasis by pressure.
- Axillary cannulation can also be done in the same way, and is useful option in the patient with peripheral vascular or aortic disease
- As large a venous cannula as possible (24–28F) is inserted into the femoral vein using the same modified Seldinger technique.
- The cannulas are carefully de-aired and connected to the circuit, which has also been fully de-aired, bypass is discontinued and the ECMO pump is slowly increased to flows of 4–6L.

Venovenous ECMO

- Percutaneous insertion is generally used, one cannula in each femoral vein: the largest possible venous cannula (24–28F) is directed into the RA under TEE guidance.
- A smaller cannula returns oxygenated blood from the ECMO circuit.

Management

- Oxygenation is dependent on blood flow in venovenous ECMO: near maximum flow rates may be required.
- LV function may worsen: ECMO does not offload the LV as effectively as an LVAD, and progressive low cardiac output may result in LV distension, pulmonary hypertension, and eventually catastrophic pulmonary hemorrhage.
- Inotropes and an IABP may be indicated, along with LV decompression (percutaneous balloon atrial septostomy).

Basic transplant immunology

Allorecognition is a by-product of a system that evolved to recognize and eliminate infectious agents, by identifying peptide fragments as 'self' or 'non-self'. The mammalian immune system is conventionally considered in two parts: innate and adaptive. Allorecognition is a function mainly of the adaptive immune response.

Allorecognition

Allorecognition depends on two main processes. Firstly, alloantigen must be taken up and complexed with surface MHC molecules on antigen presenting cells (APCs). Direct recognition is where donor APCs within the allograft perform this function. Indirect recognition is where host APCs do this. Secondly, antigen-specific host T cell receptors must bind to the peptide fragments of alloantigen complexed with the MHC molecules on APCs, which include B cells, dendritic, and Langerhans cells.

B- and T-cell diversity

APCs are able to identify, take-up, and present alloantigen because of the presence of B-cell receptors (BCRs) specific for each alloantigen. Similarly T-cell receptors (TCRs) are specific to each alloantigen. The production of a huge number of receptors (approximately 2.5×10^7), each specific to a particular peptide fragment, is possible because of the millions of potential combinations of the thousands of TCR and BCR gene segments. The TCR gene segments are located on chromosomes 14 and 7; the BCR gene fragments are on chromosome 14.

T-cell activation

When the TCR binds to antigen complexed with MHC molecules a chain of reactions between intracellular signalling molecules leads to cell apoptosis unless CD4 or CD8 also binds to the MHC. There are a number of other co-stimulatory molecules. Binding of the TCR as well as CD and co-stimulatory molecules with the MHC leads to T-cell activation, differentiation and clonal expansion. This results in the rapid production of large numbers of cells able to coordinate and effect destruction of tissues bearing the specific alloantigen: this manifests clinically as rejection.

Rejection

There are several types of rejection:
- *Hyperacute rejection* (HAR) is mediated by preformed antibodies that bind to antigens of ABO blood groups, non-self HLA, and xenografts similar to antigens found on bacteria and viruses, and results in immediate tissue edema, hemorrhage, and thrombosis.
- *Acute rejection* is a function of both the innate and the adaptive immune system, triggered by the recognition of foreign MHC and foreign peptides presented by self-MHC, by T cells, and results in tissue destruction over days to many months after transplant.
- *Chronic rejection* is a poorly understood vasculopathy which occurs over years: it is probably a function of the adaptive immune system mediated predominantly through indirect recognition.

A glossary of terms in transplant immunology

Adaptive immunity: learned response to specific non-self antigens.

Allo-: tissue from a genetically different member of the same species. Alloantigen: antigen from a genetically different member of the same species. Allogenicity: ability of tissue to provoke an immune response when transplanted into genetically different member of the same species. Allorecognition: recognition of alloantigen as non-self.

Antigen: cell surface glycoproteins.

Antibody: specific proteins produced by B cells in response to non-self antigen, consisting of two light and two heavy chain proteins, composed in a constant and a variable region. The variable chain region binds with the antigen that triggered the response, and the constant region coordinates the cellular response.

APC (antigen presenting cells): these cells ingest and process antigen, then present it bound to surface MHC to T cells. APCs are most commonly found B cells, but other leukocytes can act as APCs.

B cells: B cells mature in bone marrow. They are APCs which can produce antibodies. In response to antigen they undergo clonal expansion, triggered and coordinated by T-helper cells.

Cellular immunity: adaptive immunity.

CD: cellular differentiation molecule (followed by a number, e.g., CD4).

Clonal expansion: production of large numbers of identical cells.

Co-stimulatory molecules: molecule receptors that must be activated, in addition to a main receptor, for a process to happen.

Direct recognition: donor APCs present alloantigen to host T cells.

Indirect recognition: host APCs present alloantigen to host T cells.

Innate immunity: instant inbuilt response to certain non-self proteins.

HLA (human leukocyte antigen): human MHC.

Humoral immunity: innate immunity.

MHC (major histocompatibility complex): glycoproteins expressed on the surface of all cells, unique to that individual, coded for by the MHC genes on chromosome 6. Alloantigen must be bound to MHC for T cells to recognize it. There are two classes of MHC. Class I (HLA molecules A, B, and C) is present on all cell membranes. Class II (HLA molecules DP, DQ, and DR), also known as minor histocompatibility complex, is present on only certain cell types. Class II is less allogeneic.

Rejection: destruction of tissue by host immune response (📖 p502).

T cells: T cells mature in the thymus. T cells that bind to thymic tissue (self) are destroyed. T-helper cells, which are CD8 +ve, coordinate and T cytotoxic cells (CD4 +ve) effect the response.

Patient selection

Key facts

The following guidelines for patient and donor selection are taken from the International Society of Heart and Lung Transplantation (ISHLT) Recommendations for Donor Heart Selection 2010.

Indications for heart transplantation

- Refractory heart failure (stage D).
- Ischemic heart disease with intractable angina not amenable to revascularization or responsive to maximal medical therapy.
- Intractable arrhythmia not amenable to ablative therapy, not responsive to maximal medical therapy.
- Hypertrophic cardiomyopathy that has failed maximal medical and surgical therapy.
- Congenital heart disease.
- Cardiac tumor confined to myocardium without metastases.

Contraindications to heart transplantation

- Age >70 years.
- Fixed pulmonary hypertension.
- Life threatening, life-limiting illness, e.g., HIV, malignancy.
- Sepsis including endocarditis.
- Active peptic ulcer.
- Continued abuse of alcohol or other drugs.
- Irreversible secondary organ failure not appropriate for combined transplant.
- Diabetes with end-organ dysfunction.
- Multisystem SLE/sarcoid.
- Psychiatric history likely to result in non-compliance.
- Severe peripheral or cerebrovascular disease.
- Malignancy (except cardiac with low probability of metastasis).
- Lack of psychosocial support.

Patient assessment

Once a patient has been referred assessment normally takes place in two main stages: an initial detailed outpatient assessment designed to avoid invasive and costly investigations in a patient who is clearly unsuitable for transplantation, followed in appropriate cases by a 2–4-day inpatient assessment. The goals of the inpatient assessment are:

- To assess the patient's clinical, psychological, and social suitability.
- To ensure that the patient and relatives are fully informed about all aspects of being on the transplant list, the procedure, and aftercare.
- To familiarize the patient with the transplant unit and staff.
- To optimize the patient's clinical, psychological, and social condition.

Accepting a patient on to the transplant list

The results of these investigations are considered at a multidisciplinary meeting attended by cardiothoracic surgeons, cardiac anesthesiologists, cardiologists, respiratory physicians, transplant coordinators and nurses, dieticians, and physiotherapists. This is usually after the patient's discharge. The patient is informed of the decision and receives:

- A detailed explanation of the waiting list procedures (including their responsibility to be available for potential transplant at all times, and duty to inform the transplant team of any changes in their health, circumstance, medication, and planned holidays).
- A booklet describing this in more detail, and explaining what to do when called for surgery, the operation, accommodation for partners, publicity and the media, wards, and departments after surgery.

Routine investigations in transplant assessment

- A detailed history and physical examination.
- CXR, lung function testing, chest CT if >65 years.
- Cardiovascular evaluation:
  - 12-lead EKG, Holter, echo.
  - Thallium, PET or MRI for viability.
  - Right and left heart catheterization.
  - Exercise stress with VO_2max.
  - Myocardial biopsy for CHF of unknown etiology.
- FBC, ESR, APTT, PT, INR, fibrinogen, reticulocytes.
- Plasma viscosity.
- U&Es, creatinine, creatinine clearance, urate, calcium, phosphate, liver enzymes, cardiac enzymes, fasting blood glucose and lipids, amylase.
- Screening for malignancies: PSA, mammogram, PAP smear, endoscopy as indicated.
- MSU, urinalysis, nose swab and MRSA screen.
- 24h urine, creatinine clearance, renal function, urinalysis, ultrasound and pyelogram as indicated.
- Full dental assessment and repair, bone densitometry.
- Serology for Hep B/C, HIV, syphilis, rubella, EBV, herpes varicella and zoster, CMV, toxoplasma, fungal, parasites.
- AMF, anti DNA, SCAT/LATEX.
- HLA typing, lymphotoxic and blood group antibody screen.
- Neuropsychiatric assessment.
- Physiotherapy and social work assessment.

Donor selection and matching

Key facts

- Donor hearts are ideally from patients aged <45 years, with LVEF >40% on minimal inotropic support, with absence of structural or functional valve disease (including endocarditis) and no coronary disease.
- The alternate list provides less optimal donor hearts: from patients >55 years of age, with valve disease that can be treated by bench repair or replacement, or coronary disease that could be bypassed.
- An estimated ischemic time of <4h is preferable.
- The donor body weight should not be <30% of the recipient's weight in females (20% in males), and hearts must be ABO compatible.

Donor selection

Patients are considered for organ donation if there is evidence of brainstem death (apnea, absent papillary reflexes, irreversibility over 24h, and absence of reversible causes) and prior consent. Potential donors undergo a review of their history and clinical examination, EKG, CXR, ABGs, ABO typing, testing for HIV, hepatitis C and B, HCV and CMV, and echocardiography. The shortage of donor organs means the criteria for donor suitability are elastic:

- *Age <45* ideal, 45–55 years acceptable. >55 years in specific situations.
- *LVEF >40%*, no major regional wall motion abnormalities, no intractable arrhythmias, no excessive inotropes. Absence of EKG findings of LVH, wall thickness<14mm on echo.
- *Valves*: absence of structural or functional valve disease (bench repair most commonly of tricuspid valve and replacement acceptable).
- *Coronaries*: absence of obstructive disease of major coronary arteries (concomitant CABG can be considered for alternate list).
- *Estimated ischemic time*: <4h preferable, but can be more when other conditions favourable, and in sparsely populated areas, e.g., in Canada longer ischemic times are the norm.
- *Toxins:* cocaine use OK if cardiac function acceptable, and no LVH. History of alcohol abuse usually not acceptable. Poisoning acceptable if all other parameters OK.
- *Sepsis:* acceptable if recent cultures negative after treatment with antibiotics according to sensitivities, and no evidence of endocarditis. HIV is an absolute contraindication; Hep B and C are relative contraindications.
- Absence of prolonged cardiac arrest, prolonged ↓↓BP, pre-existing cardiac disease, chest trauma, or intracardiac drug injection, extracerebral malignancy.

Matching donors and recipients

The shortage of donor organs led to the formation of authorities designed to coordinate the transplant recipient list and donor availability, so that organs are allocated to the most suitable recipient, e.g., UNOS (United Network for Organ Sharing) in the US, UK Transplant in the UK. The following factors are taken into account:

Logistics

Geographical limitations are important to minimize ischemic time to <4h wherever possible.

Priority

In patients listed for heart transplant the *UNOS status* is used to prioritize management:

- *Status 1A:* patient admitted in listing transplant centre with at least one of the following:
  - VAD ≥30 days, or TAH, IABP or ECMO.
  - Mechanical circulatory support <30 days, but device-related complications.
  - Mechanical ventilation.
  - High-dose or multiple inotropes, or continuous hemodynamic monitoring.
  - Life expectancy <7 days.
- *Status 1B:* VAD <30 days without complications, or continuous iv inotropes.
- *Status 2:* all other actively listed patients.

Histocompatibility

ABO compatibility

Donor and recipient must be ABO compatible: hyperacute rejection (HAR) occurs in ABO incompatible patients. Flow cytometry ABO testing is more sensitive than cytotoxic testing. In infants, with underdeveloped complement system and low levels of isohemagglutinins, ABO mismatched transplants have been carried out without *HAR* and with good long-term outcomes. Some have extended use to children 2 years of age.

HLA typing

Although hearts are amongst the least allogeneic organs, and a HLA mismatch is not a contraindication to transplantation, HLA-A$_2$ or A$_3$ mismatch has been associated with chronic rejection, and some centers choose to avoid this. HLA typing is important as it guides immunosuppression postoperatively. Pre-formed antibodies in the recipient sera are detected by adding patient sera to a panel of 40–60 HLA antigens. This is called a *lymphocyte toxicity screen*. If more than 10% show reactivity a lymphocyte cross-match between recipient candidate to donor must be performed, as pre-formed antibodies mediate hyperacute rejection. A positive lymphocyte cross-match means a high probability of hyperacute rejection, and the donor is rejected for that recipient.

Virology

CMV +ve hearts are given preferentially to CMV +ve patients, and CMV −ve hearts are ideally given to CMV −ve patients.

Size

Recipient and donor should be a similar size (see 📖 p506).

Donor preparation

Management of the organ donor

In order to optimize donor organs, the donor should have invasive monitoring with a radial arterial line, central venous line, and urinary catheter, pulse oximetry and EKG monitoring. Hypotension, hypothermia, and diabetes insipidus frequently accompany brain death. In addition to continued mechanical ventilation, it is often necessary to carry out large-volume fluid resuscitation, active warming, and inotropic support.

Organ procurement

Harvest of multiple organs is common: liver and heart teams both want to maximize the length of IVC they procure, the same if lungs are being harvested. Inotropic, volume, and respiratory support is continued until the thoracic viscera are excised.

Prior to incision

- A final check of donor identity, UNOS ID, organ donation consent, brain death certification, and serology is made.
- The donor chart is read for history and investigations. The CXR, EKG, cardiac cath, and echo are reviewed; donor hemodynamics are discussed with the anesthesiologist.
- The plan/timings discussed with the abdominal procuring teams, and confirmed with the recipient surgeon (to ensure arrival of donor heart coordinates with timing of recipient cardiectomy).

Technique of donor cardiectomy

- A midline incision from sternal notch to pubis is made.
- A median sternotomy is made with liberal use of bone wax and cautery to minimize bleeding, pericardium opened and hitched to the skin.
- The **heart is carefully examined** for evidence of trauma, regional wall motion abnormalities, including palpation for aortic or coronary calcification, and thrills.
- Findings are discussed with the recipient transplant surgeon and the heart is accepted, and timing of cross-clamping agreed.
- Once the abdominal teams have finished their preliminary dissection, the aorta is mobilized as far as the innominate artery and a cardioplegia purse-string placed, and the SVC is mobilized, avoiding the SA node.
- When all teams are ready **30 000U of heparin** iv is given centrally.
- The central line is withdrawn so that the **SVC can be clamped** as far distally as possible, the **azygos ligated**, and the IVC is partially divided anteriorly: make sure you have adequate length as the liver team will try to take this up to the RA.
- The **right superior pulmonary vein is opened** to vent the left heart.
- The cardioplegia tubing is carefully de-aired, connected to the cannula, aorta is cross-clamped, and 1L **cold crystalloid cardioplegia** (Celsior low to moderate K⁺, high sodium extracellular in adults, Del Nido in children taking care to avoid overdistension of the root) infused.
- The pericardial sling is filled with ice-cold saline: palpate the heart frequently to ensure root pressure adequate and heart decompressed.

- The *IVC incision is completed*, the *right and left pulmonary veins are divided* at the pericardial reflection (Fig. 11.6).
- The heart is pulled down, the *clamp removed and the aorta is divided* as high as possible (in paediatric transplants the aortic arch, innominate vein, and pericardium are taken), *pulmonary arteries are divided* at the pericardial reflections, and the *SVC divided* below the tie.
- Finally the connective tissue at the pericardial reflection behind the left atrium is divided, allowing the *heart to be removed* from the chest.
- The heart is immediately immersed in cold isotonic solution.
- It is *inspected carefully* for any injuries (e.g., laceration to coronary sinus) and congenital anomalies.
- The chambers are irrigated with cold isotonic solution and the heart placed in three serial sterile plastic bags containing cold saline and ice without air, and transferred to an ice chest.
- If *lungs harvested* vent heart through LA appendage instead of RSPV, divide PA at bifurcation, and divide LA leaving atrial cuff and pulmonary veins with lungs.

Organ preservation

Preservation means ischemic times up to 6h may be tolerated, but the key to minimizing ischemic injury remains minimizing ischemic time. A variety of storage solutions are used at temperatures of 4–10°C. Two categories exist: intracellular solutions characterized by high K^+ and low Na^+, e.g. Bretschneider (HTK), or extracellular with low to moderate K^+ and high Na^+, e.g. St Thomas' cardioplegia solution. Intracellular solutions may offer better protection against cellular edema; extracellular solutions may reduce cellular damage associated with hyperkalemia.

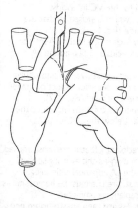

Fig. 11.6 Donor heart harvest. Division of the great vessels: leave as much length on the heart as possible in all cases.

Orthotopic cardiac transplant

Key facts

There are several techniques of orthotopic heart transplantation:

- *Original Shumway technique* where donor LA is anastomosed to recipient LA, and RA to RA.
- *Wythenshawe bicaval technique*: separate SVC to SVC and IVC to IVC anastomoses, instead of single right atrial anastomosis.
- *Total technique*: bicaval end-to-end anastomoses, and bilateral pulmonary venous cuffs of recipient anastomosed to right and left half of donor LA.
- Anastomosing atria to atria is technically less demanding than bicaval anastomosis, or the total technique, but total technique reduces atrial redundancy and tricuspid regurgitation, improving atrial function, and reduces postoperative arrhythmias including need for PPM.

Bicaval anastomosis technique

Recipient cardiectomy

The recipient procedure is timed so that the recipient cardiectomy can be performed at the time of donor heart arrival: it is occasionally necessary to ask the procurement team to delay clamping the aorta if resternotomy and mediastinal dissection takes longer in complex reops.

- Midline sternotomy.
- Aortobicaval CPB with IVC and SVC cannulated directly and snared, and vacuum-assisted venous return.
- The *donor heart is inspected* before recipient cardiectomy proceeds.
- The *aorta is cross-clamped*.
- The *RA is incised* parallel to the AV groove, extending the incision towards the LA superiorly and medial to the IVC inferiorly.
- The heart is lifted up to expose the *LA which is incised* so that the incision extends towards the RA incision (Fig. 11.7).
- The *septum is divided* between the two incisions, and the LA incision continued in front of the left pulmonary veins and behind the LA appendage.
- The *aorta and pulmonary trunk are divided* just above the sinotubular junction and retracted inferiorly so that the superior aspect of the left atrium is exposed and the *atrial incisions continued* (Fig. 11.7).
- The *right atrium is divided* so that a generous cuff remains above the IVC cannula, and the SVC is divided far below the SVC cannula.

Donor heart implantation

- *Left atrial anastomosis*: the donor and recipient left atria are anastomosed with continuous 3/0 Prolene, taking 1cm margins and everting so that intima is opposed to intima, starting at the LA appendage, finishing laterally over the pulmonary veins. This suture line must be hemostatic as it is relatively inaccessible once the transplant is completed.
- *Great vessels*: the donor and recipient PAs are then anastomosed end to end with 4/0 Prolene, followed by anastomosis of the aorta.
- To minimize ischemic time the aorta can be anastomosed immediately after the LA, and the clamp removed, allowing the heart to reperfuse while the right-sided anastomoses are completed.

- *Caval anastomoses*: the end-to-end anastomoses of the *IVC and SVC* are performed next with 4/0 Prolene: the IVC is first as this has the least possibility for adjustment, whereas both recipient and donor SVC are long enough to be tailored.
- *High-dose (1g) methylprednisone is given before reperfusion.*
- The heart is de-aired, the anastomoses secured, and after placing an aortic root vent, the cross-clamp is removed and the heart reperfused.

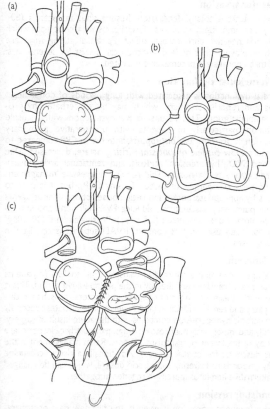

Fig. 11.7 Orthotopic heart transplantation. (a) Recipient for bicaval anastomosis. (b) Recipient for classic anastomosis. (c) Left atrial anastomosis being performed during bicaval technique.

Transplant care on ICU

Key facts

- Transplant patients face the same problems and receive the same management as patients who have undergone cardiac surgery.
- *Immunosuppression, rejection* (📖 p514), and *sepsis* (including atypical organisms such as CMV and fungus) are specific to transplant patients.
- Complications more commonly seen in cardiac transplants than other cardiac surgery patients include *sinus node dysfunction*, *RV dysfunction* which may be severe, and *renal dysfunction*.

Cardiac denervation

The donor heart is totally denervated. Resting sinus tachycardia (80–110bpm) is common because of loss of vagal parasympathetic input which normally has negative chronotropic effect. Epicardial pacing wires are routinely employed. Sinus node dysfunction can persist for several days, beyond that a permanent pacemaker is indicated.

Right ventricular dysfunction

Myocardial dysfunction is associated with long periods of donor heart ischemia and reperfusion injury, which may be exacerbated by protamine administration. This results in RV dysfunction with tricuspid regurgitation, particularly in patients with preoperative pulmonary hypertension. It presents as a *disproportionate rise in CVP* compared to PA pressures, *low cardiac output state* (rising lactate, decreased urine output and SVO_2, hypotension, acidosis, and ventricular arrhythmias). Echocardiography is diagnostic. This requires aggressive management (including early recognition of cause of rising CVP): but it is best to avoid this by appropriate donor and recipient selection. Various agents dilate the pulmonary vasculature, reducing PVR: milrinone and inhaled NO have already been discussed (📖 p191). Prostaglandin E (30–50ng/kg/min) has been used in this context. RVAD support is required in refractory cases.

Renal function

Renal failure is common after cardiac transplant: up to 15% of patients will require renal replacement therapy in the perioperative period. This is because firstly, there a number of common risk factors for ischemic cardiomyopathy and renal dysfunction (age, hypertension, diabetes); secondly because chronic hypoperfusion combines with the acute insult of surgery; and thirdly and importantly nephrotoxic drugs, particularly ciclosporin, are a mainstay of treatment of transplant patients. Renal management is the same as described for cardiac surgery. Additionally a rise in creatinine normally responds to lowering ciclosporin dosage, which can be changed for an alternative immunosuppressive regimen altogether.

Immunosuppression

High-dose immunosuppression is given in the first few days postoperatively and reduced to maintenance doses. A standard regimen for the first 24h postoperatively includes ciclosporin 2mg/kg/day iv (or tacrolimus if renal function is adequate), methylprednisolone 125mg iv three times daily, and azathioprine 2mg/kg iv 6-hourly, or mycophenolate mofetil 1.5gm iv 12-hourly. OKT3 may be used instead of ciclosporin.

Antibiotic prophylaxis

As a result of early high-dose immunosuppression the patient is vulnerable to infection in the early postoperative period. Standard antibiotic prophylaxis lasts for 48h (flucloxacillin 1g 6-hourly iv). Nystatin or amphotericin are given orally for 4–6 weeks to prevent oral candidiasis. Trimethoprim 200mg 8-hourly po is given for prevention of *Pneumocystis jiroveci (carinii)* infection. CMV −ve blood products or leukocyte-depleted blood should be given to CMV −ve recipients. If the donor heart was CMV +ve then ganciclovir should be given for 2 weeks postoperatively.

Sepsis

Common within the first 3 months, or after treatment of acute rejection. Commonest organisms are *E. coli*, *Pseudomonas* spp, *Staphylococcus* spp. Aggressive treatment with antimicrobials and reduction in immunosuppression may be required.

Lung and heart–lung transplantation

In lung and heart–lung transplantation ventilatory management is the most significant challenge. This is primarily dependent on the quality of the donor organ, the duration of the ischemic time, and the quality of preservation. Respiratory dysfunction in the early postoperative period is the result of a number of processes:

- Ischemia/reperfusion injury as a result of long ischemic times and inadequate preservation leads to increased capillary permeability.
- Impairment of lymphatic drainage may exacerbate pulmonary edema.
- In bilateral sequential lung transplant the first implanted lung receives all the cardiac output while the second lung is being implanted: edema is normally more pronounced in this lung.
- Other causes of impaired respiratory function include subclinical disease in the implanted lung, shock, sepsis, multiple transfusion, and LV failure.

Positive pressure support is normally required for several days, but early extubation reduces the pressure on suture lines and negative effects on right ventricular function. Respiratory management aims to use the lowest FiO_2 to produce a PaO_2 >10kPa to minimize the risk of barotrauma. Peak inspiratory pressures are kept low by increasing respiratory rate rather than tidal volumes to achieve optimal minute volumes. Minute volumes are high to achieve relative hypocapnia which helps reduce pulmonary vascular resistance. PEEP is not used in patients with COPD in residual native lung as hyperinflation results. Great care must be taken to avoid volume overload and consequent pulmonary edema.

Rejection

The goal of immunosuppression is to inhibit the immune response to alloantigen, while preserving the immune response to infection and malignancy. Immunosuppression consists of a short, intense induction phase followed by a permanent maintenance phase. A careful balance is maintained between therapeutic and toxic doses of immunosuppression: this is achieved by combining drugs with different mechanisms of action.

Immunosuppressive agents

Corticosteroids
Corticosteroids inhibit the immune response at many levels. They decrease production of λ-interferon and interleukins which would normally cause upregulation of the lymphocyte response; and reduce macrophage function.

Ciclosporin (CYA)
Ciclosporin is a calcineurin inhibitor: it inhibits the production of IL-2 by T-helper cells, selectively reducing the cytotoxic T-cell response.

Tacrolimus (FK506)
Tacrolimus is also a calcineurin inhibitor with a similar profile.

Mycophenolate mofetil (MMF)
MMF inhibits purine synthesis in lymphocytes, reducing clonal expansion, and lymphocyte counts.

Azathioprine (AZA)
Azathioprine causes dose-related bone marrow suppression by suppression of purine synthesis.

Sirolimus (rapamycin)
Sirolimus stops IL-2 triggering clonal expansion of T lymphocytes.

Daclizumab, basiliximab
IL-2 receptor blockers which prevent clonal expansion of T cells.

OKT3
OKT3 is a monoclonal antibody produced in mice that binds the CD3 receptor site on cytotoxic T cells, preventing antigen recognition and clonal expansion.

Polyclonal antibody (e.g., antithymocyte globulin)
These are produced by animals after immunization with HLA: they attach to most circulating lymphocytes effecting a reduction in cell counts to less than 10% of normal.

Simvastatin
• Simvastatin has a moderate protective effect against chronic rejection: it suppresses T-cell function.

Acute rejection

Diagnosis

Clinical features include low-grade fever, malaise, reduced exercise tolerance, pericardial rub, supraventricular arrhythmias, low cardiac output, and signs of congestive cardiac failure. Blood tests reveal a lymphocytosis. As all patients are on immunosuppression, symptoms may be minimal until rejection is quite advanced, so routine surveillance is undertaken. Hemodynamic measurements with a PA catheter may be helpful, but the gold standard diagnostic tool is RV endomyocardial biopsy: usually via a right internal jugular percutaneous approach. This is carried out every 7–10 days for a month, tapering to 2–6-month intervals. Lymphocyte infiltration and myocyte necrosis is used to grade the severity of cellular rejection. Biopsy-negative cardiac dysfunction raises the possibility of accelerated coronary artery disease or vascular rejection.

Management

- Asymptomatic mild rejection is monitored but not routinely treated.
- Myocyte necrosis is a definite indication for increased immunosuppression, but intermediate grades are treated according to clinical context.
- 3 days iv methylprednisolone 1000mg/day for acute rejection within 3 months of transplant, or for severe episodes.
- 100mg/day po methylprednisolone on a reducing dose over several weeks for all other episodes.
- Repeat endomyocardial biopsy after 7–10 days: repeat steroid course if no improvement, or give rescue therapy if hemodynamically unstable.
- Rescue protocols include methylprednisolone + OKT3, or methotrexate.
- Total lymphoid irradiation and photophoresis has been used in refractory rejection.
- Retransplantation is no longer performed in many centres for refractory rejection as results are extremely poor.

Chronic rejection

Chronic rejection manifests as allograft CAD, detectable in over half of cardiac transplant patients within 5 years of transplantation, and within months in a few patients. Other processes that have been associated with allograft coronary disease include increased donor age, hyperlipidemia, and CMV infection. Ischemia is frequently silent as the heart is denervated. The clinical picture includes ventricular arrhythmias, congestive cardiac failure, and sudden death. Coronary angiography is the gold standard investigation but may underestimate the extent of the disease as the morphology is diffuse, smooth, intimal proliferation. There is no effective treatment apart from retransplantation. Prophylaxis centers on the same risk reduction strategies used in native ischemic heart disease.

Heart transplantation results

Infection

Non-specific suppression of lymphocyte activation, differentiation, proliferation, and function by immunosuppression means that transplant patients are particularly prone to infection which may be life threatening. The use of more selective immunosuppressive agents such as ciclosporin and tacrolimus, and a more conservative approach to treating low-grade, asymptomatic rejection, mean that the frequency and severity of infection post-transplant have fallen in the last few years (Table 11.1).

- CMV, *Toxoplasma gondii*, HBV, HCV, and HIV may be transmitted to the recipient from the graft.
- Infections in first month are most commonly nosocomial, months 1–6 opportunistic, after 6 months community acquired or opportunistic.

Table 11.1 Infections post transplantation

Infection/site	Organism	Treatment
Within 30 days		
Pneumonia	Gram −ve bacilli	Imipenem, ceftazidime
Sternal wound	*Staphylococcus epidermidis*, *S. aureus*,	Flucloxacillin, vancomycin
	Gram −ve bacilli	Imipenem, ceftazidime
Line associated	*S. epidermidis*, *S. aureus*,	Flucloxacillin, vancomycin
	Gram −ve bacilli	Imipenem, ceftazidime
	Candida albicans	Fluconazole,
Urinary tract	Gram −ve bacilli, *Enterococcus*	Imipenem, ceftazidime
	Candida albicans	Fluconazole
Mucocutaneous	Herpes simplex virus,	Aciclovir
	Candida sp.	Fluconazole
After 30 days		
Pneumonia	*Pneumocystis jiroveci (carinii)*	Trimethoprim
	Cytomegalovirus, herpes simplex virus	Ganciclovir, aciclovir
	Haemophilus influenzae,	Augmentin
	Cryptococcus, *Aspergillus*, *Myocbacterium* spp.	Amphotericin
		Isoniazid, rifampicin
CNS	*Toxoplasma gondii*, *Aspergillus*, *Cryptococcus*, *Listeria*	Daraprim
		Amphotericin
GI tract	*Candida albicans*, herpes simplex virus, *Aspergillus*,	Fluconazole Aciclovir
Cutaneous	Herpes simplex virus, varicella-zoster, *Candida*, *Mycobacterium*	

Renal failure

Cardiac and renal disease frequently coexist because they share common etiologies. Up to 70% of patients awaiting heart transplantation suffer from diabetes and atherosclerosis in addition to low cardiac output states, which predispose to renal impairment. Progression of renal failure is common in the later stages of cardiac disease: many patients develop end-stage renal failure while on the waiting list for heart transplantation. Native renal function may also be compromised after heart transplantation by factors including perioperative low cardiac output states, nephrotoxic antibiotics, and immunosuppressive regimens particularly calcineurin inhibitors which cause irreversible interstitial fibrosis. Although renal function can improve dramatically after restoration of blood flow, a minority of patients develop dialysis-dependent renal failure following transplantation. The survival of such patients is dramatically reduced: a creatinine clearance <40mL/min is therefore an accepted contraindication to heart transplantation. Frequent monitoring of ciclosporin levels with dose titration, and avoidance of hypovolemia are important adjuncts in the prevention of renal failure.

Hypertension

The majority of heart transplant recipients develop severe to moderate hypertension that is usually refractory to single therapy management. The etiology is poorly understood, but it is thought to include a combination of fluid retention as a result of ciclosporin-induced nephrotoxicity, and sympathetic-mediated vasoconstriction.

Hyperlipidemia and glucose intolerance

Hyperlipidemia and glucose intolerance develop in most patients as a result of immunosuppressive regimens. Both are treated aggressively to reduce the risk of early CAD. Simvastatin is used for both its lipid lowering effect and its ability to suppress T-cell function and the onset of chronic rejection.

Malignancy

The incidence of malignancy is 100× greater in heart transplant patients than in the general population: the majority of neoplasias are lymphoproliferative disorders and cutaneous carcinomas. The reason for this is this decrease in the T-lymphocyte response to EBV as a result of immunosuppression. In addition to conventional therapies for malignancy (chemotherapy, radiotherapy, and resection), immunosuppression may be reduced, and EBV treated with ganciclovir.

Other complications

Osteoporosis, avascular necrosis, biliary stasis and cholelithiasis, and obesity are common.

Results of cardiac transplantation

- UK 30-day mortality is 4%.
- 1-year survival is 82%.
- 5-year survival is 75%.

Heart–lung transplantation

Key facts

- Heart–lung transplantation is not performed often: in 2008 only 73 such transplants were performed worldwide.
- This is because as results of single and double lung transplantation have improved, the indication for heart–lung transplant has reduced. At the same time pressure on donor organs means that organ blocs are usually divided to ensure maximum benefit to the greatest number of high-priority recipients.
- The *domino procedure*, where a heart–lung transplant was performed for septic lung disease and the healthy explanted heart then transplanted into a second recipient, is now rarely performed.

Indications

Patients are in end-stage cardiopulmonary disease with a life expectancy of 18–24 months. Congenital heart disease with secondary pulmonary hypertension or Eisenmenger syndrome (30%) is the commonest indication. Primary pulmonary hypertension with right-sided heart failure (cystic fibrosis, COPD, idiopathic pulmonary fibrosis) is the second commonest indication, but these cases are increasingly treated by lung transplant as native RV function often recovers.

Contraindications

- Significant multisystem disease.
- Renal dysfunction.
- Malignancy.
- HIV, hepatitis B, hepatitis C with biopsy-proven liver disease.
- Infection with resistant respiratory flora.
- Mechanical ventilation.
- Relative contraindications include age >50, active extrapulmonary infection, peptic ulcer disease, continued smoking, high-dose steroids.

Investigations and management of the recipient

The panel of investigations listed on p504 is carried out, additionally:

- Sputum for Gram stain, AFB and bacterial, mycobacterial, and fungal cultures.
- Thoracic measurements.
- Cystic fibrosis patients require specialist management including endoscopic maxillary antrostomies for sinus irrigation to decrease the bacterial load in the upper respiratory tract.

Matching donor to recipient

Donor organs are matched to recipient on the basis of:

- Strict ABO compatibility.
- Donor and recipient height so that lung sizes are appropriate.
- HLA matching is not necessary but improved graft survival is associated with matching HLA-B, HLA-A, and HLA-DR loci.
- Lymphocyte toxicity screen <25% reactive.
- Negative donor–recipient cross-match if the screen is >25%.

Technique of donor procurement

- The set-up is similar to that described for cardiectomy on 📖 p508.
- Median sternotomy.
- The inferior pulmonary ligaments are divided.
- The pericardium is opened and hitched to the skin, dissected off the ascending aorta, vena cavae, PA, and trachea, and excised to the hilum.
- Cardioplegia is infused into the aortic root, pulmonoplegia infused into the PA (📖 p508), and topical cold poured over the heart.
- The SVC is ligated as high up as possible, the IVC divided. And the left side of the heart vented through a cut in the LA appendage.
- The heart–lung bloc is dissected from the esophagus from diaphragm to carina, and the posterior hilar attachments divided.
- Lungs are inflated and the trachea stapled at least four rings above the carina, divided superiorly, and the heart–lung bloc is removed.

Organ preservation

Ischemia and reperfusion injury is minimized by limiting ischemic time to a maximum of 6–8h, maintaining hypothermia at 0–10°C, intra- and extracellular cardioplegia and pulmonoplegia solutions, PGE_1 which reduces pulmonary vasoconstriction, and pretreatment with iv steroids.

Heart–lung implantation

- Median sternotomy.
- Anterior pericardium is excised, the aorta and cavae are taped.
- The right phrenic nerve is separated from the hilum.
- CPB is instituted via high aortic cannula and direct caval cannulas.
- Left and right pneumonectomies are performed by dividing left and right inferior pulmonary ligaments, PA, and veins and main bronchi.
- The heart–lung bloc is placed in the chest, with the lungs passed under the phrenic nerve pedicles.
- The tracheal anastomosis is performed with continuous 3/0 Prolene, the caval and aortic anastomosis with continuous 4/0 Prolene.

Postoperative management

Early postoperative management centres on maintaining a balance between adequate perfusion and gas exchange, while minimizing fluid load, cardiac work and barotraumas. Cardiovascular management and complications are very similar to those outlined on 📖 pp512–513.

Results for heart–lung transplantation

- 1-year survival is 64%.
- 5-year survival is 49%.

Congenital surgery

Overview of congenital surgery

Key facts

Congenital cardiac defects are infinitely variable and fascinating, and provide the surgeon with continuing intellectual challenges. The surgical therapy of these defects is technically enjoyable, and the postoperative care rewarding. There is no opportunity for complacency, as each operation brings new and often unexpected demands on the surgeon's abilities.

- Congenital heart disease is one of the commonest congenital defects with an incidence of 0.8%.
- Away from the operating room and the ICU, the results of surgery on very heterogeneous groups of patients must be analysed to improve procedures and decision-making pathways.
- In order to compare surgical results on small numbers of patients, a common nomenclature and risk stratification tools are required in order to pool the small groups of patients from various units.

Anatomical nomenclature

Congenital heart disease involves abnormalities in form, spatial relationships, interconnections, and physiology. It can be classified in terms of presentation (📖 p527), physiology (📖 p527), anatomy (📖 p526), outcome (📖 p523), aim (e.g., palliative or corrective), by type of correction (anatomical or physiological), and by technical aspects (first time, redo primary correction).

Controversies

Early primary repair versus staged palliation and repair

The principle of palliating a small infant to allow them to grow enough to reduce the risk of corrective or definitive surgery has been increasingly superseded by early primary repair, where children undergo the definitive repair at the first operation, reducing the number of operations needed, and eliminating morbidity associated with palliative procedures, e.g., pulmonary artery stenosis after systemic-pulmonary artery shunt. Other advantages include normalization of volume load on the heart, elimination of cyanosis, normal organ development in infancy, reduced mortality from one operation compared to two or three. But a staged approach is used in many types of anomaly, e.g., early primary repair in cyanotic tetralogy of Fallot may be associated with stormier postoperative course.

Other controversies in congenital cardiac surgery

- Long-term mechanical support as bridge to recovery or transplantation.
- Fenestrations connecting the systemic venous circulation to the atrium in the Fontan circulation.
- Type of shunt that is optimal for use in the Norwood stage I operation.
- Cardiac MRI as a substitute for cardiac catheterization.
- Use of selective cerebral perfusion and low flow cardiopulmonary bypass instead of deep hypothermic circulatory arrest.

Risk stratification

This enables clinicians to predict outcomes and compare results between surgeons and centers. It is difficult in congenital cardiac surgery because:
- The defects treated are rare.
- Patients with similar diagnoses may be treated in a variety of ways.
- Several techniques may be used in one operation.
- A single 'repair' may require several admissions/operations.
- Large variation in age and weight.
- Confounding variables, e.g., chromosomal abnormalities, prematurity.

Basic Aristotle Complexity Score

This reflects complexity as a composite of mortality, morbidity and technical difficulty, of 145 procedures rated by 50 surgeons who were required to arrive at a consensus 'complexity score' from 3 to 14.5. If a further 248 variables are rated, both procedure-dependent and independent, a 'comprehensive' score from 3 to 25 may be derived. It is a subjective score, and was not designed or validated to predict the three main outcomes.

Risk Adjustment in Congenital Heart Surgery (RACHS-1)

A consensus panel of 11 experts subjectively rated the risk of postoperative mortality for 207 surgical procedures, arriving at 6 risk categories. This was validated against 2 datasets and found to be effective.

Morphology

Key facts

- Sequential segmental analysis is a morphological approach to the heart that allows cardiac malformations to be described in a logical and straightforward way.
- It is based on the observation that all hearts are built from three segments: the atria, the ventricular mass, and the arterial trunks, with the atrioventricular and ventriculo-arterial junctions joining them.
- Sequential segmental analysis describes these segments and their relationships to each other.

Clinical nomenclature

Congenital heart disease is normally described in the following order:
- *Cardiac position.*
- AV connection (segmental notation).
  - Atria and systemic venous drainage (visceroatrial).
  - Ventricles.
  - Great arteries.
- Chamber, valve, and vessel abnormalities including coronary arteries.
- Physiological diagnoses including arrhythmias.
- Surgical corrections and persistent problems.

Describing chambers and great vessels

In the normal heart, there are left- and right-sided versions of each segment. In abnormal hearts, segments and structures may not be in the expected position, or may be absent or duplicated, so it is necessary to recognize the chambers. When cardiac chambers are described, the terms 'right' and 'left' refer to normal *morphological* characteristics, e.g., the right atrium is the atrium with a wide-based appendage. When describing structures according to where they lie within the body the terms 'right-sided' and 'left-sided' are used.

Morphologically right atrium
- Broad triangular appendage.
- Terminal crest (crista terminalis).
- Extensive pectinate muscles.
- Muscular rim of fossa ovalis.
- Sinus node.

Morphologically left atrium
- Narrow tubular appendage.
- No terminal crest.
- Limited pectinate muscles—smooth internal surface.
- Flap valve of fossa ovalis.
- No sinus node.

Morphologically right ventricle
- Coarse apical trabeculation.
- Septal leaflet of the tricuspid valve attached to the septum.
- Moderator band.

Morphologically left ventricle
- Fine apical trabeculations.
- Mitral valve leaflets all attached to the papillary muscles.
- No moderator band.

Pulmonary trunk
- Bifurcates into left and right.
- No coronary arteries.

Aorta
- Arch giving rise to head and neck vessels.
- Coronary arteries.

Atrial arrangement
- Four possible atrial arrangements:
- *Situs solitus*: usual atrial arrangement. Morphologically right atrium on the right, morphologically left atrium on the left.
- *Situs inversus*: mirror-image arrangement. Morphologically left atrium on the right, morphologically right atrium on the left. Associated with mirror-imagery of other organs, such as liver, spleen.
- *Right atrial isomerism*: both atrial appendages are morphologically right. Associated with isomerism of bronchi, and variable arrangement of abdominal organs, often with **asplenia** (heterotaxy).
- *Left atrial isomerism*: both atrial appendages are morphologically left. Associated with isomeric left bronchi and variable arrangement of abdominal organs, often with multiple spleens (heterotaxy).

Atrioventricular connections
Atrioventricular connections may be **biventricular** or **univentricular**:
- Biventricular: each atrium is connected to its own ventricle:
    - *Concordant:* right atrium to right ventricle, left atrium to left ventricle.
    - *Discordant:* right atrium connected to left ventricle, left atrium connected to right ventricle.
    - *Ambiguous:* in the case of atrial isomerism, e.g., right atrium to right ventricle, and right atrium to left ventricle.
- Univentricular connections: one of the ventricles has a double inlet, with both atria opening into it. The right-sided or left-sided atrioventricular connection is absent, leaving only one remaining atrioventricular connection.

Ventriculo-arterial junction
- *Concordant*: right ventricle to pulmonary artery, left ventricle to aorta.
- *Discordant*: right ventricle to aorta, left ventricle to pulmonary artery.
- *Double outlet*: both great arteries, or >50% of both great arteries arise from one of the ventricles, e.g., in double outlet right ventricle: the pulmonary artery and >50% of the aortic circumference arise from the right ventricle.
- *Single outlet*: only one arterial trunk is connected to the ventricular mass.

Classification systems

Key facts
- This physiologically and anatomically heterogeneous group of conditions is difficult to classify.
- Physiologically the lesions can also be classified according to whether they are cyanotic or not.

Morphological classification

Anomalies with normal segmental connections:
- Septal defects.
- ASDs.
- VSDs.
- AVSDs

Malformations of the atrioventricular valves:
- Over-riding of the AV junction and straddling mitral or tricuspid valves.
- Mitral stenosis.
- Ebstein malformation of the tricuspid valve.
- True 'clefts' of anterior mitral leaflet.
- Parachute mitral valve.

Malformations of the arterial valves and outflow tracts:
- Aortic valve stenosis, bicuspid aortic valve, left ventricular outflow tract obstruction.
- Aortic valve regurgitation.
- Right ventricular outflow tract obstruction.
- Tetralogy of Fallot, absent pulmonary valve syndrome.
- Pulmonary atresia with VSD.
- Pulmonary atresia with intact ventricular septum.
- Congenital pulmonary valvular insufficiency.

Anomalies with abnormal segmental connections
- Double inlet ventricle.
- Tricuspid and mitral atresia/absent right or left atrioventricular connection.
- Transposition of the great arteries/discordant ventriculo-arterial connection.
- Congenitally corrected transposition of the great arteries/ discordant atrioventricular and ventriculo-arterial connections.
- Double outlet ventricle.
- Truncus arteriosus/common arterial trunk.

Anomalies of the great vessels
- Anomalous systemic venous drainage.
- Anomalous pulmonary venous connection.
- Anomalies of the aorta:
  - Coarctation and hypoplasia.
  - Interruption.
  - Vascular rings.
  - Sinus of Valsalva aneurysm.

- Pulmonary arterial abnormalities:
  - Anomalous origin, vascular sling.
  - Persistent arterial duct.
  - Aortopulmonary window.

Anomalies of the coronary arteries

- Anomalous origin.
- Anomalous course.
- Anomalous communications.

Physiological classification

Cyanotic lesions

- Tetralogy of Fallot.
- Transposition of the great arteries.
- Congenitally corrected transposition of the great arteries.
- Tricuspid atresia/absent right atrioventricular connection.
- Total anomalous pulmonary venous connection.
- Common arterial trunk.

Obstructive lesions

- Pulmonary stenosis with intact ventricular septum.
- Pulmonary atresia with intact ventricular septum.
- Left ventricular outflow tract obstruction.
- Coarctation of the aorta/hypoplastic aortic arch.
- Interrupted aortic arch.

Left-to-right shunt defects

- ASD.
- VSD.
- Patent ductus arteriosus.
- Partial anomalous pulmonary venous connection.
- Aortopulmonary window.

Other

- Congenital mitral valve disease.
- Cor triatriatum.
- Double inlet left ventricle.
- Double outlet right ventricle.
- Coronary artery anomalies.
- Hypoplastic left heart syndrome.
- Ebstein anomaly.
- Vascular rings/slings.

Embryology of heart and lung

The highly specialized four-chambered heart develops in a complex, set sequence of events (Fig. 12.1). Embryonic development begins with fertilization between a **spermatocyte** and a secondary **oocyte** within the fallopian tube, resulting in a **zygote**: a diploid cell with 46 chromosomes. The zygote undergoes rapid mitotic cell divisions as it passes into the uterine cavity, to produce a solid sphere of 12–16 cells to form the **morula**. Fluid spaces start to appear and coalesce inside the morula, which is now known as a **blastocyst**. This implants into the uterine wall by day 7. The spaces are reorganized into a larger space on the uterine wall side which will become the **yolk sac**, and a smaller space which becomes the **amniotic sac**, separated by a **trilaminar disc**. The **vascular plate** consists of a germ layer of mesenchymal tissue on the yolk sac of the disc.

Cardiogenic mesenchyme

The cardiovascular system arises from the vascular plate. The mesodermal layer forms into blood islands which evolve into four simple tubes (two anterior and two posterior). The two anterior tubes become the **ventral aortas** which fuse to form the **cardiac tube**—a single-chambered heart. The two posterior tubes become the two **dorsal aortas**. **Six paired arches** communicate between ventral and dorsal aortas. The cells between the dorsal and ventral aortas eventually form lung tissue, pulmonary veins, and foregut.

Chamber formation

By 23 days the **cardiac tube** lies within the embryo's pericardial cavity. The tube has three cell layers: an inner structureless mass of cells known as the **cardiac jelly**, the second layer which will give rise to the endocardium, and a third layer which gives rise to the myocardium known together as the **cardiac mantle**. The heart tube pumps blood in two parallel circulations by week 4. The heart tube is divided into three regions: the cranial portion (**conus truncus**), the caudal portion (**sinus venosus**), and the mid portion (**bulbus cordis**).

Folding of the heart tube

As the heart grows longitudinally it bends to the right: this is called **d-looping**. The cardiac jelly acts as a valve controlling direction of blood flow. By day 24 the cardiac jelly contains **trabeculae**. Differential growth of the proximal ventricle causes the folded heart tube to rotate counterclockwise. The conotruncal region rotates centrally to produce the curves of the aorta and PA. Bulboventricular looping is essential in establishing normal hemodynamic patterns.

Embryology of the lung

Development begins early in week 4 of embryonic development and continues up to around 8 years old. There are four phases of development.

Embryonic phase: weeks 4–8

The tracheo-esophageal groove appears in the cranial ventral foregut by invaginating ridges of the endoderm known as tracheoesophageal folds. These unite in the midline to form the dorsal esophageal lumen and the ventral laryngotracheal primordial. The intervening tissue degenerates

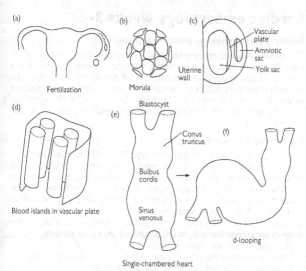

Single-chambered heart

Fig. 12.1 Simple representation of the sequence of main events in the formation of the primitive heart during days 1–24 of gestation.

forming two separate tubes, the esophagus and the trachea, surrounded by mesenchyme derived from the splanchnic mesoderm. The primordial lung bud develops from the caudal end of the trachea. Shortly afterward right and left bronchial buds form. Axial growth and dichotomous division of the airways continue to produce the secondary bronchi.

Pseudoglandular phase: weeks 8–17
Bronchi continue to grow and branch forming the bronchopulmonary segments. Mesenchyme develops into vascular and stromal connective tissue elements. Cartilaginous rings develop.

Canalicular phase: weeks 17–26
Capillarization and morphogenesis of the pulmonary acini (a terminal bronchiole, 2–4 respiratory bronchioles, and 4–7 saccules per respiratory bronchiole). The distal bronchioles terminate in closely arranged buds with air spaces surrounded by abundant connective tissue. This tissue thins and elastic tissue forms around air spaces. Capillaries move towards adjacent air spaces and acinal endothelium differentiates into type I (specialized for gas exchange) and II (production of surfactant) pneumocytes.

Terminal sac phase: weeks 24 to birth
Respiratory saccule development. Respiratory bronchi develop from each terminal bronchiole and develop into respiratory saccules. These saccules become septated, the walls thin, and they mature into alveoli. After birth total alveolar surface area continues to increase by means of maturation of diverticula found on terminal bronchioles until 8 years of age.

Cardiac embryology weeks 3–5

Endocardial cushion growth and fusion

The *endocardial and conus cushions* are areas of mesenchymal proliferation. The endocardial cushions form a partition between the atrium and ventricle in the heart tube, to create the *AV canals*. Proliferation of the fibrous skeleton and fusion of the cushions forms the *mitral and tricuspid valves*. The conus cushions divide the outflow region of the ventricles from the great vessels. The *truncus cushions* divide the aorta from the pulmonary artery.

Interatrial septum formation

The interatrial septum forms between days 27–37. The *sinus venosus* consists of a transverse portion with *two sinus horns*. Each horn receives blood from three veins: the *umbilical* draining the chorionic villi, the common or *cardinal veins* draining the cranial region of the body, and the *vitelline veins* draining the yolk sac. The left sinus horn is obliterated leaving the *oblique vein* of the LA and the *coronary sinus*. The junction between right sinus venosus and atrium folds to form the *right sinus valve*, which is large in the embryo and directs blood from IVC across the interatrial septum.

- The *septum primum* grows downwards from the atrial wall.
- The hole between the growth edge of the septum primum and the fused endocardial cushions is the *foramen primum*.
- The growth edge fuses to the endocardial cushions.
- Apoptosis in the superior part of the septum primum forms a new opening, the *foramen secundum*.
- The left sinus valve grows down as a *septum secundum*.
- Fusion of the septum secundum to the endocardial cushions leaves an opening known as the *foramen ovale*, and the superior part apoptoses, creating a one-way flap valve (Fig. 12.2).

Interventricular septum formation

The interventricular septum begins to develop around day 27. It is the final event in separating aortic and pulmonary outflow, and it occurs at the same time as aorto-pumonary septum formation. The septum is characterized by two portions, made up of three structures. The *muscular portion* is formed from the opposing walls of the growing ventricles which fuse, and grow up towards the fused endocardial cushions. The *membranous portion* is composed of the fused endocardial cushions and the descending truncus cushions.

Aorto-pulmonary septum formation

The truncus arteriosus divides into aorta and pulmonary artery from distal towards the conus cordis. The septum results from the growth of the bulbar cushions. The truncal swellings develop into pulmonary and aortic valves cusps. The intercalated swelling also contributes to the cusps of both valves.

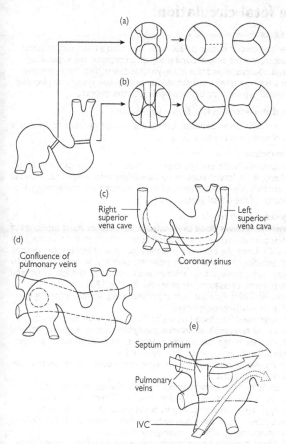

(a)

(b)

(c)

Right
superior
vena cava

Left
superior
vena cava

Coronary sinus

(d)

Confluence of
pulmonary veins

(e)

Septum primum

Pulmonary
veins

IVC

Fig. 12.2 Simple representation of the formation of the cardiac chambers and valves. (a) Endocardial cushions and formation of AV valves. (b) Conus cushions and formation of semilunar valves. (c) The left SVC disappears and the coronary sinus is absorbed into the AV groove. (d) The left atrium is formed in part from the confluence of pulmonary veins which are absorbed into the posterior wall of the heart. (e) Formation of the interatrial septum.

The fetal circulation

Key facts

- The fetal cardiac output is ~300mL/kg/min, with a heart rate of about 140bpm, and the systemic and placental circulations are in parallel.
- *Hematopoiesis* takes place in the yolk sac rather than bone marrow.
- *Gas exchange* takes place at the interface between fetus and placenta: so blood bypasses the developing lungs in the embryo.

Main differences in the fetal circulation

The main differences between fetal and postnatal vasculature arise as a result of three main factors:

Hematopoiesis

Hematopoiesis in the embryo takes place on the surface of the yolk sac. Blood enters the fetal circulation via the **vitelline veins** which drain into the sinus venosus. The yolk sac receives blood from the vitelline artery, which is a branch of the dorsal aorta.

Oxygenated blood supply

The embryo receives blood oxygenated at the placenta in the capillaries of the chorionic villi, via a single **umbilical vein** which enters the sinus venosus (📖 p530). Once the heart is partitioned into four chambers, oxygenated blood entering the right atrium from the umbilical veins is diverted by the sinus venosus through the patent foramen ovale to the left atrium and hence systemic circulation, bypassing the RV (Fig. 12.3).

- About 40% of the cardiac output perfuses the placenta, returning to the fetus relatively oxygenated.
- Deoxygenated fetal blood passes to the placenta, where gas exchange occurs, via **two umbilical arteries**, arising from the internal iliac arteries.
- After gas exchange, oxygenated blood returns to the fetus via a single **umbilical vein**, which drains into the fetal IVC.
- The oxygen saturation in the umbilical vein is 80%, the highest found in the fetal circulation.
- About 50% of this blood supplies the **liver**, the rest bypasses the liver via the venous duct, draining into the IVC, where it meets deoxygenated blood returning from the lower fetal extremities.
- The better-oxygenated blood streams posteriorly in the IVC, to a large extent not mixing with the deoxygenated blood.
- IVC blood enters the right atrium, where the **eustachian valve** directs the streams so that the posterior, leftward stream (more oxygenated) crosses the oval foramen into the left atrium. The oxygen saturation in the left atrium is 70%. This relatively oxygenated blood is ejected by the left ventricle into the ascending aorta and arch, thus supplying primarily the **heart and brain**.
- The anterior, less-oxygenated rightward stream enters the right atrium, and thus the right ventricle, along with the coronary sinus blood and the blood returning from the upper body via the superior caval vein. RV oxygen saturation is ~50%.
- The RV ejects into the pulmonary artery, which is connected by the **ductus arteriosus** to the descending thoracic aorta and **lower body**.

Only 8% of the right ventricular ejection passes to the pulmonary circulation, as the pressure of this vascular bed in the fetus is very high: the pressure in the pulmonary circulation is higher than the systemic circulation by about 1–2mmHg, and right atrial pressure >left atrial.

Proliferating tissue

Proliferating tissue (especially brain and liver) has a high O_2 demand: brain and liver see proportionately higher cardiac output with the highest O_2 saturation.

Differences in fetal hemoglobin

- 75% of fetal hemoglobin is hemoglobin F (HbF) with a higher overall hemoglobin concentration (18g/dL) than in the adult.
- HbF has lower affinity for 2,3-diphosphoglycerate (2,3-DPG).
- The oxygen dissociation curve for HbF is shifted leftward compared with that of adults, i.e., at a given PaO_2, the amount of oxygen bound to hemoglobin (O_2 saturation) is higher. This favours uptake of O_2 by the fetus at the placental interface with the mother.

Development of the venous circulation

The development of the venous system takes place via a complex system of shunts and folding, evolving from a symmetrical arrangement of paired veins to an asymmetrical arrangement that reflects visceral asymmetry.

Shunts

The brachiocephalic veins form between right and left cardinal veins. The ductus venosus forms between the left vitelline vein and the right umbilical vein. The portal vein is created by the fusion of the vitelline veins.

Involutions

- The SVC is formed from right anterior cardinal veins.
- The IVC is formed from the right common cardinal veins.
- The azygos vein is formed from the right posterior cardinal vein.
- The coronary sinus is formed from the left horn of the sinus venosus.
- The left posterior cardinal vein disappears.
- The left anterior cardinal vein disappears proximally, becomes the left first intercostal vein proximally, and contributes to the brachiocephalic.
- The umbilical veins mostly disappear into the ligamentum teres.
- The ductus venosus becomes the ligamentum venosum.

Development of the arterial system

Blood from the heart flows into paired aortic arches then the paired dorsal aortas. Tissues are supplied via segmental arteries. This symmetrical paired system evolves into the asymmetrical adult system:

- The first aortic arch becomes the maxillary artery and external carotid.
- The second aortic arch becomes the stapedial artery.
- The third aortic arch becomes the common and internal carotid.
- The fourth left arch becomes the ascending aorta and arch, and the 4th right contributes to the right subclavian.
- The fifth aortic arch involutes.
- The sixth left aortic arch becomes the left PA and the ligamentum arteriosum, the sixth right becomes the right PA.

Circulation after birth

Changes in the circulation at birth

Three main cardiopulmonary adaptations occur within a short time of birth to transfer gas exchange from the placenta to the lungs.

Change from placental to pulmonary gas exchange

- At birth the placental blood flow is interrupted. The decrease in oxygen saturation and the increase in carbon dioxide in the infant circulation triggers inspiration.
- When the lungs expand, there is a reduction in hypoxic vasoconstriction and pulmonary stretch receptors are stimulated, contributing to a dramatic fall in pulmonary vascular resistance and pulmonary arterial pressure.
- There is a resultant increase in blood flow into the pulmonary vasculature via the pulmonary arteries, and this in turn leads to a rise in the pulmonary venous return to the LA.

Closure of the foramen ovale

The increase in volume of blood returning to the LA means that LA pressure rises, forcing the flap covering the foramen ovale against the interatrial septum, finally completely separating the right and left atria.

Closure of fetal vessels

- The ductus arteriosus closes almost immediately after birth due to muscular contraction mediated by bradykinin released from the lungs after the first breath.
- The umbilical arteries close shortly after birth as a result of smooth muscle contraction triggered by the changes in oxygen tension. Fibrous proliferation results in their obliteration over the next few months.
- The umbilical vein and ductus venosus close after the umbilical arteries. The delay allows placental blood to flow into the infant circulation until the umbilical cord is divided. The ductus venosus forms the ligamentum venosum.
- The fall in blood flow through the IVC and venous duct causes the venous duct to close over the next 3–10 days.

Later changes

- Over the next few weeks, the RV wall thickness reduces, the LV wall thickness increases, and the muscle within the walls of the pulmonary arterial system reduces.
- Intimal hyperplasia obliterates any residual lumen of the ductus arteriosus.

Persistent fetal circulation

- This is a pathophysiological state that occurs when the neonate reverts to a fetal type circulation.
- It occurs in the presence of pulmonary arteriolar vasoconstriction, favouring a right-to-left shunt, and causing the oval foramen and the arterial duct to stay open.
- It may be caused by hypoxia, hypercarbia, acidosis, or hypothermia.

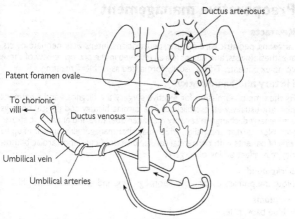

Fig. 12.3 Fetal circulation.

Preoperative management

Key facts

Surgeons, pediatric cardiologists, pediatricians, intensivists, neonatologists, anesthesiologists, and nurses are all involved in the pre-op review of these complex patients. This is usually formalized as an MDT meeting.

History and examination

By the time of admission for elective surgery the diagnosis and treatment plan are usually well established. The cardiac history and clinical findings are reviewed: change in severity may alter operative and anesthetic strategies. Non-cardiac anomalies, which may alter management, appear in up to 25% of patients with congenital cardiac disease. Acute non-cardiac pathology may affect timing of surgery.

Background
Note the primary cardiac condition, age, sex, and gestation of the child.

Symptoms
- Blue baby, pale.
- Failure to feed, failure to thrive, fatigue, poor exercise tolerance.
- Dyspnea, recurrent chest infections.
- Squatting, 'tet' spells (📖 p616), blackouts, mental obtundation.

History of presenting complaint
- Coexisting medical problems.
- Previous surgery, percutaneous procedures.
- Summary of known anomalies with relevant investigations.
  - EKG and CXR.
  - Echocardiography, cardiac catheterization, angiography, MRA.

Previous medical history
- Previous PICU/SCBU admissions and treatment.
- Meconium aspiration, pneumothorax, chest and upper respiratory tract infections, respiratory syncytial virus (RSV), asthma.
- Intestinal malrotation, herniation, atresia, necrotizing enterocolitis.
- Asplenia and athymia.
- Vitamin K deficiency, metabolic derangements.
- Exposure to infection.
- Allergies and current medication.

Signs
- Dysmorphic or syndromic features, small for age.
- Cyanosis, anemia, clubbing, mottled extremities, peripheral edema.
- Tachycardia, arrhythmia, hypertension, hypotension.
- Radio-femoral delay, reduced femoral pulses, upper limb hypertension.
- ↑JVP, hepatomegaly, ascites, added heart sounds, murmurs.
- Tachypnea, tracheal tug, wheeze, crackles.

Investigations
- Hematology: CBC, APTT, PT, (elevated in cyanosis), sickle cell.
- Biochemistry: Chem 7, BUN calcium, glucose, drug levels, urinalysis.

Preparation for surgery

Prostaglandin E1

Infants with cyanotic lesions may be dependent on a patent ductus arteriosus for survival. Prostaglandin E_1 (PGE_1) is given (5–100ng/kg/min iv) to prevent closure of the ductus. PGE_1 is a potent vasodilator, and volume resuscitation and inotropic support are frequently necessary. PGE_1 reduces the urgency of surgery, allowing more complete preoperative resuscitation. Lesions benefiting from pre-op PGE_1 infusion include:

* Lesions with inadequate pulmonary blood flow in neonates:
  * Tetralogy of Fallot.
  * Pulmonary atresia.
  * Tricuspid atresia.
* Lesions with inadequate systemic blood flow in neonates:
  * Coarctation.
  * Interrupted aortic arch.
  * Critical aortic stenosis.
  * Hypoplastic left heart syndrome.
* Lesions with inadequate mixing in neonates:
  * Transposition of the great arteries.

Ordering blood and products

* Neonates 2 units packed RBCs or fresh whole blood.
* Infants and children: 3 units packed RBCs or fresh whole blood, 2 units platelets, 2 units FFP, and 2 units cryoprecipitate.

Medication

* Preoperative cardiac medication is not given on the day of surgery.
* Vitamin K (0.25mg/kg by slow iv bolus) may be given in infants with deranged clotting.

Antibiotics

* Vancomycin 40mg/kg/24h iv on induction *or*
* Cefotaxime 50mg/kg/24h iv on induction, 8-hourly until lines out.

Starving

* Stop solids or milk 6h, breast milk 4h, clear fluids 2h before surgery.
* Iv maintenance fluids (5% dextrose 2mL/kg/h) should be given if oral fluids are withheld >4h as cyanosis is associated with polycythemia, and dehydration can result in systemic thrombosis.

Consent

For most procedures the parents will have had the opportunity for discussing the options, risks, and benefits of surgery with the operating surgeon. Signing the consent form the night before surgery should therefore be a chance to review the important issues.

Adjuncts to surgery

Do any of the following need to be ordered in advance?
* Homograft: what type, what size?
* Synthetic conduit: what size, valved or unvalved?

Postoperative cardiac management

Key facts

- Principles of cardiovascular management after surgery for congenital heart disease are similar to those in Chapter 8, with several key differences, including the normal hemodynamic parameters (Table 12.1), dose ranges of vasoactive drugs (Table 12.2), and residual pathology.
- Management of low cardiac output and arrhythmias in pediatric population is dealt with in more detail on 📖 p542.

Hemodynamic monitoring

Monitoring

- Arterial lines are placed immediately pre-op.
- PA catheters are not used routinely because small hearts with highly abnormal anatomy make percutaneous insertion inappropriate.
- RA, LA, and PA catheters can be inserted at surgery and provide information on ventricular filling and function.
- SvO_2 and transoesophageal Doppler help assess cardiac output.
- Normal pediatric hemodynamic parameters are listed in Table 12.1.

Table 12.1 Pediatric reference table for hemodynamic variables

Age	Systolic (mmHg)	Diastolic (mmHg)	Heart rate (bpm)
Birth (<1kg)	40–60	15–35	85–205
Birth (3kg)	50–70	25–45	
Neonate (1–28 days)	60–80	20–50	
Infant (1–12 months)	80–105	50–65	100–190 (to 2 years)
Child and adolescent (1–18 years)	Median systolic BP = 90mmHg + (2 × age)		60–140 (to 10 years) 60–100 >10 years

Residual lesions

Many lesions are associated with specific cardiovascular problems postoperatively: these are dealt with in turn under the description of individual defects and operations. The following generalizations apply:

- Pulmonary hypertension and RV dysfunction, outflow tract obstruction, valvular incompetence, and intracardiac shunts, may occur postoperatively.
- Acute low-output states may result from thrombosed shunts, intracardiac shunts, valvular incompetence, or outflow tract obstruction.

Extracorporeal membrane oxygenation

Also known as extracorporeal life support (ECLS), ECMO can be used in children above 2.5kg as mechanical assistance during cardiac or pulmonary failure, for up to 30 days. It is indicated for acute, severe, reversible cardiac or respiratory failure where oxygenation and/or cardiac output cannot maintain life despite optimal conventional treatment. ECMO may

Table 12.2 Commonly used vasoactive drugs

Drug (range = micrograms/kg/min)		Comments
Epinephrine	0.01–0.1	Beta-adrenergic, first-line inotrope
	>0.1	Beta- and alpha-adrenergic, strong inotropic and vasoconstrictive effects
Dopamine	1.0–10.0	Dopaminergic inotrope, arrhythmogenic
	>10.0	Also vasoconstriction
Dobutamine	1.0–20.0	Beta-adrenergic inotropic, vasodilating, arrhythmogenic
Milrinone	0.3–0.9	Inhibits cAMP breakdown by phosphodiesterase, mild inotrope, synergy with beta-adrenergic, decreases SVR and PVR
Norepinephrine	0.01–0.5	Mainly alpha-adrenergic vasoconstriction, some beta-adrenergic inotropic effect
SNP	0.5–5.0	Smooth muscle dilator, easily titrated
Vasopressin	0.0003–0.002 units/kg/min	V1 receptor activation, potent pure vasoconstrictor

be venovenous (VV), (usually for pure respiratory failure), or venoarterial (VA), for cardiac failure or respiratory failure where there is cardiac compromise. VV ECMO does not provide cardiac support to assist the systemic circulation, and maintains pulmonary blood flow. The ECMO circuit consists of an oxygenator (silicone membrane oxygenator, hollow fibre oxygenator), a pump (centrifugal or roller pump), and a heat exchanger. There are bubble detectors, in-line blood gas and saturation monitors, and flow measurement devices.

Indications for ECMO for neonatal respiratory failure
- Congenital diaphragmatic hernia.
- Meconium aspiration syndrome.
- Primary pulmonary hypertension of the newborn.
- Group B streptococcal sepsis.
- Respiratory distress syndrome.

Venovenous ECMO cannulation
- Infants <10kg: double-lumen cannula in the internal jugular vein.
- Children >10kg: two separate cannulas to drain from femoral vein, and reinfuse into jugular vein (the reverse sometimes more efficient).

Venoarterial ECMO cannulation
Mostly cannulation is through the jugular vein and common carotid artery by cut-down in the neck. If VA ECMO is required for failure to wean from bypass, or soon after cardiac surgery, the CPB cannulation sites may be used. Venting of the left heart may be achieved through an ASD, or a vent placed through the RSPV or LAA.

Complications
- *Mechanical*: clots or air in circuit, oxygenator failure, pump failure.
- *Cannula*: mediastinal bleeding, carotid artery, and aortic dissection.
- *Neurological*: thromboembolic, intracranial bleeds, seizures.
- Pneumothorax, tamponade, cardiac ischemia, overwhelming sepsis, coagulopathy, infection, renal failure, GI hemorrhage, or ischemia.

Outcomes
Current survival rate after ECMO for neonatal respiratory failure is 77%, pediatric respiratory failure 56%. eCPR is the use of ECMO to salvage patients with cardiorespiratory arrest. In children survival to hospital discharge is 40%.

Low cardiac output

Low cardiac output

Key facts

- Low cardiac output state is when cardiac function is so poor that delivery of oxygen and substrates to the organs is impaired: the measured *cardiac index* <2L/min/m². In children this is associated with a elevated SVR and PVR, and can result in multiorgan failure.
- Clinical indicators include hypotension, slow capillary refill time (>2s), elevated core–peripheral temperature gradient (toe–core gap), oliguria (<2mL/kg/h), irritability or confusion, metabolic indicators, e.g., lactate >2mmol/L, BE <−2, arteriovenous O₂ difference >25% (SaO₂ − MVO₂).

General management of low cardiac output

Principles are similar to adults (📖 p184), i.e., optimizing preload (via measuring filling pressures and response to fluid boluses), afterload, contractility and rhythm, with continuous reassessment. Differences include:

- *Pulmonary hypertension* is more common cause of RV failure.
- Negative pressure ventilation (Hayek jacket) may help in RV dysfunction following Fallot repair, and in the Fontan circulation.
- Cooling is a useful adjunct to reduce O₂ consumption.
- Keep an open mind about possible residual pathology.

Low cardiac output scenarios

Bleeding

Excessive blood loss from surgical site may be due to inadequate hemostasis or clotting abnormalities, e.g., incomplete heparin reversal or rebound (📖 p116), dilution/consumption of clotting factors, platelet dysfunction (long CPB run, ECMO, sepsis, antiplatelet drugs). Bleeding may cause low cardiac output. If blood loss >10% of blood volume in 1h, or 20% in 4h, re-explore. Treat with transfusion, and correct coagulation (📖 p146). Tranexamic acid is useful during and after surgery (📖 p147). Children with cyanotic conditions, impaired coagulation, hepatic congestion, post deep hypothermic circulatory arrest, and post redo surgery are at increased risk of bleeding.

Cardiac tamponade

Hemorrhage may compress the RA and LA reducing filling and cardiac output (📖 p144). Even small collections may cause tamponade in small chests. Always exclude a pericardial collection in post-op LCOS by TEE. Worsening LCOS requires re-exploration of the chest.

Acute pulmonary hypertension

Patients with large, chronic left-to-right shunts frequently have hyperreactive pulmonary vasculature with a tendency to paroxysmal acute pulmonary hypertensive episodes characterized by rapid desaturation, arrhythmias, and hypotension.

- Triggers include hypoxia, hypercarbia, sympathetic activation, e.g., pain.
- Manually hyperventilate with 100% O₂.
- Give NaHCO₃ to induce an alkalosis which will reduce PVR.
- Sedate with opioids (fentanyl 2–5 micrograms/kg/h) and paralyze.
- Pulmonary vasodilators: NTG, PGE₁, milrinone, and inhaled nitric oxide.

Arrhythmias

- Occur in 10–20% of patients postoperatively.
- The aim is to restore a physiological heart rate and AV synchrony. Temporary epicardial pacing wires are placed on the RA and RV intraoperatively. When tachyarrhythmias are difficult to control and cause significant deterioration in cardiac output, a period of **mechanical support** (📖 p539) may be required.
- **Junctional ectopic tachycardia**/His bundle tachycardia: a malignant arrhythmia originating near the AV node, associated with significant morbidity and increased ICU length of stay. Most commonly requires treatment postoperatively. Loss of AV synchrony leads to further deterioration in cardiac output.
  - Surface cooling to 34–35°C to lower metabolic rate and O_2 demand.
  - Intravenous amiodarone (25 micrograms/kg/min for 4h, then 5–15 micrograms/kg/min). Overdrive pacing.
- **Atrial ectopic tachycardia**.
- **Ventricular tachycardia** (rare, associated with ALCAPA repair, Fallot repair, LVOTO relief):
  - DC cardioversion.
  - Amiodarone, lidocaine, Mg^{2+} if no hemodynamic compromise.
- **Atrial flutter** (rare), associated with RA dilatation, e.g., large ASD.
  - DC cardioversion. Overdrive pacing.
- **AV node dysfunction**: occurs in 2–3% of congenital cardiac surgery, associated with LVOTO relief, tricuspid surgery, VSD closure, Fallot repair, in ccTGA. 70% recover conduction, by day 9 postoperatively.
  - Permanent pacemaker should be planned after this period.
- **Sinus node dysfunction**: usually transient, associated with sinus venosus ASD repair, Mustard or Senning operations.
  - Atrial pacing resolves the bradycardia.

Management of life-threatening arrhythmias

Life-threatening arrhythmias in children are usually secondary to low cardiac output or respiratory compromise, not the primary event.

Bradycardia, asystole, pulseless EMD
- Bradycardia (<80bpm in infants, <60bpm in children) is a life-threatening arrhythmia, and is treated in the same way as asystole.
- Secure the airway and hyperventilate with 100% O_2.
- Single hand/two-finger cardiac massage at 80–100/min.
- Pacing at 100bpm if epicardial leads are present.
- Epinephrine (0.01mg/kg iv or 0.1mL/kg of 1:10,000 solution).
- Atropine 0.02mg/kg (maximum dose 0.5mg for child).

Ventricular fibrillation, pulseless ventricular tachycardia
- Defibrillate with 2J/kg once, then 4J/kg twice.
- Cardiac massage and ventilate as for bradycardia.
- Epinephrine (0.01mg/kg iv or 0.1mL/kg of 1:10,000 solution).
- Repeat defibrillation with 4J/kg after every 60s.
- Look for and treat airway compromise, tension pneumothorax, cardiac tamponade, metabolic derangements.

Postoperative fluid management

Key facts

- The inflammatory response to CPB causes fluid shifts and capillary leak. Neonates and infants are particularly at risk. Initial postoperative fluid intake from all sources is restricted to 50% of daily requirements.
- Pediatric patients are generally filtered on pump to try and avoid arriving on ICU in a state of fluid and salt overload.

Pediatric daily fluid and electrolyte requirements

- Fluids:
  - <10kg: 100mL/kg/day.
  - 10–20kg: 1000mL + (50mL/kg over 10kg).
  - >20kg: 1500mL + (20mL/kg over 20kg).

Target serum electrolytes
- Sodium: 135–140mmol/L.
- Potassium: 3.5–4.5mmol/L.
- Magnesium: >0.8mmol/L.

Types of fluid

- *Blood products* (including human albumin solution) should only be used for clearly defined indications. Cyanotic patients require a higher hemoglobin.
- *Colloid solutions*: although there is little evidence to support the use of colloids over crystalloids, colloids may be given if there is a risk of severe capillary leak.
- *Crystalloids*: higher volumes of crystalloids may be required to maintain plasma volume expansion.

Renal management

Oliguria

Oliguria is a urine output <1mL/kg/h. Management follows the same principles as outlined in adults (📖 p234), with the following differences:
- Furosemide is given at a dose of 0.5–1mg/kg iv, to a maximum of 3mg/kg.
- Mannitol is given at a dose of 0.5g/kg iv over 20min.

Renal failure

The management of renal failure follows the same principles as that outlined in 📖 pp236–237 for adults. Treatment of hyperkalemia and metabolic acidosis differs only in the doses of drugs used:
- $NaHCO_3$ mEq/kg iv over 15min, or 0.3 x wt (kg) x base deficit.
- Calcium gluconate 20mg/kg iv over 5min (0.2mL/kg of a 10% solution).
- 25% glucose 1–2g/kg iv (4–8mL/kg) followed by insulin 0.3U/kg iv.
- Hyperventilation to induce respiratory alkalosis.
- Dialysis (📖 pp236–237). In nenonates peritoneal dialysis is efficient and readily available.

Metabolic management

Cardiac arrest can be caused by hypoglycemia, hypocalcemia, and hypomagnesemia in pediatric patients.

Hypoglycemia

Hypoglycemia is a BM <4.0 in neonates, or <6.0 in children.
• Give 0.25–0.5 g/kg (1–2mL/kg) 25% dextrose iv over 5min, and then maintenance 10% dextrose in 0.25% normal saline, with hourly blood glucose measurements.

Hpocalcemia

Hpocalcemia is an ionized calcium <1mmol/L.
• Give calcium gluconate (10mg/kg or 0.1mL/kg of a 10% solution iv slowly) or equivalent dose of calcium chloride.

Hypomagnesemia

Hypomagnesemia is a serum Mg <1.5mEq/L.
• Give magnesium sulphate 1mL/kg iv.

Bleeding and transfusion

Normal bleeding post operatively should be no more than 1mL/kg/h. Hemoglobin should be maintained above 9.0g/dL in patients with continued cyanotic lesions, and at above 8.0 g/dL with no cyanosis. In neonates pericardial collections as small as 10mL may cause hemodynamic compromise. Re-exploration should be considered for bleeding rates >5.0mL/kg/h. Children with cyanotic conditions, impaired coagulation, hepatic congestion, post-deep hypothermic circulatory arrest, and post redo-surgery are at increased risk of bleeding. Within the parameters listed, the principles of managing mediastinal bleeding are similar to those described on 🕮 pp144–145 with the following differences:
• Administration of product is modified according to coagulation screens, including TEG.
• Transfusion of RBCs is either matched to the previous hour's mediastinal drainage, or guided by the difference between the actual and the desired hematocrit (δHCT) according to the formula:

$$\text{ML packed cells transfused} = \text{wt (kg)} \times \delta\text{HCT}$$

• FFP is given at a dose of 10mL/kg.
• Platelets are given at a dose of 0.2U/kg.
• Cryoprecipitate is given at a dose of 1U/kg.
• Desmopressin is given at a dose of 0.3 micrograms/kg iv in 50mL normal saline.
• Antifibrinolytics may be given (🕮 p147).
• All products should be warmed before transfusion.
• Ionized calcium levels must be corrected: calcium gluconate 20mg/kg iv over 5min (0.2mL/kg of a 10% solution).

Postoperative considerations

Key facts

- Respiratory, cardiovascular, renal, and bleeding complications are outlined on 🕮 pp542, 545 and 549.
- Most of the postoperative complications described in Chapters 5 and 6 occur after congenital heart surgery. The complications described here have certain features unique to congenital heart surgery.

Cyanosis

Cyanosis is blue discoloration of the skin due to increased amount of deoxygenated hemoglobin. Cyanosis may occur despite relatively high oxygen saturations in children with polycythemia: conversely in anemia, cyanosis may not be evident until oxygen saturations are extremely low.

- **Peripheral cyanosis** is limited to fingers and toes: arterial saturation is normal but sluggish flow through capillaries results in high oxygen extraction. Causes include:
  - Hypothermia.
  - Vasoconstrictors.
  - Low cardiac output.
- **Central cyanosis** includes fingers, toes, and mucous membranes. There are two categories:
  - **Cardiac:** caused by intracardiac right-to-left shunt (pulmonary hypertension, RVOT obstruction, aortopulmonary shunt occlusion), and usually not improved by ↑FiO_2.
  - **Pulmonary:** caused by inadequate oxygenation (usually VQ mismatch: pulmonary edema, atelectasis, pneumonia, PE), and improves with ↑FiO_2.

Shunt occlusion

This may be complete or partial. It may occur as a result of acute thrombosis. Occasionally a shunt will have no blood flow despite being patent: a non-functioning shunt. Signs include:

- Cardiopulmonary collapse, cyanosis.
- Decreased central and peripheral oxygen saturations.
- Loss of shunt murmur.
- TTE, TEE, or cardiac catheterization is diagnostic.
- Treatment includes:
  - Immediate iv heparinization which may reverse shunt thrombosis.
  - Cardiac catheterization with a view to percutaneous reopening.
  - Redo surgery may be necessary.

Chylothorax

This is seen as a result of extensive dissection in the region of the thoracic duct in the posterior mediastinum in, for example, formation or take-down of Blalock–Taussig shunts or coarctation of aorta repair. Diagnosis and management are discussed on 🕮 p737, although intercostal drain technique differs in infants:

- Because there is less soft tissue, drains are often tunnelled to avoid pneumothorax on removal.

- The largest drains range from 12F in premature infants to 16F in infancy. The liver and spleen are relatively higher relative to the costal margin in children than they are in adults.
- Remove drain when drainage <2mL/kg/24h.
- Medium chain triglyceride (MCT) diet for 6–8 weeks, diuretics.
- Remove with weekly radiograph or US after finishing MCT diet.

Neonatal sepsis

Many infants have high temperatures postoperatively: this may be from an inflammatory response, atelectasis, or immature thermoregulation. Fever increases cardiac output requirements as a result of increased metabolic demand:

- Thermoregulation is an important feature of pediatric care:
  - Paracetamol 10–20mg/kg/dose reduces pyrexia.
  - Cooling blanket or surface cooling with tepid water may be used.
  - Glucocorticoids also reduce pyrexia.
- In the neonate signs if sepsis are subtle, and in addition to the usual signs described in adults (📖 p239) include:
  - Lethargy, agitation, seizures.
  - Apneic spells, tachypnea, tachycardia.
  - Decreased as well as increased temperature.
  - Persistent jaundice.
- Late features suggesting septic shock include:
  - ↓GCS.
  - Hypotension.
  - Reduced filling pressures.
  - Fall in cardiac output.
  - Decreasing urine output.
  - Coagulopathy.
- The following sites should be routinely cultured if sepsis is suspected (temperature after postoperative day 3–5):
  - Indwelling cannulas.
  - Umbilicus/umbilical lines (common cause).
  - Blood, urine, and stool.
  - Wounds.
  - Drain fluid.
  - Nasopharyngeal, CSF.

Nutrition and gut

The aim of ICU nutrition is to promote anabolism and growth and reduce the effects of catabolism and hypermetabolism due to stress. Feeds should commence as soon as the patient is hemodynamically stable, preferably enterally. Many children are nutritionally impaired before surgery. Enteral feeding should start within 12h of PICU admission. Contraindications to enteral feeding include:

- Necrotizing enterocolitis.
- Severe low cardiac output.
- Reduced splanchnic perfusion (e.g., coarctation of the aorta).
- Parenteral feeding is only used if enteral contraindicated or not tolerated, as it is expensive, requires central venous access, increases risk of line sepsis, thrombosis, gut mucosal atrophy, biochemical abnormalities.

Postoperative respiratory management

Key facts

- Normal respiratory parameters are different in infants and adults; and in all patients with cyanotic defects with persistent shunts (see Box 12.1).
- Choice of anesthetic agent and ventilatory management reflects the presence of shunts: changes in PVR and SVR affect oxygenation.
- Infants are more prone to both barotrauma and atelectasis (below).
- Hypoxic, pulmonary hypertensive crises are more common in patients with pulmonary hypertension.
- Nasal intubation is used routinely in infants (see below).
- Small infant ET tubes are more prone to obstruction (see opposite).
- After extubation, children commonly require a further period of non-invasive positive pressure support. Nasal CPAP may be delivered to neonates and infants via nasal cannulas or short nasopharyngeal tubes (short-tube CPAP). Older patients may have CPAP via face mask.

Modes of ventilation

Ventilatory management is about treading a fine line between barotrauma and atelectasis. Basic ventilator settings for SIMV (□ p158) on admission to ICU are outlined in Box 12.1.

- Postoperatively, the most common ventilator strategy in children is positive pressure ventilation via an ET tube.
- Neonates and infants, who are susceptible to barotrauma, may be managed on pressure-limited ventilators which provide an inspiratory volume determined by a preset peak airway pressure.

PEEP in children

- PEEP opens collapsed alveoli, increasing functional and residual capacity, compliance, and PaO_2. PEEP can be used to treat pulmonary shunting. In certain circumstances PEEP may over-distend alveoli, decreasing compliance: the beneficial effects are then outweighed by the negative effects.
- Pulmonary vascular resistance is increased.
- Shunting of blood to underventilated alveoli is increased and PaO_2 falls.
- Cardiac output may be decreased by the fall in venous return.
- Pneumothoraces may result from barotrauma.

Box 12.1 Normal pediatric respiratory parameters

- *Normal respiratory rates:* neonates, 40–60rpm. 1–12 months, 30 rpm. 1–2 years, 26rpm. 2–6 years, 22–24rpm. 6–14 years, 20–18 rpm.
- *ET tube* is estimated by the formula (age + 16)/4 = tube size in mm. Size range: 2.5–3.0 uncuffed in 1kg, to 6.5–7.0 cuffed in 16-year-olds.
- *Ventilator settings:* initial FiO_2 = 1.0 reducing to 0.40, tidal volume = 6–8mL/kg, peak pressure <20cm H_2O, PEEP = 2–5cm H_2O, rate (see earlier), I/E ratio = 1:2 in children, 1:1 in neonates and infants.
- Normal pO_2 is >10.0kPa (75mmHg) in total physiological correction, and pO_2 6–8kPa (45–60mmHg) with oxygen saturations of 75–85% in cyanotic defects with persistent shunts.

Weaning

Children undergoing simple repairs such as PDA ligation or ASD closure may be extubated in the OR. Pre-term infants, children with large left-to right shunts, pulmonary hypertension, or complex cardiac repairs are usually weaned over several days using SIMV, progressing to CPAP in older but not younger children. Weaning is slower than in adults as small changes in ventilating volumes result in large changes in blood gases, and small reductions in PEEP or CPAP can result in massive atelectasis. Criteria are:

- Adequate level of consciousness, hemodynamic stability, normothermia.
- Mediastinal bleeding <1mL/kg/h.
- PaO_2 >10.0kPa (6.0kPa in cyanotic lesions) on FiO_2 0.40.
- $PaCO_2$ <6.0kPa.
- pH 7.35–7.45.
- Vital capacity >10–15mL/kg.

Extubation

- Stomach contents are emptied by aspiration of the NG tube.
- 0.5–2mL saline are instilled, followed by 2min of manual ventilation.
- ET suctioning and suctioning of the oropharynx.
- Ventilation and removal of the ET tube during peak inspiration.
- Repeat suctioning of the oropharynx.
- Steroids may be required to reduce tracheobronchial edema and stridor after traumatic or prolonged intubation.

Respiratory failure

In addition to ↓PaO_2, signs include cyanosis, hypotension, ↓↑BP, agitation, tachypnea, intercostal and subcostal retraction, and nasal flaring.
Causes of respiratory failure on the ventilator include:

- ET misplacement, obstruction, or kinking.
- The distal lumen of smaller (3.5–5mm) ET tubes may become obstructed by dried blood or secretions: this should be prevented by regular saline irrigation and suctioning.
- Ventilator malfunction.
- Increased oxygen demand, e.g., pain, agitation
- Pulmonary problems such as pneumothorax, hemothorax, chylothorax (☐ p737), atelectasis, pulmonary edema, aspiration, pneumonia.
- Pulmonary hypertension, shunt occlusion, low cardiac output.
- Phrenic nerve palsy, abdominal distension.

Management of acute respiratory failure

- Manually ventilate with 100% O_2.
- Auscultate for bilateral breath sounds: if there is doubt that the ET tube is patent or in the correct position it may be necessary to remove it and ventilate using a mask and oropharyngeal airway.
- Irrigate the ET tube with 1mL saline and suction.
- Get an immediate portable CXR.

Principles of bypass in children

Key fact

Children are not small adults.

Differences between children and adults

- *Molecular and cellular*: immature myocytes and immature calcium metabolism lead to higher intracellular calcium concentrations after ischemia/reperfusion; this in turn leads to decreased levels of ATP, and also to abnormal activation of various enzyme systems causing cellular damage.
- *Metabolic*: the immature myocardium can use anerobic glycolysis more efficiently than mature myocardium, making it more resistant to ischaemic injury.
- *Physiological*: smaller circulating volume, thus more hemodilution by priming the circuit, increased edema, coagulopathy, transfusion requirements. Higher oxygen consumption rates of neonates and infants leads to higher flow requirements on bypass (Table 12.3).
- *Pathology*: intra- and extracardiac shunts and more reactive pulmonary vascular bed lead to differences in bypass strategy and the response to bypass, presence of cyanosis.

Bypass circuit and techniques

- *Prime*: composition varies and subject of debate and strong opinions.
  - Aim for hematocrit 20–35% depending on temperature.
  - Colloidal solutions: human albumin, FFP, synthetic colloids; avoid glucose.
  - Mannitol and bicarbonate.
  - Keep volume small (1m of 1/4 inch tubing = 32mL).
- *Venous reservoirs:* two main types:
  - Hard-shell with air–blood interface; allows vacuum assistance and easily handles entrained air.
  - Soft-shell without air–blood interface; may be associated with less bleeding and inflammatory response.
- *Pumps*: either roller pumps or centrifugal pumps.
- *Oxygenators*: hollow-fibre membrane oxygenators are used most commonly for routine bypass cases. Silastic oxygenator is used where longer-term perfusion is required, i.e., for ECMO.

Effects of CPB in children

Many effects are similar to those described in adults (□ pp106–107).
- *Inflammatory response*: this is more pronounced in children, leading to increased capillary permeability and interstitial edema, pulmonary dysfunction, and renal impairment. The inflammatory response is inversely proportional to the patient's age.
- *Disordered glucose metabolism*: hyperglycemia may be implicated in adverse neurological outcome after bypass; hypoglycemia is a common complication due to decreased glycogen stores in small children/infants, and impaired hepatic function.

Table 12.3 Flow rates on cardiopulmonary bypass in children

Patient group	Pump flows
Neonates	120–200mL/kg/min
Infants <10kg	100–150mL/kg/min
Children	80–120mL/kg/min
Adults	2.4L/min/m²

- *Hematological effects*: platelet activation, tissue factor release, and thrombin release; this may lead to positive feedback activation of the coagulation and inflammatory cascades.
- *Stress response*: catecholamine, cortisol, growth hormone, ACTH, TSH, endorphin release. ↓TSH up to 48h after bypass.
- *Cardiac effects*: improved tolerance to ischemia.
- *Neurological effects*: central injury after routine CPB is uncommon, but risk is increased if DHCA used, with up to 25% of infants manifesting some sign of CNS injury, e.g., seizures, changed tone, motor disorders, choreoathetosis. Higher intracellular calcium may promote generation of free radicals and thus cell injury/death.
- *Lung injury*: leukocyte and complement activation cause an inflammatory response, while mechanical effects may lead to atelectasis and surfactant loss; these effects lead to lung edema and increased pulmonary vascular resistance.
- *Renal effects*: 8% have acute renal insufficiency, defined as oliguria and increased serum creatinine.

Moderating the response to bypass in children

- *Corticosteroids*: iv methylprednisolone pre- and postoperatively may reduce the inflammatory response to bypass—there is some evidence of reduced post-CPB edema, lung injury, and ICU stay.
- *Serine protease inhibitors*: may reduce postoperative bleeding and inflammation; in children there is no association between use and increased rates of renal failure, neurological complications, or mortality.
- *Leukocyte depleted blood*: may reduce the immunomodulatory effects of graft-vs.-host reactions of leukocytes in transfusion products.
- *Leukocyte filters*: leukocyte filtration during bypass may reduce the inflammatory response post-bypass.
- *Biocompatible circuits and oxygenators*: some evidence of improved postoperative outcomes with heparin-coated circuits, but these results have not been widely reproduced.
- *Miniaturized circuits*: reduced length and diameter of tubing, pump designed to allow pump-heads to be closer to operating table; the aim is to reduce prime volume and thus hemodilution.
- *Vacuum-assisted drainage*: this allows further miniaturization, as smaller diameter tubing may be used.
- *Modified ultrafiltration (MUF)*: see p553. Studies show decreased postoperative edema, intubation times, postoperative bleeding and pleural effusions, and increased ventricular systolic function, cerebral blood flow, pulmonary function; overall shorter hospital stay.

Conduct of bypass in children

Key facts

Anticoagulation: heparin at 3mg/kg, maintain ACT >450s. Reversed with protamine at 1.5mg per 1mg of circulating heparin.

Blood gas management: alpha stat versus pH stat

With body cooling, gas solubility increases, with lower $PaCO_2$, higher pH and leftwards shift of the oxygen-dissociation curve (📖 p152). During hypothermia or deep hypothermic circulatory arrest, blood gas measurements can either be corrected to patient temperature (*pH stat*) or not (*alpha stat*). pH stat is increasingly seen as beneficial in DHCA.

- With pH stat management, the pH is maintained at 7.4 by manipulating $PaCO_2$ to counteract some of the changes occurring due to cooling (Table 12.4).
- About 50% of centers use the pH stat strategy. In many centres, for DHCA, pH stat is used during cooling, converting to alpha stat during the arrest period and rewarming.

Table 12.4 Differences between pH stat and alpha stat

pH stat	Alpha stat
Temperature-corrected acid–base management	Non-temperature corrected acid–base management
CO_2 added to maintain temperature corrected pH at 7.4 and $PaCO_2$ at 40mmHg	pH allowed to drift up with cooling. pH neutral only at normothermia
Cerebral perfusion pressure autoregulation lost, cerebral blood flow becomes pressure dependent. Excess cerebral blood flow allows more uniform cooling but may increase microemboli in cerebral circulation	Cerebral perfusion pressure autoregulation maintained, even at lower pressures
Lower intracellular pH suppresses cellular function and metabolism—may delay cerebral metabolic recovery when rewarming, but may also reduce reperfusion injury	More normal transmembrane pH gradients, protein and enzyme functions, leading to better metabolic recovery
Leftward shift of O_2 dissociation curve counteracted—more O_2 uptake by tissues during cooling when brain still relatively warm	
Animal studies show better cerebral protection during DHCA, and there is evidence of improved short-term outcomes in infants undergoing DHCA	

Myocardial preservation

As in adults this is usually achieved by initiating diastolic arrest using high concentrations of potassium, with hypothermia and ventricular decompression. Neonatal hearts are more resistant to hypoxia, but less able to cope with increased myocardial edema from repeated doses of crystalloid cardioplegia, thus operations may be performed with a single dose of

crystalloid cardioplegia. 30mL/kg is a standard dose of crystalloid cardioplegia, usually delivered into the aortic root or directly into the coronary
ostia. There is no evidence that blood cardioplegia is superior in infants
and neonates; theoretical advantages are:
• Better oxygenation of myocytes during arrest.
• Improved buffering.
• Reduced risk of reperfusion damage.

Other adjuncts and strategies
Induced ventricular fibrillation without aortic cross-clamping may be used
in some circumstances: care must be taken not to allow distension of the
heart (e.g., if the aortic valve is incompetent, or there are extracardiac
shunts, e.g., a PDA).

Neuroprotection

Deep hypothermic circulatory arrest (DHCA): See also 📖 p124. At 18°C,
metabolic activity is reduced sufficiently to allow circulatory arrest for
40min without organ damage; it is thought that children may be protected
for longer periods at equivalent temperatures. For DHCA, bypass with
cooling should continue for at least 20min before arresting the circulation,
perhaps longer in cyanotic patients with extensive aortopulmonary collaterals, to ensure uniform cooling.

Alternatives to DHCA
• *Low-flow CPB*: low temperatures reduce cerebral metabolic activity,
allowing periods of low flow. Alternatively, DHCA may be interrupted
intermittently with periods of bypass, even at low flow, to improve
cerebral recovery.
• *Selective antegrade cerebral perfusion*: when DHCA is utilized for
surgery on the aortic arch, selective antegrade cerebral perfusion may
be achieved with direct cannulation of the carotid artery, cannulation
of the innominate artery via a Gore-tex tube, or by advancing the
aortic cannula up into the innominate artery. One-third to one-half of
estimated full flow should maintain adequate cerebral blood flow, and
often maintains a satisfactory femoral pressure as well (📖 p125).

Other aspects of bypass

• Mechanical ventilation is usually discontinued during bypass, and should
be restarted as soon as possible during rewarming to allow time to
reverse atelectasis, high pulmonary vascular resistance, and accumulated
extravascular fluid, which are more problematic in children than adults
• *Ultrafiltration*: two types:
  • Conventional ultrafiltration: a filter within the bypass circuit filter
  blood throughout bypass or during rewarming, thus removing
  excess water from the circuit.
  • *Modified ultrafiltration:* the circuit is modified slightly (or not at all)
  to allow blood to be removed from the arterial cannula at the end
  of bypass, filtered, and returned via the venous cannula. This can
  take 10–15min, or continued to a target hematocrit. It is used in
  small children and neonates.
• *Hemodilution*: allows the use of hypothermia by reducing blood
viscosity; minimizes exposure to donor blood.

Basic operative technique

Opening

- Spend time ensuring hemostasis at all stages: small amounts of blood loss have a much larger impact in children.
  - Arterial collaterals are enlarged in coarctation of the aorta.
  - In any cyanotic condition venous collaterals are prominent; they may require ligation rather than cautery.
- There is much less soft tissue, bone is less calcified, and cardiac structures and abdominal viscera may be disproportionately enlarged:
  - Set the cautery at half what you would use in adults.
  - Avoid subxiphisternal dissection prior to sternotomy.
- The thymus is much more prominent: a subtotal thymectomy improves exposure, and may facilitate subsequent resternotomy.
- If pericardium is needed for reconstruction, open the pericardium to one side so that you can harvest a large patch: some surgeons like this to be placed in 0.6% glutaraldehyde, fixing it, to reduce later shrinkage.
- Some surgeons open both pleura, to reduce the risk of postoperative cardiac tamponade by allowing mediastinal blood to enter the pleurae.

Cannulation and venting

- Cannulation must provide adequate flow, unobstructed venous drainage, perfusion of all organs, unobstructed operative field.
- Arterial: in small patients place longitudinal aortic purse-string sutures to avoid stenosis.
- Venous: usually bicaval venous cannulation; if circulatory arrest planned then atrial cannulation.
- Venting: decompressing the left heart during bypass; vent should be introduced after clamping the aorta to minimize the risk of entraining air into the left side of the heart.
  - RSPV/through the atrial septum—facile way to decompress the LA.
  - Pulmonary artery—decompresses both sides.
  - LV apex—rarely used.

Bypass

Pediatric heart surgery presents challenging problems to perfusionists.

- Circulating volume is much less:
  - Priming volume is kept to a minimum to avoid hemodilution.
  - Blood may be used to prime the circuit.
  - Changes in even small volumes can have profound consequences.
  - Albumin and FFP may be added to prime to counteract the reduction in colloid osmotic pressure and fibrinogen concentrations that results from hemodilution.
- In infants a larger percentage of venous return is via the SVC.
- Pediatric patients are often cooled to lower temperatures than adults: the brain receives 1/3 of cardiac output in children (much higher than in adults) and procedures are more complex and more likely to need circulatory arrest.
- Termination of bypass is challenging because of anatomic and physiological defects, as well as the small circulating volume.

Blood conservation
- Meticulous hemostasis is key. Tranexamic acid is increasingly used, and despite withdrawal from adult market aprotinin is also used in some countries as evidence of adverse sequelae in children not established.
- Cell salvage is routinely used in all patients.

Closure
Once again, meticulous hemostasis is key:
- If re-sternotomy is anticipated the pericardium is closed with 3/0 Prolene with an interrupted suture. A pericardial substitute, e.g., Gore-tex membrane, is used in the absence of pericardium.
- Pacing wires should be placed routinely in all except the simplest cardiac repairs and extracardiac defects as dysrhythmias are common.
- Extracardiac pressure lines may be placed in the RA, LA, and occasionally PA (which requires pledgetted purse-string):
  - The sternum is closed with wire, Ethibond, or Vicryl: sutures may be less likely then sternal wires to 'cheese-wire' through the sternum. Steel wires carry lower risk of stitch sinuses.
- In sick and unstable infants chest closure may cause unacceptable hemodynamic and respiratory compromise: it is not unusual in these cases to leave the chest open with a Bogota bag (📖 p151).

Special circumstances

Shunts
Shunts must be identified and mobilized pre-bypass, and controlled once on bypass in order to avoid massive run-off into the pulmonary circulation during bypass. Similarly, during repair of common arterial trunk, the pulmonary arteries must be controlled.

Persistent left superior vena cava (📖 pp121, 537)
These are present in perhaps 2% of congenital cardiac cases, and are usually identified on preoperative imaging. In adults they may not be spotted until the intraoperative TEE (classic features include an enormous coronary sinus on TEE, and the surgeon may find that the innominate vein is absent). In adults they can be ignored (it is not possible to give retrograde cardioplegia). In children they may be snared:
  - If there is an innominate vein draining the LSVC into the RSVC, the LSVC may be snared without the need for cannulation.
  - If there is no innominate vein, and the pressure in the LSVC on snaring it is >20mmHg, the LSVC must be cannulated to drain it. It may be cannulated directly to ensure a blood-free operative field, or may be drained via a pump sucker in the coronary sinus.

Redo surgery for congenital heart disease
It is vitally important to have a clear idea of what previous surgery has been carried out. Preoperatively identify the details of:
- Previous incisions and whether the pericardium was closed.
- Previous shunts and conduit, previous cannulation sites.
- Whether shunts and conduits are patent: exposing and previous shunts is an important part of redo surgery.
- Groin or neck (<2 years) should be prepared for peripheral cannulation.

Materials

Key facts

- Congenital cardiac surgery involves much surgical reconstruction, for which additional material may be required.
- The advantages and disadvantages of the available options are outlined as follows:

Patches and baffles

Autologous pericardium

Available, sterile, non-antigenic, hemostatic, little adjacent reaction; however, may thicken, fibrose, contract, or dilate. This is addressed to a certain extent by glutaraldehyde fixation which strengthens it helping to reduce the risk of aneurysmal dilatation and slowing the onset of calcification.

Cryopreserved homograft pericardium

Rarely used as it is expensive, with all the disadvantages of fresh autologous pericardium.

Glutaraldehyde-treated xenograft/heterograft pericardium

Usually bovine or equine; rapidly available, but develops severe calcification.

Cryopreserved homograft arterial wall

Hemostatic, handles nicely and conforms to contours; however, risk of disease transmission, expensive, requires time to thaw, may stretch/dilate, risk of calcification.

Dacron (polyethylene terephthalate)

Synthetic polymer. Stable, but stimulates inflammatory reaction causing adjacent fibrosis. Inelastic, does not conform to shape required; probably not suitable for complex baffles in small spaces.

Gore-Tex/Impra (expanded poytetrafluoroethylene, ePTFE)

This microporous synthetic polymer, derived from PTFE, was developed specifically as a biomaterial. The pores allow ingrowth of pseudointima. Less fibrous reaction than Dacron, thus advantageous for baffles, though as a VSD patch may allow the persistence of needle-hole leaks. Conforms better than Dacron, thus a good material for pulmonary artery reconstruction. There may be problems with needle-hole bleeding when used in high-pressure settings.

Valves

These are divided into biological and mechanical prostheses (🕮 p364).

Autografts

The autograft is the patient's own pulmonary valve. The commonest use is in the **Ross procedure** as an aortic valve replacement (🕮 p369, 🕮 p388). The autograft grows with the child. However, there is a tendency for the neoaortic root to dilate when the pulmonary autograft is implanted as a root; this may be reduced with the early technique of subcoronary implantation.

Homografts

Aortic and pulmonary roots are available; in the pediatric population there is aggressive calcification when used in the aortic position, leading to early failure/stenosis. In the pulmonary position they may last longer.

Bioprosthetic valves

Stented porcine, stented bovine pericardial, stentless porcine. These are unsuitable for pediatric patients due to the accelerated calcification that occurs up to the age of about 25 years.

Mechanical valves

Bileaflet pyrolytic carbon valves—most commonly used, available down 19mm, newer modified versions 'equivalent' to 17mm.

Valved conduits

- Homograft—pulmonary or aortic.
- Bioprosthetic conduit e.g.:
  - Porcine valve within Dacron tube—glutaraldehyde-fixed; (Hancock).
  - Bovine jugular vein—glutaraldehyde fixed bovine jugular vein with valve (Contegra).
- Composite mechanical valved conduit—bileaflet mechanical valve within a Dacron tube.

Atrial septal defects

Key facts

- ASDs are defects at atrial level leading to shunting of blood between left and right atria. They constitute 10–15% of congenital cardiac defects, and up to 40% of congenital defects presenting in adulthood.
- The commonest defects are of the septum *secundum*, the 'true' septum, these constitute >80% of ASDs. Female:male=2:1.

Anatomy

There are four types of ASD:
- *Ostium secundum* defects (70–80%): commonest type of ASD. They involve the fossa ovalis. Should not be confused with a patent foramen ovale which occurs in 25% of adults, where septum primum lying to the left of the foramen ovale fails to fuse with its sides postnatally, leading to 'probe patency'. Secundum ASDs may extend to the IVC.
- *Ostium primum* defects (20%): form of AV defect (see 📖 p 568) and as such are by definition associated with cleft mitral valve.
- *Sinus venosus defects* (10%): majority are superior sinus venosus ASDs, at the mouth of the SVC, associated in 90% of cases with *partial anomalous pulmonary venous drainage (PAPVD)* of anomalous right upper pulmonary vein from the upper ± middle lobe draining into this junction.
- *Coronary sinus defects* (<1%): varying communications between the coronary sinus and the LA, also known as *unroofed coronary sinus*, almost always associated with persistent left SVC.

Pathophysiology

ASDs permit left-to-right shunting, causing volume overload of the right heart and increased pulmonary blood flow. The magnitude and direction of flow through any ASD depends on the size of the ASD and the relative diastolic filling properties/compliance of the ventricles. In children, the shunt in isolated ASD is left-to-right. With time (rarely in childhood), pulmonary overcirculation leads to pulmonary vascular occlusive disease, with raised PVR, pulmonary hypertension, and eventually decreased RV compliance and reversal of the shunt. When blood shunts from right to left secondary to RV failure, causing cyanosis, this is called *Eisenmenger syndrome*, and has a very poor prognosis. A significant shunt has a Qp:Qs >1.5:1, or is associated with right heart dilatation. The chronic atrial dilatation leads to the development of atrial arrhythmias, usually after the third decade.

Natural history/long-term sequelae

In patients operated on before the age of 25, long-term survival is normal, but after this age, mortality is higher than in healthy controls. When ASDs are closed in childhood, the long-term risk of arrhythmias is not much higher than the general population, but after the age of 11 this risk increases, so that about 50% of 60-year-olds with ASD have flutter or fibrillation or sinus node dysfunction.

Presentation and initial management

ASDs rarely cause symptoms in children, and are usually found incidentally. The majority of children with PAPVC are asymptomatic throughout childhood, presenting in their third/fourth decade with fatiguability and reduced exercise tolerance. Rarely, if the defect is very big, there may be heart failure and failure to thrive (1% of patients). In older children and adolescents, there may be reduced exercise tolerance in comparison to peers. Patients are pink, with normal respiratory rate. (Infants may be tachypneic.) If desaturated, indicates right-to-left shunt, and should be further investigated before surgery. Parasternal heave at LLSE suggests RVH. PA systolic impulse at ULSE. Systolic ejection murmur over left second intercostal space—pulmonary flow murmur. Second heart sound is split, with no respiratory variation (*fixed splitting*). Diastolic murmur LLSE—tricuspid flow murmur.

Investigations

* EKG normal in 20–40% of children. May show right axis deviation, rSR′ or rsR′, RA enlargement (tall p wave, prolonged PR).
* CXR shows ↑RA, RV, PA, and pulmonary vascular markings.
* Echo is diagnostic and identifies RA, RV, and PA enlargement, septal defect and associated anomalies. Sinus venous ASDs may be difficult to visualize, requiring TEE or MRI to delineate the associated pulmonary venous anomalies.
* Catheterization is not indicated in the routine management of secundum ASD. It is necessary if there are concerns about pulmonary hypertension, to measure pulmonary vascular resistance and its reversibility with vasodilators. Older adult patients require coronary angiography.

Percutaneous options

Defects up to 40mm within the fossa ovalis, with a 5mm rim between the defect and AV valves/major veins, can be closed percutaneously in the cath lab. The device is placed across the atrial septum via a catheter in the femoral vein, under TEE guidance. Success depends on the anatomy of the defect, but this is becoming the standard treatment for suitable defects. *Complications:* incomplete defect closure, device migration or erosion, local vascular complications.

Surgical management

Up to 40% of small and moderate sized ASDs close spontaneously by age 4, although this becomes rare after age 2. Secundum ASDs still present after this time should be closed.

Indications

* In adults ASDs should be closed to prevent pulmonary hypertension.
* In older patients with pulmonary hypertension, if PVR <10U/m^2, the outcomes are good; but with 15U/m^2 or higher, the mortality is high.
* In infants, a large shunt with failure to thrive, recurrent respiratory tract infections or signs of heart failure. Evidence of RV or LV volume overload. Secundum ASDs should be closed electively in 3–5-year-olds.
* Paradoxical embolus causing TIA/stroke.

Atrial septal defect repairs

Key facts

- ASDs account for 10% of open congenital heart defect surgery. The classification of ASDs and indications for repair are outlined on 📖 p558 (see also Fig. 12.4).
- ASDs are usually repaired with a patch closure technique through a median sternotomy (or right anterolateral thoracotomy), via a right atriotomy, on bypass. Associated defects that require surgical repair include **PAPVD**.
- PAPVD involves anomalous connection of at least one but not all four pulmonary veins with the right atrium or its systemic tributaries.

Set-up

- Asymmetrical pericardiotomy so that a large patch of pericardium can be harvested. This is placed in 0.6% glutaraldehyde.
- Median sternotomy, heparinization at 300U/kg.
- Standard CPB with distal ascending aortic cannula, bicaval venous cannula (for sinus venosus ASDs), SVC cannula must be placed high, at the junction with the innominate vein). Cool to 32–34°C.
- Antegrade cardioplegia with cross-clamp: or if fibrillatory arrest planned, care must be taken to leave the LA filled with blood.

Procedure

Repair of secundum atrial septal defects

The anatomy of the SVC, IVC, tricuspid valve, coronary sinus are noted. If the hole is small–moderate, it can be directly sutured with continuous 5/0 or 4/0 Prolene. If >1–2cm, a suitably sized pericardial patch may be sutured to the edges of the defect with continuous 5/0 or 4/0 Prolene.

Repair of superior sinus venosus atrial septal defects

The anatomy of the right pulmonary veins and their relation to the SVC and RA must be determined by careful mobilization of these structures. >90% of defects involve one or two right upper pulmonary veins draining into the RA or SVC. Most can be redirected when closing the ASD with a patch of Gore-tex/bovine pericardium through a slightly higher RA incision anterior to the insertion of the pulmonary veins, crossing into the SVC/RA junction. Care must be taken not to injure the SA node. The defect is patched to redirect the pulmonary veins to the LA. The incision is closed with a patch of autologous pericardium to prevent SVC stenosis. If a pulmonary vein drains high into the SVC (PAPVD), the **Warden procedure** may be used: the SVC is transected just distal to the highest PV, and proximally oversewn. Through a RA incision, the ASD is closed with a patch, redirecting PV flow to the LA. The distal SVC is now anastomosed to the RA appendage, restoring normal systemic venous return.

Repair of inferior sinus venosus atrial septal defects

Rare. The pulmonary veins are inspected to exclude anomalous drainage, from the outside of the heart, and on opening the RA. The defect is closed with a patch of pericardium, taking care not to obstruct the IVC.

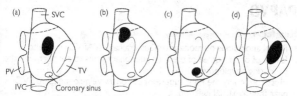

Fig. 12.4 Types of ASD. (a) Secundum ASD. (b) Sinus venosus ASD. (c) Coronary Sinus ASD. (d) primum ASD.

Repair of coronary sinus atrial sepal defects

The repair of unroofed coronary sinus is simple in the absence of a persistent LSVC: the septum between the CS and the oval fossa is excised and the defect closed with a patch of autologous pericardium, committing the CS to the LA. If there is a LSVC draining into the CS, then this flow must be rerouted to the RA. If there is a good-sized innominate vein accepting flow from the LSVC, the LSVC can be ligated distal to its insertion into the innominate. Even if there is no innominate vein, the LSVC can be clamped and pressure measured in the cranial end of the LSVC—if this is below 30cmH$_2$O, the LSVC can be safely ligated. However, in the absence of an innominate vein, most authorities advise the LSVC should be baffled into the RA and the defect closed. This is usually done using autologous pericardium, and can be complex. If complex repair of unroofed LSVC is high risk then LSVC may be anastomosed to the LPA.

Closure

- Just before the final closure of the ASD, the anesthesiologist should expand the lungs a few times, forcing blood into the LA, and air out of the LA into the RA, de-airing the left side of the heart.
- The RA can now be closed, and after further de-airing, the clamp removed, or the heart defibrillated.

Specific complications

- The aortic root lies just posterior to the superior end of a secundum ASD, so care must be taken when suturing the patch in this area.
- Residual leaks should not require surgery; if significant they can be closed with a device.
- Late pericardial effusions are common (15%), and tamponade (1.5%) can be fatal: routine opening of the right pleura may reduce risk.
- ASD predisposes to development of atrial arrhythmias, whether operated on or not. Atrial flutter and re-entrant tachycardias may occur around the patch or atriotomy scar. AF is the dominant arrhythmia in later life, and in untreated ASDs, sick sinus syndromes may develop.

Outcomes

Survival after interventional or surgical closure of all ASDs is now >99%. In older age groups, results are good if PVR<10U/m^2 at time of surgery.

PAPVD

Key facts

- Partial anomalous pulmonary venous drainage (PAPVD) is due to failure of one to three of the four pulmonary veins to connect with the LA during development.
- Most commonly the right superior pulmonary vein connects to SVC near the cavoatrial junction.
- 90% of PAPVD are associated with an ASD.

Set-up

- Median sternotomy.
- Standard aorto-atrial cardiopulmonary bypass.
- The ductus arteriosus is ligated before initiation of CPB.

Repair of drainage of right pulmonary veins to right atrium

The RA is opened (below and parallel to the AV groove), and the ASD closed with a patch baffling the right pulmonary veins into the LA. If the ASD is restrictive it can be enlarged by extending its inferior margin towards the IVC orifice (dashed line). The atrial septum can be opened in such a way as to create a flap of septal tissue, which can then be sutured to the lateral wall to baffle the pulmonary veins posteriorly into the LA. This flap can be augmented, or replaced, with a patch of autologous pericardium. Damage to the conduction tissues is avoided by taking shallow sutures around the anterior rim of the coronary sinus.

Repair of drainage of the right pulmonary veins to the IVC

The pulmonary veins form a curved channel that drains to the IVC above or below the diaphragm (also known as *Scimitar syndrome*). This is often associated with hypoplasia of the right lung, which may be supplied by MAPCAs from the descending aorta, and other major cardiac anomalies. There is usually pulmonary venous obstruction. The anomalous venous channel is exposed by lifting the heart out of the pericardial well and incising the posterior pericardium. There are two techniques to correct the anomalous venous drainage:

- *Tunnelling*: the RA is opened and the ASD inspected and, if necessary, enlarged inferiorly. During a period of DHCA, the IVC cannula is removed and the atrial incision extended into the IVC. The hepatic vein, IVC, and anomalous pulmonary vein can now be identified, and a channel created with a patch to baffle the pulmonary venous flow across the ASD to the LA.
- *Reimplantation*: if the anomalous vein joins the IVC very low below the diaphragm then the vein can be ligated and divided, and then reanastomosed to the LA. The vein may be anastomosed to the LA in a side-to-side fashion for a long anastomosis, or end-to-side with a wide, spatulated anastomosis.

Pulmonary venous anastomoses have a tendency to shrink and stenose, therefore the tunnelling technique is preferred.

Repair of drainage of left pulmonary veins into the innominate vein

If the left upper lobe alone drains anomalously, this does not have to be corrected. However, when the whole left lung drains into the innominate vein, usually in the context of mixed type of total anomalous pulmonary venous drainage, it must be repaired. This is done through a median sternotomy using cardiopulmonary bypass: the vertical vein is ligated close to its insertion into the innominate vein, and then anastomosed to the LA or the LA appendage (Fig. 12.5). This procedure can be performed through a left thoracotomy without cardiopulmonary bypass.

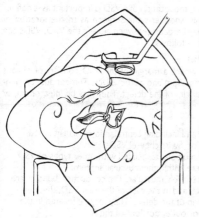

Fig. 12.5 Anastomosing vertical vein to left atrial appendage in repair of drainage of left pulmonary veins into the innominate vein.

Ventricular septal defects

Key facts

- A VSD is a congenital, abnormal defect in the ventricular septum allowing communication of blood between the ventricles.
- They occur as isolated lesions, or in combination with other anomalies constituting 25% of all defects: the commonest congenital heart defect.
- Prevalence increasing over the last three decades with the improvement of imaging technology, and associated with maternal drug and alcohol abuse.

Morphology

From a surgical standpoint, the location of a VSD is important as it defines the approach to closing it, and alerts the surgeon as to the location of conduction fibres that may be damaged when closing the VSD. VSDs can most simply be classified as follows:

Perimembranous (70–80%)

Perimembranous VSDs: where a margin of the VSD consists of fibrous continuity between the tricuspid and aortic valves. The conduction bundles run along the inferior rim of the defect. They may be *inlet, outlet, or inlet–outlet VSDs*.

Muscular (5–10%)

- Also called *trabecular* and including central, mid-muscular, apical, marginal, and multiple or 'Swiss cheese' VSDs.
- They may be single or multiple, associated with other types of VSD and may occur anywhere within the muscular septum.
- The rim of the VSD is entirely muscular. The conduction bundles are remote from the defect, and in the case of the inlet VSD, they run near the superior margin of the defect. They may be located in the inlet, apicotrabecular, or outlet portions of the RV.

Juxta-arterial (5–10%)

- Also called *conal septal, supracristal, infundibular, subpulmonary, doubly committed sub-arterial (DCSA) VSDs*.
- The conjoined leaflets of aortic and pulmonary valves form rim of VSD.
- The conduction bundles are remote from the defect.
- They extend up to the aortic and pulmonary annuli, and result in aortic valve prolapse in up to 50% of cases.

Low infundibular pulmonary stenosis and VSD

This is also known as double-chamber RV. It consists of an intraventricular stenosis separating the inflow from the outflow tract, usually associated with a VSD. The obstructing muscle band is excised, taking care to preserve tricuspid papillary muscle attachments, and the VSD is repaired, either through a right ventriculotomy or right atriotomy.

Pathophysiology

May be *restrictive defect*: small defects, presenting resistance to flow across the defect, with Qp:Qs <1.5, or *non-restrictive defect*: where the cross-sectional area of the defect is equivalent or larger than that of the aortic annulus—there is no resistance to flow across the VSD, RV, and LV pressures approach parity, and Qp:Qs is inversely proportional to the ratio of PVR to SVR.

- Three hemodynamic consequences: (1) LV volume overload, (2) increased pulmonary blood flow, (3) reduced systemic cardiac output.
- The magnitude and direction of shunting across the defect depends on the size of the defect and the compliance of the distal vascular bed.
- Unrestricted left-to-right shunting leads to pulmonary overcirculation and LV volume overload, causing CHF acutely and irreversible pulmonary hypertension and pulmonary vascular disease in the long term.
- In untreated patients, raised PVR and high right-sided pressures can lead to shunt reversal and cyanosis in about 10% of patients in the third and fourth decades (*Eisenmenger syndrome*).

Presentation

Larger defects present in infancy with CHF, recurrent chest infections, failure to thrive; Qp:Qs >2 is poorly tolerated. Smaller defects may be entirely asymptomatic. Bacterial endocarditis is a risk. DCSA and outlet VSDs may present with AI with the RCC prolapsing through the VSD. Examination shows failure to thrive (FTT), tachypnea, and recession.

Investigations

- EKG shows LV and RV hypertrophy.
- CXR may show increased vascular markings.
- Echo is diagnostic, and defines the location and size of the defect, the extent of the hemodynamic consequences, and associated anomalies.
- In cases where pulmonary vascular disease is suspected, or there are multiple VSDs, cardiac catheterization may be required.

Natural history

- 30–40% of all VSDs close spontaneously. Up to 70% of small VSDs close spontaneously (50% of small PM VSDs close spontaneously in the first 2 years). Inlet perimembranous VSDs and DCSA VSDs do not close spontaneously, and are candidates for early closure.
- 10% of infants with large untreated VSDs die within first year of life.
- Eisenmenger syndrome may be complicated by fatal hemoptysis, polycythemia, cerebral abscess or infarction, and RV failure.

Percutaneous closure

VSDs can be closed by percutaneously placed devices—these are mainly used to close muscular defects, and smaller perimembranous defects. In the latter there is a high incidence of AV node block, up to 10%.

Surgical closure

Operative mortality for VSD closure in pediatric setting is <1%.

Indications

- Moderate to large VSD after age 1 year.
- Congestive cardiac failure resistant to medical therapy in infants.
- Elevated pulmonary vascular resistance after the age of 6 months.
- Evolving aortic regurgitation in outlet VSDs.
- Multiple muscular VSDs (Swiss cheese defects) with significant shunt undergo PA band (📖 p598).

Ventricular septal defect repair

Key facts

- VSDs are usually repaired with a patch closure technique via the tricuspid valve through a right atriotomy, and occasionally via a right ventriculotomy depending on location.
- VSD repair is indicated for severe symptoms during the first 6 months, or electively after the first 6 months based on the assessment of pulmonary vascular disease (🕮 p565).
- Associated defects that commonly need surgical correction include PDAs (🕮 p572), coarctation of the aorta (🕮 p578), aortic regurgitation, straddling, and over-riding AV valve.

Set-up

- Standard invasive monitoring and general anesthesia.
- Median sternotomy, heparinization at 300U/kg.
- Standard aorto-bicaval venous cannulation, and patient cooled to 30–32°C. Antegrade cardioplegia.

Procedure

- Incisions used to approach VSDs are shown in Fig. 12.6.

Repair of perimembranous ventricular septal defects

- These are best repaired via a right atriotomy across the tricuspid valve.
- If the defect cannot be fully seen the septal leaflet is retracted or occasionally detached.
- A Gore-tex, Dacron, or bovine pericardium patch is sewn using continuous or interrupted pledgetted sutures parachuting the patch down, depending on how friable the tissues are.
- Sutures are placed around the rim of the defect avoiding the **conduction tissue** at the inferior rim (the right-hand side of the VSD from the surgeon's view: Fig. 12.6).

Repair of muscular ventricular septal defects

- Inlet and trabecular muscular defects are approached as previously described through the RA: apical trabecular muscular defects may need to be approached through a right ventriculotomy, in extreme cases with multiple apical VSDs through a left ventriculotomy; and outlet VSDs may be approached through the MPA, through a right ventriculotomy, through the RA or through a combination of approaches.
- Trabeculations that may obscure the lower rim may be divided.
- Multiple, small muscular VSDs may be closed by a singled pledgetted mattress suture.
- A single patch may be used to close multiple defects, e.g., when a muscular VSD coexists with a perimembranous VSD, or when there is a cluster of muscular VSDs.
- 'Swiss cheese' septum may only be correctable via a left ventriculotomy and single patch placed over the entire muscular septum.
- The conduction bundle in inlet VSDs lies along the superior margin (left hand of surgeon's view).

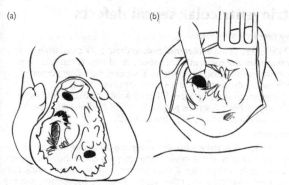

Fig. 12.6 Ventricular septal defects. (a) Types of VSDs. (b) Surgical approach through the tricuspid valve via right atriotomy to a perimembranous VSD showing retraction of the septal leaflet, and location of the conduction tissue.

Repair of juxta-arterial or DCSA defects

- These are approached through a pulmonary arteriotomy, across the pulmonary valve, with some sutures anchoring the patch through the base of pulmonary valve leaflets.
- A patch is used to close these defects.
- The conduction axis is remote from the margins.

Closure

- The right atriotomy is closed and the heart de-aired in the usual way.
- Cross-clamp is removed, caval tapes are released, and the heart is filled.
- TEE is used to assess residual shunts, and any aortic or tricuspid regurgitation requiring correction.
- If the result is satisfactory bypass is discontinued.
- The chest is closed in the usual manner.

Specific complications

- Mortality is <1% in isolated VSD; up to 8% in Swiss cheese defects or with other anomalies.
- Residual VSD (1/2%), may be due to missed defects, incomplete closure, reopening of defect.
- Conduction disturbance:
    - RBBB common; complete heart block 1%.
    - In the long term, 4% get sick sinus syndrome, 6% need reoperations, 15% develop aortic regurgitation.
- Persistent PAH and poor RV now unusual, due to earlier intervention.
- Acute pulmonary hypertensive crises (📖 p542).

Atrioventricular septal defects

Key facts

- AVSDs, also called *endocardial cushion defects, AV canal defects,* or *atrioventricular communis*, are a spectrum of defects resulting from incomplete development of the atrial septum, the inflow portion of the ventricular septum, and the atrioventricular valves.
- These defects make up about 5% of congenital cardiac anomalies.
- Congenital heart disease is present in 45% of children with Down's syndrome, and 45% of these have an AVSD.

Anatomy

In all AVSDs the atrioventricular valves are abnormal, and cannot be termed tricuspid or mitral valves, rather they are called the right and left atrioventricular (AV) valves. If the common valve is predominantly centered over 1 ventricle, the other ventricle may be *hypoplastic* and the AVSD is *'unbalanced'* and may not be amenable to biventricular repair. There is a wide spectrum of lesions involving atrial, ventricular, and valvar components of the AV canal, but they are broadly classified as:

Partial AVSD (primum ASD)

Inferior ASD immediately superior to the separate left and right AV valves; the left AV valve is trileaflet, and in 10% it is incompetent.

Complete AVSD

Single AV valve common to the right and left atrioventricular junction; an *ostium primum defect* (🕮 p561) above the valve leaflets and a *ventricular septal defect* (🕮 p564) below. The common AV valve has four leaflets: the superior bridging leaflet, lying across the crest of the ventricular septum, the inferior bridging leaflet, also lying across the crest of the septum, the left mural leaflet, and the right mural leaflet. A bare area of ventricular septum can be seen lying under the bridging leaflets.

Intermediate AVSD

In this form there is a *primum ASD* (🕮 p561) the superior and inferior bridging leaflets may meet and be attached to the underlying ventricular septum thus forming two AV valves, and there is a variable VSD.

Further characteristics of hearts with AVSD

- Aortic valve displaced anteriorly, superiorly, and rightward.
- Inlet of LV deficient relative to outlet, leading to long, horizontally oriented outflow tract, the *'gooseneck' deformity.*
- The AV node is displaced inferiorly and posteriorly toward the coronary sinus; the His bundle courses along the leftward aspect of the crest of the VSD.
- There are several commonly associated lesions:
  - In unbalanced AVSD, **RV hypoplasia** may be associated with tetralogy of Fallot (🕮 p616), pulmonary stenosis/atresia (🕮 p622). When there is non-dominant LV or *LV hypoplasia*, associated lesions include LVOTO (5%), aortic coarctation (🕮 p576).
  - 10% have tetralogy of Fallot (🕮 p616), 10% PDA (🕮 p572).

Pathophysiology and natural history

Partial AVSD

As with ASD, the long-term complications arise due to decades of right-sided volume overload, with dilatation leading to arrhythmias, ventricular dysfunction, and potential pulmonary vascular disease.

Complete AVSD

There is left-to-right shunting across ASD and VSDs with RV and LV pressures equivalent. This leads to pulmonary overcirculation and CHF. Irreversible pulmonary vascular disease may develop rapidly due to the large shunt: up to 90% of untreated patients develop pulmonary vascular disease by 1 year, with life expectancy <2years. Pulmonary disease develops earlier in Down's syndrome.

Presentation

Routine echo screening in Down's syndrome.

Partial AVSDs

In partial AVSD (as with ASD) in the 10% with LAV valve regurgitation, there is so-called LV–RA shunting, which may lead to earlier presentation with congestive heart failure. The latter may also occur in the presence of associated left-sided lesions such as coarctation, LVOTO. Partial AVSD may present very late, e.g., in adulthood with recurrent chest infections, a murmur, or congestive cardiac failure secondary to the shunt and left AV valve regurgitation. PVR >10 Wood units is a contraindication to surgery. Examination findings are similar to those in ASD (📖 p558): active precordium, pulmonary outflow murmur, fixed split second heart sound.

Complete AVSDs

Complete AVSD usually presents early with CHF. Examination reveals hyperactive precordium with thrill, systolic murmur LSE, apical systolic murmur of LAVVR; split first heart sound indicates elevated PVR.

Investigation

- EKG shows left axis deviation, prominent P waves demonstrating enlarged atria, prolonged PR interval.
- CXR shows cardiomegaly, increased pulmonary vascular markings.
- Echo is diagnostic and delineates the anatomy of the AV valves, the size of the septal defects, and the susceptibility of the LVOT to the characteristic gooseneck deformity that can cause obstruction. It is important to characterize the L AV valve, the size of the mural leaflet, so as to estimate the chances of successful repair.
- Cardiac catheterization is only required rarely, if AVSD is part of a more complex constellation of anomalies, or assess raised pulmonary vascular resistance, e.g., in children, >1 year with complete AVSD, or adults with partial AVSD.

Indications for surgery

- Partial AVSD: similar to ASD (📖 p558)—repair between ages of 2 and 4.
- Complete AVSD: surgical repair should take place between 3–6 months of age, but earlier if heart failure cannot be controlled: failure to thrive, intractable respiratory symptoms.

Atrioventricular defect repairs

Key facts

- A single or double patch technique is used to repair the VSD followed by the ASD.
- The size and shape of the patch is key in restoring competence to both AV valves, which may need to be replaced if significant regurgitation remains.
- **PA band** (📖 p598) is performed instead to palliate symptoms of heart failure and pulmonary overcirculation if the clinical condition precludes major cardiac surgery, in unbalanced VSD when the ultimate aim is a univentricular circulation, or if there are complex anomalies.

Set-up

- Standard invasive monitoring and general anesthesia.
- Median sternotomy, heparinization at 300U/kg.
- Asymmetrical pericardiotomy so that a large patch of pericardium can be harvested: this is placed in 0.6% glutaraldehyde.
- Standard CPB with distal ascending aortic cannula, bicaval venous cannula, and patient cooled to 28–32°C, antegrade cardioplegia.

Procedure

Access is via a right atriotomy Fig. 12.7b.

Partial AVSD

- Fill the ventricles with cold saline to inspect the valve.
- Pass buttressed mattress sutures through the base of the R AV valve.
- Pass these sutures through an autologous pericardial patch and tie it down securely, using the outer sutures to secure the patch to the remaining margin of the defect.
- Close the 'cleft' in the L AV valve with interrupted 6/0 Prolene sutures.
- The coronary sinus may be left behind the patch draining to the LA to protect the conduction system close to the CS (except if there is a persistent LSVC to coronary sinus).

Complete AVSD

- Fill the ventricles with cold saline to inspect the valve in the closed position, and identify the point of coaptation of the superior and inferior bridging leaflet above the crest of the ventricular septum—approximate them at this point with a 6/0 Prolene suture; this marks the point of separation of left and right AV valves.
- A hemi-oval patch is now sutured to the ventricular septal crest below the valves, either with continuous or interrupted sutures.
- Horizontal mattress sutures are placed through the superior straight edge of the patch, and then through the bridging leaflets, thus defining the separation of left and right AV valve leaflets.
- These sutures are then passed through the pericardial patch to be used to close the ASD, and tied down.
- Now the left AV valve is inspected, and the inferior and superior bridging leaflets approximated with 6/0 Prolene single sutures along their line of apposition up to the insertion of the chords.

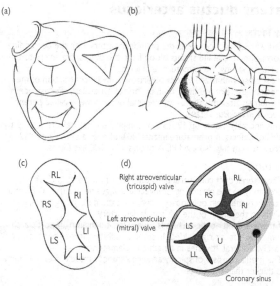

Fig. 12.7 Atrioventricular sepal defects (AVSDs). (a) Mitral tricuspid relationship. In the normal heart the valves are separated by the fibrous skeleton of the heart. (b) Surgical approach and patch closure of ostium primum ASD. The LS and RS are the superior bridging and the RI and LI are inferior bridging leaflet. (c) Complete AVSD. AL, Anterior; PL, posterior; SL, septal; LS, left superior; RS, right superior; RL, right lateral; RI, right inferior; LI, left inferior; LL, left lateral. (d) Partial AVSD.The mitral and tricuspid valves are fused but there is no interventricular communication.

- Finally, the pericardial patch is secured to the edges of the ASD with continuous 6/0 Prolene as for partial AVSD, leaving coronary sinus to drain into the RA or LA.
- Good results have also been reported with single patch techniques, where the VSD component is small.

Complications

- In those children repaired after 6 months, there is a risk of postoperative pulmonary hypertensive crises. Those at risk may be kept paralysed, treated with inhaled nitric oxide, milrinone, enoximone, high FiO_2; vasoconstricting agents and acidosis must be avoided.
- Significant AV valve regurgitation in 10–15%, reoperation in 10%.
- Permanent complete AV block in 1%, right bundle branch block in 20%.
- Down's syndrome patients may have lower mortality, lower reoperation rate, less pre-op AV valve regurgitation.

Patent ductus arteriosus

Key facts

- The arterial duct connects the pulmonary artery with the descending aorta, and in fetal life shunts blood from the pulmonary artery to the aorta, bypassing the immature fetal lungs.
- Most close within 2–3 weeks of birth, initially by contraction of the medial muscle of the duct, then by intimal hyperplasia. Persistence of the lumen after this time, with reversal of the flow, is called *patent ductus arteriosus (PDA)*.
- This anomaly makes up 12–15% of congenital heart defects, and up to 30% of defects in premature infants. 80% of premature infants <1200g present with this. Isolated PDA occurs 1 in 2000 live births.

Anatomy

- The arterial duct runs parallel to the arch of the aorta in close proximity to the recurrent laryngeal and vagus nerves (Fig. 12.8), and connects the main pulmonary artery with the descending aorta, just distal to the origin of the left subclavian artery.
- If there is a left aortic arch, it is usually left-sided; in right aortic arch it may be left- or right-sided. In some conditions, it may be absent, or rarely, bilateral. It varies in length and diameter.
- The media consists of spirally arranged smooth muscle, and the intima is thicker than the aorta.

Physiology

The PDA is closed by 8 weeks in 88% of children with a normal cardiovascular system (📖 p534). Closure occurs in two stages, and is mediated by increased oxygen tension and prostaglandin levels (PGE_1, PGE_2, and PGI_2). First, smooth muscle contraction within 10–15h of birth produces shortening, thickening, and functional closure. The second stage occurs over 2–3 weeks. It involves fibrous proliferation of the intima, associated with medial necrosis producing the fibrous ligamentum arteriosus.

- Pathophysiology depends on the size of the left-to-right shunt.
- When the PDA is large, aortic and PA pressures are equal, and the magnitude and direction of shunting depends on the PVR.
- As neonatal PVR falls the left-to-right shunt increases and congestive cardiac failure ensues.
- Pulmonary vascular changes may lead to irreversible pulmonary hypertension and reversal of the left-to-right shunt (Eisenmenger syndrome) which has a very poor prognosis, even though the initial reduction in the left-to-right shunt leads to a brief improvement in the clinical picture (see also 📖 p565).
- In moderate PDAs the size of the shunt is proportional to the size of the PDA, and LV hypertrophy usually compensates.
- A small PDA does not produce HF until the fourth or fifth decade.

Presentation

Presentation depends on the size of the PDA.

- Large PDAs present with symptoms of severe heart failure in preterm babies, a wide pulse pressure, ↑JVP, and a systolic murmur.

- The findings are similar in smaller PDAs but develop later; additionally the ductus may be calcified.
- Premature infants with this defect may be ventilator-dependent, or require long periods of non-invasive ventilation.
- Many children may be asymptomatic. Large shunts may present as congestive heart failure early in life.

Examination
- Bounding pulses due to wide pulse pressure.
- In premature infants, there is usually a systolic murmur at the second left intercostal space; with increasing size of the shunt, this murmur may extend into diastole and become the classic harsh, continuous 'machinery' murmur.

Investigations
- The EKG shows left and sometimes right ventricular hypertrophy.
- CXR may be normal, or show cardiomegaly, an enlarged PA, and pulmonary congestion in large shunts.
- Echo is diagnostic, demonstrating the shunt flow from descending aorta to pulmonary artery, and enlarged left-sided chambers. Associated anomalies must be carefully excluded.
- Cardiac catheterization is not usually required, but catheter closure is usually possible in infants >2kg.

Management
Indomethacin and ibuprofen are equally effective in closing the patent duct in pre-term infants, and improve outcomes even in asymptomatic pre-term infants. They are contraindicated in renal insufficiency or intracranial hemorrhage. The use of these drugs has reduced the need for surgical closure from 30% to 5% of hemodynamically significant ducts. If medical therapy fails, surgical ligation is considered for all symptomatic infants, and in all infants in whom the duct has not closed after 3 months. All ducts should be closed to prevent the risk of bacterial endocarditis. In patients with pulmonary vascular resistance >8U/m², duct closure is contraindicated. PDA surgical and catheter closure techniques are described on 📖 p574.

Indications for closure
- Persistent PDA is an indication for elective closure.
- Urgently if there is evidence of cardiac failure.

Contraindications to closure
PVR >8U/m².

Outcome
- Death rate falls and is 0.5% per annum after the first year, but increases after the third decade and 60% of patients are dead by the age of 45.
- Spontaneous closure occurs in 0.6% of patients per year.
- Operative mortality of isolated PDA closure is <1%.
- Recurrent laryngeal nerve palsy in 30%, permanent in 5%.

Closure of PDA

Key facts

- If medical therapy fails, surgical ligation is considered for all symptomatic infants, and in all infants in whom the duct has not closed after 3 months.
- All ducts should be closed to prevent the risk of bacterial endocarditis.
- In patients with pulmonary vascular resistance >8U/m², duct closure is contraindicated.

Set-up

- This procedure is often done on the ICU with pressure cuff monitoring of the right arm, and O_2 saturations monitored in the lower limb.
- Left side up with roll under ribs.

Operative technique

- Small left anterior thoracotomy through the 4th intercostal space.
- Lung gently retracted medially.
- Posterior pleura incised.
- Identify left vagus nerve (enters thorax between left subclavian and left common carotid arteries, crossing aortic arch and ductus arteriosus) and left recurrent laryngeal nerve (curves around ductus arteriosus and extends back up into the neck) to avoid injury. The vagus nerve may be reflected medially or laterally (Fig. 12.8).
- Dissect above and below the ductus, staying in plane near the aortic wall.
- When dissection is deep enough, right-angled instrument passed beneath the duct to allow passage of thick silk ligature.
- Trial occlusion of the duct (should note rise in systemic BP, no drop in lower limb O_2 saturations).
- Duct is doubly ligated.
- In premature infants, the duct may be ligated with titanium vascular clips. In some centers, this is achieved thoracoscopically. In larger patients, the duct may be divided between vascular clamps and both ends oversewn.
- The duct is often closed during median sternotomy for other procedures. This is usually achieved with a silk ligature just after commencement of cardiopulmonary bypass.

Coil occlusion

Transcatheter occlusion of patent ducts with coils are performed in patients >6kg in size, and can be done in >2kg.

Complications

Very rarely, hemorrhage and death, <1%, although in extremely premature infants 30-day mortality may be as high as 20%. Recurrent laryngeal nerve palsy may be as high as 30%, but is usually transient.

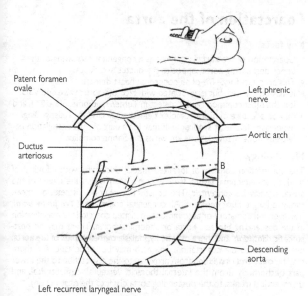

Fig. 12.8 Surgical anatomy of the ductus arteriosus. (A) This incision line is used if the vagus nerve is to be retracted medially. (B) This incision is used if the vagus nerve is to be retracted laterally.

Coarctation of the aorta

Key facts

- Coarctation of the aorta is defined as a congenital narrowing of the upper descending aorta, opposite the ductus arteriosus.
- This accounts for 5–8% of all congenital heart defects.
- It may be isolated, but is associated with bicuspid aortic valve and VSD. It is the most common cardiac defect in **Turner syndrome**. (15–20%), and may be a feature of more complex defects such as TGA, Taussig–Bing, hypoplastic left heart syndrome. It may form part of the constellation of left-sided obstructive lesions known as the Shone complex.

Morphology

The constriction consists of localized medial thickening with infolding of medial and neointimal layers. It may form a **shelf** within the lumen of the aorta, or may be **concentric**. The constriction may be discrete, or, more rarely, a long tubular segment. All congenital coarctations are **juxtaductal**; however, inflammatory or autoimmune-mediated coarctations may develop in the descending thoracic aorta or abdominal aorta. There may be **post-stenotic dilatation**, and there may be hypoplasia of the isthmus of the aorta, just proximal to the coarctation. The arch may be hypoplastic, and there may be **collateral circulation** from proximal to the coarctation to the lower part of the body (from the internal thoracic, vertebral, costocervical, and thyrocervical trunks, to the descending aorta distal to the obstruction).

Pathophysiology

- The hemodynamic consequences are high afterload on the LV, increasing LV wall stress and causing **LV hypertrophy**.
- Systemic perfusion depends on ductal flow. In neonates with severe coarctation, there may be circulatory collapse when the duct closes.
- In less severe coarctation, there is a slower evolution, with LV failure, mitral incompetence, left-to-right shunt, and pulmonary congestion.
- After infancy, CHF rarely occurs before the age of 20; these children may be asymptomatic until hypertension is noted.
- **Hypertension** develops due to the mechanical obstruction and possibly, renin–angiotensin-mediated pathways.

Presentation and natural history

- Depends on the existence of coexisting abnormalities, as well as the location and severity of the location:
- **Neonates**: collapse, acidosis, hypotension, heart failure; absent femoral pulses on routine review.
- **Infancy**: upper extremity hypertension with absent/reduced femoral pulses; congestive heart failure causing dyspnea and failure to thrive.
- **Children/young adults**: headaches, lower extremity weakness, exertional dyspnea, fatigue; hypertension.
- Examination findings also depend on the age and presentation:
  - In the shocked neonate, all pulses may be weak; however, absent femoral pulses should not be disregarded.

- There may be differential cyanosis, with the duct supplying the lower body, and the aorta supplying the upper body, demonstrated with preductal and postductal oxygen saturation readings.
- Systolic murmur in the left infraclavicular or infrascapular area.
- In older children, BP reading should be made in all limbs, and discrepancies of >20mmHg between upper and lower are significant. There may be a systolic murmur in the left infrascapular region, or a continuous murmur in the presence of collaterals.
- Uncorrected coarctation leads to a curtailed life expectancy of 30–40 years, with causes of death including aortic rupture, intracranial hemorrhage, cardiac failure, bacterial endocarditis. Beyond infancy, even after correction there is a lifetime risk of hypertension and its sequelae. After correction, freedom from death or complication or hypertension is only 20% at 25 years.
- Patients can die from cardiac failure, aortic rupture, infective endocarditis, or intracranial hemorrhage. Untreated isolated coarctation has a 1-month mortality of 10%, 1-year mortality around 30%.

Investigation

- EKG: LV hypertrophy.
- CXR: in sick children, cardiomegaly, pulmonary congestion. Later, there may be a classic '3' hourglass sign of coarctation along the upper descending aorta, and rib-notching from collaterals in children >10 years.
- Echo: shows the arch, and the coarctation shelf is usually visible just distal to the subclavian origin. Doppler measures velocity across the coarctation, enabling estimation of pressure gradient. Colour flow mapping demonstrates the diastolic 'tail' of flow in the descending aorta.
- MRI/CT useful in older patients or reoperations to plan approach.

Management

Neonates

In the shocked neonate, the initial management is supportive, improving peripheral perfusion by **reopening the duct** if possible, correcting the acid and electrolyte disturbances, and supporting the circulation and ventilation as necessary prior to undertaking corrective surgery. In neonates who are stabilized within 24h of presentation, surgical repair can be carried out urgently. In those not responding to treatment of acidosis/anuria, earlier surgery may be required. In infants not critically ill, but with hypertension and cardiomegaly, repair is the nonetheless urgent, but can be performed semi-electively on the same admission.

Older children

Balloon angioplasty of the coarctation is now the first-line treatment. Hypertension should be treated, usually with β-blockers, but intervention should not be delayed while waiting for normotension.

Indications for surgery

Isolated coarctation is an indication for surgical repair, once critically ill infants have been stabilized, and within 4–6 weeks of presentation in stable children.

Coarctation of the aorta repair

Key facts

- Symptomatic neonates and infants should undergo surgery as soon as they are stabilized. Older children and adults may undergo surgery electively, even if they are asymptomatic. It is preferable to treat this lesion before the age of 5, to reduce the risk of residual hypertension.
- Isolated coarctation are usually approached via a left thoracotomy and repaired without bypass.
- Coarctation with associated defects, e.g., VSD, interrupted aortic arch are approached through a median sternotomy using DHCA (⌑ p552).
- A small *concomitant VSD* will probably close spontaneously and does not need intervention. There are three main options for moderate or large concomitant VSDs: (1) PA band at the time of coarctation repair via a thoracotomy, (2) repair via median sternotomy on bypass during coarctation repair, (3) a staged procedure.

Set-up

- PGE$_1$ infusion.
- Left lateral thoracotomy for isolated coarctation.
- Collateral vessels temporarily ligated with clips.
- Spinal cord protection: surface cooling, short clamp time, avoid acidosis, measure distal aortic pressure after clamping to avoid paraplegia.

Procedure

There are several ways of repairing the coarctation:

End-to-end anastomosis

- This is used for discrete coarctations.
- The descending aorta, the LSCA, LCCA, and the arch are mobilized.
- Vascular occlusion clamps are placed either side of the coarctation.
- If the coarctation extends into the arch clamps are placed across the LSCA and LCCC, and the ductus arteriosus is ligated.
- The coarctation segment is completely excised, and the two ends are anastomosed together (Fig. 12.9). If the transverse arch is hypoplastic the incision can be extended into the proximal arch with a counter incision in the descending aorta in order to form an extended end-to-end anastomosis.

Subclavian flap repair

- This once popular technique has been largely superseded.
- The subclavian artery is divided and turned down as a flap, and used instead of a prosthetic patch to repair the coarctation.
- If there is a hypoplastic arch, the flap can be used to augment the arch.
- The repair is associated with the same frequency of recurrent coarctation, as well as problems due to division of the subclavian artery including long term weakness, subclavian steal and occasionally ischemia.

Prosthetic patch aortoplasty

- This is rarely used due to aneurysm formation at the suture site.
- Vascular occlusion clamps are placed either side of the coarctation.
- The ductus arteriosus is ligated, an incision is made longitudinally across the coarctation and a patch of Dacron or Gore-tex is used to augment the diameter of the aorta at the site of coarctation.

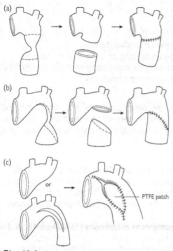

Fig. 12.9 Coarctation of the aorta repair. (a) End to end anastomosis.
(b) Bevelled end-to-end anastomosis. (c) Prosthetic patch aortoplasty.

Interposition graft
This technique is rarely used as it results in a fixed stenosis.

Complications

- *Early*: rebound hypertension in 30%, bleeding, paraplegia 0.4%
  (associated with long cross-clamp times and division of collaterals), renal
  failure in sick infants, abdominal symptoms from mesenteric arteritis
  including pain, ileus, rarely necrotizing enterocolitis—risk reduced if
  hypertension controlled, chylothorax, recurrent laryngeal nerve injury.
- *Late*: aneurysm—this is most common after patch repair, which is
  therefore rarely performed now.
- *Recoarctation* is the main long-term complication and is reported in
  10–45% of patients. It may be due to technically inadequate repair,
  hypoplasia of the arch proximal to the repair, or anastomotic stricture.
  Reintervention is usually transcatheter in the first instance, with
  freedom from reintervention after balloon dilatation up to 75% at 12
  years and is indicated if resting gradient >20mmHg. Balloon dilatation
  is method of choice to abolish gradient, and in children older than 12,
  stenting may be considered.

Outcomes

Coarctation of the aorta, although apparently a simple technical problem,
has continuing long-term sequelae in spite of repair. Only 20% of patients
are alive and free from hypertension or a complication at 25 years. Repair
before the age of 5 years may reduce the risk of hypertension later; however, even with early repair the life expectancy is reduced.

Vascular rings

Key facts

- These constitute <1% of congenital cardiac defects.
- Abnormal development of the embryonic aortic arches produces vascular rings or slings that partially or completely encircle the trachea and/or esophagus, causing compressive symptoms.

Morphology

These anomalies occur early in the development of the aortic arch and vessels: they result from incomplete regression of one of the six embryonic branchial arches. Rings usually surround the trachea and esophagus. There are two main categories:

Complete rings

- **Double aortic arch** (50%) is due to failure of involution of distal right 4th arch—the right and left arches encircle the trachea and esophagus. One is usually smaller, less dominant, and in 30% this is atretic. The RCCA and RSCA come off the right arch, the LCCA and LSCA come from the left arch.
- **Right aortic arch with left ligamentum arteriosum** (45%). Left 4th arch involutes, right 4th arch remains—in combination with left arterial ligament or aberrant LSCA. The right arch gives off the LCCA first, then the RCCA, the LSCA, with the duct originating at the base of the LSCA to the LPA.
- **Right aortic arch with mirror image branching** (<1%). Partial resorption of the left 4th arch.
- **Left aortic arch** with retroesophageal right subclavian artery, right-sided descending aorta and right ligamentum arteriosum (<1%). Left aortic arch with right descending aorta and right arterial ligament
- Anomalous left pulmonary artery or **pulmonary sling**. Abnormal 6th arch development—anomalous origin of the LPA from posterior aspect of RPA—LPA swings over the RMB, around the trachea between trachea and esophagus, to the left lung. 50% are associated with tracheal stenosis due to complete tracheal rings and 20% have other cardiac anomalies.

Incomplete vascular rings

- 'Anomalous' innominate artery: the innominate artery arises more leftward on the arch than usual possibly causing tracheal compression.
- Retro-oesosophageal right subclavian artery (**arteria lusoria**).

Pathophysiology

These anomalies are associated with chromosome 22q11 deletion, anomalies of the aortic arch, and other cardiac defects. 30% of patients with tetralogy of Fallot have a right aortic arch.

Presentation

Symptoms and signs are primarily those of airway and/or esophageal compression. The majority present in infancy. Symptoms include:
- May be asymptomatic.

- Stridor, respiratory distress or apnea.
- Characteristic high-pitched 'brassy' cough.
- Asthma, recurrent chest infections.
- Dysphagia and difficulty in feeding are more common in late presentations.

Investigations

- CXR commonly performed because of presentation.
  - Identifies pulmonary complications, e.g., atelectasis, hyperinflation.
  - May identify position of aortic arch, tracheal compression.
- TTE and TEE help identify any concomitant cardiac defects, but are not good at identifying the ligamentum arteriosum, and compressed structures in the midline, and are diagnostic of double aortic arch.
- Angiography, MRA, or CT angio are mandatory to define anatomy.
- Bronchoscopy is mandatory where presentation is with respiratory symptoms, and is needed to diagnose tracheomalacia or stenosis (📖 p750).
- Barium swallow may delineate esophageal compression, which is more common in adults.

Surgical management

Left posterolateral thoracotomy (or occasionally median sternotomy) and cardiopulmonary bypass are used for surgical division of most arches. Sternotomy and bypass are required for pulmonary artery sling and tracheal reconstruction. Although configurations associated with a right descending thoracic aorta may be approached via a right thoracotomy.

Indications for surgery

Symptoms, particularly those of upper airway obstruction.

Contraindications

Asymptomatic patients may be managed expectantly.

Surgical techniques

- Double aortic arch: division of the non-dominant arch.
- Right aortic arch with ligamentum arteriosum: division of the ligament.
- Right aortic arch with mirror image: division of the duct and Kommerll's diverticulum if present.
- Left aortic arch: aortopexy (median sternotomy), division and reimplantation of RSCA.
- Pulmonary artery sling: division and translocation of the LPA ± repair of the trachea via left thoracotomy/median sternotomy with CPB.

Complications

- Injury to the vagus, phrenic, and recurrent laryngeal nerves.
- Chylothorax from injury to the thoracic duct.
- Tracheomalacia and bronchomalacia.
- Late vascular complications such as subclavian steal.
- The risk of death is low if surgery is for isolated vascular ring, i.e., <1%. If combined with tracheal surgery, the results are not as good.
- There is evidence of persistent airway obstruction in about 50% of patients postoperatively.

Interrupted aortic arch repair

Key facts

- Interrupted aortic arch is defined as an interruption of lumenal continuity between the ascending and descending aorta. There are three types.
- It is rare, comprising <1% of congenital cardiac defects.
- The PDA is the only supply of blood to the descending aorta and neonates present in circulatory shock when the duct closes.
- Repair is indicated as a single or staged procedure: under DHCA, the descending aorta is transected from its anomalous origin from the PA trunk, and anastomosed directly to the ascending aorta.

Anatomy

- Interrupted arch is commonly associated with other defects: VSD 80–90%, bicuspid aortic valve 60%, subaortic stenosis 20%, common arterial trunk 10%. There are three possible points of interruption, correlating with the different embryonic derivations of the aortic arch:
- Type A (25–35%): at the isthmus, just distal to the LSCA origin.
- Type B (60–70%): between the LCC and LSCA: often associated with aberrant RSCA and subaortic stenosis.
- Type C (5%): between the innominate and LCC arteries.

Pathophysiology and natural history

The patent arterial duct is the only source of blood supply distal to the interruption. Ductal closure thus leads to systemic hypoperfusion, acidosis, renal failure, necrotizing enterocolitis, hepatic ischemia, heart failure.

Presentation

Neonates present when the duct closes with circulatory shock and congestive cardiac failure. They must be resuscitated, with prostaglandin infusion, inotropes if necessary, and intubation and ventilation to allow easy manipulation of the pulmonary vascular bed, and thus ductal flow. There may be abnormal pulse patterns depending on the site of interruption.

Investigations

- CXR: cardiomegaly and pulmonary vascular congestion.
- EKG: RV hypertrophy may be evident.
- Echo is diagnostic, showing narrow ascending aorta, absent arch, descending aorta continuing from the duct.

Surgery

Single-stage complete repair

The commonest presentation of interrupted arch with VSD is most commonly repaired completely in the neonatal period through a median sternotomy using cardiopulmonary bypass. This approach can also be used for interrupted arch in conjunction with anomalous pulmonary artery, A-P window, common arterial trunk, TAPVC, TGA, Taussig–Bing.

- Median sternotomy, and cannulation of both the ascending aorta and the duct if temperature >28°C at onset of bypass
- Cool to 20°C, mobilize the head–neck vessels and arch while cooling
- Arch repair during DHCA, or more frequently now with antegrade cerebral perfusion during aortic arch exclusion for repair.

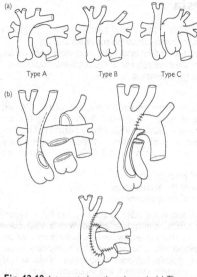

Fig. 12.10 Interrupted aortic arch repair. (a) Three types of interrupted aortic arch. (b) Repair of type B interrupted aortic arch.

- Duct is divided, ductal tissue excised, descending aorta anastomosed to the distal ascending aorta (7/0 Prolene).
- The left common carotid artery or left subclavian artery may be turned down as a flap to reconstitute the arch, with the distal left carotid anastomosed to the RCC to secure antegrade flow.
- Prosthetic tube grafts have been used in the past to achieve tensionless anastomosis, but this inevitably leads to the need for reoperation to upsize the graft, and is usually unnecessary.

Staged repair

The interrupted arch may be repaired through a thoracotomy, and the main PA banded to prevent pulmonary overflow in cases such as double inlet LV. Again, it is best to avoid prosthetic tube grafts. The left subclavian artery or left common carotid artery may be used to augment the repair, with or without a pericardial patch.

Specific complications

Mortality for single-stage repair is 10–20%. Risk of reoperation is no higher than with staged repair. 5-year survival is 65–70%; late survival is less with LVOTO. 10-year freedom from reoperation is 50%. Mortality for repair via thoracotomy with PA banding is low, but long-term reinterventions are as previously described. Anastomotic obstruction is common, with 25–40% requiring further arch intervention. Recurrent laryngeal and phrenic nerve damage and tracheal compression are also potential complications.

Tricuspid atresia

Key facts

- Absent right AV connection or tricuspid atresia comprises 1–3% of congenital cardiac defects; it is the third most common cyanotic heart defect.
- It results from failure of the development of the atrioventricular valve between the right atrium and ventricle.

Anatomy

Most commonly, there is an atretic tricuspid valve, hypoplastic RV, and restricted pulmonary blood flow and an ASD, leading to right-to-left shunting and cyanosis. There is usually a VSD, often restrictive. The ventriculoarterial arrangement is usually normal, and these patients usually have obstructed pulmonary flow, but in about 20% the great arteries are related abnormally.

- Type I: normally related great arteries.
- Type II: D-transposition of the great arteries.
- Type III: L-transposition of the great arteries.

Blood flows from the RA across the ASD to the LA. The RA is hypertrophied. The RV is hypoplastic and muscle bound, with a VSD communicating with the RVOT. There is usually, in 70%, pulmonary outflow obstruction, with a restricted infundibulum, and also pulmonary valvar stenosis/atresia or MPA hypoplasia. Left-sided obstructive lesions such as coarctation of the aorta, subaortic stenosis, and interrupted aortic arch are not uncommon.

Pathophysiology

The LA and LV support both systemic and pulmonary circulations and are therefore chronically volume overloaded. In neonates with pulmonary atresia, severe *cyanosis* develops with closure of the arterial duct; in those with unobstructed pulmonary flow, there is pulmonary overcirculation, pulmonary hypertension and heart failure.

Presentation and natural history

This is usually in the neonatal period with cyanosis. There may be heart failure in those with unrestricted pulmonary blood flow. 50% of patients have symptoms on the first day of life. The VSD causes a harsh ejection systolic murmur at the left sternal border; a cardiac murmur is present in 80% of cases. Without treatment survival beyond infancy is 10–20%.

Investigation

- EKG: characteristic notched P wave. LV hypertrophy.
- CXR: this is variable. There may be a boot shaped heart if there is pulmonary atresia/hypoplasia, or 'egg-on-a-string' if there are transposed great arteries; pulmonary vascularity may be decreased or increased.
- Echo: this is diagnostic, revealing difference in ventricular sizes, absence of the tricuspid valve, ASD with right-to-left flow. Relationship of the

great arteries, VSD, PDA, coarctation must all be assessed. The size of the ASD must be determined.

- Cardiac catheterization: this is recommended for operative strategy, determining the source and adequacy of pulmonary supply, measurement of the pulmonary artery pressure, pulmonary vascular resistance, left ventricular pressure, shunt fractions, and assessment of the pulmonary artery tree.

Management

Neonates presenting with severe cyanosis should be treated with PGE$_1$ to maintain ductal patency, those in heart failure should be treated with diuretics. However, most infants require some form of palliative surgery within the first year of life.

Surgery

Surgical management consists of initial palliation to achieve unobstructed systemic outflow and appropriate pulmonary blood flow.

- If the ASD is restrictive, a balloon atrial septostomy may be performed
- If the pulmonary blood flow is restricted, a systemic-pulmonary shunt, usually a BT shunt, is performed.
- If there is pulmonary overcirculation, a PA band is performed.

Subsequent definitive procedures aim to establish systemic venous return directly to the pulmonary arteries, thus bypassing the right heart altogether. This is the **Fontan circulation** (📖 p592) and tricuspid atresia provides the paradigm for this type of circulation.

- Bidirectional superior cavopulmonary shunt (📖 p601) to direct superior caval return to the right pulmonary artery (at about 6 months of age).
- Completion of total cavopulmonary connection with extracardiac tube graft draining the inferior caval vein flow to the right pulmonary artery, thus redirecting all systemic venous return directly to the lungs, bypassing the RV (2–4 years of age).

Outcomes

The overall mortality through all stages to completion of the Fontan circulation is <10% for this condition, and the 1-year survival after Fontan completion is 85%; the procedure should eliminate cyanosis, polycythemia and ventricular volume overload, improving prognosis.

Congenital tricuspid valve stenosis

Isolated congenital tricuspid stenosis and incompetence are exceedingly rare. Congenital tricuspid stenosis is usually due to hypoplastic annulus and forms part of the spectrum of tricuspid atresia, hypoplastic RV. Isolated tricuspid incompetence may be due to agenesis of one or two leaflets, annular distension, or absence of papillary muscles; surgery may be undertaken in older children.

Hypoplastic left heart syndrome

Key facts

- Hypoplastic left heart syndrome (HLHS) is a spectrum of left-sided cardiac malformations characterized by marked hypoplasia of the LV and ascending aorta (Fig. 12.11).
- It comprises 7–10% of congenital cardiac defects of the neonate.
- More common in Turner, Noonan, and Smith–Lemli–Opitz syndromes. 25% of infants have chromosomal abnormalities on karyotyping.

Morphology

Highly variable (Fig. 12.1). Hallmarks include:

- Aortic valve hypoplasia or stenosis.
- Ascending aorta hyoplasia or atresia, arch hypoplasia, coarctation.
- LV absence, atresia or hypoplasia.
- Associated mitral valve atresia, hypoplasia or stenosis.
- Ventricular septum usually intact (ASD necessary for viability).
- Systemic circulation is by necessity supplied by a large PDA.

Physiology

- Fully saturated pulmonary venous return to the LA cannot flow to the LV, and must cross the ASD to the RA, where it mixes with systemic venous return. Any restriction in the PFO/ASD is equivalent to pulmonary venous obstruction.
- As a result both systemic and pulmonary venous return are directed through the RV. The RV pumps blood to:
  - The lungs via the pulmonary arteries.
  - The body via the PDA which supplies the descending aorta.
  - The coronary arteries are supplied by retrograde flow of blood from the PDA down the hypoplastic ascending aorta.
- The relative flow to each circulation will depend on the relative vascular resistances in each bed (because flow is inversely proportional to vascular resistance).

After birth

After birth, a *'balanced' circulation* and maintenance of life depends on:

- Adequate interatrial communication.
- Patent ductus arteriosus.
- Pulmonary vascular resistance.

After birth, as the pulmonary vascular resistance falls, the RV will pump preferentially to the pulmonary vascular bed, thus increasing oxygen saturation, but at the expense of systemic blood flow, cerebral blood flow, and coronary blood flow. Poor systemic perfusion leads to metabolic acidosis, oliguria, and eventually collapse. Coronary and cerebral perfusion are also decreased. Conversely, increased systemic blood flow at the expense of pulmonary blood flow leads to good peripheral perfusion. However, the reduced pulmonary perfusion leads to hypoxia. Thus, a delicate balance between the two vascular beds must be maintained to ensure adequate tissue perfusion and oxygenation, and the aim of neonatal management is a 'balanced' circulation.

Presentation

HLHS is uniformly fatal in the first weeks of life without intervention. Usually presents in the first 24–48h of life. Most are term infants after a normal pregnancy. If there has been pulmonary venous obstruction *in utero* due to a restrictive ASD, the child may be born in respiratory distress. Usually, as the duct closes within the first 48h postnatally, the child becomes cyanosed, tachycardic, tachypnoeic, oliguric, acidotic, and hypothermic. There is a normal first heart sound, loud, single second heart sound, usually no murmurs, and prominent RV impulse.

Investigations

- The EKG shows RA enlargement and RV hypertrophy.
- CXR shows cardiomegaly and increased pulmonary vascular markings.
- Echo is diagnostic. Shows anatomy of left-sided hypoplasia and arch, coarctation, and adequacy of any ASD. TR predicts poorer outcomes.
- Cardiac catheterization is not normally required but may be necessary to perform atrial septostomy to relieve pulmonary venous obstruction
- Intracranial bleeds and abdominal pathology are common: US of head and abdomen is standard preoperatively.

Management

This lesion is the most frequent congenital heart lesion associated with cardiac death in the newborn. Goals of initial management include:
- Maintaining the PDA with PGE_1 infusion 0.025–0.05 micrograms/kg/min.
- Maintaining a balance between PVR and SVR to maintain flows using either CO_2 or hypoxic inhaled mixtures to maintain ↑PVR.
- The infant can usually be stabilized for a few days prior to surgery but the only definitive intervention is surgical.
- The option of **supportive therapy** only, with discharge home and eventual death, must be offered to parents. This requires an honest discussion about the mortality rates of each stage and the interstage mortality rates as well as an estimate of long-term functional outcomes.

Overview of surgical options
- The three options available are:
- **Norwood**
  - **Norwood stage I procedure** within a few days of birth (📖 p588).
  - Second stage is performed at 3–6 months to minimize the time the RV has to cope with two circulations, and consists of performing a bidirectional **Glenn shunt** (📖 p601), dividing the B-T shunt, augmenting the pulmonary arteries, addressing residual surgical issues, e.g., restrictive ASD, or recoarctation. Some units prefer to perform the **hemi-Fontan procedure** (📖 p591) at this stage instead.
  - Finally a **Fontan** (📖 pp594–595) at 2 years.
- Orthotopic cardiac transplantation.
- Stenting of the duct and bilateral PA band (hybrid procedure).

The first two of these options are the more established procedures, with equivalent long-term outcomes (75% at 5 years). The third is a recent innovation, largely restricted in its use to 'high-risk' neonates. Therefore, indications for its use have not been fully elucidated at this time.

Norwood procedure

Key facts

- The Norwood procedure is the first of a three-stage repair of *HLHS* (📖 p586) which results in a single-ventricle *Fontan circulation* (📖 p592).
- It is also used as a palliative procedure for conditions in which the morphological left heart is inadequate to maintain systemic circulation such as AV and ventriculoarterial (📖 p598) malconnections.
- The aim of the Norwood stage I is to secure systemic cardiac output and balance the pulmonary and systemic vascular beds. This is done by:
  - Atrial septectomy to ensure pulmonary venous return bypasses LV.
  - Securing the systemic output: augmenting the aortic arch, repairing coarctation, and converting the right-sided ventricle and outflow tract to a systemic ventricle and outflow tract.
  - Securing a controlled pulmonary blood supply with a B-T shunt (📖 p600) or RV-PA conduit.
- The second and third stages are described on 📖 pp590–595.

Setup

- Standard invasive monitoring, with antifibrinolytic, PGE₁ discontinued.
- Median sternotomy, heparinization at 300U/kg.
- PDA, and left and right PA, are dissected completely free, and the aorta is freed from root to head and neck vessels, mobilized and snared.
- Standard CPB with distal ascending aortic cannula (or via 3–3.5mm Gore-tex tube which may be used for later B-T shunt), single-stage venous cannula, and patient cooled to 18–20°C.
- Pulmonary blood flow may require cross-clamping or snaring the PA.

Procedure

Repair of the hypoplastic aorta and connection to the LVOT

- The main PA is transected just proximal to the main bifurcation.
- The distal PA is closed with a patch of cryopreserved homograft.
- The ductus arteriosus is transected at its entrance to the aorta, all ductal and any coarcted tissue is completely excised.
- The aorta and arch is enlarged during a period of DHCA or selective cerebral perfusion using a patch of homograft tissue, and the back wall of the aorta and distal arch are then anastomosed.
- The aorta and proximal margin of the homograft patch is anastomosed to the proximal main PA (Damus–Kaye–Stansel anastomosis Fig. 12.11d). may be made in several ways depending on the geometry of the arch. An easy way of making this anastomosis is to make an incision in the patch used to augment the arch, and anastomosing the MPA into this.
- During DHCA, the RA cannula is removed and atrial septectomy performed through the cannulation site; if necessary a separate incision may be made to achieve this.

Formation of shunt to restore pulmonary blood

- Pulmonary blood flow is secured with an RV-PA conduit, usually a 5mm Gore-Tex tube, from the right ventricle to the left (Sano) or right (modified Sano) pulmonary artery.

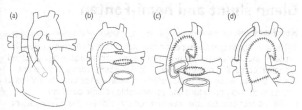

Fig 12.11 (a) Hypoplastic left heart. (b) Transected PDA, PA, and aortotomy. (c) Patch augmentation of aorta. (d) Anastomosis between aorta and PA, and B-T shunt.

- Alternatively a systemic to pulmonary artery shunt is constructed by anastomosing a 3–4mm PTFE graft between the innominate artery and the right PA, restoring flow to the pulmonary arteries.

Closure

Standard closure with epicardial pacing wires, LA catheter, meticulous hemostasis (blood products usually mandatory) and Ethibond to sternum.

Specific complications

- ↑PVR reduces pulmonary blood flow causing hypoxemia.
- ↓PVR increases pulmonary blood flow, reducing systemic cardiac output, and causing myocardial ischemia, acidosis, and cardiac arrest.
- Pulmonary venous hypertension.
- Right ventricular failure.

Outcomes

Mortality after the Norwood stage I varies from 5 to 30% between centers. Risk factors for poor outcomes include weight <2.5kg, no ASD at presentation, small ascending aorta, TR, late presentation, prematurity, mitral stenosis with aortic atresia. There is substantial mortality between stages, with mortality of 5–15% between stage I and II. The best centers achieve an 80% survival to completion of the Fontan circulation, usually performed at 4–5 years. 80% of children who reach school age are developmentally normal. Neonatal transplant is performed at a few centres worldwide for this condition, with a surgical mortality of 14%, and a further mortality of 20% of those waiting for transplant. The scarcity of donors makes this an option only in a few centers.

BT shunt vs. RV PA (Sano) conduit

Over the last 5 years, use of the RV to PA (Sano) shunt has increased due to apparently better outcomes. However, large centers with previously good results using B-T shunts have not shown reproducible benefit, and a multicenter trial from the USA has not shown benefit of one over the other. Postoperatively, RV-PA conduits may allow a more stable course and easier manipulation of competing vascular beds; however, an appropriately sized BT shunt should not lead to difficulties in this matter.

Glenn shunt and hemi-Fontan

Key facts

• These are both types of superior cavopulmonary anastomosis (see 📖 p600), and they are usually performed as an intermediate stage in staged surgical correction of a single ventricle (📖 p586), usually 3–6 months after the Norwood stage I (📖 p588) to minimize the time the RV has to cope with two circulations and considerable volume overload.

• The bidirectional superior cavopulmonary (bidirectional Glenn) shunt consists of an anastomosis between the SVC and the pulmonary circulation, with the proximal pulmonary artery oversewn.

• It can be performed without bypass off-pump, under cardioplegic arrest, or DHCA.

• The hemi-Fontan procedure, which involves anastomosis of the RA to the right PA, with the proximal PA oversewn and the SVC outlet oversewn, is rarely used today—it is a staging procedure for the lateral tunnel fenestrated Fontan which itself is not commonly used.

Set-up

• Triple lumen lines are not placed in the upper great veins because of the risk of thrombosis of the cavopulmonary anastomosis or PA; however, a single lumen SVC monitoring line is necessary.

• Standard preparation for resternotomy is used, including external defibrillator paddles and preparation of the groin or neck (<2 years).

• The bidirectional Glenn shunt and hemi-Fontan procedures are performed via a median sternotomy.

• Standard aorto-bicaval cannulation is used in the bidirectional Glenn procedure, and aorto-atrial cannulation is used in the hemi-Fontan.

• Right atrial cannulation with DHCA may be used to avoid trauma to the SVC.

• Bypass is commenced, the heart vented, and the patient cooled.

• The pulmonary artery, branch arteries, aorta, SVC, and RA are completely dissected, and the azygos vein is ligated.

• If a left SVC is present it is dissected free, so that a left cavopulmonary anastomosis can be performed.

Procedure

Bidirectional Glenn shunt

• This is the first stage of a TCPC (📖 p592), and the second stage of the Norwood sequence of operations (📖 p588). It prepares the way for the final completion of the total cavopulmonary connection, the currently favored form of Fontan circulation (📖 p592).

• As a stage II Norwood operation, the B-T or RV-PA shunt must be ligated and divided, any residual pulmonary artery stenoses or hypoplasia must be augmented, and lesions such as restrictive ASD, recoarctation or AV valve regurgitation addressed.

• If this is the first stage of a Fontan operation for other anomalies, lesions such as AV valve regurgitation or outflow tract obstruction must be repaired. If the MPA has forward flow it may be ligated at this stage.

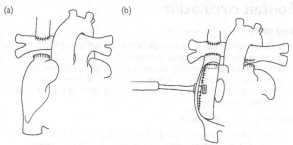

Fig. 12.12 Superior cavopulmonary anastomosis. (a) Bidirectional Glenn shunt. (b) Hemi-Fontan.

- The SVC is transected at its junction with the RA; the RA is oversewn.
- The SVC is then anastomosed to a longitudinal incision in the RPA, establishing continuity between the SVC and both PAs (Fig. 12.12).
- The PAP measured in the SVC must be <20mmHg postoperatively, and the transpulmonary gradient should be <10mmHg (PAP-CVP).

Hemi-Fontan

- If deep hypothermic circulatory arrest is used CPB is discontinued at 20°C and the patient exsanguinated into the venous reservoir.
- The dissection is completed.
- The main PA is divided, and the proximal end oversewn.
- The RA is opened towards the IVC, and an ASD created.
- The superior cavoatrial junction is opened and extended up the SVC.
- The right PA is incised inferiorly and superiorly so that the opening in the cavoatrial junction can be anastomosed to these incisions.
- A piece of homograft is used to close the SVC orifice into the RA.
- If a left SVC is present this is divided and anastomosed to the left PA.

Closure

- Atrial and ventricular temporary epicardial pacing wires are placed.
- Ventilation is resumed, the heart is de-aired and weaned from bypass.
- After placing mediastinal and pleural drains, and securing hemostasis, and patch closure of the pericardium, the chest is closed.

Classic Glenn shunt

The classic Glenn shunt is no longer used, but it is still encountered in adult patients. It was performed via a right–left posterolateral thoracotomy in the fourth intercostal space. The right PA was divided along the medial border of the SVC, and the proximal PA stump oversewn. The distal end of the right PA was anastomosed to the SVC.

Fontan circulation

Key facts

- A '*Fontan circulation*' is the physiological end result of staged procedures for univentricular hearts where the systemic veins are anastomosed directly to the pulmonary circulation, in an attempt to separate the systemic and pulmonary circulations which are otherwise mixed.
- The circulation completely depends on blood crossing a low-gradient pulmonary vasculature.

Indications for a Fontan

It is indicated for any lesion with only one well-developed ventricle:

- Tricuspid atresia/absent right AV connection (📖 p584) or mitral atresia/absent left AV connection.
- Double inlet left ventricle/double inlet right ventricle.
- Hypoplastic left heart syndrome (📖 p586).
- Unbalanced AVSD (📖 p568).
- Straddling left or right atrioventricular valves.
- Pulmonary atresia with intact ventricular septum and small right ventricle (📖 p614).

Principles of the Fontan circulation

- In a normal biventricular heart, the systemic and pulmonary circulations are in *series*: each one is supported by a ventricle.
- In patients born with a single ventricle, the two circulations are in *parallel*: systemic and pulmonary venous blood mixes.
- In the Fontan circulation, the systemic and pulmonary circulations are *separated* and placed in *series* without the interposition of a ventricle (*Fontan operation*): there are three types:
  - Atriopulmonary connection (📖 p590), e.g., *hemi Fontan*.
  - Intracardiac total cavopulmonary connection (📖 p594).
  - Extracardiac total cavopulmonary connection (📖 p594).

Technical overview

The Fontan circulation is achieved in two stages (in hypoplastic left heart (📖 p586) a *Norwood procedure* precedes the two other stages):

- *Bidirectional Glenn shunt,* bidirectional superior cavopulmonary shunt (📖 p601): the systemic venous drainage from the *upper body*, i.e., via the superior caval vein(s), is disconnected from the RA and anastomosed to the right PA (in the case of bilateral SVCs, bilateral CP shunts are constructed, with the LSVC to the LPA).
- *Fontan operation,* completion of total cavopulmonary connection (📖 p594): the systemic venous return from the *lower body*, via the inferior caval vein, is redirected to the pulmonary circulation by disconnecting it from the RA and directing it to the right PA via an extracardiac conduit (usually Gore-Tex tube), or from within the RA using native tissue or a patch to baffle flow (lateral tunnel). If a connection is made between systemic venous circulation and pulmonary venous circulation, this is called a fenestration. The need for a fenestration in the Fontan circuit is controversial (📖 p522).

Physiological considerations

In the Fontan circulation, pulmonary blood flow is dependent on the passive return of systemic venous blood into the pulmonary vasculature, rather than by the RV. This is only possible if:

- Pulmonary vascular resistance is low (mean PAP≤15mmHg).
- Ventricular function is good.
- Atrioventricular valves are competent.
- There are no obstructive lesions in the circulation.
- There are no shunts (e.g., large collaterals, previous B-T shunt).

Requirements for a Fontan circulation to work

The original '10 commandments' indicating suitability for Fontan procedure (now not so rigidly applied) are listed here: the two current mandatory criteria are asterisked.

- Age >4.
- Sinus rhythm.
- Normal caval drainage.
- Normal volume RA.
- *Mean PAP≤15mmHg.
- PVR <4 units/m².
- PA diameter: aorta diameter ≥0.75.
- *LV ejection fraction ≥0.6.
- Competent atrioventricular valve(s).
- No shunts.

One-stage versus two-stage procedures

Two stages have lower mortality and morbidity than if the cavopulmonary connections are completed in a single operation; this may be because the first operation reduces the volume load on the single ventricle, allowing some of the resulting hypertrophy to regress, and diastolic function to improve, before the final operation. The bidirectional superior cavopulmonary connection can only be undertaken after 3 months of age when the neonatal pulmonary vascular resistance will definitely have fallen—with a higher pulmonary artery pressure the cavopulmonary shunt will fail. Thus, many neonates require a palliative operation before they can undergo staged Fontan.

Systemic-pulmonary versus cavopulmonary shunts

- Cavopulmonary shunts redirect venous, desaturated blood into the pulmonary circulation; systemic-pulmonary shunt redirects arterial, saturated blood into the pulmonary circulation.
- CP shunts divert 30–50% of systemic venous blood from the heart to the lungs, thus **reducing** the volume load on the heart; systemic-pulmonary shunts add to the pulmonary circulation, thus **increasing** the volume load on the heart.

Fontan operation

Key facts

- The Fontan operation has been described as, 'the surgical endpoint for patients whose cardiac anomalies do not allow two ventricle circulation.' It is the final stage of the three-stage repair of hypoplastic left heart syndrome (📖 p586).
- All forms of the Fontan operation aim to divert systemic (with or without coronary sinus) venous return to the pulmonary circulation.
- There are many modifications, but currently the extracardiac total cavopulmonary connection is most widely used.
- Only pulmonary venous (with or without coronary sinus) blood returns to the common atrial chamber and single ventricle.
- The entire cardiac output is provided by one ventricle, with the separated pulmonary and systemic circulations in series rather than in parallel.
- Pulmonary blood flow is dependent on CVP and outflow resistance.
- The lateral tunnel Fontan is usually performed with cardioplegic arrest, whereas the external conduit Fontan can be performed on the warm beating heart or off-pump.

Setup

- Standard invasive monitoring and general anesthetic, with antifibrinolytic.
- Median sternotomy, heparinization at 300U/kg.
- An atrial catheter is inserted directly into the common atrium via the right atrial wall or RSPV.
- Standard CPB with distal ascending aortic cannula, bicaval cannulation with the caval purse-strings as far distal as possible, and patient cooled to 32°C.
- The right and left PA are completely dissected free before CPB.
- If required the aorta is cross-clamped and cold blood cardioplegia given.

Procedure

Lateral-tunnel fenestrated Fontan operation

- The pulmonary trunk is transected and the ends oversewn, if this has not already been performed in previous surgery (hemi-Fontan 📖 p590, or Norwood 📖 p588).
- The RA is opened.
- The SVC is divided, and the distal portion anastomosed to the superior aspect of the right PA, and the proximal portion anastomosed to the inferior aspect of the right PA.
- If the Fontan procedure follows a previous Glenn shunt procedure the proximal SVC will have been oversewn: this is opened up, and enlarged if necessary onto the roof of the RA.
- A large ASD is created avoiding the conducting tissues.
- A PTFE baffle is sewn to channel IVC blood into the SVC and right PA.

- Typically a fenestration is placed on the edge of the lateral tunnel using a 4mm aortic punch: a purse string may be placed around this and brought out through the RA so that the size can be adjusted.
- The right atriotomy is closed.

Extracardiac conduit fenestrated Fontan operation

- May be performed off-pump, with CPB on the beating heart, or on the arrested heart.
- Usually the previous operation of a bidirectional Glenn also includes any other repairs/modifications needed, so that this final stage need only establish continuity between the inferior caval vein and the pulmonary circulation.
- A 20mm Gore-tex tube is first anastomosed to the inferior RPA.
- The IVC is transected at its junction with the RA, the RA is oversewn.
- The other end of the Gore-tex tube is anastomosed to the IVC.
- A fenestration may be formed by anastomosing a punch-hole in the Gore-tex tube to the RA wall. The need for a fenestration in the Fontan circuit is controversial—many authorities feel it is unnecessary if patient selection is optimal, however many centers continue to add a fenestration as routine.
- Chest drains are placed in both pleural cavities and the mediastinum.
- An atrial pressure monitoring line must be placed through the RA wall to allow fluid management ('CVP' lines no longer measure atrial pressure).

Closure

- An atrial catheter and atrial and ventricular temporary epicardial pacing wires are placed.
- Ventilation is resumed, the heart is de-aired and weaned from bypass.
- After placing mediastinal and pleural drains and securing hemostasis, the chest is closed with Ethibond sutures to the sternum.

Care after Fontan operation

Key facts

Monitoring of the common atrial pressure and the PAPs is mandatory in the first 24h. The difference between these is the transpulmonary gradient. The PA pressure and the transpulmonary gradient usually fall after extubation.

In the immediate postoperative period

- Blood loss causes profound hemodynamic instability—hemostasis must be meticulous.
- May need aggressive filling to maintain BP.
- Avoid the use of vasoconstrictors: elevated PVR will cause Fontan circulation to fail as minimal resistance across pulmonary bed is required given absence of chamber functioning as RV.
- Maintain sinus rhythm.
- Aim to extubate early to improve Fontan hemodynamics (positive pressure ventilation reduces systemic venous filling of pulmonary circulation).
- Respiratory failure and acidosis cause pulmonary vascular resistance to rise, therefore 'early' extubation must be rationally performed.
- The chest drains should not be removed in the first 48h.
- Atrial line can be removed on day 1 postoperatively.
- Heparinize when bleeding has stopped.

Hospital course

- The patient should be anticoagulated after the acute postoperative period, once the intracardiac lines and pacing wires have been removed.
- The chest drains will often continue to drain for several days, and may drain for weeks. Effusions are usually serous, occasionally chylous. If they drain for >2 weeks, the patient may be carefully assessed with cardiac catheter and any pathway obstructions corrected. Longer drainage may necessitate:
  - Cardiac catheter intervention: enlarge/create fenestration, stent PA stenoses.
  - Total parenteral nutrition.
  - Regime of fluid restriction, diuretics, pulmonary arterial vasodilators, ACE inhibitors, continuous oxygen administration, aggressive mobilization.
  - Intravenous ocreotide—only anecdotal evidence.
- Reversal of the Fontan circulation—this is high risk, particularly if the decision to undertake this management is delayed.

Early complications

- Elevated Fontan pathway pressure.
- Ascites, hepatomegaly, pleural effusions from high CVP required to generate pulmonary blood flow.
- Poor pulmonary blood flow secondary to ↑PVR, positive pressure ventilation, loss of sinus rhythm.

- LV dysfunction.
- Extremely poor hemodynamics requiring surgical reversal or fenestration of the circuit.

Long-term outcomes
- Atrial or Fontan pathway thrombosis.
- Patient should be maintained on anticoagulation for life.
- 5- and 10-year survival with modern techniques of Fontan completion are in the order of 95% and 90%.

Late complications
- Atrial arrhythmias: probably lower incidence with lateral tunnel and extracardiac conduit TCPC.
- Protein-losing enteropathy: loss of protein from the GI tract—unknown cause—debilitating and life threatening, occurs in up to 15%.
- Thromboembolic complications—up to 20%.
- Development of collateral vessels.
- Ventricular failure.
- Plastic bronchitis with bronchial casts—these may cause airway obstruction.
- 'Failing' Fontan—inability of the circulation to deliver adequate cardiac output—if heart transplantation undertaken for this, mortality is up to 65%.

Pathophysiologic sequelae
- Fontan circulation has the following pathophysiological sequelae:
  - Acute increases in PVR can decrease systemic venous return, particularly impeding portal venous flow.
  - High venous return causes increased lymph production, and contributes to impaired lymph reabsorption.
  - Chronic lymphatic hypertension contributes to protein losing enteropathy and plastic bronchitis.
- Aortopulmonary collaterals develop and may result in large left-to-right shunts contributing to ventricular volume overload.

Pulmonary artery banding

Key facts

- This is a palliative operation that aims to limit pulmonary blood flow by reducing the circumference of the main PA. Its indications have reduced over the years.
- A band is placed around the PA trunk, via either a left thoracotomy or median sternotomy. The band is sequentially tightened while PA pressures are monitored, until the PA pressure is <50% of the systolic pressure, or the lowest possible PA pressure with acceptable SaO_2 is achieved.

Indications

Pulmonary artery banding was first used for children with single ventricles, or large left-to-right shunts, e.g., VSD, AV canal, and truncus arteriosus. Improvements in surgical techniques and myocardial preservation mean that most of these disorders can be corrected, and PA banding is now reserved for a few defects:

- **VSD**, multiple VSD, coarctation aorta with large VSD, large VSD with major non-cardiac malformation.
- In **late presentation TGA** (🕮 p624) to prepare the LV for arterial switch.
- After **Mustard/Senning**, to prepare the LV prior to converting to arterial switch (🕮 pp626–629).
- Double inlet ventricle and no PS.
- Tricuspid atresia with no PS.
- AVSD unsuitable for repair (pulmonary hypertension, AV discordance, recent RSV bronchiolitis).
- HLHS—bilateral PA bands in combination with arterial duct stenting and atrial septostomy.
- ccTGA with TR.

Contraindications

- In single-ventricle anomalies where the aorta arises from muscular infundibulum, (e.g. DILV, TA with TGA), there is a potential for subaortic obstruction, and PA banding may hasten this. These patients should have Damus-Kaye-Stans Norwood (🕮 p588).
- Not recommended in common arterial trunk.

Setup

- Standard invasive monitoring and general anesthesia, avoid inotropes to reduce acute changes in SVR and PVR.
- Median sternotomy or left thoracotomy with pericardium opened anterior to the phrenic nerve, and LA appendage retracted with a stay suture. Rarely, anterior extrapleural approach.

Procedure

The band may be a 3mm cotton tape, thick braided silk, 2mm strip of Gore-Tex, silk tape, or siliconized silk tape.

Placement of PA band

- As the PA may be dilated and extremely thin-walled, the safest method of encircling the PA is to place the band around both PA and proximal aorta, then develop the plane between aorta and PA, through which the free edge of the band may be pulled.
- The band is sequentially tightened and may be secured with Ligaclips so that it can be released later with angioplasty.

Degree of banding

- This is a clinical judgement based on:
- Systemic pressure.
- PAP.
- Echo appearance of the septum.

The degree of banding depends on the underlying lesion—the principle is to balance the systemic and pulmonary blood flow. Trusler and Mustard calculated optimal length of the band using the patient's weight:

- Biventricular heart: 20mm + weight in kg.
- Complex malformations with mixing: 24mm + weight in kg.
- Malformations proceeding to Fontan circulations: 22mm + weight in kg.

This formula can be used as a guide when banding, but must be adjusted according to the conditions found at operation, e.g., in VSD aim to reduce PAP to near normal, i.e., 30mmHg, with near normal O_2 sats.

Removal of PA band

- This is normally performed through a median sternotomy with CPB as dictated by the planned surgical repair (Fontan or arterial switch).
- All the band must be removed as adherent fragments cause strictures.
- The area banded is either opened and patched anteriorly or excised, anastomosing the PA trunk in an end-to-end fashion.
- The manner in which the chest is closed depends on the nature of the surgical correction performed at the same time.

Complications

These patients may be very unstable postoperatively, and some centers advocate deep sedation and paralysis for the first 24h. If there is sudden hemodynamic instability with loss of cardiac output, the safest option on the PICU is reopening of the chest and release of the band.

- RVOT obstruction.
- Severe right PA stenosis and left PA hypertension if the band migrates.
- Congestive cardiac failure if the band is too loose.
- Hypoxemia and shunt reversal if the band is too tight.
- Pulmonary valve damage.

Shunts

Key facts

- Systemic–pulmonary shunts provide a source of blood flow to the pulmonary arterial system from the systemic circulation, thus improving the oxygen saturations in cyanotic heart disease. They may facilitate pulmonary artery growth where these are hypoplastic.
- Indications include tricuspid atresia, tetralogy of Fallot, hypoplastic PAs, anomalous coronary artery with associated complex cardiac anomalies, pulmonary atresia with intact ventricular septum, pulmonary atresia with VSD, Ebstein anomaly, single-ventricle anomaly with pulmonary or aortic atresia.
- The ideal systemic–pulmonary artery shunt has several features:
  - Technically simple to perform.
  - Provide adequate but not excessive pulmonary blood flow.
  - Good long-term patency.
  - Causes no cardiopulmonary abnormalities.
  - Technically simple to close.

Historical

- **Blalock–Taussig–Thomas shunt** involved connecting the subclavian artery directly to the PA, thus sacrificing subclavian artery flow. Pulmonary blood flow was limited by the size of the subclavian artery, and the shunt grew with the child.
- **Waterston shunt** consisted of anastomosis of the ascending aorta directly to the right PA. Shunt size was difficult to regulate, with the risk of pulmonary overflow and the development of pulmonary vascular disease. The right PA was often distorted by this anastomosis. It may be difficult to close these shunts.
- **Potts shunt** connected the descending aorta directly to the left PA. This also raises the risk of over-shunting, and led to left PA distortion

Commonly used shunts in the modern era

Modified Blalock–Taussig shunt (mBT shunt)

- These are now the most commonly performed systemic-pulmonary artery shunts, with a resurgence in their use as part of the Norwood stage I procedure.
- An ePTFE (Gore-tex) tube is anastomosed end-to-side to the subclavian artery without dividing it, and end-to-side to the PA.
- Approach: either via lateral thoracotomy on the side of the innominate artery (i.e., on side opposite arch), or via a midline sternotomy in very small neonates, or when cardiopulmonary bypass may be required (if the child is hemodynamically unstable)if the duct has to be closed.
- 3.5–4mm shunts in neonates; flow regulated by size of subclavian artery.

Central shunt

- A short PTFE tube is used between the ascending aorta and the main PA, both anastomoses performed end-to-side.
- Particularly useful with small branch pulmonary arteries, encouraging their growth, useful in small infants
- Prevents distortion of the branch pulmonary arteries, equal blood flow to both lungs, low occlusion rate, easily closed.
- Performed through a median sternotomy.

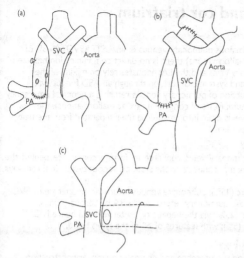

Fig. 12.13 Aortopulmonary shunts: (a) Blalock–Taussig. (b) Modified Balock–Taussig. (c) Cooley.

Melbourne/Mee shunt
The anastomosis of diminutive main PA end-to-side to ascending aorta to promote growth of PA in pulmonary atresia/VSD/MAPCAs.

Cavopulmonary shunt/bidirectional Glenn shunt
- This is the anastomosis of the superior caval vein to the right PA (and/or LSVC to LPA) (see also 🕮 p590).
- PVR must be low, therefore contraindicated under 3–6 months.
- Does not increase volume load on the heart, commonly used as the first stage of a total cavopulmonary connection, or Fontan circulation.

Sano shunt
- PTFE tube connecting the RV to the left PA as part of the Norwood stage I operation, instead of a modified BT shunt.
- Prevents the low diastolic pressure and poor coronary perfusion seen with 'classical' Norwood stage I with mBT shunt
- Appears to lead to more stable immediate postoperative hemodynamics, and may reduce the mortality 'between stages'.
- 4mm shunt in neonates <2.5 kg, 5mm >2.5kg.
- Requires a right ventriculotomy, becomes obstructive over 3 months.
- When the shunt is taken from the RV to the RPA (Birmingham modification), it is easier to access at the second stage.

Complications of shunts
Sudden death, occlusion—patients should remain on aspirin ± dipyridamole until shunt takedown, infection, PA distortion/stenosis up to 30%, false aneurysm formation with rupture, phrenic nerve injury (left mBT shunt), Horner's syndrome, seroma formation from leak through the porous PTFE tube.

TAPVD and cor triatrium

Key facts

- In total anomalous pulmonary venous drainage (TAPVD) (1–3% of congenital malformations) there is no direct communication between the pulmonary veins and the LA: neonates rely on mixing of the pulmonary and systemic circulation through an ASD for survival.
- Total obstruction of pulmonary venous return is a neonatal emergency
- In cor triatrium, (0.1% of congenital cardiac malformations), the pulmonary veins drain into an antechamber separated from the true LA by a diaphragm.

Morphology

In TAPVD pulmonary veins converge to form a confluence behind the pericardial sack that connects to the systemic venous system in three ways (Fig. 12.14).

- *Supracardiac* (45%): pulmonary venous return via innominate or SVC.
- *Cardiac* (25%): pulmonary return via the RA or coronary sinus.
- *Infracardiac* (25%): via the hepatic or portal vein and hence IVC.
- *Mixed type* (5%): with features of >1 of the types listed.

Pathophysiology

This depends on the presence and degree of pulmonary obstruction.

- Non-obstructed TAPVD is effectively a large left-to-right shunt, with greatly increased pulmonary blood flow, and RV volume overload, resulting in ↑ PVR, RVH, CCF.
- Cyanosis occurs because fully oxygenated pulmonary venous blood mixes with desaturated systemic venous return, the resultant mix reaches the left side of the heart via an ASD or PFO, which is mandatory for survival, and the ductus arteriosus while patent.
- Obstruction to pulmonary venous flow in TAPVD, which is a common feature of infracardiac TAPVD results in pulmonary edema, ↑↑PVR, and severe cyanosis, although RV volume overload is less marked.
- It is common for the blood in all four chambers to have the same oxygen saturations because of mixing.

Presentation

Infants with non-obstructed TAPVC (uncommon) present a few months after birth with mild cyanosis and signs of heart failure, a systolic murmur, and loud second heart sound with fixed splitting. Infants with obstructed TAPVC, in contrast, present with profound cyanosis and signs of severe heart failure within hours to days of birth.

Investigations

- The CXR in non-obstructed TAPVD shows increased pulmonary vascularity, a prominent pulmonary border, enlarged right heart border and after 6 months in supracardiac TAPVD a 'figure of 8'.
- In obstructed TAPVD the cardiac and pulmonary shadows are normal in size, but the lung fields show signs of severe pulmonary venous obstruction.
- TTE and TEE are diagnostic.

- Cardiac catheterization is only required if there are associated cardiac anomalies, or to examine individual pulmonary vein anatomy and identify obstructions.

Surgical management

TAPVD repair is described on ▢ p604.

Indications for surgery

- Obstructed TAPVD is a surgical emergency, even within the first few weeks of life.
- Non-obstructed TAPVD is an indication for urgent surgery.

Outcome

The hospital mortality of TAPVD repair is 5–10%.

Cor triatrium

In cor triatrium the pulmonary venous collecting chamber is *intrapericardial* and lies superior and posterior to the LA, from which it is separated by a *fibromuscular diaphragm*. There may or may not be a communication between the two chambers; the RA may communicate with one or both chambers. The true LA contains the LA appendage and the mitral valve. Pulmonary venous flow reaches the left side of the heart by passing across the diaphragm into the LA, and thus is subject to obstruction at this site. If the collecting chamber communicates with the RA but not the LA, then the results are similar to TAPVC.

Presentation and investigation

Depending on the size of communication between the chamber, LA, and RA this may present like a large ASD, or like obstructed TAPVD. Echo is diagnostic: should delineate the pulmonary venous anatomy, as well as differentiating between cor triatrium and supramitral membrane, where the membrane lies between the mitral valve and the LAA: in cor triatriatum, the mitral valve and the LAA are on the same side of the diaphragm.

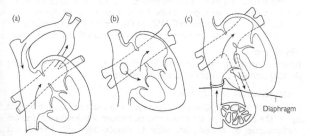

Fig. 12.14 The three types of anomalous pulmonary venous connection. (a) Supracardiac. (b) Cardiac. (c) Infracardiac.

Repair of TAPVD

Key facts
- Pulmonary venous obstruction is a surgical emergency in most neonates with TAPVD.
- Surgical technique is dictated by the anatomy (📖 p602).

Set-up
- Median sternotomy.
- Standard aorto-atrial cardiopulmonary bypass and DHCA.

Supracardiac TAPVC
- The heart is elevated out of the mediastinum to the right, to expose the LA and the pulmonary venous confluence behind the posterior pericardium (Fig. 12.15).
- The vertical vein is identified and either ligated and divided to provide mobility to the confluence, or left intact as a pressure vent for the non-compliant LV after surgery.
- Incisions are made in the pulmonary venous confluence and the base of the LA appendage, and the two anastomosed with 7/0 Prolene.

Infracardiac TAPVC
- This usually presents in the neonatal period with a shocked patient.
- The confluence behind the heart is exposed as previously described.
- The confluence and the LA appendage are incised and anastomosed together (Fig. 12.15).
- The vertical vein may be ligated or left open as previously described.

Intracardiac TAPVC
- This is performed under cardioplegic arrest.
- The RA is opened.
- If the pulmonary venous confluence opens directly into the RA, if the ASD is large enough, a patch is sutured around the defect and the pulmonary venous orifice, thus channelling pulmonary venous blood to the LA through the ASD.
- If the ASD is too small, it can be enlarged before this patch is applied.
- If the pulmonary veins drain to the RA through the coronary sinus, a cutback is made from the PFO/ASD to the coronary sinus, partially unroofing it. The defect and the coronary sinus are then patched over.

Mixed type
Repair depends on the anatomy. Most often there is a mixture of veins draining into the coronary sinus and elsewhere.

Postoperative management
In neonates following emergency surgery, it is advisable to leave the chest open. The pulmonary vasculature may be treated with milrinone, sodium nitroprusside, or inhaled nitric oxide to reduce the PAPs. The LV will be restrictive initially, and LA and PA pressures should be monitored. To reduce the risk of pulmonary hypertensive crises, patients should be paralyzed.

Complications
Early: pulmonary hypertensive crises, pulmonary edema, phrenic nerve injury. **Late**: pulmonary venous obstruction, pulmonary vein stenosis, anastomotic stricture.

Outcomes
Pulmonary venous stenosis usually develops within the first postoperative year, and occurs in 10–20% of patients in reported series. The mortality after surgical reintervention is in the order of 25%, with risk factors being early representation and bilateral stenotic disease.

Management of cor triatrium

If the patient presents acutely with pulmonary venous obstruction, the aim of management is to stabilize the patient with a view to performing surgery urgently. When there is good communication across the diaphragm, elective repair is sufficient. Surgical repair is performed using cardiopulmonary bypass and cardioplegic arrest. The RA is opened, and the PFO or ASD enlarged to allow access to the LA. The diaphragm is visualized, and the LA appendage and mitral valve identified. The diaphragm is then resected, and the position of the pulmonary veins ascertained. The ASD is closed either directly or with a patch if necessary. The outcome from surgery depends on associated defects, and therefore ranges from 5 to 25% in published series.

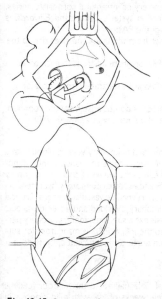

Fig. 12.15 Correction of total anomalous pulmonary venous drainage.
(a) Intracardiac. (b) Infracardiac.

Truncus arteriosus

Key facts

• There is a single arterial trunk arising from the ventricles, with a single valve with semilunar leaflets, and a subvalvar VSD. The PAs and the aorta both arise from this single arterial trunk (Fig. 12.16).
• This comprises 3% of congenital cardiac anomalies. 30–40% of patients with common arterial trunk have microdeletions in chromosome band 22q11.2 and have DiGeorge syndrome or velocardiofacial syndrome.

Morphology

The valve between the ventricles and the trunk is called the *truncal valve* and may be tricuspid (60%), bicuspid (25%), quadricuspid (10–15%), or, rarely, unicuspid. This valve is usually dysplastic. There is always continuity between the truncal valve and the mitral valve. The truncal valve overrides the VSD and in 50% is equally committed to both ventricles, in the remainder usually arises predominantly from the RV. The LV is relatively normal, but the RV is nearly always hypertrophied. The **VSD** is subarterial, with its roof made from the truncal valve, and its posterior border muscular (80%) or perimembranous (20%). The coronary arteries are often displaced caudally, and occasionally arise from the PA. The aortic arch may be left (60%) or right-sided. There may be arch interruption (10%), usually type B (between LCCA and LSCA). There may be coronary artery anomalies, such as single coronary artery or intramural coronary arteries. The most commonly used classification system, *Collett and Edwards*, is based on the pattern of the origin of the PAs:

• Type I (60–70%): a single PA arises from the trunk and gives rise to the left and right branches.
• Type II (20%): the left and right PAs originate adjacent to each other from the trunk.
• Type III (10%): the left and right PAs arise separately from the lateral aspects of the trunk.
• Type IV: where the pulmonary arteries do not arise from the common trunk; now recognized as a form of pulmonary atresia with VSD.

Pathophysiology

There is complete mixing of systemic and pulmonary venous blood with a left-to-right shunt at the ventricular level leading to cyanosis, and pulmonary volume overload. AS the PVR falls in the weeks after birth pulmonary overload worsens, resulting in CHF, and eventual pulmonary hypertension in survivors by 6 months as a result of irreversible vascular changes. Truncal valve insufficiency exacerbates pulmonary overload and adversely affects survival, whereas pulmonary stenosis has a survival benefit. Coronary perfusion is jeopardized by run-off into the PA. A PDA is mandatory for survival in patients with an interrupted aortic arch. Untreated, most do not survive beyond 6 months.

Presentation

Patients present with symptoms of CHF (failure to thrive, poor feeding, tachypnea, sweating) in the first few weeks of life, with mild cyanosis in

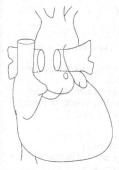

Fig. 12.16 Truncus arteriosus.

1/3 of cases which increases in frequency and severity with age. Older children may present with worsening cyanosis as a result of Eisenmenger syndrome (📖 p558). On examination a collapsing arterial pulse, left parasternal systolic murmur and single second heart sound are features.

Investigations

- EKG shows RVH and LVH with right axis deviation and P pulmonale.
- CXR shows cardiomegaly, absent pulmonary trunk, and increased pulmonary vascularity.
- Echo is diagnostic. The pulmonary artery origins should be elucidated and there should be an attempt to characterize the truncal valve and its function. The coronary pattern may be determined. The arch must be investigated for hypoplasia or interruption.
- Cardiac catheterization is not necessary unless there is late presentation, in which case the aim is to measure PVR of both pulmonary vascular beds (they may differ). Pulmonary vascular resistance of >10U/m² is a contraindication to surgical repair.

Management

In patients who present subacutely with CHF, initial treatment is with diuretics. In patients presenting with circulatory collapse, there is usually associated aortic arch interruption, and a prostaglandin infusion is commenced to maintain the PDA, along with other supportive measures. Surgery should be performed soon after presentation, and urgently in the patient with uninterrupted arch.

Outcome

Early mortality after surgery is now in the order of 5–10%. Risk factors include arch interruption, severe truncal valve regurgitation, and coronary artery anomalies. In the longer term, the RV–PA conduit requires intervention as the child grows.

Truncus arteriosus repair

Key facts

- Truncus arteriosus is an indication for urgent operation to prevent pulmonary vascular disease.
- The PAs are removed from their origin from the arterial trunk, which is committed to the LV when closing the VSD.
- The PAs are then connected to the RV either via a valved conduit such as a homograft, or by anastomosing the PAs directly to the right ventriculotomy and completing the repair with a patch.

Set-up

- Standard invasive monitoring and general anesthesia.
- Asymmetrical pericardiotomy so that a large patch of pericardium can be harvested: this is placed in 0.6% glutaraldehyde.
- Median sternotomy, heparinization at 300U/kg.
- PDA, left and right PA and aorta dissected free. The RPA and LPA are taped so that they can be occluded as soon as CPB is commenced to prevent pulmonary flooding and systemic hypoperfusion.
- Standard CPB with distal ascending aortic cannula, two-stage venous cannula, RSPV vent and patient cooled to 20°C if DHCA planned.

Procedure

Division of the pulmonary arteries from the truncal root

- The right and left PA are excised from the truncal root, taking care not to damage the coronary arteries (Fig. 12.17).
- The defect in the truncal root is closed with a pericardial patch, or if small, by primary anastomosis.

VSD repair

- A vertical right ventriculotomy is made and the VSD is closed with a patch of bovine pericardium/Gore-tex/glutaraldehyde fixed autologous pericardium.
- The right ventriculotomy will be used to recreate the RVOT later.

ASD repair

- The ASD can be repaired wither via a right atriotomy or through the right ventriculotomy and tricuspid valve.
- It is closed with a pericardial patch, and the atriotomy is closed.

Reconstruction of the RVOT

The RVOT is reconstructed by anastomosing a valved conduit (homograft or bovine jugular) to the PA bifurcation distally, and then to the right ventriculotomy proximally. The PAs may be directly anastomosed to the RV with anterior augmentation with a patch if a valved conduit is unavailable.

Closure

- The heart is de-aired in the usual fashion (📖 p114).
- The patient is rewarmed and weaned from bypass, PA, LA, and RA catheters are placed.
- TEE may be used to assess residual shunts
- The chest is closed in the standard fashion.

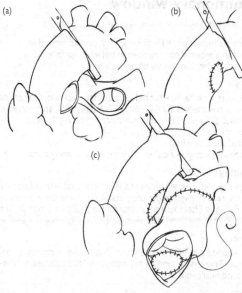

Fig. 12.17 Truncus arteriosus repair. (a) Division of pulmonary arteries from the truncal artery. (b) Closure of the defect in the trunal artery primarily, and with a patch. (c) VSD patch closure, and reconstruction of the RVOT with a pulmonary homograft.

Specific complications
- Truncal valve regurgitation and LV failure.
- Persistent left-to-right shunts.
- Conduit failure.
- Pulmonary hypertension and RV failure.

Aortopulmonary window

Key facts
- This is a rare malformation: <1% of congenital cardiac anomalies.
- It consists of an abnormal communication between aorta and pulmonary artery distal to the semilunar valves.

Morphology
Associated defects include interrupted aortic arch, anomalous origin of right or left coronary artery, VSD (📖 p564), PDA (📖 p572), aortic atresia, tetralogy of Fallot (📖 p616). Divided into three types (Fig. 12.18):
- Type I: proximal.
- Type II: distal, close to RPA.
- Type III: anomalous origin of either PA from the ascending aorta.

Pathophysiology
There is a high-flow, left-to-right shunt at the arterial level with pulmonary over-circulation, resulting in rapidly progressive CHF and early development of high PVR and Eisenmenger syndrome. Survival past 1 year is rare if untreated.

Presentation
Heart failure secondary to left-to-right shunt. Wide pulse pressures, systolic flow murmur. There is pulmonary hypertension, loud pulmonary component to second heart sound.

Investigation
- EKG: right axis deviation, biventricular hypertrophy.
- CXR: cardiomegaly, plethoric lung fields, pulmonary edema.
- Echo should be diagnostic, but may be difficult to see. The differential diagnoses of VSD, PDA, and common arterial trunk should be excluded.

Management
Infants in heart failure should be treated medically, and if this fails to stabilize them, early surgery is warranted. If heart failure can be controlled, surgery can be performed electively, but as the development of pulmonary vascular disease is unpredictable, still early.

Surgery
Set-up
- Median sternotomy, pericardium opened towards the right.
- Anatomy of the window, right PA and coronary arteries identified.
- Systemic heparinization.
- Aortic cannula placed close to innominate artery origin.
- Bicaval cannulation if there is no VSD or ASD, otherwise aorto-bicaval cannulation, caval snares, RSPV vent.
- Complete dissection of ascending aorta, and pulmonary arteries so they can be snared with silastic loops immediately after CPB commenced to prevent flooding the pulmonary circulation.
- Clamp aorta distal to the defect, arrest heart with cardioplegia.

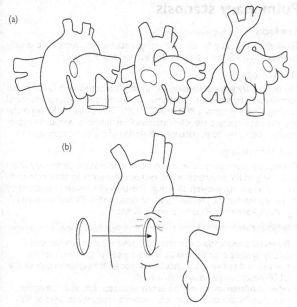

Fig. 12.18 Aortopulmonary window. (a) Spectrum of abnormalities.
(b) PTFE sutured to posterior, superior, and inferior walls of the defect and then incorporated into the suture line closing the incision.

Procedure

- Vertical incision in the anterior portion of the window or aorta.
- Identify the defect, the coronary arteries and the origin of the branch PA.
- Close defect with a patch of Gore-tex, close aortotomy, rewarm, de-air, reperfuse, and come off bypass.
- Other less favoured techniques include the double sandwich technique with a patch of Gore-tex, ligation, clamping and division, and division and suture. There are a few case reports of catheter occlusion.
- Bypass is weaned using hypocarbia and pulmonary vasodilators such as SNP, milrinone, and inhaled nitric oxide to reduce PVR.
- The chest is closed in the usual fashion with a mediastinal drain.

Outcomes

Repair of simple AP window has low mortality, but in association with other complex defects, surgical mortality is up to 20%.

Specific complications

- Pulmonary artery stenosis.
- Residual aortopulmonary defects.

Pulmonary stenosis

Key facts

This defect makes up 8–10% of all congenital cardiac defects, and usually involves valvar PS, but includes subvalvar and supravalvar PS.

Morphology

The *pulmonary valve is stenotic*, and usually is tricuspid with fusion of the commissures, thus producing a dome-like structure with a variable central opening. There is often a *PFO or ASD* (40%). There may be *RV hypertrophy*, even at birth, and *subvalvar stenosis* from infundibular muscle hypertrophy. There may be *poststenotic dilatation* of the pulmonary arteries.

Pathophysiology

The stenotic pulmonary valve impedes blood flow to the pulmonary arteries, leading to RV hypertrophy and cyanosis. If there is an atrial communication, there is *right-to-left shunting*. The level of stenosis is assessed by measuring the systolic pressure gradient between the RV and the main PA; a gradient >50mmHg is considered significant.

Presentation

- *Neonatal presentation*: neonates with severe pulmonary stenosis usually present critically unwell within a week of birth with severe cyanosis and tachypnea, a systolic murmur with an ejection click at the ULSE, hepatomegaly due to severe TR.
- *Infants/children*: these may be largely asymptomatic, with a murmur picked up incidentally. However, moderate stenosis may lead to RV hypertrophy, with increasingly inadequate pulmonary blood flow leading to exertional dyspnea.

Investigation

- EKG: RA dilatation and RV hypertrophy.
- CXR: there may be moderate cardiomegaly, prominent main PA from poststenotic dilatation, and, if severe PS, oligemic lung fields.
- Echo is diagnostic, showing a stenotic, dysplastic, sometimes hypoplastic pulmonary valve, RV hypertrophy, and tricuspid valve incompetence. The gradient across the RVOT may be measured, as well as RV pressures. The size of the tricuspid valve, the RV cavity must be assessed in order to plan management.
- Cardiac catheterization is not indicated in mild stenosis, but is an essential prelude to interventional balloon dilatation of the stenotic valve. An accurate peak-to-peak gradient can be measured, the size of the RV assessed, and the distal pulmonary vasculature imaged. The RV pressure may be measured.

Management

Trivial (<25mmHg) or mild (<50mmHg) gradients across the pulmonary valve do not require intervention, but must be followed up regularly.

Balloon valuloplasty

Pulmonary stenosis that is **moderate (50–79mmHg) or severe (>80mmHg)** both in the critically ill neonate and in the less symptomatic child is largely managed with interventional cardiological techniques. The critically ill neonate will require resuscitation, with the use of PGE_1 to maintain pulmonary blood flow, before transfer to the cath lab or operating room. **Balloon pulmonary valvuloplasty** has superseded the use of surgery to achieve an unobstructed RVOT in cases of isolated pulmonary stenosis with normal pulmonary valve annulus size. The aim is to achieve a gradient <30mmHg. If there is subvalvar stenosis secondary to muscle hypertrophy, this often recedes in the months following valvotomy. β-blockers may be used if infundibular stenosis is >50mmHg immediately after balloon valvuloplasty.

Surgical valvuloplasty

If the pulmonary valve annulus is small and the RV cavity appears small, surgery may be chosen in order to augment the annulus with a **transannular patch**. Similarly, if there is fixed infundibular stenosis, the infundibulum may be augmented with this patch, having **divided obstructing muscle bundles**, and extending the transannular incision further into the RVOT.

Adults

In adults with PS, the long-term outcomes may be good without intervention, but there is a trend towards intervention in those with moderate to severe PS in order to prevent RV dysfunction in the long term, due to lowered pre- and post-exercise cardiac indices and to prevent exercise-induced hemodynamic abnormalities.

Complications

- Residual/recurrent valve stenosis (10% at 6 months, but late recurrence is 1–2%).
- Persistent postoperative hypoxia.
- Pulmonary valve regurgitation (up to 80% at 10 years).
- The need for reintervention is higher after balloon valvuloplasty in neonates, with up to 25% of patients requiring reintervention for PS or associated defects compared to 8–10% of older children.

Outcomes

Mortality from balloon or open valvotomy is in the region of 1–3%, with RV size approaching normal in 90% of patients. 5- and 10-year freedom from reintervention is in the order of 88% and 84% respectively.

Pulmonary atresia with intact ventricular septum

Key facts

- Pulmonary atresia with an intact ventricular septum is a rare defect characterized by variable RV development in association with an imperforate pulmonary valve.
- There may be extensive right ventriculocoronary connections.
- It makes up about 1% of congenital cardiac defects.

Morphology

The pulmonary valve is *completely atretic*, replaced by an *imperforate fibrous membrane*, with *thick RV hypertrophy* and *infundibular stenosis* or atresia. The main and branch pulmonary arteries are usually of good size with variable poststenotic dilatation. The RV and tricuspid valve have variable degrees of hypoplasia. There is always an *interatrial communication*. A substantial number of patients (50–60%) have *fistulous communications* from the hypertrophied RV to the coronary arteries. The *coronary arteries may be disconnected* from the aorta, and intimal fibromuscular dysplasia may develop in these abnormal connections causing stenosis.

Pathophysiology and natural history

The atretic or stenosed pulmonary valve restricts blood flow into the pulmonary arteries, causing *hypoxia*, with the arterial duct being the only source of blood. *Cyanosis* becomes worse as the duct closes. When the *coronary circulation is RV-dependent* (20%), coronary perfusion is dependent on the hypertensive RV, thus there will be coronary steal into the RV during diastole when the RV pressure falls. Stenoses within the fistulas may also lead to *myocardial ischemia*. If pulmonary blood flow can be maintained by ductal patency until surgical intervention, the 1- and 5-year survival is up to 80% and 75%. Sudden death, angina, ventricular arrhythmias, congestive heart failure, and the consequences of prolonged hypoxia are all risks for these patients.

Presentation

Most of these patients present in the neonatal period with worsening cyanosis and tachypnea as the arterial duct closes. Examination reveals central cyanosis, normal arterial pulses, single first and second heart sounds, pansystolic murmur of tricuspid regurgitation.

Investigation

- EKG usually shows sinus rhythm, ↓RV forces, LV dominance.
- CXR shows mild cardiomegaly and oligemic lung fields.
- Echo is diagnostic. The diameter of the tricuspid valve, the size of the RV cavity, TR, and the adequacy of the interatrial communication must be assessed. Ventriculocoronary connections may be identified.
- Cardiac catheterization is required to identify ventriculocoronary connections, and RV-dependent coronary circulations. The RV size and morphology may be further studied, and pressure measured.

Management

Percutaneous intervention

In some cases, an attempt may be made to cross the atretic valve using laser or radiofrequency and perform balloon valvuloplasty. The rate of complications is high, and often these patients will require further intervention to establish adequate pulmonary blood flow.

Surgery

The aim of management is to restore flow through the RV to the pulmonary circulation in order to decompress the RV and allow it to grow. However, the adequacy of the RV for two-ventricle repair is difficult to assess, and is generally based on the size of the tricuspid valve, as this correlates well with an adequate ventricular cavity.

In general, a tricuspid valve measuring at least three standard deviations of the mean normal valve should be able to support the pulmonary circulation (z score up to −3). These patients can undergo treatment to restore pulmonary blood flow, either by interventional cardiological techniques or surgery, with the aim of a two-ventricle circulation.

If the RV is hypoplastic with a small tricuspid valve and ventriculocoronary connections, pulmonary blood flow should be improved with systemic-pulmonary artery shunt; a transannular patch may be performed if there is hope that the RV may grow. These patients will probably require transplantation or Fontan palliation in the future.

Outcomes

Neonatal palliation

This may be surgical, with pulmonary valvotomy and systemic–pulmonary shunt, or RVOT patch; or by catheter intervention, decompressing the RV by radiofrequency ablation of the pulmonary valve with balloon dilatation. Any of these initial palliations may be followed by further interventions, surgical or catheter based. Mortality rates for these procedures are high, with mortality approaching 40% for surgical palliation and 20% for percutaneous intervention. In selected patients, without RV-dependent coronary circulations, RVOT patch has a low mortality.

Repair

The largest multicenter studies suggest that about 50% of children presenting with this condition should be suitable for a two-ventricle repair, with the remainder requiring Fontan palliation (📖 p594) or transplant (📖 pp504–519), with survival rates of about 60% at 15 years.

Tetralogy of Fallot

Key facts

- ToF makes up 10% of congenital heart defects and is the commonest cyanotic lesion. 25% of patients have DiGeorge syndrome or deletion/ abnormalities of chromosome 22.
- It is usually an isolated defect, and is characterized by four lesions caused by anterior deviation of the outlet septum:
  - Pulmonary stenosis (at the infundibulum, valve or the PA).
  - RV hypertrophy.
  - Overriding aorta.
  - VSD.
- Children present soon after birth with cyanosis, depending on the severity of the pulmonary stenosis, and are usually managed with surgical correction.

Morphology

- The underlying morphological abnormality causing the features of tetralogy is anterior and leftward deviation of the outlet septum.
- There is a large perimembranous outlet VSD.
- Hypoplasia of the RVOT causing obstruction at multiple levels (10% pulmonary valve stenosis, 50% infundibular stenosis, 30% combined).
- The pulmonary valve is usually involved, and is bicuspid in 60% of ToF, with a hypoplastic annulus; however, it is usually not the narrowest point of the outflow tract. In 7% of patients with ToF there is complete pulmonary atresia; in 5% the pulmonary valve is completely absent and the PAs are aneurysmal.
- In about 5% of patients the LAD arises from the right coronary artery, crossing the right outflow tract just below the pulmonary valve annulus to achieve its interventricular course.
- There is a right arch in 25%.

Pathophysiology

The RVOT obstruction **reduces pulmonary blood flow** and also increases the RV pressure causing **a right-to-left shunt** across the large, unrestricted VSD. Both these effects cause **cyanosis**. Immediately after birth, the ductus arteriosus supplies blood to the pulmonary vasculature, but after it closes there may be a sudden onset of cyanosis, and the RV will start to hypertrophy. In a small subset, the RVOT obstruction is so mild as to avoid cyanosis: *'acyanotic' or 'pink' tetralogy*. The pulmonary vasculature is protected from the effects of the VSD by the outflow obstruction, and some patients may be well balanced for years.

Presentation and natural history

In children with a very hypoplastic annulus, the presentation is usually soon after birth, with cyanosis due to the obstruction in pulmonary blood flow and thus increased flow across the VSD from right to left. In children with a larger pulmonary valve annulus, where obstruction is muscular at the infundibular level, presentation is usually later, and may be with 'tet spells'—cyanotic episodes that occur when there is muscular spasm causing acute obstruction to RV outflow and reversal of the shunt (also due to falling SVR with exercise). 'Squatting' is a characteristic compensatory maneuver, seen in right-to-left shunts developing on exercise. Hemoptysis may be present late. Examination shows RV heave and a systolic ejection murmur. The degree of RVOT obstruction is the main determinant of outcome in untreated ToF: most children develop signs and symptoms by 6 months of age, and <10% survive to the age of 21 without surgical intervention. 25% of untreated patients die within 1 year of life, 40% of untreated patients die within 4 years, and 95% of untreated patients die within 40 years.

Investigations

- EKG shows right-axis deviation, RVH and RA hypertrophy.
- CXR shows a 'boot-shaped' heart as a result of RVH and the small or absent MPA; and decreased pulmonary vascularity, ↑RA.
- Echo is diagnostic, and defines the severity and extent of the RVOT obstruction, the size of the pulmonary valve annulus, the size and position of the VSD, the coronary artery arrangement, and any associated anomalies.
- Cardiac catheterization is used if there is a need to further image the coronary arteries, or if there are concerns about the size or arborization of the pulmonary arteries.

Surgical management

There is an increasing trend towards earlier complete repair, but there is still a place for early palliation with a *systemic–PA shunt* (📖 p600) followed by repair at a later stage. A sensible approach is to aim to repair all tetralogies between 3–6 months. If they present with cyanotic spells they can be repaired earlier, or if institutional policy dictates, undergo a *B-T shunt* (📖 p601) with elective repair when they are bigger.

Palliative procedures

- Modified B-T shunt (📖 p601): this is an interposition shunt, usually a Gore-tex tube, placed from the subclavian artery to the left or right PA. It may be performed through a thoracotomy or a sternotomy. Many centers no longer perform palliative surgery such as the modified B-T shunt on symptomatic infants with ToF, instead opting for complete repair.
- RVOT patch or conduit: if the PAs are too small to accept a B-T shunt, flow to the PAs may be secured with an outflow tract patch or with a limiting RV-PA conduit, e.g. 5mm Gore-tex tube.

Tetralogy of Fallot repair

Key facts

- To repair this defect, the VSD must be closed, and the RVOT obstruction must be relieved. The RVOT obstruction may be at several levels: muscular infundibular stenosis, pulmonary valvar stenosis, small pulmonary annulus, small main pulmonary artery.
- There is some evidence that the need for future reoperation may be less if the pulmonary valve annulus is preserved.
- A patch across the RVOT acts as an akinetic, dilated area in the RV that does not contribute to useful function: the aim should be to preserve the PV annulus where possible, and limit as much as possible the size of the RVOT patch.
- Variations in morphology which impact on surgical technique include:
  - Right, left, and bifurcation PA stenosis.
  - Anomalous origins of the coronary arteries.
  - Pulmonary atresia.
  - Absent pulmonary valve.

Set-up

- Standard invasive monitoring, general anesthesia.
- Median sternotomy, heparinization at 300U/kg.
- Asymmetrical pericardiotomy, pericardial patch harvested and treated in 0.6% glutaraldehyde.
- PDA and left and right PA are dissected completely free, and the aorta is freed from root to head and neck vessels.
- If the PDA is patent it is ligated.
- Standard aorto-bicaval CPB, patient cooled to 25°C.
- The aorta is cross-clamped and cold cardioplegia given into the root.

Procedure

To repair this defect, the VSD must be closed, and the RVOT obstruction must be relieved. The RVOT obstruction may be at several levels: muscular infundibular stenosis, pulmonary valvar stenosis, small pulmonary annulus, small main PA. There is some evidence that the need for future reoperation may be less if the pulmonary valve annulus is preserved. Similarly, a patch across the RVOT acts as an akinetic dilated area in the RV that does not contribute to useful function. In operating, the aim should be to preserve the PV annulus where possible, and limit as much as possible the size of the RVOT patch.

Right atriotomy

- VSD closure through RA (📖 p566). Care is taken to avoid the conduction tissues by placing sutures into fibrous tissue rather than muscle tissue.
- There are frequently multiple VSDs, most frequently in the muscular portion anterior to the septal band: these are closed with patches.
- Resection/division of muscular obstruction through the RA, and assessment of tricuspid valve.

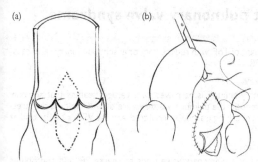

Fig. 12.19 Enlargement of the pulmonary annulus. (a) With a homograft monocusp. (b) With a pericardial patch.

RVOT reconstruction

- Open the MPA to inspect the valve and the RVOT through the valve.
- If PV annulus adequate, preserve the valve and patch the infundibulum and/or the MPA.
- If the PV annulus is too small, the PA incision is taken across the annulus and into the RVOT if necessary—the whole can be patched over with autologous pericardium, bovine pericardium, Gore-tex, 'monocusp' patch with some form of valvar substitute (Fig. 12.19).
- In principle, as small a patch as possible is used on the RV aspect in order to preserve RV function.
- In principle, leave the annulus intact if at all possible, even if this means going back on bypass to redo it if the RV pressures are too high at the end of the operation.

Closure

- After the VSD is closed the right heart is filled with saline, the atrial cannula replaced, and bypass recommenced.
- The patch on the RVOT can be sutured to the PA and right ventriculotomy during rewarming.
- RV pressure measurement can be performed at the end of the procedure with a pressure transducer. Generally, if RV pressure is 80% or less, this can be tolerated. Above this pressure, further RVOT obstruction relief may be necessary.

Specific complications

The operative mortality from repair of ToF is 1–2%. The early outcomes for repair of ToF are now excellent. However, in the long term, pulmonary insufficiency causing RV dilatation and dysfunction may cause symptoms, and increase the risk of sudden death due to malignant arrhythmias. Early pulmonary valve replacement, before the development of symptoms, may protect against irreversible RV dilatation.

- Early complications: bleeding, heart block, 1%, restrictive RV physiology and RV dysfunction requiring ITU support.
- Late complications: residual/recurrent RVOT obstruction, pulmonary regurgitation, RV dilatation and dysfunction.

Absent pulmonary valve syndrome

Key facts

This is a variant of ToF, with rudimentary or absent pulmonary valve causing severe PR.

Morphology

The pulmonary annulus is narrowed with vestigial leaflets that are only minimally stenotic, the pulmonary arteries are often dilated placing pressure on the underlying tracheobronchial tree, and the VSD is similar to that in TF with PS.

Pathophysiology

The absence of a pulmonary valve leads to severe PR, and contributes to the massive PA dilatation. There may be airway compression from the dilated branch pulmonary arteries, but even deeper in the lung there may be small airway obstruction from abnormal pulmonary vasculature. Although there is usually some pulmonary stenosis, in this condition there is usually a net left-to-right shunt.

Presentation

These patients can be broadly categorized into two groups:
• Very sick infants or neonates with severe bronchial compression, with signs and symptoms of respiratory distress: tachypnea, wheeze, cyanosis, air-trapping, respiratory failure.
• Older children with less severe respiratory symptoms where the intracardiac manifestations of ToF are the dominant pathology.
There may be mild cyanosis. There is a hyperactive precordium. The first heart sound is normal, the second single due to absent pulmonary component, and there is a to-and-fro murmur over the pulmonary area. There may be atelectasis, hyperinflation, or consolidation of the lungs.

Investigations

• Echo is diagnostic, but may be difficult due to distortion of the cardiac anatomy by the huge PAs. Other anomalies must be identified.
• CT scan may delineate airway compression by the PAs, and identify intrapulmonary vascular abnormalities.
• Bronchoscopy or bronchogram are often necessary in those patients with a long postoperative ICU course due to difficulties weaning from respiratory support.

Management

In asymptomatic patients, surgery is deferred until later childhood. If there are significant airway problems, earlier surgery is necessary, but outcomes may be worse in this subgroup. Preoperative intubation and ventilation is a risk factor for poor outcome, and repair in the critically ill neonate has a high mortality rate.

Surgical strategies

Closure of the VSD and relief of RVOT obstruction as for isolated ToF (□ p616).

- It may be necessary to plicate or resect pulmonary arterial wall in order to reduce their size and propensity to compress the airways.
- Alternatively, the *Lecompte maneuver* (□ p626), in which the pulmonary arteries are brought anterior to the aorta, may be performed.
- There is debate about how to reconstruct the RVOT, with many centres advocating the insertion of a valved conduit to prevent the severe PR seen with the relatively high pulmonary resistances seen in this condition.

Complications

Morbidity arises mainly from the effects of airway compression. Many of these children have a prolonged postoperative course on the ICU, requiring invasive and non-invasive positive pressure ventilation. If a valved conduit is used in the reconstruction of the RVOT, then further intervention will be mandatory as the child grows. In neonates with APV, the postoperative mortality is 20–60% in historical series, although in older children the mortality is closer to that for ToF repair. There may be continuing respiratory symptoms in spite of adequate surgery. As with ToF, there must be continuing surveillance.

Pulmonary atresia with VSD

Key facts

- This cyanotic congenital cardiac anomaly is characterized by an underdeveloped RVOT, atretic pulmonary valve, a VSD with variable aortic override, and variable development of the PAs.
- It makes up about 3% of all congenital cardiac anomalies.
- There is a spectrum of severity dictated by the degree of PA development. 35% of these patients have 22q11.2 deletion, while 65% of patients with PA/VSD/MAPCAs have this anomaly.

Morphology

There is *absence of continuity between the RV and the PA*, and the pulmonary artery development varies from normal-sized to entirely absent. The RV may be entirely disconnected from the MPA, connected by an atretic valve, or obstructed by infundibular muscle. Blood flow to the lungs may be from a *PDA*, or from *MAPCAs*. These patients are more likely to have more severe PA hypoplasia, and pulmonary vascular arborization abnormalities. The *VSD* is outlet, and the aortic override may be more than 50% (i.e., DORV) in 26–50%. There is a right aortic arch in 25–50%. RV is usually hypertrophied; LV and coronaries normal.

Pathophysiology

Good-sized, confluent pulmonary arteries supplied by a PDA

Intrapulmonary vascular patterns should be normal; when the duct closes, an alternative pulmonary inflow is needed, e.g., a systemic–PA shunt.

Hypoplastic pulmonary arteries or absent PDA

Intrapulmonary arborization is abnormal. Collateral supply to lungs may come from MAPCAs from the descending thoracic aorta, systemic arteries such as the subclavian or intercostals, bronchial arteries, or coronary arteries. These collaterals have a tendency to stenose: *there may be different sources of blood for different segments of lung, all with different pressures*. The intrapulmonary vasculature may have abnormal distribution and distal stenoses. Even after reconstruction of the pulmonary arteries and reconnection to the RV, the distal vasculature may be so abnormal that if the VSD is closed, RV pressure would be too high to be sustainable, causing RV failure and circulatory collapse.

Presentation

Most patients present in the neonatal period with cyanosis and hypoxia as the duct closes. If there are well-developed collateral arteries, presentation may be delayed as these children may have good SaO_2, and hypoxia only occurs as growth outstrips pulmonary blood supply. Rarely, there may be CHF in the case of a large PDA or multiple large MAPCAs.

Examination

There may be central cyanosis, worse after ductal closure. There may be signs of *DiGeorge/velocardiofacial syndrome*, developmental delay, or growth retardation. First heart sound is normal, single second heart sound, continuous murmurs in the case of PDA or MAPCAs.

Investigation

- CXR: normal sized, boot-shaped heart, absent MPA shadow.
- Echo: this is diagnostic and quantifies size of the PAs and their blood supply. It is unable to define the course of collateral arteries adequately, and the intrapulmonary vascular arborization cannot be defined.
- If PAs are large and confluent, supplied by a PDA, catheterization is unnecessary. There are hypoplastic PAs with undefined or variable blood supply. It is also required after systemic–PA shunt to define the PA anatomy and diagnose damage or distortion by the shunt.
- MRI/CT: these define collateral arteries within the chest, and the size and distribution of the PAs, allowing the surgeon to plan incorporation of MAPCAs into the native pulmonary circulation.

Management

Good-sized, confluent pulmonary arteries supplied by a PDA

The adequacy of the pulmonary arteries may be determined using the **McGoon ratio or Nakata index**. Repair is performed by closing the VSD and placing a valved conduit from the RV to the PA, or it may be staged by performing a palliative systemic–pulmonary artery shunt and then a repair when the child is bigger, allowing placement of a more satisfactory conduit from the RV to the PA. Mortality is 15%, and 5-year survival is 75%.

PA/VSD with hypoplastic central pulmonary arteries, no MAPCAs

Systemic–pulmonary artery shunt from the ascending aorta to the PAs via a direct connection (**Watterston shunt**) or a Gore-tex tube—this promotes growth of the central PAs. An RVOT patch may be used, or a limiting RV-PA conduit. Repair may only be possible after reconstruction of the central PAs, either with patches or with an interposition tube in the case of non-confluent PAs. The VSD can be closed once the PA reconstruction is adequate; however, if it is left open, a restrictive RV to PA conduit may be used to prevent overflow of blood to lungs.

PA/VSD/MAPCAs

Many children are stable, with good SaO_2, and repair may require several operations and reinterventions. However, MAPCAs and dependent lung territories may change, with stenoses in the MAPCAs and PVR changes in the lungs, leading to deterioration. The aim of surgery is to unifocalize the sources of supply to each lung, centralize those to the native central pulmonary arteries if possible, and connect these to the RV via a valved conduit. If the reconstructed pulmonary arteries supply adequate segments of lung, the VSD can be closed. This can be done as a single procedure, with a thoracotomy on the side of the descending aorta to mobilize the MAPCAs, then a sternotomy to perform the repair. VSD closure may be performed if there is perfusion of 15 lung segments.

Outcomes

10-year survival is roughly 80%, and freedom from reintervention at 10 years is <50%.

Transposition of great arteries

Key facts

- TGA is a congenital cardiac anomaly in which the aorta arises from the RV and the pulmonary trunk arises from the LV.
- Complete TGA is the most common cyanotic lesion presenting in the neonatal period, and makes up 5% of congenital cardiac lesions. In 90% it is isolated, with no associated extracardiac malformations.
- Infants present with cyanosis and in the absence of an ASD or VSD infants die within a few hours of closure of the ductus arteriosus.
- A corrective arterial switch procedure can be performed in neonates with low mortality.

Morphology

In simple TGA, the ventricular septum is intact (70%); however, a VSD is present in 30%. In 1/3 the coronary anatomy is abnormal, the commonest aberrant pattern is the left circumflex arising from the right coronary (22%). However, the coronary arteries arise from the 'facing' sinuses in 99%. There is LVOTO (pulmonary or subpulmonary) in 10% of simple TGA and 30% of TGA with VSD.

Pathophysiology and natural history

- TGA results in the systemic and pulmonary circulations operating in parallel rather than in series: i.e., non-oxygenated venous blood passes through the RV into the aorta, while oxygenated pulmonary blood passes through the LV back to the pulmonary circulation.
- Mixing between the two circulations is mandatory for survival: this may occur through an ASD, PFO, VSD, or PDA.
- Inadequate mixing leads to cyanosis, acidosis, and death in the neonatal period.
- The LV ejecting to the low-resistance pulmonary bed does not develop its muscle mass in the normal manner, and after a few weeks loses the ability to produce normal cardiac output against systemic resistance.
- Patients with a VSD maintain this ability, as the LV pressure and volume load is closer to systemic values, and they also have better SaO_2 because of greater mixing of cardiac blood, but may have CHF, and in the long term develop irreversible pulmonary vascular disease.
- Untreated TGA causes death in 30% in the first week, 50% in the first month, and 90% by the first year. In long-term survivors, the complications of cyanosis develop: polycythemia, hyperviscosity, thrombocytopenia with bleeding complications.

Presentation

Male to female ratio is 2:1. Neonates present with cyanosis: if a VSD is present cyanosis is not so severe, but there may be signs of heart failure. Unless there is a shunt at the atrial or ventricular level, infants collapse within a few hours of ductus arteriosus closure. In the first 3 weeks as pulmonary resistance falls leading to overcirculation, signs of CHF dominate (failure to thrive, tachypnea, sweating). Examination in TGA without VSD may be normal apart from cyanosis. In TGA/VSD: mild cyanosis, increased RV impulse, prominent grade 3–4/6 holosystolic murmur, third heart sound, mid-diastolic murmur, gallop rhythm, with hepatomegaly.

Investigations

- EKG shows RV hypertrophy in isolated TGA, and LVH if patent VSD.
- CXR: with intact septum there may be classic '**egg-on-a-string**' cardiac silhouette (narrow mediastinum and enlarged heart), with VSD present, there may be cardiomegaly and increased pulmonary vascularity.
- Echocardiography is diagnostic demonstrating the bifurcating pulmonary artery arising from the LV. The echo should further delineate the relationship of the great arteries, the presence and adequacy of shunts such as ASD, VSD, PDA, the coronary anatomy, and other malformations, such as coarctation.
- Cardiac catheterization is occasionally useful to characterize VSDs, or to improve mixing, e.g., for balloon atrial septostomy. In older children, it may be required to assess PVR, or to test the adequacy of left ventricular preparation for a late arterial switch operation.

Surgical management

Surgical repair (📖 pp626–629) is well established, effective and mandatory for TGA, and ideally performed within the first few weeks of life.

Congenitally corrected transposition

Congenitally corrected transposition of the great arteries (ccTGA) is a very different problem to TGA, with a more insidious course, and no well-defined surgical solution.

- The main abnormality is reversed morphology of the RV and LV. As in TGA the aorta arises from the RV and the pulmonary trunk from the LV, but there is atrioventricular discordance, i.e., the RA connects with the LV and the LA connects with the RV. The pulmonary and systemic circulations are therefore in series (rather than in parallel as in TGA).
- In the long-term the RV is unable to sustain a normal cardiac output against systemic vascular resistance and RV failure occurs in the third or fourth decade.
- Associated lesions which may pose additional problems include VSD (📖 p564), pulmonary atresia (📖 p612), and tricuspid regurgitation.
- Patients usually present late in their first decade with exercise intolerance. Bradycardia caused by complete heart block may be present.
- EKG may show AV block. Cardiac catheterization quantifies shunts and delineate anatomy, particularly when associated with pulmonary atresia.
- Management is controversial: PA banding early in life may preserve morphological LV function, restore septal symmetry and reduce systemic AV valve (tricusid) regurgitation. Results of the double switch or Senning-Rastelli operation to "correct" the anatomy are best in the first decade of life.

Arterial switch (Jatene)

Key facts

- This is the operation of choice for neonates presenting with TGA/IVS or TGA/VSD, and the related DORV with subpulmonary VSD.
- It is a single-stage anatomical correction consisting of transection of the aorta and PA, anastomosis of the PA to the aortic root, anastomosis of the ascending aorta to the pulmonary root, with both coronary arteries reimplanted into the neo-aorta, and closure of the ASD (Fig. 12.20).
- After balloon atrial septostomy, if the neonate is well palliated, the operation is performed electively in the first 2 weeks of life. If BAS does not solve hypoxia, prostaglandin is restarted and the operation should be performed within the next 24–48h.

Contraindications

- Intramural coronary arteries were historically a contraindication.
- LV outflow obstruction.
- Abnormal pulmonary valve (may require Ross + switch).
- Late presentation with deconditioned LV.

Set-up

- Standard invasive monitoring and general anesthesia.
- Median sternotomy, heparinization at 300U/kg.
- Asymmetrical pericardiotomy so that a large patch of pericardium can be harvested: this is placed in 0.6% glutaraldehyde.
- Aorta, head/neck vessels, and PAs mobilized to hilum.
- Aortic cannulation high, RA cannula; if VSD, bicaval cannulation.
- Duct ligated and divided after establishment of bypass.
- PA branches snared with silastic loops.
- RSPV vent, patient cooled to 20–25°C.

Procedure

Division of PDA and aorta

- PDA ligated and divided and both ends are oversewn.
- Distal ascending aorta is clamped and cold blood cardioplegia given into the root.
- The aorta is transected about 3–5mm above coronary ostial bulge.

Coronary transfer and reimplantation of coronaries

- Coronary ostia excised (right first) with surrounding button of aortic wall, mobilized, and the resultant deficiency in the aortic sinuses repaired with harvested pericardium to form the neo-MPA.
- MPA transected just proximal to bifurcation.
- 'Trapdoor' incisions made in the facing sinuses of this neo-aorta, to receive the coronary buttons.
- Coronary buttons sutured to the trapdoor incisions (left first).

Lecompte manoeuvre and aortic anastomosis

- **Lecompte manoeuvre** brings the neo-MPA anterior to the neo-aorta. This maneuver avoids the need for an interposition graft to connect the new pulmonary root to the pulmonary bifurcation, by bringing the pulmonary bifurcation anterior to the ascending aorta.
- The neo-aortic root is anastomosed to the ascending aorta.

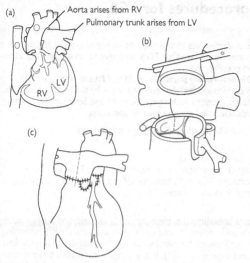

Fig. 12.20 Arterial switch (Jatene) operation. (a) Anatomy of TGA. (b) Division of the pulmonary trunk, aorta and coronary buttons. (c) Completed operation.

ASD repair and reconstruction of RVOT

- Bypass is discontinued, the atrial cannula is removed, and the ASD closed primarily through the right atriotomy which is then closed.
- The venous cannula is replaced, bypass resumed at full flow, rewarming commenced, the cross-clamp removed and the RSPV vent turned on.
- The neo-PA trunk is anastomosed to the PA bifurcation.
- TEE or epicardial US is mandatory post CPB, LA catheter is placed via LAA or RSPV.

Specific complications

- LV failure due to ischemia (due to coronary kinking/malposition) or inability to support the systemic vascular resistance: any evidence on post-bypass TEE of ischemia must be addressed, with a coronary bypass graft if the coronary implantation cannot be revised.
- Renal failure requiring peritoneal dialysis.
- Supravalvar pulmonary and/or aortic stenosis.
- Aortic root dilatation and regurgitation.

Outcomes

Surgical mortality for simple TGA with the commonest coronary patterns is 2%. Intramural coronaries, single coronary, or a long tortuous LMS are risk factors for a higher mortality. Overall mortality for all arterial switch operations is 10%. There is concern about the function of the neo-aortic valve in the long-term: incidence of AI is still 5–7%.

Other procedures for TGA

Key facts
- A number of alternatives to the single-stage Jatene arterial switch (📖 p624) may be indicated for TGA according to anatomy, associated lesions and presentation.
- Palliative **Blalock–Taussig shunt** (📖 p600) and **PA banding** (📖 p598) which may be followed later by complete repair by the Rastelli operation.
- Atrial switch operations such as the **Mustard** and **Senning procedures**.
- The **Nikaido operation** and the **Rastelli operation**.

Atrial switch: Mustard or Senning operations

Indications
- Previously for TGA ± VSD.
- Now as part of the double switch operation for ccTGA (📖 p625).
- Late presentation TGA unsuitable for LV preparation (see 📖 p624), e.g., pulmonary vascular disease.

Technique
In the Mustard operation, the atrial septum is excised, and a large patch of autologous pericardium is used to form an intra-atrial baffle, directing systemic venous flow to the mitral valve and the pulmonary venous flow to the tricuspid valve (Fig. 12.21). In the Senning operation, there is redirection of systemic and pulmonary venous pathways by cutting and folding of the native atrial tissues, usually without the use of extraneous material.

Complications
- Mustard: constriction of the venous pathways, baffle leaks, sinus node dysfunction, atrial arrhythmias.
- Senning: systemic venous pathway obstruction.

Outcomes
Surgical mortality is <5% for both these procedures. 20-year survival in the order of 80–90% for both these operations; VSD at time of surgery is a risk factor for late reoperations. Senning probably has a higher reintervention-free survival at 20 years.

PA band for TGA
In infants presenting late with TGA, where there is involution of LV muscle, the LV can be 'prepared' to support the systemic circulation with a PA band. This is combined with a systemic-pulmonary shunt, e.g., modified B-T shunt (📖 p600), in order not to limit pulmonary blood flow. Although the LV may be prepared within 2 weeks, it may be more practical to perform the PA band and shunt with elective switch operation in the following 3–6 months.

Nikaido operation
This operation is used for TGA with pulmonary stenosis or pulmonary annular hypoplasia. The aortic root is excised from the RVOT, requiring explantation, mobilization, and reimplantation of the coronary arteries. The outlet septum is excised and the aortic root is translocated posteriorly to lie over the morphologic LV. The VSD is closed, and an RV-PA conduit used.

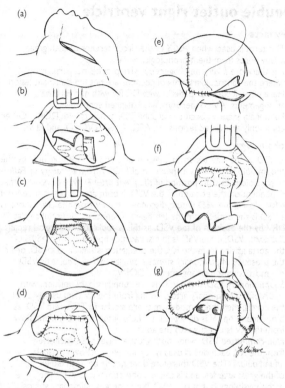

Fig. 12.21 Atrial switch operations. (a–e) Completed Senning procedure showing baffle created by septal flap redirecting IVC and SVC blood via the enlarged ASD into the left atrium, and hence LV and pulmonary arteries. Pulmonary vein inflow is directed across the tricuspid valve into the RV and aorta. (f) Mustard procedure showing baffle sutured via enlarged ASD around pulmonary veins. (g) Completed baffle will direct IVC and SVC blood in the atrium and hence pulmonary arteries. Pulmonary vein inflow is directed across the tricuspid valve into the RV and aorta.

Rastelli operation

This is a single-stage repair of d-transposition of the great arteries (d-TGA) which is used instead of the *Jatene arterial switch* (🔲 p626) when the pulmonary valve is hypoplastic and there is a VSD. The VSD is not closed—rather a pathway from the LV to the aortic valve is baffled through the VSD with a patch of Dacron. This is easiest when the VSD is a large outlet perimembranous VSD. The RV is then connected to the PA with a valved conduit (homograft, bovine jugular vein, Hancock valved conduit). The RV-PA conduit will is changed when the child outgrows it, or earlier if there is conduit stenosis.

Double outlet right ventricle

Key facts

- This term is used when >50% of the circumference of each great artery arises from the morphologically RV.
- It is therefore a very heterogeneous group of hearts, particularly where the ventriculoarterial connections are not the dominant lesion.
- Here we will consider patients with DORV with normal atrial arrangements, AV connections, and balanced ventricles
- Pulmonary stenosis occurs in around 50% of hearts with DORV. Other commonly associated lesions are ASD, AVSD, LVOTO, and PDA.

Morphology

The *VSD* is the key lesion in these hearts and its position defines the pathophysiology. There is a spectrum of DORV from **tetralogy of Fallot**-type physiology to **transposition of the great arteries** type physiology that is dependent on the position of the VSD. If both great arteries arise from the RV, closing the VSD would disconnect the LV from the circulation, as the VSD is the outlet from the left heart. Therefore, it is useful to classify DORV by the position of the VSD, as this is applicable to surgical repair:

- *Subaortic VSD*: if the VSD is in a subaortic in position, with >50% of the aorta arising from the RV, the circulation is similar to a VSD, or in the presence of pulmonary stenosis, similar to ToF. Subaortic VSD is the most common arrangement in DORV.
- *Subpulmonary VSD*: if the VSD is in a subpulmonary position, with >50% of the pulmonary artery arising from the RV (and usually all of the aorta), then the hemodynamics are similar to TGA with VSD, as blood from the LV is directed into the pulmonary arteries, and flow from the RV is directly into the aorta.
- *Non-committed VSD*: when both great arteries arise exclusively from the RV, each one is usually supported on its own muscular infundibulum. The VSD therefore does not lie beneath either of the great arteries, and is called a non-committed VSD. The pathophysiology is that of a VSD, but if there is pulmonary stenosis, there is right-to-left shunting causing cyanosis.
- *Doubly committed VSD*: when there is an absence of RV outlet septum, the VSD is committed to both great arteries and is said to be doubly committed. The pathophysiology is then similar to a doubly committed VSD. If there is pulmonary stenosis, there is right-to-left shunting causing cyanosis.

Presentation and natural history

This depends on the anatomic arrangement. If there is no pulmonary stenosis, there is heart failure and pulmonary hypertension. If pulmonary stenosis is present, there is cyanosis. Due to the heterogeneity of this condition, it is difficult to compare series of cases and surgical approaches. Overall 15-year survival for DORV with or without repair is approximately 60%, with 15-year survival after repair of non-complex DORV of 95%, and after repair of DORV/subpulmonary VSD of 90%.

Investigation

- EKG: RV hypertrophy.
- CXR: cardiomegaly. If there is pulmonary stenosis, there are diminished pulmonary vascular markings; if not, these may be increased.
- Echo is diagnostic, and additional information necessary for surgical decision-making includes location and margins of the VSD, straddling of the atrioventricular valves, the sizes of the great arteries and their relationship, distance of the tricuspid valve from the pulmonary valve, the presence of pulmonary stenosis, chordal connections of the tricuspid valve to the outlet septum, coronary anatomy, and arch abnormalities.
- Cardiac catheterization is useful at the more complex end of the spectrum to delineate the relationship of the VSD with the great arteries, the coronary artery anatomy, and the exact hemodynamics.

Management

Medical management depends on the anatomy. If there is inadequate pulmonary blood flow, the PDA must be kept open with PGE_1; conversely, if there is CHF, diuresis and management of the pulmonary overflow with manipulation of ventilation may be needed. Indications for surgery depend on anatomy. Across the spectrum of DORV, from VSD to ToF to TGA, indications for surgery are similar to these conditions.

Taussig–Bing anomaly

This is a form of DORV with **subpulmonary VSD** and **malposed great arteries** that is associated with **subaortic stenosis, aortic arch abnormalities, and unusual coronary patterns**. (Taussig–Bing anomaly is often used to describe any DORV with subpulmonary VSD).

- The principles of repair are as previously described, with arterial switch and intracardiac baffle to direct ventricular flow into the neo-aorta.
- Outcomes are not as good as for uncomplicated DORV, with 15-year survival after surgery in the region of 90%.

Repair of DORV

- Surgical approach to **DORV** varies according to the location of the VSD:
- **Subaortic VSD**: the intraventricular shunt should be closed early with an intraventricular baffle if there is a large shunt with pulmonary hypertension, CHF, failure to thrive. In the presence of pulmonary stenosis, decision-making is similar to ToF (📖 p616).
- **Subpulmonary VSD**: this requires an arterial switch operation with closure of the VSD. There may be arch abnormalities, which can be corrected at the same operation. If there is pulmonary stenosis, intraventricular tunnel repair with **Rastelli operation** (📖 p629).
- **Doubly committed VSD**: intraventricular baffle to close the intraventricular shunt and connect the LV to the aorta.
- **Non-committed VSD**: often, palliation with PA band is performed to allow growth and re-evaluation of the intracardiac anatomy. If possible, the LV is baffled to the aorta with an intraventricular baffle, with or without an arterial switch operation. The baffle will be long and large, and the VSD may need to be enlarged. It may not be possible to repair this defect, and some of these are palliated with a Fontan circulation.

LVOT obstruction

Key facts

- LVOT obstruction occurs at the subvalvular, valvular, and supravalvular level, and repairs must be tailored to the specific morphology.
- Generally operation is performed in the presence of symptoms, or an asymptomatic but significant (>50mmHg) gradient.
- LVOT obstruction may be associated with obstructive lesions of the left heart such as coarctation or interruption of the aorta, mitral stenosis, or parachute mitral valve; it is also associated with VSD, AVSD, pulmonary stenosis, PDA.

Subvalvar stenosis

This is an acquired lesion (it rarely occurs at birth or in the first year of life, is usually associated with other lesions, and has a high recurrence rate after surgery) and may be caused by abnormal flow patterns resulting from abnormal angulation of the LVOT. Exceptions include patients with **Shone complex** or interrupted aortic arch, where it may be present at birth. It makes up about 15% of fixed LVOTO lesions. There are four anatomic forms: the first two account for 80% of subaortic stenoses and may involve the AMVL or the base of the aortic valve cusps:

- A *discrete* membrane of endocardial fold and fibrous tissue.
- A *fibromuscular ridge* at the crest of the septum.
- A *diffuse*, tunnel-like narrowing of the LVOT consisting of circumferential fibromuscular hypertrophy with bulging of the septum and dynamic obstruction due to abnormal systolic anterior motion of the AMVL.
- *Accessory or anomalous mitral valve* tissue (this form of LVOTO is usually progressive, and leads eventually to aortic and mitral valve abnormalities, with 65% of patients developing AR).

Valvar aortic stenosis

This is the result of valvular maldevelopment. There are three types:

- *Bicuspid* aortic valve (70%): there are two leaflets instead of the usual three, they are usually thickened, with one leaflet having a fibrous ridge or raphe. There is usually some degree of commissural fusion, although this is not necessary for stenosis to occur.
- *Tricuspid* valve: there are three leaflets, they may be thickened and unequal, with variable degrees of commissural fusion. Usually this type of valve 'domes' in systole, with a central orifice, and is most amenable to valvotomy.
- *Unicuspid* valves are rare, and usually very stenotic.

Supravalvar stenosis

This comprises <10% of congenital LVOT obstruction and involves the aorta distal to the STJ. Most commonly it occurs sporadically (>50%), but it may occur as a part of Williams syndrome or in a familial form inherited in an autosomal dominant fashion. It is associated with coronary abnormalities such as diffuse narrowing of the left coronary, obstruction due to leaflet fusion with the ridge, and narrowed left coronary ostium. There are two types:

- **Discrete** (75%): stenosis is usually due to an annular ridge within the lumen of the aorta, with a normal or reduced outer diameter. The aortic cusps are abnormal in about 30% of cases, and may adhere to the ridge, thus impairing filling of the coronary arteries. Other associations include peripheral pulmonary artery stenoses; when part of Williams syndrome it is associated with elfin facies, hypercalcemia, and severe developmental delay.
- **Diffuse** (<25%): the ascending aorta and origins of the head and neck vessels may be involved, with an abnormally thick-walled aorta due to intimal thickening and medial hypertrophy with increased fibrous and elastic tissues.

Presentation and management

Supra- and subvalvar stenosis

- Catheter peak-to-peak gradients of >50mmHg across the LVOT is an indication for surgical repair.
- Gradient of 30–50mmHg with symptoms, progression, ST/T wave changes at rest or exercise, or the Doppler peak systolic gradient is more than 50mmHg may indicate need for earlier surgery.

Valvar stenosis

In 10% this presents in the first year of life, usually as critical stenosis requiring urgent treatment, and with worse lifelong outcomes. In older children and adults the mortality arising from this diagnosis is low, with less need for urgent intervention. The neonate with critical aortic stenosis may present collapsed, with severe LV dysfunction, and will require a period of resuscitation with PGE_1, inotropes, and mechanical ventilation before intervention on the valve. In older patients, valve intervention may be performed in line with guidelines developed in the adult population.

LVOT obstruction repair

Valvar stenosis

Balloon valuloplasty

This is the mainstay of treatment of critical AS in neonates and infants, the goal being to relieve obstruction without causing AI. Balloon diameters of 80–100% of the valve annulus are used, aiming to reduce the peak-to-peak gradient by 50%.

Surgical valvuloplasty

Some centres continue to prefer surgical valvotomy, hoping to achieve a better result with fewer incidences of AI and longer reintervention-free survival. Where there are associated lesions requiring surgery or there is concern about the adequacy of the LV, surgery is preferred. Surgery involves CPB, an oblique aortotomy, and valvuloplasty consisting of **commissurotomies and thinning of the leaflets where necessary**.

Aortic valve replacement

In children this is reserved for those in whom balloon valvotomy and surgical valvuloplasty has failed, or where intervention has caused significant aortic incompetence. Where there is residual significant stenosis there may be an inadequate aortic annulus, and valve replacement (📖 p378) may be combined with root enlargement (📖 p392 and p635). Valve substitutes in small children are not available, thus making the **Ross operation** (📖 p388) the procedure of choice. In older children and young adults, usually a **mechanical valve** is the appropriate choice, due to the rapid degeneration of tissue valves in the young.

Supravalvar stenosis

- Hypothermic aorto-bicaval CPB and cardioplegic arrest.
- Incise across the localized stenosis into the non-coronary sinus and enlarge incision with a patch.
- **Brom aortoplasty**: transect ascending aorta, excise the whole ridge, enlarge all three sinuses with patches.
- If supravalvar stenosis is diffuse and extending into head and neck vessels, extensive reconstruction may be warranted, using DHCA, and reconstructing the aorta and arch with homograft, bovine pericardium or Gore-tex.

Subvalvar stenosis

- Hypothermic aortocaval CPB and cardioplegic arrest.
- Antegrade cardioplegia into root, or if AI, directly into coronaries.
- Oblique aortotomy into non-coronary sinus.
- RCC retracted anteriorly to expose subvalvular area.
- Fibrous shelf resected with knife, or peeled off with help of Watson–Cheyne dissector.
- Peel off the underside of the valve leaflets, release the fibrous trigones.
- Avoid area of membranous septum, below commissure between non-coronary and right coronary cusps.
- If necessary perform septal myotomy/myectomy—from below the commissure between RCC and LCC to below the body of the RCC.

Small aortic roots and tunnel-like LVOT obstruction

Where there is a small aortic root and diffuse narrowing of the LVOT, the outflow tract can be enlarged prior to inserting an aortic valve substitute:

Nick's aortic root enlargement (📖 p392)

Oblique aortotomy incision into the non-coronary sinus is extended across the aortic annulus, and a patch sutured into this defect to enlarge the root.

Manouguian aortic root enlargement (📖 p393)

The aortotomy is directed towards the commissure between the LCC and NCC, and extended across the fibrous continuity between the aortic and mitral valves—patch inserted.

Konno aortic root enlargement

The aortotomy is made longitudinally towards the commissure between the RCC and the LCC, avoiding the RCA. A transverse incision is made proximal to the pulmonary valve in the RVOT; then with scissors, one blade in the LV the other in the RV, the interventricular septum is opened. The aortic valve is removed, then a patch used to reconstruct the septum to the desired width. An aortic valve substitute is then inserted. This method of enlargement may be easily performed during a Ross operation, the **Ross–Konno operation**.

Extracardiac valve conduit

Extracardiac valved conduit from LV apex to ascending, descending or abdominal aorta have been used to bypass very narrow tunnel-like LVOTs in the past.

Outcomes

Valvular stenosis

- Neonatal aortic valve stenosis: mortality for balloon aortic valvotomy is ~10%, with risk of significant AI ~15%. The mortality risks are similar with surgical valvotomy, with less incidence of AI. 25–40% need reintervention by 5 years.
- Early degeneration/calcification/structural failure of heterograft substitutes have lead to discontinuation of their use in children. Homografts are slightly better, with 10-year freedom from reoperation about 40–50%, and are also not commonly used.
- Mechanical valves have low postoperative mortality, 2–3%, and good long-term outcomes, but in smaller children may have to be up-sized. At 20 years, freedom from thromboembolism is ~93%, from reoperation ~87%.
- The early mortality from the Ross operation is <2%, freedom from reoperation of 90% at 7 years.

Subaortic stenosis

Low early mortality, but recurrence rates up to 35% have been reported.

Supravalvar stenosis

Early mortality is up to 10%, with recurrence rates up to 25% reported, with no differences between the surgical techniques.

Ebstein anomaly

Key facts

- This rare malformation accounts for <1% of congenital cardiac anomalies, and is characterized by abnormalities of the tricuspid valve and RV.
- 10–20% have Wolff–Parkinson–White (WPW) syndrome, 25–30% have accessory pathways on EPS, and up to 25% have pre-excitation on the surface EKG.

Morphology

Very variable. Posterior and septal tricuspid leaflets are displaced inferiorly into the RV with associated RV hypoplasia and 'atrialization,' tricuspid incompetence, and ASD. The displaced leaflets are usually hypoplastic and tethered. The functional RV lies beyond the apically displaced coaptation point, and proximal to this the RV is 'atrialized.' The anterior leaflet is a 'sail like' structure (Fig 12.??), and tethering of this leaflet can cause RVOT obstruction. Lungs are hypoplastic in severe cases. WPW syndrome is present in 14%.

Pathophysiology

Pathophysiology depends on the severity of the RV hypoplasia, tricuspid valve abnormalities, and WPW syndrome. At birth the PVR is close to systemic pressures and as a result of tricuspid regurgitation and functionally small TRV, right-to-left shunting occurs resulting in cyanosis. The PVR falls after birth. If the RV is adequate then shunting and cyanosis reduce. If TR and RV pressures are high, cyanosis persists.

Presentation

Depending on the severity of the anomalies, patients may present with any of the following symptoms and signs at any stage of childhood:

- Cyanosis.
- Cardiomegaly and congestive cardiac failure.
- Malar flush, systolic murmur along LLSE, diastolic murmur.
- Hepatomegaly, ascites and peripheral edema.
- Paroxysmal supraventricular and ventricular tachyarrhythmias.
- Paradoxical embolus, cerebral abscess, sudden death.

Investigations

- EKG shows right bundle branch block, RA hypertrophy, and type B WPW in 14%.
- CXR shows marked cardiomegaly.
- Echocardiography is diagnostic and shows apical displacement of the septal leaflet >8mm/m², abnormalities of the leaflets and their septal attachments, dilated RA, dilated RV with reduced contractile function, delayed closure of the tricuspid valve (>65ms after MV) paradoxical septal motion: echo is also used to assess functional RV size (<35% of total RV size is poor prognostic indicator), degree of leaflet displacement, tethering, deformity, severity of TR and RVOT.
- Cardiac catheterization is sometimes used to quantify shunts and delineate anatomy.

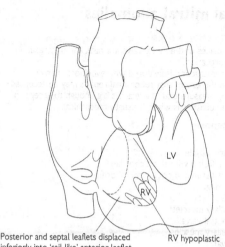

Posterior and septal leaflets displaced
inferiorly into 'sail-like' anterior leaflet

RV hypoplastic

Fig. 12.22 Ebstein anomaly.

Surgical management

Neonates

Just over a half of neonates will need surgical intervention. Neonates dependent on PGE$_1$ require early intervention. If stable with good SaO$_2$ and no CHF, a systemic–pulmonary shunt may be adequate palliation. If on PGE$_1$, oxygenation is adequate but CHF is present, then tricuspid repair or replacement is required if the RV is adequate, or tricuspid valve closure (right ventricular exclusion) and B-T shunt if not. In severe cases, transplant may be the only option (📖 pp504–519).

Older children and adults

May become symptomatic with onset of arrhythmias. Subtle decline in exercise tolerance must be anticipated with regular exercise testing. Tricuspid repair for all but the most severe forms should be attempted; surgical outcome is dependent on the size and function of the right RV. Techniques include: detachment of the anterior and some of the inferior leaflet to allow mobilization of the tethered leaflet tissue, plication of the atrialized chamber and right atrium, annuloplasty (with a ring if adequate siize), repositioning of the anterior and inferior leaflets at the repaired annulus. If repair fails, replacement with a biological prosthesis has acceptable results. If the RV of inadequate size or function, tricuspid repair may be combined with a cavopulmonary shunt to ensure off-loading of the right heart. In severe RV hypoplasia, total cavopulmonary connection may have to be considered

Outcomes

In neonates, survival 1 year after surgery is about 65%. In older patients, postoperative mortality is about 10%.

Congenital mitral anomalies

Key facts

- Congenital anomalies of the mitral valve are rare, and may result in stenosis or regurgitation.
- Mitral valve reconstruction is favoured wherever possible over replacement, to the extent that suboptimal repairs may be accepted as a temporizing measure until the infant is big enough to accept an adequately sized prosthesis which is usually mechanical.

Mitral valve stenosis

Anatomy

- Normal papillary muscles:
  - Commissural fusion with short chordae.
  - Excess valvar tissue and double mitral orifice.
  - Supravalvar ring.
  - Small annulus.
- Abnormal papillary muscles:
  - Parachute mitral valve.
  - Absent papillary muscles.
  - Hammock valve.

Pathophysiology and presentation

Results in pulmonary venous hypertension and presents with features of pulmonary hypertension, e.g., RV heave, prominent S2, mid-diastolic flow murmur.

- EKG: LA enlargement and RV hypertrophy.
- CXR: enlarged LA, increased pulmonary vascular markings.
- Echo: this is diagnostic and some time and effort should be spent in analysing the mechanism of valve dysfunction. Associated lesions must be sought.

Management

Surgery is best not undertaken in the first 6 months of age unless absolutely necessary. However, severe pulmonary hypertension may necessitate early surgery, which is high risk. Techniques employed include papillary muscle splitting, commissurotomies, resection of secondary chordae, chordal fenestration, resection of supravalvar fibrous rings. Mitral valve replacement can often be avoided.

Mitral valve regurgitation

Anatomy

This classified according to Carpentier's classification (🕮 p400):

- Type I (normal leaflet motion):
  - Annular dilatation and deformation.
  - Cleft leaflet.
  - Leaflet defect.
- Type II (excessive leaflet motion):
  - Elongated chordae.
  - Elongated papillary muscle.
  - Absent chordae.

- Type III restricted leaflet motion:
  - Normal papillary muscles: commissural fusion or short chords.
  - Abnormal papillary muscles: parachute or hammock mitral valve.

Pathophysiology

Results in progressive pulmonary venous hypertension, LV volume over-load, and eventually CHF (📖 p401).

Management

Techniques to *repair* these defects include the use of annular rings, triangular resections, annular plication, commissuroplasties, leaflet extension, suture closure of clefts, chordal transposition, chordal shortening, papillary muscle sliding plasty, papillary muscle plication.

If *mitral valve replacement* is required, this usually necessitates the use of mechanical valves in small sizes, with significant morbidity in children aged <6. Outcomes are better when the prosthesis is implanted in the anatomical position, rather than in the supra-annular position, and when there is less mismatch in size between the native annulus and the replacement. A strategy of palliative mitral valve repairs accepting a suboptimal result until the patient is big enough to undergo replacement with a reasonable sized prosthesis may have to be considered.

Outcomes

Mortality for surgery for true congenital mitral valve anomalies is 5% for mitral regurgitation and 25–30% for mitral stenosis, with 10-year survival in the order of 50–60%. Mortality of mechanical valve replacement in children <2 years old is >30–40%.

ALCAPA

Key facts

- Anomalous origin of the left coronary artery from the pulmonary artery (ALCAPA) is rare condition in which the whole or one branch of the left main coronary artery (LMCA) arises from the main pulmonary artery, or occasionally from the right pulmonary artery.
- It leads to early symptoms in infancy, with heart failure although it can present for the first time in adulthood.
- Coronary artery reimplantation is the procedure of choice.

Morphology

The left coronary artery usually arises from the left-sided sinus of the main pulmonary artery, then assumes the normal course of the LMCA.

Pathophysiology

In the neonate with high PVR, the pressure within the coronary artery is adequate for coronary perfusion. As PVR falls, perfusion pressure within the coronaries falls as well, and myocardial oxygenation depends on collaterals. Thus during increased myocardial oxygen demand, the low-pressure, low-oxygen blood supply may lead to anterolateral LV free wall ischemia and *infarction*—the latter causes mitral valve papillary muscle dysfunction and **MR**.

Presentation

Symptoms may begin soon after birth or within the first 3 months as the PVR falls. There is heart failure with dyspnea; poor feeding, failure to thrive, sweating, and tachycardia are common. 85% of patients present within the first 2 months of life. When symptoms are delayed, presentations may be in later years, and adult patients may remain asymptomatic for many years. Sudden cardiac death may be the mode of presentation at any stage.

Investigation

- EKG may show Q-waves and ST elevation in the anterolateral leads.
- CXR: will show cardiomegaly.
- Echo shows a dilated and poorly contracting LV, with mitral regurgitation, and the appearances must be distinguished from dilated cardiomyopathy. The anomalous coronary artery should be demonstrable on echo, with colour-flow Doppler showing retrograde flow from the coronary into the PA.
- Cardiac catheterization is unnecessary in infancy, but show the anomalous origin, a step up of oxygen saturations in the PA, and only the RCA arising from the aorta.

Surgical management

Surgery is indicated in the infant as they are at risk of sudden cardiac death. Infants in heart failure with diffuse myocardial fibrosis and severe mitral regurgitation may require transplantation. In all other patients, surgery should be undertaken to provide a coronary supply arising from the systemic circulation.

Mitral regurgitation improves after coronary artery reimplantation, but may require further intervention if it remains significant. Usually, mitral valve repair is not performed at the first operation. Surgical techniques include ligation of LMCA if there is a good collateral circulation, subclavian-coronary anastomosis, CABG, intrapulmonary tunnel by creating an AP window and baffling the coronary through the MPA to the aorta. The operation of choice currently is coronary artery reimplantation.

Coronary artery reimplantation
- Standard aortocaval bypass via a median sternotomy.
- Snare the PAs to prevent 'steal' from the LCA.
- Cardioplegia into the aortic *and* pulmonary roots, and LCA origin once the MPA opened.
- Button of PA around the LMCA ostium excised, mobilized, anastomosed to aortic root.
- If far from aorta, posterior PA wall harvested with the coronary, and this is used as a tube to extend the LCA towards the aorta.
- A minority of patients require postoperative mechanical support.

Outcomes

Early postoperative mortality is in the order of 5–10%. Late deaths are rare since the adoption of coronary artery reimplantation. Late patency of the reimplanted coronary artery has been shown to be excellent.

Chapter 13

Assessment and anesthesia for thoracic surgery

Anesthetic considerations

Key facts

* Specific anesthetic considerations in thoracic surgery include the need for accurate assessment of the airway, need for lung isolation and bronchoscopy prior to procedure, increased use of epidural anesthesia, and greater need for invasive monitoring, particularly arterial blood gases and pressures, with location depending on procedure.
* The *Mallampati classification* is used to identify patients who may have difficult airways.
* Bronchoscopy is routinely performed after intubation, and may impact on conduct of anesthesia in several ways.
* Tracheal reconstruction has several unique anesthesia issues.

Preoperative assessment

Prior to anesthetic for an operation the global function of a patient is described by assigning one of the *American Society of Anesthesiologists (ASA) Physician Status Classes*. If the procedure is an emergency, than the letter E is added to the class description (📖 p89, Box 3.1).

Evaluation of the airway

* Factors that determine whether a patient has a difficult airway include:
  * Trauma to the head, neck, or face.
  * Ability to open mouth, micrognathia, obstructive teeth, short 'bull' neck, morbid obesity.
  * Diminished cervical spine mobility.
* The airway can be categorized using the *Mallampati classification* which determines the degree at which the base of tongue may obstruct a potential view of the vocal cords, prior to intubation. It is assessed by having the patient sit upright with their head in the neutral position, the mouth maximally opened, and the tongue protruded anteriorly. Class I is the easiest potential intubation.
  * Class I: faucial pillars, soft palate, and uvula are visible.
  * Class II: faucial pillars and soft palate are visible, but the uvula is obscured by the base of the tongue.
  * Class III: only the soft palate is visible.
* Class III airway predicts a difficult intubation.

Hemodynamic monitoring

* Basic hemodynamic monitoring should include frequently cycled BP, pulse oximetry, continuous EKG, and occasionally CVP.
* A radial arterial line should be used in any major thoracic surgery procedure, not only for BP monitoring (particularly in patients with epidurals), but also to measure frequent ABGs, especially in single-lung ventilation.
* The arterial line should be placed in the dependent arm when the patient is in the lateral decubitus position.
* For tracheal surgery (📖 pp750–757) or mediastinoscopy (📖 p662), the arterial line should be placed in the left arm, to avoid inaccurate readings during compression of the innominate artery.

Anesthetic considerations for key procedures

Flexible bronchoscopy

- Most flexible bronchoscopy can be performed with topical analgesia with 2–4% lidocaine sprayed onto the vocal cords.
- Conscious sedation can be used with benzodiazepines and narcotics.
- If performed under general anesthetic, a >7.5mm ET tube is needed to allow for comfortable manipulation of the bronchoscope.
- Most common complication of flexible bronchoscopy is *hypoxia* from excessive suction aspiration; therefore 100% oxygen should be used.

Rigid bronchoscopy

- General anesthesia required: hypoxia and hypercapnia may complicate procedure.
- Most rigid scopes have a sidearm to allow positive pressure ventilation.
- While anesthesiologists are accustomed to this mode of ventilation, it has to be suspended while the surgeon is working.
- *Intermittent jet O_2 ventilation* may be used: this entrains oxygenated air via a Venturi effect with the advantage that ventilation is not interrupted. Disadvantages are: (1) an iv anesthetic is required as volatile agents are unpredictable given the high gas flow rates, and (2) the anesthesiologist may not be familiar with this type of ventilation.

Mediastinoscopy

BP measurements in the right arm may become inaccurate or unavailable if the innominate artery is intermittently compressed by the mediastinoscope. Therefore arterial lines should be placed in the left arm and a pulse oximeter on placed on the right hand. If the pulse oximeter loses its tracing, the surgeon should be warned that the innominate artery is being occluded.

Tracheal resection and reconstruction

- Airway with critical stenosis may make induction anesthesia difficult.
- Muscle relaxants should be avoided, as the patient may need spontaneous efforts.
- If the stenosis is too narrow to intubate, the surgeon can core out the stenosis with a rigid bronchoscope, or the patient may be intubated above the stenosis and jet/spontaneous ventilation used to proceed.
- Once the trachea is divided, the surgeon can intermittently intubate the distal trachea with a sterile armored *Tovell tube*, while the ET tube is retracted to the proximal airway.
- Just before completion of the tracheal anastomosis, the ET tube is advanced beyond the repair.

Thymectomy for myasthenia gravis

- Patients with MG have autoimmune antibodies to the acetyl-cholinesterase receptor (AChR), and may be overly sensitive to non-depolarizing muscle relaxants.
- Anticholinesterase medications should be avoided, and patients may require plasmapheresis preoperatively to clear anti-AChR antibodies.
- Non-depolarizing muscle relaxants should be avoided.
- Patients may require a short duration of mechanical ventilation postoperatively secondary to muscle weakness.

Single-lung ventilation

Key facts

- Many thoracic surgical procedures require the surgical lung to be non-ventilated, with selective ventilation of the non-operative lung, with a *double lumen endotracheal tube (DLT)*.
- A *bronchial blocker* is an alternative for lung isolation when placement of a DLT would be too difficult, in a patient that is already intubated with a single lumen ET tube or a tracheostomy.

Oxygenation and ventilation

- Oxygenation may be affected by shunting of pulmonary blood flow through the non-ventilated lung.
- Oxygenation should be carefully monitored with measurements of ABGs.
- Tidal volumes of 10–15mL/kg should be used to achieve desired minute ventilation volumes.
- The respiratory rate can be increased to achieve CO_2 levels appropriate for two-lung ventilation.
- Peak airway pressure should be monitored to avoid hyperinflation of the ventilated lung.

Troubleshooting

- *Isolated lung fails to deflate*: suction secretions from the ET tube, confirm appropriate tube position with a pediatric bronchoscope.
- *Oxygenation is inadequate*: suction secretions from the ET tube, confirm appropriate tube position with a pediatric bronchoscope.
  - Add PEEP to the ventilated lung.
  - Increase the fraction of inspired oxygen (FiO_2) to 100%.
  - Briefly inflate the non-ventilated lung.
  - The surgeon can clamp the pulmonary artery of the non-ventilated lung to limit ventilation–perfusion mismatch.
- *Hypercapnia*: briefly inflate non-ventilated lung.

Double lumen endotracheal tubes

- Double lumen tubes are fitted to either the right main stem bronchus (right-sided DLT) or the left main stem bronchus (left-sided DLT). DLT have separate channels to ventilate both the main stem bronchus and the trachea. The right-sided DLT has a 'Murphy's eye' to allow for ventilation of the right upper lobe (Fig. 13.1a).
- Sizing DLT: 39–41F for a man and 35–37F for a woman.
- Left-sided DLTs are adequate for most lung isolation needs, and are easiest to place.
- Right-sided DLTs are harder to place secondary to the need to align the Murphy's eye with the orifice of the RUL bronchus. However, right-sided DLTs are ideal for left pneumonectomy left main stem bronchoplasty procedures and left lung transplants.

Placement of a DLT

- The DLT is inserted with the point of the distal curve facing anteriorly.
- The stylet is removed when the tube enters the trachea.

- Tube is rotated so the bronchial lumen is towards the intended side.
- The tube is advanced until resistance is felt.
- The tracheal cuff is inflated, and the patient is ventilated, allowing for bilateral chest expansion. If satisfactory, then the tracheal side is clamped and tracheal lumen is opened to air, and the bronchial cuff is inflated and the chest is auscultated. Selective ventilation is confirmed.
- Correct positioning is confirmed with a pediatric bronchoscope, immediately after tube placement, and again after positioning patient.
- For a left-sided DLT, the bronchoscope is inserted through the tracheal lumen. The bronchial cuff should be just past the carina in the left main stem. The right upper lobe orifice is identified.
- For right-sided DLT, the bronchial cuff should be just past the carina in the right main stem. The bronchoscope is then inserted down the bronchial lumen, and the Murphy's eye is confirmed to be positioned at the right upper lobe orifice.

Common problems

- Common errors include advancing the tube too far, not far enough, not aligning the Murphy's eye with the right upper lobe bronchus, overinflating the bronchial cuff causing herniation, displacement of the tube with patient positioning.
- Complications of placement include airway injury, pneumothorax, and esophageal intubation.

Bronchial blocker

- Involves placement of a Fogarty type balloon through a single lumen ET tube to selectively occlude an airway.
- Can be used for lung isolation when placement of a DLT would be too difficult, a patient is already intubated with a single lumen ET tube, or a tracheostomy.
- Arndt wire-guided bronchial blocker (Fig. 13.1c): a Fogarty type balloon is attached to a 5–9F catheter with one 1.4mm inner lumen.
- The catheter has a guidewire that passes through the lumen, which can be coupled to a flexible bronchoscope.
- The bronchoscope, with the wire looped, guides the catheter to the correct position, and the balloon is inflated to occluding one bronchus.

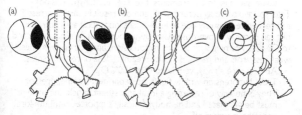

Fig. 13.1 (a) Left-sided, (b) right-sided double-lumen ET tube. (c) Bronchial blocker in right mainstem. Inserts are bronchoscopic views at each level.

Thoracic analgesia

Key facts

- *Epidural analgesia* provides excellent analgesia via administration of opioids (e.g., fentanyl) or local anesthetics (e.g., bupivacaine) via a catheter inserted into the epidural space usually before surgery.
- *Total spinal block* is a potentially fatal complication of epidural anesthesia.
- *Intercostal blocks* provide shorter-term local anesthesia by infiltration of the intercostal nerves above and below a thoracotomy incision: these can be performed at completion of a procedure or postoperatively.

Epidural analgesia

- Thoracic epidural is beneficial in patients undergoing thoracotomy as well as upper abdominal surgery.
- Local anesthetic is continuously applied through a flexible catheter into the epidural space, accessed via a lumbar puncture.
- Anesthetic solution into the pleural space affects the spinal nerve roots by entering the CSF via the dura.
- Epidural infusions include bupivacaine and fentanyl.

Complications

These include complications from placement and side effects of the infusion and inadequate analgesia.

- Placement complications include headache, epidural abscess, and epidural hematoma.
- Infusion side effects include urinary retention, pruritus, hypotension, respiratory depression, and CNS depression.
- *Hypotension:* this is due to vasodilation because of loss of sympathetic vascular tone, and in the case of a complete spinal block (see 'Total spinal block', next bullet point) bradycardia, hypercapnia, and hypoxia. Treat isolated hypotension by:
  - Checking level of block to ascertain it is no higher than dermatome (nipples): if higher reduce infusion rate or discontinue.
  - Giving iv fluid bolus (e.g., 250–500mL normal saline).
  - Start pressor infusion, e.g., 0.03–0.05 micrograms/kg/min norepinephrine (with bolus, e.g., 1mg metaraminol in 10mL normal saline, given in 1mL increments if severe, acute hypotension).
- *Total spinal block:* may occur rapidly and can result in cardiac arrest if not recognized. Usually due to inadvertent intrathecal administration, but can occur with overdose via epidural route causing block to ascend to C8–C4. Warning signs include hypotension, bradycardia, numbness/weakness arms and hands, difficulty breathing, loss of consciousness.
  - ABC: secure airway, ventilated with 100% O_2.
  - Treat hypotension with iv fluids, epinephrine, atropine, pressor.
  - They is no way of reversing a local anaesthetic block: the patient must be ventilated and hemodynamically supported until the local anaesthetic wears off.
  - Naloxone (0.2–0.4 mg iv) reverses effects of opiate analgesia.

- *Epidural headache*: usually postural—worse with standing, relieved by lying down, may be associated with signs of meningism (stiff neck, photophobia, nausea, vomiting, dizziness) and is thought to be due to CSF leak causing traction on the meninges.
  - Small needles and meticulous technique help reduce incidence.
  - Patient can lie down if appropriate.
  - Fluid resuscitation: iv if not tolerating oral fluids.
  - Simple analgesia (acetaminophen, aspirin) and sumatriptan.
  - Caffeine: cola drink or coffee.
  - Blood patch if severe/prolonged: 15–20mL patient's own blood is injected into epidural space to seal CSF leak.
- *Urinary retention*: most thoracic surgery patients will have a Foley catheter in situ, which is discontinued after the epidural.
- *Epidural abscess*: potentially fatal complication. Epidurals are normally discontinued after 3–5 days. Check site daily if kept for longer for inflammation, cellulitis, or pus, particularly if patient develops signs of sepsis postoperatively. If you see these, the anesthesiologist who placed the epidural should be informed, the epidural should be removed, and broad-spectrum iv antibiotics should be started.
- Side effects can be managed by turning the rate of the epidural down or administering naloxone (0.2–0.4mg IV) if the epidural contains an opiate, e.g., fentanyl—naloxone has no ability to reverse the effects of local anesthetic-based epidurals.

Troubleshooting inadequate analgesia
- The anesthesiologist can bolus the epidural to gauge a patient response to determine if it is working.
- The solution concentration, type of analgesia given, and rate may be increased.

Intercostal rib blocks
- Rib blocks are performed at the level of the incision, as well as 2–3 ribs above and below the level of incision.
- Using a 22-G needle, anesthetic agent is administered at the inferior edge of the rib, after an aspiration negative for blood or air.
- Flexible fine-bore catheters can be inserted in the intercostal space at the time of surgery and continuous infusion of local anesthetic (usually bupivacaine) run for several days postoperatively, with the option for bolus top-ups.

Patient-controlled analgesia
- PCA use patient-controlled administration of narcotics such as morphine, fentanyl, hydromorphine, and pethidine (meperidine).
- The computerized system has a loading dose, a timed lockout range in minutes, an hourly limit range in mg, and a potential for a basal rate in mg/h.
- The basal rate option should be avoided in elderly patients or those in an unmonitored unit.

Risk assessment

Key facts

- Performance scores help quantify a patients overall function.
- Major and intermediate cardiovascular risk factors necessitate additional preoperative investigation.
- Postoperative predicted FEV_1 and DLCO are the best indicators for a patient's ability to undergo pulmonary resection.
- The ability to climb a flight of stairs without significant dyspnea is a good surrogate for cardiopulmonary exercise testing.

Major predictors of postoperative complications

- Extent of resection, increased age, pre-existing cardiovascular disease, emergency procedure, immunocompromised patient, current or recent smoker, multiple comorbidities.
- Vital capacity decreases by 25% following a thoracotomy without lung resection, and takes 4–6 weeks to return to preoperative levels.

Performance or Zubrod scores

Performance scores are used to measure and quantify a patient's overall performance status and ability to perform activities of daily living:

- 0: asymptomatic.
- 1: symptomatic but completely ambulatory.
- 2: symptomatic, <50% in bed during the day.
- 3: symptomatic, >50% in bed, but not bedbound.
- 4: bedbound.
- 5: dead.

Assessment of cardiovascular risk

- In patients at risk for coronary artery disease (CAD), a small sub-population of patients with heart failure, exercise-induced arrhythmia, or myocardial ischemia may be identified by non-invasive testing.
- Per 2002/2006 ACC/AHA perioperative clearance guidelines thoracic surgery is an intermediate risk procedure with a 1–5% cardiac risk.
  - In patients with no cardiac history, risk of perioperative MI is 0.07–0.13%.
  - In patients with prior history of MI, risk of a perioperative MI is 2.8–17%.

Initial history and examination

- Includes physical exam, baseline EKG, determine cardiac risk factors by identifying history of CAD, valvular disease, heart failure, arrhythmia.
- Minor risk factors:
  - Diminished activities of daily living such as inability to climb a flight of stairs.
  - Age.
  - Abnormal EKG.
  - AF or other abnormal rhythms that are controlled.
  - Hypertension.
  - History of stroke.

- *Intermediate risk factors:*
  - Canadian class I or II angina.
  - Compensated CHF.
  - Chronic renal insufficiency.
  - Diabetes mellitus.
  - Prior MI.
- *Major risk factors:*
  - MI within 30 days.
  - Unstable or Canadian class III or IV angina.
  - Decompensated CHF.
  - Significant arrhythmias, including AF with rapid ventricular response, AV block.
  - Severe valvular disease.

ACC/AHA guidelines

- Patients with no cardiovascular risk factors do not require additional cardiovascular testing. For patients with minor or intermediate risk factors additional cardiovascular testing may be warranted, on a case-by-case basis.
- Patients with minor risk factors may proceed to surgery without additional cardiovascular testing.
- Patients with intermediate risk factors but good exercise capacity (e.g., can walk up a flight of stairs without dyspnea), can proceed with out additional cardiovascular testing.
- Patients who have undergone surgical or procedural revascularization within 5 years and who are asymptomatic may proceed without additional cardiovascular testing.
- Patients with one or more major risk factors require additional cardiovascular testing.

Cardiovascular investigations

- In patients where significant coronary artery disease is the main concern, non-invasive tests include myocardial perfusion stress/rest imaging (☐ p28), and stress echocardiography (☐ p25). Areas of reversible ischemia require invasive coronary imaging.
- Coronary catheterization identifies significant coronary stenoses, which would need treatment regardless of planned pulmonary resection. For lesions than can be treated with PCI, *bare metal stents* are favoured in this context, because of the potentially catastrophic sequelae of stent thrombosis associated with stopping antiplatelet therapy remains a risk for much longer with drug-eluting stents:
  - Clopidogrel increases bleeding risk: although surgery can be carried out safely, most surgeons prefer to discontinue clopidogrel for 5–10 days preoperatively.
  - It is usually safe to do this 6 weeks after angioplasty or bare metal stent, but probably not for ≥1 year after drug-eluting stent.
  - Planned thoracic surgery should be delayed 6 weeks after CABG.

Pulmonary assessment

Key facts

Pulmonary function testing allows for the assessment of lung volume, air flow, lung mechanics, and gas exchange.

Spirometry

- Measures expiratory airflow volume over time.
- 'Normal' reference values are based on age, gender, and height.

Forced vital capacity and forced expiratory volume in 1s

- FVC and FEV_1 are probably the most important measurements for assessing risk of postoperative pulmonary insufficiency.
- Most commonly used spirometry tests.
- Value after bronchodilator therapy should be used.
- % predicted (predicted value based on age, gender, and height) is better representative of pulmonary function than absolute value.
- Obstructive conditions (see Table 13.1) result in reduced FEV_1, reduced FEV_1/FVC is indicative of obstructive lung disease secondary to a larger total lung capacity from air trapping, and reduced elastic recoil of the lung.
- Restrictive lung disease (see Table 13.1) results in reduced FVC and FEV_1 and possible preserved FEV_1/FVC ratio.
- FEV_1 of 2L, or >80% predicted is suitable for pneumonectomy, and FEV_1 >1.5L is suitable for lobectomy.

Predicted postoperative (ppo) FEV_1 and DLCO

- If either the FEV_1 or DLCO is <80% predicted, postoperative lung function should be predicted through additional calculation or testing.
- Ppo FEV_1 and ppo DLCO values are more accurate in predicting operative risk.
- Ppo FEV_1 and DLCO are calculated by estimating the quantity of lung parenchyma lost after surgical removal.
- For lobectomy, counting the number of anatomic segments removed is used for calculation, whereas lung perfusion measured by quantitative radionuclide perfusion should be taken into account in borderline cases and in pneumonectomy (Box 13.1).

Table 13.1 Pulmonary disorders

Obstructive disorders	Restrictive disorders
Asthma	Sarcoidosis
Chronic bronchitis	Congestive heart failure
Emphysema	Pulmonary fibrosis
Cystic fibrosis	Fibrosing alveolitis
Bronchiolitis obliterans	Thoracic deformities
Eosinophilic granulosa	Interstitial pneumonitis
Lymphangiomyomatosis	

Gas exchange
- Gas exchange tests measure alveolar oxygen exchange.
- Diffusing capacity of the lung for carbon monoxide (DLCO) Identifies patients with restrictive lung disease such as interstitial lung disease and other parenchymal abnormalities.

Predicting postoperative FEV₁

$$\text{ppo FEV}_1 = \text{Pre-op FEV}_1 \times \frac{(19 - \text{number of segments to be resected})}{19}$$

$$\text{ppo FEV}_1 = \text{Pre-op FEV}_1 \times (1 - \text{fraction of total perfusion for resected lung})$$

- DLCO has been demonstrated to be a predictor of postoperative morbidity and mortality.
- Low preoperative DLCO correlates with hospital readmission and poorer quality of life indexes.
- On average the right lung contributes 55% of perfusion and the left lung 45%.
- ppo FEV₁ or DLCO <40% indicates an increased risk for perioperative and cardiopulmonary morbidity after pulmonary resection. Patients should undergo additional exercise testing to confirm inoperability.
- A ppo FEV₁ or DLCO <30% may be a better threshold.

Cardiopulmonary exercise testing (CPET)
- CPET records the exercise EKG, heart rate response, minute ventilation, and maximal oxygen consumption (VO₂max).
- A VO₂max of 10–15mL/kg/min indicates an increased risk of morality after pulmonary resection.
- For patients with a VO₂max of <10mL/kg/min or <15mL/kg/min and a ppo FEV₁ and/or DLCO <40%, non-operative therapy is recommended.[1]
- Stair climb of 1 flight (4m) is a good surrogate.
- Inability to climb a flight of stairs without dyspnea corresponds to a VO₂max of <10mL/kg/min.[2]
- Combined lung volume reduction surgery (LVRS) and cancer resection.
- LVRS has shown to be effective in patients with heterogenous emphysema and upper lobe predominance and poor exercise capacity (📖 p726).
- For patients with poor lung function, upper lobe cancer, and upper lobe predominant emphysema, combined LVRS and lung cancer resection should be considered if the FEV₁ and/or DLCO are >20% predicted.[1]

References
1. Colice GL et al. Physiologic evaluation of the patient with lung cancer being considered for resectional surgery. Chest 2007; **132**:161S–77S.
2. Pollock M et al. Estimation of ventilatory reserve by stair climbing. A study in patients with chronic airflow obstruction. Chest 1993; **104**(5):1378–83.

Flexible bronchoscopy

Key facts

- Flexible bronchoscopy is the evaluation of the bronchial airways, for diagnostic or therapeutic purposes, using a flexible bronchoscope equipped with fiberoptic bundles, or with new-generation scopes, a charge coupled device at the end of the scope for improved optics.
- Flexible bronchoscopy can be readily accomplished with topical analgesia (awake patient) and therefore allows assessment of vocal cords and laryngeal function, and tracheomalacia (📖 p750), in addition to tracheobronchial toilet and biopsy.
- The most common complication of bronchoscopy is hypoxia from excessive suction aspiration.

See Fig. 13.2 for bronchial anatomy.

Procedure

- Flexible bronchoscopy can be performed via general anesthesia (7.5 ET tube or larger for standard adult scope), conscious sedation, or topical analgesia.
- The scope can be introduced through the nose, mouth, ET, or tracheostomy tube or stoma, or a rigid bronchoscope and can visualize the airway down to subsegmental bronchi.
- If you are doing this for the first time, familiarize yourself with the flexion and extension position, and the up, down, and neutral positions.

Setup

- There should be a nurse or other clinical assistant present.
- You need a clean bronchoscope, image processor, and light source (bronchoscope stack), aerosolized local anesthetic for awake patients and adequate sedation on board for intubated patients (for whom you also need the ET tube adaptor so they can still be ventilated during the procedure), 1L sterile normal saline, and a 10mL syringe with a straight nozzle for flushing, suction and suction tubing, specimen trap, flexible biopsy forceps, needle, and specimen pots.
- In case of emergencies have readily available equipment to perform bag and mask ventilation, and 1:10 000 epinephrine to control endobronchial bleeding.
- In awake bronchoscopy the upper airway is anesthetized by spraying 1–2% lidocaine aerosol into the nostril and onto posterior oropharynx. A bite block should be used if the oral route is planned.

Airway inspection

- Introduce scope and visualize vocal cords: in awake bronchoscopy spray lidocaine via bronchoscope which will induce coughing but eventually suppress the cough reflex.
- Instruct patient to take a deep breath and pass scope through open cords in trachea.
- Maintain orientation at all times: the soft, flat membrane is posterior.
- Systematically inspect the trachea, mainstem bronchi and segmental bronchi for size, patency, erythema, thrombi, secretions, masses.
- It is vital to use a system to ensure that each segment is correctly identified and none are missed.

Diagnostic applications

- *Brushing*: brush enclosed within a flexible catheter is advanced out of the sheath once near the lesion, which is then briskly rubbed a few times, retracted, and washed in saline/smeared on a microscopy slide.
- *Bronchoalveolar lavage*: a specimen trap is attached to the suction port on the handle of the scope which is advanced into the subsegmental bronchi, 10–20mL of sterile saline flushed down the scope and then aspirated into the trap, and sent for cytology. The difference between this and bronchial washings, is that the scope is wedged in a small airway in BAL to increase the specificity of the sample to the distal airway (washings are contaminated with oral flora).
- *Endobronchial biopsy*: flexible biopsy forceps advanced onto lesion under bronchoscopic vision, closed, and pulled quickly back.
- *Transbronchial biopsy*: this is a method of blindly sampling lung parenchyma using biopsy forceps. The patient is instructed to take a deep breath, the forceps are opened at the limit of the airway, the patient exhales, the forceps are closed, and if the patient does not complain of pain (indicating that the visceral pleura has been breached, risking pneumothorax) the forceps are tugged back.

Therapeutic applications

Aspiration of secretions, laser treatment, photodynamic therapy (PDT), argon plasma coagulation (APC), cryotherapy, stent placement, foreign body retrieval, and Wang needle transbronchial needle aspiration (TBNA).

Complications

- The most common complication during flexible bronchoscopy is hypoxia from suction aspiration.
- Other complications are rare, and include bleeding, pneumothorax, and respiratory failure (~0.1–0.2% each)
- The incidence of pneumothorax is ~4% in transbronchial biopsy.
- Self-limiting fever is not uncommon after BAL.

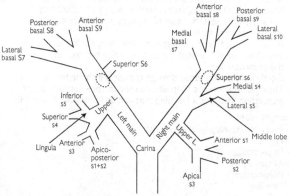

Fig. 13.2 Bronchoscopic anatomy.

Rigid bronchoscopy

Key facts
- Rigid bronchoscopy involves a stainless steel tube equipped with a removable lens that can allow for direct visualization, or insertion of a Hopkins's telescope for magnified camera visualization.
- Rigid bronchoscopy is best performed with general anesthesia.
- The rigid bronchoscope is useful for diagnostic and therapeutic interventions. As a flexible bronchoscope can be inserted down a rigid bronchoscope, all the therapeutic and diagnostic manoeuvres of a flexible bronchoscope can be performed through a rigid bronchoscope.
- Endobronchial ultrasound transbronchial needle aspiration (EBUS-TBNA) is an adjunct to mediastinoscopy, although cervical mediastinoscopy is the gold standard for evaluation of nodal tissue and other pathology of the superior and middle mediastinum.

Procedure

Set-up
- It is generally performed under general anesthesia, and it is inserted under direct visualization through the vocal cords (Fig. 13.3).
- The patient can be ventilated via intermittent insufflations through a side port, or Venturi (jet) ventilation (📖 p159).
- Sedate and preoxygenate the patient using bag and mask ventilation.
- Protect patient's eyes, lips, and teeth with eye pads and mouth guard.
- Place the patient's head in the sniffing position, standard for intubation.

Rigid bronchoscopy intubation
- Insert scope into mouth, advance under direct vision posterior to the tongue.
- The upper row of teeth is protected by the examiner's thumb at all times: resist any temptation to lever the scope against the teeth.
- By elevating the tongue the epiglottis is identified (Fig. 13.3).
- Raise the tip of the epiglottis anteriorly with the bronchoscope to visualize the posterior part of the vocal cords. Alternatively a laryngoscope can be used.
- Advance the bronchoscope towards the visual cords and turn the bronchoscope 90° to align the vertical orifice between the cords with the bronchoscope.
- Gently advance the scope through the cords into the trachea.
- The rigid bronchoscope can also be used to core out tumours or granulation tissue, or a flexible scope can be introduced (📖 p654).

Complications
- Injury to oropharyngeal structures.
- Hypoxia.
- Hypercapnia.
- Airway injury.
- Pneumothorax.
- Bleeding.

Endobronchial ultrasound

- EBUS-TBNA offers a minimally invasive approach to biopsying mediastinal nodal tissue and other pathology adjacent to the airways.
- EBUS-TBNA may not be ideal for diagnosis of lymphoma given the small amounts of tissue obtained.
- Current EBUS specialty bronchoscopes have a 7.5MHz convex array linear US probe. When the linear probe is coupled with the bronchial wall, 5cm penetration depth US images are obtained.
- EBUS scopes have a 2mm biopsy channel, with 35° oblique view.
- TBNA utilizes a 22G needle (Wang) suction aspirator system passed through the scope working channel.
- When aspirating a lymph node, lymphocytes must appear in the specimen for the sample to be considered diagnostic.
- Diagnosis of lymphoma may be problematic, given the small-gauge needle and need for a large tissue sample.
- Complications are the same as for flexible bronchoscopy TBNA.

Outcomes

EBUS-TBNA offers 89–99% sensitivity and diagnostic accuracy 85–99%, although a negative predictive value around 90%.

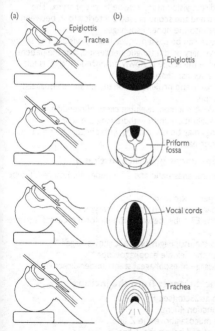

(a) Epiglottis
Trachea

(b) Epiglottis

Priform fossa

Vocal cords

Trachea

Fig. 13.3 Rigid bronchoscopy. (a) Position of scope. (b) Views as scope enters airway.

Esophagoscopy

Key facts

- Used for investigation of hematemesis, foreign bodies, esophageal strictures, dysphagia, non-cardiac chest pain, symptoms of gastro-esophageal reflux disease, recurrent aspiration pneumonia, odynophagia, abnormal esophageal shadow on chest radiograph.
- May be diagnostic, identifying esophagitis and malignancy, achalasia, webs, diverticula, rings, strictures.
- May be therapeutic, dilating strictures, arresting sites of bleeding, removing foreign bodies, allowing dilation and relief of obstruction.
- There are two main types:
  - Rigid: requires general anesthetic.
  - Flexible: may be performed under sedation as an outpatient procedure.

Flexible esophagoscopy under sedation

Patient must be starved for 6–8h prior to procedure to ensure complete gastric emptying.

- Patient placed in left lateral decubitus position or supine if under general anesthesia.
- Scope is passed by direct vision along tongue to oropharynx. The epiglottis is identified and the scope passed posterior to it, between the piriform recesses into the upper esophagus
- Alternatively the scope can be passed under indirect vision. The scope is placed into the oropharynx, the tongue depressed, and the patient asked to swallow while the scope is slowly advanced. A 'give' is felt when it enters the upper esophagus.
- The esophagus, stomach, and proximal duodenum can be visualized using the flexible scope.
- Scopes may have a double lumen, useful in cases of bleeding.
- Ensure continued visualization upon withdrawing the scope.
- Biopsies and brushings may be taken along with photographs and video recording of any abnormality.

Rigid esophagoscopy under general anesthesia

Patient undergoes general anesthetic and ET intubation. Ensure ET tube is securely fastened.

- Patient supine with neck extended.
- Scope is passed under direct vision into oropharynx.
- It is passed behind the ET tube, between the piriform recesses into the upper esophagus.
- The scope visualizes the esophagus only but allows larger instrumentation than the flexible esophagoscope.
- It also allows the passage of esophageal stents under direct vision.

Normal endoscopic distances from the incisors

- Aortic compression at 25cm (see Fig. 13.4).
- Squamocolumnar junction 40cm:
  - Whitish smooth mucosa above the Z line.
  - Reddish mucosa at and below the Z line.

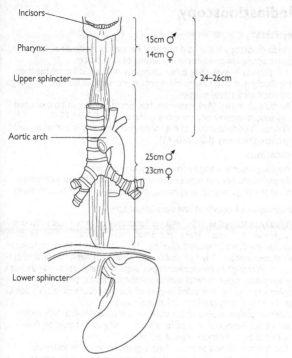

Fig. 13.4 Technique of esophagoscopy.

Labels on figure:
- Incisors
- Pharynx
- Upper sphincter
- Aortic arch
- Lower sphincter
- 15cm ♂
- 14cm ♀
- 24–26cm
- 25cm ♂
- 23cm ♀

Mediastinoscopy

Key facts

- Mediastinoscopy is the gold standard for staging mediastinal paratracheal lymph nodes in the setting of lung cancer.
- It is also key in evaluating other pathology of the middle mediastinum.
- Mediastinotomy or Chamberlain procedure is useful for biopsying large anterior mediastinal masses.
- Aortic-pulmonary (AP) artery window lymph nodes can be evaluated by mediastinotomy or now more commonly by left VATS.
- Thorough understanding of the mediastinal anatomy is critical to avoid catastrophic injury (📖 pp40–41).

Indications

- Pre-lung resection staging for primary lung cancer.
- Biopsy of mediastinal masses and lymph nodes for histological tissue diagnosis (e.g., sarcoid, lymphoma, mediastinal tumours, tuberculosis).

Technique of cervical mediastinoscopy

Originally described in 1954.[1] Allows for biopsy of lymph node stations 7 (subcarinal), 4, 2, and 1 (para- and pretracheal regions), as well as some superior mediastinal masses (see Fig. 13.5). Extended mediastinoscopy may access station 10 lymph nodes, though this carries additional operative risk. Although all mediastinoscopes allow the surgeon to look through the eyepiece, most cervical mediastinoscopy can be performed with a Hopkin's telescope, and video display of the procedure on a high-definition monitor (video cervical mediastinoscopy).

- Position patient supine with a transverse shoulder roll to fully extend the neck. The head is placed on a support ring, and should be flush with the superior most edge of the table.
- The entire neck and anterior chest is prepped, with the ability to perform a median sternotomy if necessary. Surgeon stands behind head.
- A pulse oximetry probe is placed on the right hand. If excessive levering causes occlusion of the innominate artery, the pulse oximeter will lose its tracing, alerting the surgeon to relax the mediastinoscope.
- A 1.5cm transverse cervical incision is made one fingerbreadth above the sternal notch, preferably in a pre-existing skin crease.
- The platysma is divided transversely, and the median raphe of the strap muscles are divided longitudinally and the strap muscles are retracted laterally, exposing the pretracheal fascia.
- The pretracheal fascia is divided sharply with Metzenbaum scissors, elevated, and the plane along the trachea is developed with the middle finger and extended down to the carina, with left-to-right blunt dissection of the space. In the process, the locations of the carina, innominate artery, and arch of the aorta are palpated and located.
- Pass the mediastinoscope along the anterior surface of the trachea beneath the pretracheal fascia and beneath the innominate artery which can be palpated.
- Care must be taken to clearly have the tracheal rings in view. Bluntly dissect with the suction cautery before advancing the scope. Advance the scope with two hands, to avoid sudden jerky movements. If disoriented, always return to the tracheal rings to re-establish anatomy.

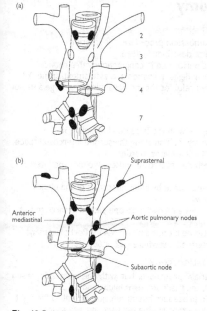

Fig. 13.5 (a) Standard lymph node stations accessible by standard cervical median-stinoscopy (2, 3, 4, and 7). (b) Lymph nodes not readily accessible by this approach.

- Prior to biopsy, identify the carina, then the right mainstem, followed by the left mainstem.
- In order of biopsy:
  - Station 2R, 4R, 4L, 2L if present, and 7.
  - Station 7 is biopsied last as there is frequently nuisance bleeding when biopsying this station. This bleeding nearly always stops with simple packing and time. Avoid cautery in this area because of the proximity of the right main PA.
- Important anatomical points to avoid injury:
  - 4R is near the azygos vein, and pleura of the lung.
  - 2R may be near the innominate artery, pleura of the lung, and the SVC.
  - 4L is near the recurrent laryngeal nerve and arch of the aorta.
  - 7 is near the right main PA and esophagus.
- Tissue is biopsied by grasping it with biopsy forceps, and gently twisting with supination and pronation and gentle traction. Never forcefully pull on tissue, as this may inadvertently avulse an adherent vessel.
- If in doubt whether a structure is vascular or solid, attempt to aspirate with a spinal needle before biopsy.

Reference

1. Harken DE *et al.* A simple cervicomediastinal exploration for tissue diagnosis of intrathoracic disease. *New Engl J Med* 1954; **251**:1041.

Medianstinotomy

Key facts

- Also known as the *Chamberlain procedure*, left anterior mediastinotomy was first described in 1966.
- This procedure may be performed in conjunction with a cervical mediastinoscopy allowing digital palpation and assessment of the AP lymph nodes. Also very useful for the incisional biopsy of large anterior mediastinal masses.

Procedure

- Position the patient supine with the left side elevated at 30°.
- Make a 4cm left transverse incision along the second intercostal space starting just lateral to the left sternal border.
- Sharp dissection through the intercostal muscle avoiding the internal thoracic vessels.
- Avoid entering the pleural space by blunt dissection of the pleura down to the AP window.
- Biopsy may be direct or via a mediastinoscope passed in through this incision.
- The AP window can also be biopsied by left VATS. Port placement and positioning are described elsewhere (📖 pp686–687).

Right anterior mediastinoscopy

Position as for Chamberlain procedure, but with the right side raised. Allows assessment of the mediastinum, right hilum, and SVC.

- As for the Chamberlain procedure but starting just lateral to the right sternal border and passing through the right second interspace.
- The right mediastinum, SVC, and right hilum can also be explored by right VATS. Port placement and positioning are described elsewhere (📖 pp686–687).

Outcomes

Cervical mediastinoscopy is very effective in staging the mediastinum and generally safe:

- Cervical mediastinoscopy in 947 patients with NSCLC. 2.1% false negative rate for accessible lymph nodes. 0.6% morbidity , 0.2% mortality.[1]

Complications of mediastinoscopy and mediastinotomy

Complications can be catastrophic.

- Tracheal injury, hemorrhage, wound infection, pneumothorax, recurrent laryngeal nerve injury (most common on left), esophageal injury (very rare).
- Azygos vein injury:
  - Usually occurs with biopsy of station 4R.
  - Often avoided by sampling indeterminate lymph nodes with a spinal needle prior to biopsy.
  - After the injury, packing the mediastinum with sponges for 10min often stops the bleeding as the azygos vein is part of a low-pressure system.

- Innominate artery, pulmonary artery, aortic or SVC injury:
  - Will not stop with packing, however, packing allows time to proceed to definitive therapy.
  - The innominate artery is often injured by excessive levering of the cervical mediastinoscope.
  - The PA and aorta may be injured during biopsy of stations 7 and 4L.
  - The SVC may be injured during biopsy of station 2R.
  - After packing, a median sternotomy is performed, providing adequate access of the earlier listed vascular structures. Repair may require establishment of cardiopulmonary bypass.
- Esophageal injury:
  - Esophageal injury may occur during biopsy of station 7. It is often identified a few days after the procedure and may present with dysphagia, odynophagia, fever and/or early sepsis.
  - Diagnosed with endoscopic evaluation and thin barium esophagram. Chest CT may identify mediastinal emphysema and an abscess.
  - The esophagus can be endoscopically stented, and the mediastinum drained via a left lateral collar incision.
- Inadvertent biopsy of the lung:
  - Often occurs on the right.

If air is leak is identified, a right chest tube may be necessary, with a Penrose drain placed in the mediastinum via the cervical incision.

Reference

1. Hammoud Z et al. The current role of mediastinoscopy in the evaluation of thoracic disease. J Thorac Cardiovasc Surg 1999; **118**:894–9.

Tracheostomy

Key facts

A tracheostomy is normally performed electively, if the patient proves difficult to wean from ventilation after 7–10 days. A tracheostomy may be performed as a formal open surgical procedure, or as a percutaneous tracheostomy using Seldinger technique and serial stoma dilation (📖 p166). A tracheostomy can be performed in the OR, or in the ICU with a skilled support team.

Indications

- Protection of the airway, i.e., from aspiratory secretions, or disrupted anatomy from trauma.
- Prolonged ventilatory support.
- Tracheobronchial toilet (particularly in pneumonectomy patients).

Contraindications

- Local sepsis and hemodynamic instability are relative contraindications.

Technique of open tracheostomy

- Most patients are able to undergo an open tracheostomy despite any body habitus. If the innominate artery is encountered, a strap muscle can be rotated to buttress the innominate artery from the tracheal stoma, and prevent the formation of a TIF.
- The patient is preoxygenated.
- With the patient positioned with the neck straight and extended, and the cuff on the ET tube deflated, the midline is carefully identified: this is critical to prevent malpositioning of the tracheostomy tube in the soft tissues adjacent to the trachea.
- The isthmus of the thyroid overlies the second to fourth tracheal rings: an approach higher than this avoids the isthmus but is associated with greater incidence of tracheal stenosis.
- Most practitioners elect to enter the trachea below the second or third ring.
- The patient's neck is extended, and a shoulder roll is used to elevate the shoulders.
- A 1–2cm incision is made about one fingerbreadth above the sternal notch.
- The platysma muscle is divided transversely and the median raphae of the strap muscles is identified and divided longitudinally.
- The strap muscles are distracted laterally, exposing the pretracheal fascia.
- If the isthmus of the thyroid is encountered, this can be divided with cautery, or suture ligated between clamps.
- The appropriate sized tracheostomy tube is selected (generally #8 or # 6 Shiley).
- The location of the stoma is chosen, and on either side of this area, traction stitches are inserted with 2/0 Prolene. This allows for elevation of the trachea into the surgical view.

- There are several techniques for creating a stoma; the author prefers removing a square segment of cartilaginous ring after cutting with a 15 blade.
- The FiO_2 is decreased at this point, to prevent blaze during cautery for hemostasis.
- After removal of the segment, the stoma can be dilated with a specialized tracheostomy spreader, or snap.
- The cuff on the ET tube is deflated, and the ET tube is backed out under direct vision from the surgical field.
- After the tip of the ET tube has passed from view of the stoma, the lubricated tracheostomy tube is inserted, the obturator removed, and the cuff inflated, and ventilator tubing connected.
- The airway can be suctioned from the field.
- 2/0 Prolene sutures are used to suture the phalanges of the appliance directly to the skin.

Inadvertent extubation and loss of airway control

- In tracheostomies over 7 days old a tract makes reinsertion of the tracheostomy tube relatively easy.
- Prior to the 7 days (including during the tracheostomy procedure itself), the tracheal stoma should not be blindly recannulated, as the tracheostomy tube has a high incidence of placement into a false passage, and consequently development of hypoxic arrest.
- The patient should be bag ventilated, and then re-intubated orally with an ET tube. If this fails, the track can be re-explored under direct vision, or a cricothyroidotomy should be performed.

Tracheoinnominate fistula (TIF)

Catastrophic late bleeding suggests formation of a TIF. It is often preceded by a small herald or sentinel bleed, and may be associated with a pulsating tracheostomy. If a sentinel bleed is suspected, the patient can be studied via a CT angiogram, or a fiberoptic and/or rigid bronchoscopy in the OR with instruments on the ready.

- To gain emergency control, the cuff of the tracheostomy tube can be overinflated, and if this fails then compress the innominate artery against the sternum by removing the tracheostomy and placing a finger inside the stoma. ET intubation must be carried out with a cuffed tube to achieve airway control.
- The patent is brought to the OR, and a median sternotomy is performed.
- The upper part of the pericardium is opened to expose the ascending aorta and origin of the innominate artery.
- The artery is controlled proximally and distally while the left innominate vein is retracted caudal.
- The innominate artery is divided proximally and distally with a running 4/0 Prolene and the tracheal defect is closed primarily with 4/0 Vicryl.
- Sternocleidomastoid, omentum, or other rotational flap is used to buttress the tracheal injury and prevent refistulization.
- Flow can be re-established to the right carotid artery with an interposition graft.

Lung and pleura

Lung cancer pathology

Key facts

- Lung cancer is divided into *small-cell lung cancer* (SCLC) (25%) and *non-small-cell lung cancer* (NSCLC) (75%): surgery is rarely indicated for SCLC, which is generally treated with systemic chemotherapy, while NSCLC in amendable to surgery as part of stage-specific therapy.
  - SCLC includes *oat cell* and *intermediate* types.
  - NSCLC includes *squamous cell* (30%), *adenocarcinoma* (35%), *bronchopulmonary neuroendocrine* tumors (BPNET), and other tumor types, e.g., *bronchoalveolar*, *adenosquamous*, and *mucoepidermoid* and *adenoid cystic* tumor (5%).
  - BPNET includes *small-cell*, *large-cell* (10%), and *carcinoid* tumors
- 1 200 000 cases diagnosed annually worldwide. In the USA there are 170 000 new cases with 160 000 deaths per year: it is the number one cancer killer of both men and women. By 2025, 80% of all lung cancers will be in Asia.
- More lung cancer deaths than colon, breast, and prostate cancer combined.
- There is a rising incidence of adenocarcinoma, and a rising incidence of lung cancer in never-smokers.

Etiology

- 87% of lung cancers are due to smoking: 90% in men and 85% in women. A smoker is defined as someone who has smoked ≥100 cigarettes in their lifetime.
- 3000 lung cancer deaths/year due to second-hand smoke.
- The lifetime risk of cancer in smokers is 17% in men and 11.6% in women: if an individual stops smoking, their chance of developing lung cancer decreases.

Pathology of small-cell lung cancer

- Bronchopulmonary neuroendocrine tumors are often centrally located.
- Considered a systemic disease, with very little role for surgery:
  - Often metastatic at the time of surgery.
  - Treated with systemic chemotherapy.
- Characterized histologically by cells with scant cytoplasm in fibrous stoma, and abundant neurosecretory granules.

Pathology of non-small-cell lung cancer

NSCLC: adenocarcinoma (35%)

- Most common lung cancer.
- Generally caused by smoking or other tobacco products.
  - New data suggests the presence of epidermal growth factor receptor mutations in never-smokers.
  - Young age, Asian, female.
- Often peripherally located, or associated with scar and fibrosis, especially in COPD (so-called *scar carcinoma*).
- Histology: acinar or glandular patterns.

NSCLC: squamous cell carcinoma (30%)

- Generally caused by smoking or other tobacco products.
- 2/3 are centrally located.
- They can obstruct airways, causing postobstructive pneumonia.
- 10–20% develop central necrosis and cavitation.
- Histology: intercellular bridge formation and keratinization.

NSCLC: bronchioalveolar carcinoma (<5%)

Adenocarcinoma *in situ* (defined by the World Health Organization).

- Occurs in non-smokers.
- Three forms:
  - Solitary (ground glass opacity).
  - Multinodular.
  - Diffuse or pneumotic.
- Only rare direct invasion or lymph node metastasis.
- Histology: spread along the alveolus without direct invasion.

NSCLC: BPNET

- Neuroendocrine origin, derived from Kulchitsky cells, with amine precursor uptake and decarboxylation.
- Three common types: *large-cell*, *carcinoid*, and *small-cell lung cancer* which is classified separately (📖 p668).

NSCLC: large-cell carcinoma (10%)

- Bronchopulmonary neuroendocrine tumor common in the periphery.
- Two subtypes:
  - Giant cell.
  - Clear cell.
- Tends to have a very aggressive clinical presentation.
- Tumors may have cavitation.
- Histology: enlarged hyperchromatic nuclei with prominent nucleoli.

NSCLC: carcinoid tumor (1%)

- BPNET often centrally located.
- Not associated with smoking.
- Carcinoid syndrome is seldom seen (<1%).
- Two subtypes:
  - *Typical:* often endobronchial, rare to have vascular invasion, 10% incidence of nodal or distant metastasis, infrequent cellular mitosis, 90% 5-year survival
  - *Atypical:* often peripheral, frequent cellular mitosis, frequent vascular invasion, 50% incidence of nodal or distant metastasis, 25–69% 5-year survival.

Metastatic disease

- 40–50% of patients with newly diagnosed lung cancer have metastatic disease at time of diagnosis.
- Modes of spread: direct invasion, lymphatics, hematogenous.
- More common sites of spread include liver, adrenal, brain, and bone. Others: skin, heart, thyroid, small intestine, ovary, spleen, kidney, parathyroid, pituitary.

Diagnosis of lung cancer

Key facts

- 95% of patients are symptomatic at diagnosis, most are male >60 years.
- Symptoms may be local, regional, or systemic (see Box 14.1).
- Chest CT, PET, brain MRI, bronchoscopy, and usually needle biopsy are necessary for diagnosis and staging, with mediastinal staging by mediastinoscopy or less invasive modalities, e.g., EBUS.

Presentation

- *Proximal tumors* tend to produce symptoms of major airway obstruction and irritation (hemoptysis, dyspnea, cough, wheezing, stridor, hoarseness, Horner's syndrome, SVC syndrome, postobstructive pneumonia, pleural effusion, *Pancoast syndrome*).
- *Peripheral tumors* are often asymptomatic or present with signs and symptoms of pleural or chest wall invasion or pleural effusion (10%) (pleuritic chest wall pain, progressive dyspnea).
- May present with symptoms and signs of *metastatic spread*: neurological—headache, blurred vision, nausea, diploplia, decreased consciousness, ataxia; bony pain and pathological fracture; liver and abdominal pain, anorexia, jaundice, ascites, liver failure, hepatomegaly; adrenal glands—symptoms of Addison's disease.
- *Paraneoplastic syndromes.*
- Always ask about history of tobacco smoking (number of pack years), asbestos exposure, employment history, unintentional weight loss >5% of body weight, and recent onset of joint pains, change in voice, chest wall pain, back pain, palpable LN.
- Examine for clubbing, palpate all lymph nodes, cutaneous lesions, pleural effusion, localize chest wall pain.

Paraneoplastic syndromes

10–20% of cases. Usually caused by SCLC and squamous cell carcinomas.

- *Metabolic:* Cushing syndrome, hypercalcemia, SIADH (see p671), carcinoid syndrome, gynecomastia, hyperthyroidism, hypoglycemia, excess growth hormone, excess prolactin, FSH, LH.
- *Neurologic:* encephalopathy, Lambert–Eaton syndrome, subacute cerebellar degeneration, peripheral neuropathy, polymyositis, autonomic neuropathy, myoclonus, optic neuritis.
- *Skeletal:* clubbing, HPOA (see p669).
- *Hematological:* anemia, thrombocytosis, thrombocytopenia, eosinophilia, red cell aplasia, leukoerythroblastosis, DIC, leukemoid reactions, migratory thrombophlebitis.
- *Cutaneous:* hyperkeratosis, dermatomyositis, acanthosis nigricans, hyperpigmentation, erythema gyratum repens, hypertrichosis lanuginose acquisita.
- *Other:* nephrotic syndrome, anorexia-cachexia, hypouricemia, secretion of VIP with diarrhea, hyperamylasemia.

Hypertrophic pulmonary osteoarthropathy (HPOA)
Periostitis of distal long bones, commonly tibia, fibula, and radius. Joint tenderness and swelling. It may involve metacarpals and metatarsals causing acute polyarthritis. Associated with clubbing. More common with adenocarcinoma. Etiology unknown.

Syndrome of inappropriate anti-diuretic hormone secretion (SIADH)
Associated with SCLC. Symptoms uncommon. Excess ADH secreted. Leads to hyponatremia, nausea and vomiting, anorexia, confusion, seizures, lethargy. Diagnosis made by low serum osmolality, high urinary excretion of sodium, and high urine osmolality.

Hypercalcemia
10% of lung cancers. ~15% of these are secondary to parathyroid hormone secretion. Most often associated with squamous cell carcinoma.

Ectopic adrenocorticotrophic syndrome
Usually occurs with SCLC. ACTH production is autonomous. <5% present with Cushing syndrome. Usual presentation is due to severe hypokalemia, hyperglycemia and metabolic alkalosis.

Neurologic paraneoplastic syndromes
Central neuropathies (brainstem encephalitis, encephalomyelitis, dementia) and many peripheral neuropathies (sensory, autonomic, and sensorimotor). Usual with small-cell lung cancer and occasionally with squamous cell carcinoma.

Peripheral neuromyopathy
The most common paraneoplastic syndrome related to lung cancer.

Box 14.1 Localizing symptoms of lung cancer
- Bronchopulmonary symptoms:
  - Cough.
  - Hemoptysis.
  - Chest pain.
  - Dyspnea.
  - Wheezing.
- Intrathoracic symptoms:
  - Pleural effusion (10%).
  - Hoarseness (recurrent laryngeal nerve).
  - SVC syndrome.
  - Chest wall pain.
  - Arm pain (brachial plexus).
  - Horner's syndrome.
  - Dysphagia.
  - Phrenic nerve paralysis.
- Paraneoplastic syndromes (2%).
- Symptoms from distant metastatic spread.

Investigation of lung cancer

Key facts

- Imaging is performed for diagnosis and staging.
- Proper staging of lung cancer includes chest CT, PET, bronchoscopy, brain MRI, and mediastinal staging.

PA and lateral chest radiograph

Allow rough localization of tumor and detection of gross hilar and mediastinal lymphadenopathy, pleural effusions, areas of consolidation, evidence of bony destruction of ribs and vertebral bodies, and elevation of the hemidiaphragm.

CT scan

- Helps define locoregional spread, invasion of local structures, synchronous lesions, and is the gold standard for determining T status.
- Allows accurate localization of primary lesion, allowing size measurements, assessment for evidence of local invasion.
- Provides detailed information regarding remaining lung parenchyma (presence of bullae, emphysema, interstitial lung disease, undiagnosed masses, pleural thickening, small pleural effusions).
- Extension into the upper abdomen should routinely be requested to allow assessment of liver and adrenal glands.
- Provides detailed information on intrathoracic lymph nodes. A positive result is one where a lymph node is >1cm in long axis.

PET scan

- Agent used is a labelled D-glucose analogue (fluorodeoxyglucose – FDG). Lesions >5mm diameter detected. False positives with granulomatous and inflammatory lesions. Useful in diagnosing mediastinal and distant metastatic disease.
- *PET/CT:* simultaneous PET scan and CT scan allowing more accurate localization of lesions including metastases when compared to either investigation alone.

MRI

- Brain MRI obtained if neurological symptoms, large tumors, or tumors with high metabolic activity on PET.
- Allows accurate assessment of spinal canal, bony lesions, and vascular structures.

Bronchoscopy

- Technique is described on 📖 pp654–657.
- Excellent modality for visualization and localization of endobronchial tumor, assessment of carina and rest of tracheobronchial tree, *direct biopsy, bronchial washings (bronchoalveolar lavage)*, and *sputum cytology*.
- Sensitivity of sputum cytology dependent on tumor size, location, and histological type. Central squamous cell tumors have highest yield. False-positive findings in up to 3%.

- Also allows **EBUS-TBNA** of lesions outside the tracheobronchial tree—subcarinal and paratracheal nodes.
- EBUS-TBNA has 69% sensitivity, 88% negative predictive value.
- A valuable tool when assessing preoperatively the extent of resection required for curative surgery as it identifies intrabronchial involvement, and possible need for bronchoplastic procedure.
- Often performed/repeated at the time of surgery.

Mediastinal staging

Mediastinoscopy

- Mediastinoscopy is the gold standard assessment of the mediastinum as it allows direct biopsy and histological assessment of mediastinal lymph nodes, hence determines presence or absence of N2/N3 disease.
- **Cervical mediastinoscopy** (📖 p660) for paratracheal lymph nodes.
- **Anterior mediastinotomy** (📖 pp662–663) (Chamberlain) or left VATS (📖 p686) for AP window station 5 and 6 lymph nodes.
- 2% false negative, 0.6% morbidity, 0.2% mortality.[1]

Thoracotomy (VATS)

Occasionally necessary for diagnosis and staging (<5% of cases). Often unable to distinguish T3 from T4 lesion prior to thoracotomy.

Reference

1. Hammoud Z et al. The current role of mediastinoscopy in the evaluation of thoracic disease. *J Thorac Cardiovasc Surg* 1999; **118**:894–9.

Staging of lung cancer

Key facts
- The TNM classification is used: 7th edition of the AJCC/IUAC cancer staging manual (2010) (see Table 14.1).
- The TNM class is based on *tumor* size and location, *node* size, and presence of *metastases* (see Table 14.2).
- Regional lymph nodes (Table 14.3 and Fig. 14.1) include double digit N1 (ipsilateral) or N3 (contralateral) nodes that are outside the pleural envelope, and single digit mediastinal N2 (ipsilateral) or N3 (contralateral).

Table 14.1 TNM classification for lung cancer

Primary tumor (T)

Tx	Primary tumor cannot be assessed
T0:	No evidence of primary tumor
Tis:	Carcinoma *in situ*
T1a:	≤2cm
T1b:	>2 , ≤3cm
T2a:	>3cm, ≤5cm
T2b:	>5cm, ≤ 7cm
T3:	>7cm; chest wall, diaphragm, phrenic nerve, mediastinal pleura, or parietal pericardial invasion; same lobe synchronous nodules; tumor in the main bronchus and <2cm distal to the carina; associated atelectasis or obstructive pneumonitis of the entire lung
T4:	Extension into mediastinal structures (e.g., heart, great vessels, trachea, recurrent laryngeal nerve, esophagus, vertebral body, carina; ipsilateral lung synchronous nodules, but different lobes

Regional lymph nodes (N)

Nx:	Regional lymph nodes cannot be assessed
N0:	No regional lymph node metastasis
N1:	Ipsilateral peribronchial, ipsilateral hilar, intrapulmonary lymph nodes
N2:	Ipsilateral mediastinal, subcarinal lymph nodes
N3:	Contralateral mediastinal, hilar, scalene (ipsilateral or contralateral), supraclavicular (unless ipsilateral superior sulcus)

Distant metastasis (M)

M0:	No distant metastasis
M1a:	Pleural effusion, pericardial effusion; synchronous nodules in contralateral lung
M1b:	Distant metastasis

Adapted from Rice TW et al. Cancer of the esophagus and esophagogastric junction: data-driven staging for the seventh edition of the American Joint Committee on Cancer/ International Union Against Cancer Cancer Staging Manuals. *Cancer* 2010; **116**(16):3763–73.

Table 14.2 Stage grouping for lung cancer

Stage	T	N	M
IA	1a	0	0
	1b	0	0
IB	1a	0	0
IIA	1a	1	0
	1b	1	0
	2a	1	0
	2b	0	0
IIB	2b	1	0
	3	0	0
IIIA	1–2	2	0
	3	1–2	0
	4	0–1	0
IIIB	1–4	3	0
	4	2	0
IV	Any	Any	1

Table 14.3 Regional lymph nodes

Superior mediastinal nodes (N2/3)	
1	Highest Mediastinal
2	Upper paratracheal
3	Prevascular and retrotracheal
4	Lower paratracheal
Aortopulmonary window nodes	
5	Subaortic
6	Para-aortic
Inferior mediastinal nodes (N2/3)	
7	Subcarinal
8	Paraesophageal
9	Pulmonary ligament (Belsey's)
N1 nodes (N3 if contralateral)	
10	Hilar
11	Interlobar
12	Lobar
13	Segmental

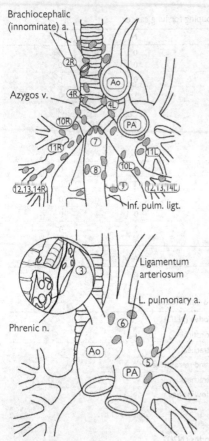

Fig. 14.1 Regional lymph nodes.

Chemoradiotherapy

Key facts
- For operable patients with stage I and II lung cancer, upfront therapy is surgical resection.
- Platinum-based adjuvant chemotherapy is reserved for pathologic node-positive stage IIA and IIB disease.

Modalities

Neoadjuvant (multimodality, chemoradiotherapy followed by surgery)
- Optimal for stage IIIA, N2 positive lung cancer.
- Superior to surgery alone.
- Multimodality therapy most beneficial for patients with single N2 station, and non-bulky (≤3cm) mediastinal lymph nodes.
- If residual N2 disease, resection is warranted if R0 resection is achievable.[1]
- High mortality if pneumonectomy is required after neoadjuvant chemoradiation:[2]
  - Regimen included two cycles cisplatin/etoposide/concurrent 45Gy XRT randomized to surgery followed by two additional cycles of cis/ etop or XRT to 61Gy followed by two additional cycles cis/etop.
  - Significant increase in progression-free survival for trimodality arm.
  - No difference in overall survival between treatment arms.
  - Subset analysis demonstrated significant 5-year overall survival advantage in the lobectomy group (36% vs. 18%) compared to chemoradiotherapy, but a non-significant disadvantage for the pneumonectomy group (22% vs. 24%) compared to definitive chemoradiotherapy.

Definitive chemoradiation
Appropriate for N3 positive stage IIIB disease, and N2 positive stage IIIA patients who are poor surgical candidates, refuse surgery, would require a pneumonectomy for R0 resection, or who have multistation N2 positive nodes, or bulky (>3cm) N2 positive nodes.

Non-small-cell lung cancer
NSCLC is relatively resistant to chemotherapy. Curative resection allows best chance of long-term survival. Surgery is normally offered to all patients with stage I and stage II disease, along with specific patients with stage III disease. Surgical principles of resection are:
- No spillage of cells from primary tumor during resection.
- Entire tumor must be resected by lobectomy, bilobectomy, pneumonectomy or extended resections along with intrapulmonary lymph nodes. Lesser resections proven to have worse outcome, only considered in high-risk patients or small tumors as part of a clinical trial.
- All accessible mediastinal lymph nodes should be excised or sampled to allow complete staging and plan for any adjuvant therapy.
- Frozen section analysis of resection margins to confirm appropriate surgical resection and complete excision of primary tumor.

Chemotherapy

To date no proven benefit from adjuvant therapy in patients with surgically resectable and potentially curative disease. Interest in neo-adjuvant therapy for locally advanced disease.

Radiotherapy

- *Upfront:* used in patients unfit or unwilling to undergo surgery. Also used in those with bulky stage IV disease. Survival benefit in non-surgical patients when combined with concomitant chemotherapy.
- *Adjuvant:* also used as an adjunct to surgery or as palliation.

Small-cell lung cancer

Small-cell lung cancer has usually metastasized by time of presentation. It is sensitive to chemotherapy. Early recurrence is common.

- The mainstay of treatment is chemotherapy.
- Surgery is indicated for very early (clinical stage I) disease.
- Surgery may be combined with chemotherapy.
- In more advanced disease multiagent chemotherapy combined with radiation therapy is indicated.
- Radiotherapy also plays an important role in palliative treatment of SVC obstruction, hemoptysis, recurrent laryngeal nerve palsy, phrenic nerve palsy, pleural effusion, bony lesions, spinal cord compression, cerebral metastases, localized metastatic lesions.

Complications of chemotherapy:

- Myelosuppression: infections, bleeding, anemia.
- Nausea and vomiting, constipation.
- Alopecia.
- Cardiotoxicity, cardiomyopathy.
- Ototoxicity, nephrotoxicity, peripheral and CNS neuropathy.
- Electrolyte disturbances.
- Mucositis.
- Pulmonary fibrosis.
- Second malignancies (acute leukemia, second lung primary).

Complications of radiotherapy

- *Thoracic:* esophagitis, pneumonitis, pulmonary fibrosis, myelitis, esophageal stricture, cardiac toxicity.
- *Cranial:* tremor, confusion, slurred speech, ataxia, memory deficits, problems with concentration, otitis, scalp erythema, dementia, dysarthria.
- *Postsurgical:* thoracotomy, incision pain, wound breakdown, bronchopleural fistulas, respiratory failure.

References

1. Martin J et al. Long-term results of combined modality therapy in resectable non-small-cell lung cancer. *JCO* 2002; **20**; 1989-05.
2. Albain et al. IASLC 2003. Intergroup 0139 Definitive chemoradiotherapy vs. neoadjuvant for stage IIIA. *Lung Cancer* 2003; **41**(Suppl 2):A#PL-4.

Pulmonary resection overview

Key facts

- Anatomic lobectomy is the standard of care for pulmonary resection of primary NSCLC.
- Lobectomy can be performed through a *posterolateral thoracotomy*, muscle sparing thoracotomy, axillary thoracotomy, or by *VATS*.
- Sublobar resection (*segmentectomy* or non-anatomic wedge) is used for patients with impaired pulmonary function, or small (<2cm) ground glass opacities such as bronchoalveolar carcinoma, or secondary or metastatic tumors to the lung as part of a metastectomy.
- Bronchoplasty or pulmonary arterioplasty (sleeve) procedures should be considered to avoid *pneumonectomy*.
- A mediastinal lymph node sampling or dissection should be performed as part of any pulmonary resection for primary lung cancer.
- VATS lobectomy is becoming more prevalent for the resection of early stage lung cancer, less so for larger and central tumors.

General principles

- Patients undergoing lung resection need additional detailed work-up (📖 p650) in addition to the extensive investigations already performed for diagnosis and staging (📖 p672).
- Lung function testing should be performed in all patients, with calculation of *predicted postoperative respiratory capacity* (📖 p652), so that resection can be modified (e.g., sublobar resection rather than lobectomy) if necessary to reduce the risk of postoperative respiratory insufficiency. Broad rules of thumb are:
  - The minimum acceptable FEV_1 after surgery is 800mL.
  - Pneumonectomy will reduce FEV_1 by around 50%, lobectomy by around 20% depending on the lobe.
  - The preoperative FEV_1 for lobectomy should therefore be >1L, and at least 2L for pneumonectomy.

Anesthesia and surgical set-up

- General ET anesthesia with invasive arterial monitoring.
- A flexible bronchoscopy (📖 p654) is performed via a single lumen tube, before lung isolation is obtained using a bronchial blocker or a double lumen tube.
- The patient is then positioned in the *lateral, decubitus position* (📖 p39) with spine parallel to and close to the edge of the table, using sandbags, or rolls and tape, usually with the upper arm positioned on a rest, the lower arm flexed in-front of the head, and the table 'broken' (a little head-down and a little feet-down) so that the hips do not obstruct VATs instruments, and the rib spaces open up a little.
- For *posterolateral thoracotomy* (📖 p39) prep and drape so that the spinous processes, ipsilateral nipple, and midaxillary line are exposed.

Mediastinal lymph node dissection and sampling

Accurate tumor staging is critical for prognosis, planning therapy, and clinical studies. Current practice in intraoperative lymph node examination ranges from simple sampling to radical mediastinal lymph node dissection (MLND), with no consensus as to best practice: lymph nodes were sampled in <50% of patients with lung cancer in the USA in one survey. The main debate is between MLND and systematic sampling.

Mediastinal lymph node dissection

- Involves complete removal of most mediastinal lymph nodes for right- and left-sided pulmonary resections.
- *Right-sided resections:* systematic removal of stations 2R, 4R, 7, 8R, and 9R for right-sided resections, with mobilization of SVC.
- *Left-sided resections:* systematic removal of stations 2L, 4L, 5, 6, 7, 8L, and 9L with mobilization of the aortic arch and left subclavian artery.
- May be higher risk of morbidity, e.g., chylothorax, phrenic or recurrent laryngeal nerve injury (beware cautery in the aortopulmonary window), increased mediastinal drainage from bleeding or lymphatics.
- No evidence that MLND contributes to tumor control or survival.

Mediastinal lymph node sampling

- Involves removal of most mediastinal lymph nodes for right- and left-sided pulmonary resections, without the goal of complete removal. All lymph nodes readily visible are removed.
- *Right-sided resections:* involves a systematic sampling of stations 2R, 4R, 7, 8R, and 9R lymph nodes without mobilization of the SVC.
- *Left-sided resections:* systematic sampling of stations 5, 6, 7, 8L, and 9L without mobilization of the aortic arch and left subclavian artery.
- Possibility of less accurate staging, with N2 disease unrecognized in up to 5% of cases.

Evidence base: ACOSOG Z0030

- Randomized 1000 patients to lymph node sampling or lymph node dissection after pulmonary resection.
- No difference in perioperative morbidity or mortality[1] nor long-term survival.

Other technical considerations

- The vessels can be divided in any order:
  - The bronchus of the diseased segment is the landmark used to guide resection: this can be most easily visualized after division of the segmental artery which usually runs alongside it.
  - Dividing the pulmonary artery before the pulmonary veins may help avoid venous engorgement of the resected section, making dissection more difficult, and reduce hematogenous tumor spread.
- Use of clamps and sutures or ligatures or staplers for vessels and bronchus is a matter of surgeon preference.
- Prior to closure the chest is filled with saline, the lung inflated and checked carefully for air leaks, which must be carefully oversewn.

Reference

1. Allen MS et al. Morbidity and mortality of major pulmonary resections in patients with early-stage lung cancer: initial results of the randomized, prospective ACOSOG Z0030 trial. *Ann Thorac Surg* 2006; **81**(3):1013–19.

Right lobectomy

Set-up

- The patient is positioned in the left lateral decubitus position, right-side up, with the right lung fully deflated (🕮 p39).
- Right posterolateral thoracotomy incision (4th ICS) (🕮 p39) or VATS approach (🕮 p686).
- Postoperative instructions and management are described on 🕮 p696.

Right upper lobectomy

Pulmonary vein division

- The lung is positioned posteriorly, the anterior hilar pleural is incised.
- The right upper lobe (RUL) pulmonary vein is identified. Care is taken to preserve the right middle lobe vein, as it takes off from the inferior border of the proximal superior pulmonary vein.
- The vein may be divided using a vascular stapler, or silk ligature

Pulmonary artery division

- The right main pulmonary artery (PA) exits posterior to the SVC. The first branch of the right main PA is the truncus anterior, which exits posterior to the SVC.
- The truncus branch is divided with a stapler or silk ligature.
- The final arterial branch of the RUL is the posterior ascending artery. It is exposed through one of three approaches.
  - **Anterior:** the upper lobe is retracted posteriorly, and after division of the right upper lobe pulmonary vein and truncus anterior, the right main PA is dissected distally as it becomes the interlobar PA, until the posterior ascending artery is identified lateral and adjacent to the RUL bronchus.
  - **Central:** the confluence of the major and minor fissures is dissected exposing the interlobar PA. The proximal take-off of the posterior ascending artery is then clearly identified.
  - **Posterior:** the RUL is retracted anteriorly, identifying the take-off of the RUL bronchus from the right main stem bronchus. The station 10R or 'sump' lymph node is removed, revealing the posterior ascending artery.

Bronchus division and completion of fissure

- After division of the vessels, the RUL is retracted anteriorly, and the RUL bronchus is identified as it takes off from the right main stem.
- Peribronchial lymph nodes are removed, and the bronchus is divided with a stapler or with a knife and closed with Vicryl sutures.
- The major and minor fissures are completed with a stapler.

Middle lobectomy

Pulmonary vein dissection

- The lung is positioned posteriorly, the anterior hilar pleural is incised.
- The middle lobe pulmonary vein (MPV) is identified as it takes off from inferior border of the SPV.
- The MPV is divided with a stapler or silk ligature.

Pulmonary artery dissection

- The middle lobe pulmonary artery (MPA) is a branch of the ILPA that is distal and opposite to the PA branch of the superior segment of the lower lobe.
- The MPA can be identified centrally by dissecting the confluence of the pulmonary fissures, or anteriorly after division of the middle lobe bronchus.

Bronchus dissection and completion of fissure

- *Central approach:* the middle lobe bronchus (MB) is identified after division of the anteriorly located MPA.
- *Anterior approach:* the MB is identified first after division of the MPV.
- The MB is divided with a stapler or cut and closed with absorbable suture. Care is taken not to impinge the lower lobe bronchus.
- The inferior major and minor fissures are completed with a stapler.

Right lower lobectomy

Pulmonary vein dissection

- The lung is retracted superiorly, exposing the inferior pulmonary ligament. The ligament is divided with cautery. The station 9 (Belsey's) lymph node will be encountered, and then the inferior pulmonary vein (IPV).
- The IPV is easily encircled and divided with a vascular stapler or silk ligation.

Pulmonary artery dissection

- The ILPA is identified after dissecting the confluence of the fissures.
- The superior segmental artery is encountered extending superiorposteriorly. This is divided.
- The MPA is preserved as it branches off of the ILPA opposite to the superior segmental artery.
- Past the MPA, the ILPA becomes the common basal artery, which is divided by a vascular stapler or silk ligature.

Bronchus dissection

- After division of the common basal artery, the bronchus is identified posterior to this vessel, and divided.
- Care is taken not to impinge the MLB.
- Completion of the fissure.
- The major and minor fissures are completed with a stapler.

Left lobectomy

Key facts
- The patient is positioned in the right lateral decubitus position, left side up, with the left lung fully deflated (📖 p39).
- Right posterolateral thoracotomy incision (4th ICS) (📖 p39) or VATs approach (📖 p696).
- Postoperative instructions and management are described on 📖 p696.

Left upper lobectomy
Left upper lobectomy is the most technically demanding of any of the lung resections because of the location of the PA in relation to the aortic arch, and the PA branches—particularly the *anterior segmental artery*.

Pulmonary vein dissection
- The lung is retracted posteriorly, and the pleura anterior to the hilum is incised, exposing the superior pulmonary vein (SPV), as it lies anterioinferior to the left main PA.
- The SPV is encircled and divided with a vascular stapler or silk ligation.

Pulmonary artery dissection
- The left main PA enters superiorposterior to the SPV, and travels superioranterior to the left main bronchus, and passes posterior to the LUL bronchus as it becomes the interlobar PA.
- There may be multiple segmental branches extending from the interlobar PA to the LUL.
- Exposure of the interlobar PA and segmental branches is performed both with dissection anteriorly after division of the SPV, and by exposing the interlobar PA by dissecting the interlobar fissure.
- The anterior segmental artery and any accessory anterior branches are divided anteriorly: the anterior segmental artery is known as the 'artery of sorrow'. It is a short but wide branch of the left main PA that can be avulsed by over-vigorous retraction, and if the tear extends proximally may force a pneumonectomy (see 📖 p690).
- The apical, posterior, lingular and other accessory arterial branches are divided after exposure of the ILPA. Care is given to preserve the posterior segmental artery of the lower lobe, branching posterior and opposite to the take-off of the lingular PA segments.

Completion of the fissure and bronchus dissection
- The superior and inferior interlobar fissure is completed with a stapler.
- After division of the vessels and fissure, the LUL bronchus is clearly identified and divided with a stapler.

Pulmonary arterioplasty
- Tumors involving the inner curvature of the interlobar PA may require a PA arterioplasty.
- The proximal and distal control is obtained of the left main PA and interlobar PA. If the distal interlobar PA cannot be controlled, the SPV is divided, and the IPV is clamped, and this should markedly reduce back bleeding.

- The tumor is sharply excised, and the PA defect is either closed primarily, or using an autologous or bovine pericardial patch.

Left lower lobectomy

Pulmonary vein dissection

- The lung is retracted superiorly, exposing the inferior pulmonary ligament. The ligament is divided with cautery. The station 9 (Belsey's) lymph node will be encountered, and then the inferior pulmonary vein.
- The inferior pulmonary vein is easily encircled and divided with a vascular stapler or silk ligation.

Pulmonary artery dissection

- The ILPA is identified after dissecting interlobar fissure.
- The superior segmental artery is encountered extending superiorposteriorly, and opposite to the lingular branches. This is divided.
- Past the lingular branches, the ILPA becomes the common basal artery, which is divided by a vascular stapler or silk ligature.

Bronchus dissection and completion of the fissure

After division of the common basal artery, the bronchus is identified posteriorly, and divided, and the fissure is completed with a stapler.

Injury to the PA during left upper lobectomy

This is a dreaded complication due to **rupture of the anterior segmental artery from the left main PA** which may lead to unplanned pneumonectomy, and rarely to the on-table death of a patient from uncontrollable hemorrhage. It can result from traction injuries, or directly from cautery, or loss of control of ligatures after branch vessel division.

- If circumferential control of the vessel was not obtained prior to injury, trying to get a clamp around a hemorrhaging left main PA will result in torrential blood loss and is not advisable.
- Attempting to get a clamp over the laceration is difficult without circumferential control of the vessel, which may tear further, and will result in torrential blood loss.
- Blindly suturing a bleeding left main PA is virtually impossible, usually resulting in further damage to the vessel and torrential blood loss.

Management

- Put a finger on the hole, gently. If the hole is much bigger than your finger, or too deep, put a folded-up sponge on a sponge holder on the hole. This will buy you an indefinite amount of time.
- Tell your anesthesiologist that you have a serious problem: do not proceed further until you have blood in the room.
- Get senior help. Once you have help extend the incision, while maintaining control of the PA, so that you have adequate access.
- Now open the pericardium and gain circumferential control of the intrapericardial portion of the left superior pulmonary artery: clamping this will allow you to divide and oversew the avulsed branch.
- Always be wary of a hematoma on this branch artery which may be the only sign of a traction injury, heralding rupture: get proximal control and divide it as described in this chapter.

VATS lobectomy

Key facts

- A spectrum of procedures are termed VATS (video-assisted thorascopic surgery) ranging from totally endoscopic approaches without a mechanical retractor or rib spreading, to those performed though a minithoracotomy, assisted by a camera.
- Some surgeons advocate simultaneous stapling of all the hilar structures, rather than anatomical lobectomy: this is not described here.
- Many centres routinely perform complete anatomic lobectomy using a thorascopic approach, with equivalent oncological outcomes to the open technique, and reduced surgical trauma, postoperative pain, length of stay, chest tube duration, preserved pulmonary function, and improved cosmesis.

Patient selection

- The indications for VATS lobectomy are the same as for the open procedure, i.e., known or suspected lung cancer amenable to lobectomy.
- Similar cardiopulmonary capacity is required (📖 p652), although it has been suggested that older, frailer patients who are not candidates for an open lobectomy may benefit from a VATs approach.
- *Contraindications:* inability to provide complete resection with a lobectomy, T3 (chest wall), and T4 tumors, N2 and N3 disease, inability to achieve or tolerate single-lung ventilation.
- If the tumor is visualized in the lobar orifice at bronchoscopy suggesting need for a sleeve resection, then most surgeons would opt for an open procedure.
- Surgeon experience dictates whether patients with prior thoracic surgery or adhesions, T3 tumors involving the pericardium or diaphragm, incomplete fissures are suitable for a VATS approach.

Procedure

Set-up

- General endotracheal anesthesia with invasive arterial monitoring.
- A flexible bronchoscopy (📖 p654) is performed via a single lumen tube, before lung isolation is obtained using a bronchial blocker or a double lumen tube,
- The patient is then positioned in the *lateral, decubitus position* (📖 p39) with spine parallel to and close to the edge of the table, using sandbags, or rolls and tape, usually with the upper arm positioned on a rest, the lower arm flexed in-front of the head, and the table 'broken' (a little head down and a little feet down) so that the hips do not obstruct VATS instruments, and the rib spaces open up a little.

Port placement

- This is very variable but generally follows similar basic principles:
- The first port is a 5–10mm port (depending on the size of camera used) for the camera, placed in the midaxillary line, in the 7th or 8th intercostal space, which gives good visualization of the hilum and a

panoramic view of the hemithorax. Always align the camera, pathology, and monitor to reduce loss of automatic hand–eye coordination.
- The second incision is a working port—usually a 3–5cm incision in the 5th or 6th intercostal space in the inframammary crease. This can be opened with a soft tissue retractor, or potentially a small rib-spreader.
- Additional 5mm incisions for instruments are sometimes placed posteriorly or in the axilla, aiming to triangulate the ports, but it is possible to complete a VATS lobectomy through those two incisions.

Equipment
- A 30° or 45° angled or flexible scope to provide a panoramic view of the operative field without competing with the other instruments.
- Conventional sponge holders, forceps, and scissors can often be used through the working port.
- Endoscopic instruments include forceps, scissors (with the option of bipolar cautery), and soft-tipped (peanut) instruments for blunt dissection, as well as endoscopic suction tips and specially designed endoscopic stapling device, e.g., EndoGIA vascular (2–2.6mm) and bronchial (3.5mm) staplers.
- The specimen pouch is a bag in which the specimen can be placed while inside the chest, facilitating removal of a bulky tissue through a small incision without seeding malignant cells into the wound.

Dissection
- Carefully confirmation of the tumor location and lobe: manual palpation is usually not possible poor alignment of camera, pathology, and monitor may disorient the surgeon, so this step is done with care.
- The pulmonary vein is mobilized using gentle blunt dissection, with the lung retracted posteriorly (and inferiorly for upper lobectomy, superiorly for lower lobectomy) under direct visualization through the working port.
- The pulmonary vein is stapled and divided, exposing the pulmonary artery which is mobilized, stapled, and divided.
- The bronchus is usually then stapled and divided and the fissure completed with staples.
- The specimen is removed using a specially designed bag, and the hemithorax irrigated with water, and the bronchial stump and fissures inspected for air leaks.

Closure
- Chest tubes are placed (one apical, one basal) via the instrument port sites, together with a costal block.
- Soft tissues are closed in layers with interrupted absorbable sutures.

Postoperative care
- Drains on −20cmH$_2$O waterseal suction, and CXR in recovery area.
- This is much the same as for open lobectomy, except epidural and other analgesic requirements are less, and patients should be able to mobilize and be discharged earlier.

Sleeve resection

Key facts

- Patients with tumor extending out from the upper lobe orifice may require a **sleeve resection** to avoid pneumonectomy.
- The patient is positioned in the lateral decubitus position, ipsilateral side up with the lung fully deflated (🕮 p39).
- Posterolateral thoracotomy incision (4th ICS) (🕮 p39).
- Postoperative instructions and management are described on 🕮 p696.

Right upper lobectomy sleeve

- After division of the RUL arteries and veins as described on 🕮 p682, the right main bronchus is divided with a knife proximal to the tumor, and the bronchus intermedius divided distal to the tumor (slightly obliquely to minimize size discrepancy between the right main bronchus and the bronchus intermedius orifices).
- Specimen is sent for frozen section pathology to confirm R0 resection.
- 2/0 Vicryl sutures are placed in the right main bronchus and bronchus intermedius.
- The two ends are reanastomosed with either interrupted or running absorbable suture (Vicryl or PDS): a hilar release may be needed to ensure a tension free reanastomosis.
- Tumors at the base of the truncus anterior may require PA arterioplasty.
- The proximal and distal control is obtained for the right main PA and interlobar PA.
- The tumor is sharply excised.

Bilobectomy sleeve

- Patients with tumor occluding the middle lobe orifice or bronchus intermedius, may require a middle and right lower lobe bilobectomy.
- After ligation of the middle lobe and right lower lobe pulmonary vessels (🕮 p682) and completion of the fissures, the lung is retracted anteriorly, exposing the right main, right upper bronchus, and bronchus intermedius.
- The right main bronchus is divided with a knife, as well as the RUL bronchus, and the specimen is removed.
- The RUL bronchus is cut slightly obliquely to minimize size discrepancy between the right main bronchus and the RUL orifices.
- 2/0 Vicryl sutures are placed in the right main bronchus and the bronchus intermedius.
- The two ends are reanastomosed with either interrupted or running absorbable suture (Vicryl or PDS).

Left upper lobectomy sleeve

- After the division of the left upper lobe arteries and veins, the interlobar PA is encircled with umbilical tape and retracted laterally.
- The left main bronchus is divided with a knife proximal to the tumor, and the left lower lobe bronchus is divided distal to the tumor.
- The specimen is sent for frozen section pathology to confirm R0 resection.
- The left lower lobe bronchus may be cut slightly obliquely to minimize size discrepancy between the right main bronchus and the bronchus intermedius orifices.
- 2/0 Vicryl sutures are placed in the right main bronchus and bronchus intermedius.
- The two ends are reanastomosed with either interrupted or running absorbable suture (Vicryl or PDS).
- A hilar release may be performed to ensure a tension-free reanastomosis, which may be covered with an intercostal muscle pedicled flap.

Left lower lobe sleeve lobectomy

- Patients with tumor occluding the lower lobe orifice approaching the left lower lobe bronchus may require a sleeve resection to preserve the left upper lobe, and avoid a pneumonectomy.
- After ligation of left lower lobe pulmonary vessels and completion of the fissures, the lung is retracted posteriorly, exposing the left main bronchus, left upper, and left lower lobe bronchus.
- The left main bronchus is divided with a knife, as well as the left upper lobe bronchus, and the specimen is removed.
- The left upper lobe bronchus may be cut slightly obliquely to minimize size discrepancy between the left main bronchus and the left upper lobe orifices.
- 2/0 Vicryl traction sutures are placed in the left main bronchus and left upper lobe bronchus.
- The two ends are reanastomosed with either interrupted or running absorbable suture (Vicryl or PDS).

Pneumonectomy

Key facts

- Right pneumonectomy carries the highest mortality, and morbidity, especially bronchopleural fistula (BPF).
- The bronchial stump should always be covered with tissue, including intercostal muscle flap, pericardial fat pad, or pleural flap.
- Left pneumonectomy carries lower mortality and morbidity compared to right, with less incidence of BPF because, although the left main bronchus is longer than the right main bronchus, the stump retracts into mediastinal tissue where it is covered by the arch of the aorta.

Right pneumonectomy

Pulmonary vein dissection

- The lung is positioned posteriorly and the anterior hilar pleura is incised.
- The inferior pulmonary ligament is divided with cautery up to the right inferior pulmonary vein.
- The right superior and inferior pulmonary veins are divided using a vascular stapler, which can be done safely without subsequent engorgement of the lung.
- If tumor approaches the veins, making division difficult, the pericardium may be opened, gaining direct access to the pulmonary veins at the exit of the left atrium. The veins can be divided at this point, or if necessary the left atrium wall may be clamped using a vascular clamp, the confluence of the veins divided, and the atriotomy closed with a running Prolene suture in two layers.

Pulmonary artery dissection

- RMPA exits posterior to the SVC, and the SVC is mobilized and retracted medially to expose the RMPA. The RMPA is carefully dissected and encircled, and doubly ligated with vascular stapler.
- If tumor is to close to the RMPA as it exists posterior to the SVC, the SVC can be mobilized laterally, and the proximal RMPA can be exposed as it exits posterior to the aortic arch, by dividing the pericardium anterior to the phrenic nerve.

Bronchus dissection

- The RMB is then stapled or divided close to the carina, to avoid a long RMB stump, and subsequent pooling of secretions.
- The bronchial stump should be covered with tissue as mentioned earlier.

Completion of the operation

- All pericardial defects should be closed primarily or with bovine pericardium or prosthetic material to prevent cardiac herniation.
- Careful hemostasis is obtained.
- A chest tube is not needed.
- Careful watertight wound closure.

Left pneumonectomy

Pulmonary vein dissection

- The SPV and IPV are divided in similar fashion as in a right pneumonectomy.

Pulmonary artery dissection

- The LMPA exits posterior to the arch of the aorta.
- The lung is retracted posteriorly, and the pleura overlying the mediastinum is divided below the aortic arch, anterior to the vagus nerve and recurrent laryngeal nerve.
- The LMPA is carefully dissected, encircled and doubly ligated.
- If the tumor extends proximally, control of the LMPA can be obtained dividing the ligamentum arteriosum, mobilizing the aortic arch superior and laterally, and incising the pericardium and controlling the intrapericardial origin of the LMPA.

Bronchus dissection

- To gain access to the LMB, the aortic arch is mobilized and retracted superiorly and laterally.
- The LMB is then stapled or divided close to the carina as possible by pushing the stapler against the aortic arch.
- The bronchial stump should be covered with tissue as mentioned previously in this chapter (📖 p690).
- Completion of the operation.
- All pericardial defects should be closed primarily or with bovine pericardium or prosthetic material to prevent cardiac herniation.
- Careful hemostasis is obtained.
- A chest tube is not needed.
- Careful watertight wound closure.

Superior sulcus tumors

Key facts

- Superior sulcus tumors are essentially apical lung tumors that invade the chest wall, and so by definition these are all T3 tumors.
- *Pancoast tumors* are superior sulcus tumors, but a superior sulcus tumor is not necessarily a Pancoast tumor.
- Curative resection involves adjuvant chemoradiotherapy and en bloc resection including chest wall resection, possible hemi-vertebrectomy, and possible excision of the T1 nerve root of the brachial plexus.

Presentation and investigation

- Presentation depends on the location of the tumor: the thoracic inlet can be divided into three compartments by the insertion of scalenus on the 1st and 2nd ribs:
    - Anterior compartment contains platysma, SCM, and omohyoid muscles; jugular and subclavian veins: symptoms include chest wall pain, hand or arm swelling from subclavian vein compression.
    - Middle compartment includes anterior and middle scalene muscle, phrenic nerve, subclavian artery and branches, brachial plexus trunks: symptoms include brachial plexus pain and paresis.
    - Posterior compartment includes spinal accessory nerves, sympathetic chain and stellate ganglion, vertebral bodies and intercostal nerves: symptoms are those of Pancoast tumors.
- This is as described for lung cancer (☐ p672). The apex of the lung is difficult to image on plain CXR, and patients whose primary complaint is shoulder pain are often misdiagnosed until CT chest is performed.
- Defining vascular and neurological invasion is essential for planning and resection and reconstruction: clinical evidence of T1 and C8 involvement suggests R0 resection may leave patient with severe ulnar paresis.
- Contraindications to resection are invasion beyond C8 and T1; multiple vertebral involvement with spinal canal invasion, N2 and N3 disease.

Pancoast tumors

Pancoast tumors are posteriorly located, and lead to *Pancoast syndrome* due to invasion into the **stellate ganglion** and **brachial plexus**:

- They are characterized by pain in shoulder extending to the ulnar aspect of the forearm and hand.
- Atrophy of the hand and arm muscles.
- Horner's syndrome (ptosis, miosis, and anhidrosis).
- Tumor spread occurs along nerve roots up to spinal canal.

Management of superior sulcus tumors

- Ipsilateral supraclavicular lymphadenopathy is considered N1 disease.
- Operative candidates should undergo the SWOG protocol: induction chemoradiotherapy (etoposide, cisplatin, 45Gy).
    - Patients with stable disease or disease regression then undergo anatomical resection, with two more cycles of adjuvant chemotherapy.
    - Around 90% of T3 and T4 tumors have R0 resection.
    - 4% operative mortality, 55% of patients had a complete pathologic response, overall 5-year survival was 41%, 53% for R0 resection.

Surgical approaches

Set-up

- General ET anesthesia with invasive arterial monitoring, and usually a wide-bore central line allowing rapid large volume infusion.
- A flexible bronchoscopy (📖 p654) is performed via a single lumen tube, before lung isolation is obtained.
- The patient is positioned and lung isolation rechecked.

Posterior approach (Shaw–Paulson)

- For posterior lesions: position patient in lateral decubitus (Fig. 14.2) with base of skull, C7 to iliac crest prepped and in field.
- Initial posterior-lateral thoracotomy (📖 p39) to ascertain resectability.
- Can be combined with chest wall resection and hemi-vertebrectomy.
- Incision is extended between lateral border scapula and spinous processes to C7 dividing trapezius along its full length, rhomboids (preserving dorsal scapular nerve). Retractor placed between interspace and tip of scapula, and subscapular muscles divided up to 1st rib.
- En bloc chest wall resection: posteriorly erector spinae incised along its length to expose angle of ribs and transverse processes which can be resected or disarticulated depending on tumor invasion.
- Bleeding from vertebral foramen is dealt with by loose packing.
- The brachial plexus and subclavian vessels are dissected: the subclavian artery may be reconstructed, whereas the vein is ligated if involved.
- Vertebrae are resected and reconstructed with methylmethacrylate and plate-and-screw locking systems; and anatomic upper lobectomy performed with the chest wall specimen still attached.

Anterior approach (Dartevelle or hemiclamshell)

- Used for anteriorly located tumors: can be combined with an anterior thoracotomy, extended into the neck anterior to the sternocleidomastoid muscle, and laterally into the deltopectoral groove.
- Sternocleidomastoid is reflected anteriorly to expose the entire neck and thoracic inlet, except structures behind medial clavicle which may be resected to improve exposure: resecting the sternoclavicular joint is avoided to preserve shoulder movement postoperatively.
- After chest wall resection an anatomic lobectomy is performed (📖 p682).
- *Chest wall reconstruction* is described on 📖 p808.

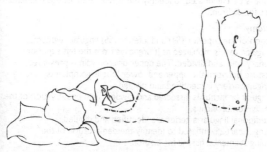

Fig. 14.2 Shaw–Paulson approach to superior sulcus tumors.

Sublobar resection

Key facts

- Sublobar resection (non-anatomic *wedge resection* or anatomic *segmentectomy*) preserve lung parenchyma in patients with small and peripheral tumors who require surgery for control, but are judged to have insufficient pulmonary reserve to tolerate lobectomy.
- Other indications include localized lesions, e.g., bronchiectasis, aspergillosis, TB, and metastatic lung lesions.
- Non-anatomical resection is an oncological compromise: around 1/3 of patients will experience local recurrence, but with careful patient selection the negative impact on oncologic outcomes may be minimal.

Principles of segmentectomy

- A wedge resection is a non-anatomic resection with a stapler, achieving wide margins. Anatomic segmentectomy is based on the segmental anatomy of the bronchial tree (Fig. 13.2, 🕮 p655).
- Generally lesions suitable for sublobar resections should be in the outer 1/3 of the lung parenchyma and <3cm in size.
- Segmentectomy is technically more demanding than wedge resection, but may be preferable for primary lung tumors because:
  - More reliable deep margins as resection extends to hilum.
  - Lymphatic drainage and interlobar nodes included.
- Wedge resection are technically easiest when the lesion is near an acute lung margin, otherwise tissue becomes too thick to staple.

Procedure

Left upper lobe apical trisegmentectomy

- Involves resection of the anterior (S3) and apicoposterior (S1+2) segments (upper division).
- The upper division vein is mobilized as it branches from the left superior pulmonary vein, and divided, the lingular vein is preserved.
- The segmental pulmonary arteries branching to the upper division are identified anteriorly, posteriorly, and within the fissure, and divided.
- The upper division bronchus is identified within the fissure, with preservation of the lingular bronchus.
- The lung is partial inflated to identify the demarcation of the segmental fissures for division.

Lingulectomy

- Resection of the superior (S4) and inferior (S5) lingular segments.
- The lingular vein is mobilized as it branches from the left superior pulmonary vein, and divided. The upper division vein is preserved.
- The fissure between the upper and lower lobe is completed.
- The lingular artery is identified and divided.
- The lingular bronchus is dissected and divided, with preservation of the upper division bronchus.
- Any additional lingular arteries are identified and divided.
- The lung is partially inflated to identify the demarcation of the remaining segmental fissure for division.

Right or left superior segmentectomy

- Involves resection of the superior segment of the lower lobe (S6).
- The major fissure is completed.
- The superior segmental artery is found within the fissure and divided.
- Posterior to the artery, the superior segmental bronchus is dissected and divided.
- The superior segment vein is identified as it branches off of the inferior pulmonary vein and divided.
- The remaining segmental fissure is identified with partial inflation of the lung, and divided.

Right upper lobe anterior segmentectomy

- Involves resection of the anterior segment (S1).
- The minor fissure is completed.
- The inferior edge of the superior pulmonary vein is dissected. The anterior segmental vein branches before the take-off of the middle lobe vein. The anterior segmental vein is then divided.
- The anterior segmental artery is then identified and divided.
- The anterior segmental bronchus is posterior to the artery. Once dissected, it is divided.
- The remaining segmental fissures are identified with partial inflation of the lung, and divided.

Oncologic outcomes for sublobar resection

- Lung Cancer Study Group randomized sublobar resection versus lobectomy for stage IA lung cancer and found a 17-fold increase in local recurrence in the sublobar cohort (17% vs. 6%).[1]
- However, tumors that are peripheral and <2cm in size appear to have oncological equivalence for sublobar resection versus lobectomy.[2]
- Segmentectomy versus lobectomy: no difference in 5-year survival for tumors <2cm, but survival advantage with lobectomy for tumors >2cm.[3]
- Outside of a clinical trial, lobectomy is the standard of care in the medically operable patient with early stage lung cancer.

References

1. Ginsberg RJ et al. Randomized trial of lobectomy versus limited resection for T1 N0 non-small cell lung cancer. Ann Thorac Surg 1995; **60**(3):615–22.
2. Okada M et al. Effect of tumor size on prognosis in patients with non-small cell lung cancer: the role of segmentectomy as a type of lesser resection J Thorac Cardiovasc Surg 2005; **129**:87–93.
3. Fernando HC et al. Lobar and sublobar resection with and without brachytherapy for small stage IA non-small cell lung cancer. J Thorac Cardiovasc Surg 2005; **129**:261–7.

Care after lung resection

Key facts

- Mortality after pulmonary resection is <2% for lobectomy and 6% for pneumonectomy.
- Morbidity for pulmonary resection is ~25% for both.
  - Perioperative morbidity is primarily cardiovascular and respiratory: pneumonia, atelectasis, supraventricular tachycardias, myocardial infarction, DVT, and PE.
  - Long-term complications include bronchopleural fistula, prolonged air leak, post-thoracotomy pain syndrome, and oxygen dependence.

Preoperative strategies to reduce morbidity

- Preoperative physiotherapy, including use of an incentive spirometer.
- Maximizing preoperative nutrition, especially for patients with preoperative cachexia and anorexia, and who have lost >10% of body weight (which is associated with increased mortality).
- Optimization of preoperative comorbidities, including glucose control for diabetics and bronchodilator therapy for patients with COPD, and smoking cessation.
- Instructing patients to walk 1–2 miles a day, to increase lower extremity circulation, and lung capacity.

Postoperative management

Monitoring

- Given the high (up to 15%) incidence of cardiac arrhythmia, all postoperative patients who do not need ICU care should be on a telemetry floor.
- In high-risk cases invasive pressure monitoring is kept for 48h.
- Patients with epidurals keep their urinary catheter, and may benefit from invasive arterial monitoring for the first 24h.
- Daily CXR: in pneumonectomy fluid level should rise, not fall.

Analgesia

- Epidural or paraspinous (🕮 p648) catheters should be used for patients undergoing thoracotomy. Hypotension, bradycardia, and low urine output may be a sign of excessive and high epidural: check sensation of dermatomes which should be intact below the nipple, and reduce or stop epidural if necessary.
- Intermittent opiates are usually sufficient for patients only undergoing VATS.
- NSAIDS such as iv ketorolac or oral ibuprofen are effective in conjunction with narcotics. Iv acetaminophen has a lower side effect profile and similar effectiveness to opiates, and is increasingly used (🕮 p648).

Antibiotic prophylaxis

- Reduces incidence of wound infections, but no proven efficacy against pneumonia or empyema.
- IV antibiotic with adequate Gram +ve and some Gram −ve coverage (e.g., cefazolin) at time of induction.
- Does not need to be continued postoperatively.

DVT prophylaxis

- Cancer patients are at high risk for postoperative thromboembolism. Generally 5000U of LMWH should be given subcutaneously prior to induction, and continued postoperatively until the patient is completely ambulatory.
- Sequential alternating leg compression devices (SCDs) can be used in conjunction with prophylactic heparin.

Respiratory physiotherapy

- Pulmonary physiotherapy is critical, including:
- Scheduled use of an incentive spirometer.
- Ambulating 4 times/day.
- Use of a pulmonary physiotherapy standardized protocol is helpful.
- **UC Davis Thoracic Pulmonary Hygiene Pathway.**
- Upon admission to the postanesthesia care unit (PACU), the respiratory therapist will begin positive airway pressure treatment, e.g., EzPAP® with 3% hypertonic saline nebulizer every 4h while in the PACU.
- Upon transfer to the thoracic surgery telemetry floor, the patient will continue with the EzPAP treatments every 6h for the first 48h.
- If the morning CXR shows increasing atelectasis than the EzPAP® will be changed to intrapulmonary percussive ventilation every 6h, which delivers rapid, percussions of oxygen into the lungs while simultaneously delivering therapeutic aerosols to loosen and help propel secretions.
- After 48h, the patient is reassessed using a cardiopulmonary therapy risk factor analysis, and their therapy is reduced as appropriate.

Fluid management

- Excess fluid restriction and administration should both be avoided in patients undergoing pulmonary resection.
- Intraoperative lung manipulation may lead to increased alveolar fluid volumes due to disruption of the alveolar capillary membranes. Excess fluid administration may result in pulmonary edema, atelectasis, and hypoxia.
- Excess fluid administration may also result in prolonged chest tube output.
- A 1500mL fluid restriction is recommended, with early oral intake, and elimination of maintenance IV fluid.

Chest tube management

- Chest tubes drain fluid and potential air leaks.
- Chest tubes are removed generally when output is <240mL/24h and there is no air leak.
- Patients with prolonged air leak (>5 days) may be discharged to home with a Heimlich valve if the lung stays expanded on water seal (see 📖 pp250–251).
- Excess fluid administration may also result in prolonged chest tube output.
- A 1500mL fluid restriction is recommended, with early oral intake, and elimination of maintenance IV fluid.

Complications after lobectomy

Key facts

These are the commonest complications and can be devastating: prevention and early treatment is absolutely key

Prevention

- Careful preoperative assessment of cardiopulmonary function, predicted postoperative respiratory capacity, and tailoring surgical resection appropriately (📖 pp652–653).
- Optimizing preoperative nutrition and respiratory status.

Reducing perioperative aspiration risk

- Meticulous attention to fasting, gastric transit, and decompression in immediate perioperative period.
- Careful operative technique avoiding direct and traction injuries of the recurrent laryngeal nerves.
- Efficient extubation in the perioperative period, close monitoring of oral diet, and sitting patient up especially when eating or drinking.
- Use of H_2 antagonists.
- Very low threshold for dysphagia diet and assessment, particularly in hoarse, elderly, and debilitated patients, and those with borderline lung function.

Reducing risk of postoperative chest infection

- Mobilize early and aggressively: the patient should not lie flat if they can sit up, not sit in bed if they can sit in a chair, and not sit in a chair if they can stand and walk.
- Good pain control, nursing, and physiotherapy, as well as patient education are key, along with being aggressive about removing lines, catheters, and drains as soon as possible.
- Daily physiotherapy, including incentive spirometry.

Pneumonia

Usually occurs within a week following surgery. Commonly Gram –ve bacilli, although others routinely colonizing the airway of patients with obstructive lung disease such as *Haemophilus influenza* and *Pneumococcus*. Covered in more detail on 📖 p268.

Diagnosis

- Usually productive cough, offensive sputum, temperature, elevated white cell count, and consolidation on CXR.
- If CXR and clinical picture unclear (patient may not have a productive cough or temperature, and the CXR may look more like a collection), CT chest without contrast will demonstrate any consolidation.

Management

- Aggressive physiotherapy, appropriate antibiotics, oxygen therapy if indicated, mobilization, adequate nutrition.
- Early bronchoscopy allows cultures to be taken and more efficient pulmonary toilet.

Respiratory failure

This is a major cause of perioperative mortality. It usually occurs within 4 days of surgery. Patients at high risk should be identified preoperatively. This is covered in more detail on 📖 p160 and 📖 pp162–163.

Management

- Postoperative chest physiotherapy decreases postoperative pulmonary complications and should be part of the normal postoperative management of thoracic surgical patients.
- Retained bronchial secretions require efficient and effective removal, sometimes necessitating the insertion of a minitracheostomy, to prevent atelectasis, hypoxia, and respiratory failure.
- Prolonged management with BiPAP or CPAP is often counterproductive: intubation and ventilation may be required.

Acute lung injury

This is a spectrum of lung injuries that includes *postpneumonectomy lung syndrome* and *adult respiratory distress syndrome* (ARDS) characterized by respiratory insufficiency and acute onset, bilateral pulmonary infiltrates, hypoxemia. It is covered in more detail on 📖 p163.

- Diagnostic criteria for ARDS: PCWP <18mmHg, non-cardiogenic pulmonary edema, PaO_2/FiO_2 <300 regardless of PEEP.
- Management: fluid restriction and diuresis, low tidal volume, high PEEP.

Arrhythmias

The most common arrhythmia following thoracic surgery is AF (📖 pp263–263). It is more common following pneumonectomy than lobectomy, and is associated with significantly increased mortality. The onset is usually within 48h of surgery. Ventricular arrhythmias are rare. Routine prophylactic administration of antidysrhythmics is not indicated.

Management

- Aim to keep potassium 4–5mmol/L.
- Administration of digoxin is the mainstay of treatment for AF. It may be given orally in patients who are hemodynamically stable or iv in those who have some degree of compromise.
- In more urgent cases administration of a 2.5–5mg iv metoprolol may produce rapid slowing of the ventricular rate.
- If hemodynamically unstable patients may require cardioversion.
- Following this digoxin should be administered to reduce the risk of recurrent AF.
- Almost all patients are back in sinus rhythm 6 weeks following surgery and medication for their dysrhythmia may then be discontinued.

Pulmonary embolism

Reported incidence is low after pulmonary surgery, but mortality is high. Thoracic surgical patients have multiple risk factors: increased age, malignancy, prolonged duration of anesthesia, smoking history, heart disease. They represent a moderate risk group for development of pulmonary embolus. Presentation and management is discussed on 📖 p476.

Outcomes of surgery for NSCLC

Key facts
- Survival after treatment for NSCLC is dependent on treatment modality and pathologic stage (Table 14.4).
- Majority of lung cancers recur within the first 3 years after pulmonary resection, and present as distant metastasis.

Recurrence
- Majority of lung cancers recur within the first 3 years after pulmonary resection, and present as distant metastasis.
- Tumors that recur after 5 years are most likely second primaries.
- The risk of developing a second lung primary tumor after pulmonary resection is 1–2% per year, with the cumulative risk 5% after 5 years and 12.6% after 10 years.

Table 14.4 NSCLC current therapy and 5-year survival[1-3]

Pathologic stage (6th and 7th AJCC)	Therapy	% 5-year survival
I	Surgery	60–75
II	Surgery	30–50
IIIA	Surgery + multimodality therapy	10–40
IIIB	Chemotherapy/radiation	<5–10
IV	Chemotherapy	<1–10

1. Mountain CF. The international system for staging lung cancer. *Semin Surg Oncol* 2000; **18**:106–15.

2. Minna JD. Neoplasms of the lung. In Kasper E (ed) *Harrison's Principles of Internal Medicine*, 16th edn. New York: McGraw-Hill, 2005.

3. Goldstraw P et al. The IASLC lung cancer staging project: proposals for the revision of the TNM stage groupings in the forthcoming (seventh) edition of the TNM classification of malignant tumours. *J Thorac Oncol* 2007; **2**(8):706–14.

Bronchopleural fistula

Key facts

- A *bronchopleural fistula* (BPF) is a communication between the bronchial airways and the pleural space, usually after pneumonectomy and in the setting of postoperative empyema.
- The incidence of **empyema** following pneumonectomy is 1%, and may develop early (within 3 months following surgery) or many years following surgery.
- The aims of treatment of both empyema and bronchopleural fistula after lung resection is to drain the fluid, and sterilize the space; and in the case of BPF to close the communication with the bronchial airways: surgery is usually required.

Empyema after lung cancer resection

Early empyema may be *primary* (bacterial contamination at time of surgery) or **secondary** (infection of pleural fluid from infected residual lung tissue or from bronchopleural fistula). Late infection is usually hematogenous in origin. Staphylococcus is the most common infection. Streptococcus and Gram–ve and anaerobic organisms also commonly cultured. Management is described in more detail on ☐ p704.

Management

- Early drainage of pleural space using tube thoracostomy, antibiotic therapy, and eventual obliteration of space.
- Bronchoscopy can confirm the presence or absence of bronchopleural fistula.
- A surgical window may be required in order to provide adequate drainage for obliteration of the space.
- Closure of window is possible following complete sterilization of the thoracic cavity.
- Other options include thoracoplasty (☐ p704) or obliteration of the empyema space.

Bronchopleural fistula

- Incidence: 1.5–6%. More common following lung resection for malignancy. Also associated with pre- and postoperative radiotherapy and pre-existing diabetes mellitus.
- More common following pneumonectomy than lesser procedures.
- Right-sided much more common than left-sided.

Prevention

- Limiting the dissection around a bronchial stump limits post-surgical ischemia, and stump breakdown.
- The bronchial stump after pneumonectomy should be covered by viable tissue, e.g., pedicled intercostal muscle, pedicled pericardial fat pad, pleural flap, omentum.
- The left pneumonectomy stump is not always covered, as it is often naturally covered by the arch of the aorta and pulmonary artery.

Diagnosis
- Patient may start expectorating foul watery fluid—most frequently after lying with operated side uppermost. Sometimes patients complain of new 'gurgling' sensation in chest. Signs of pneumonia.
- New or falling air-fluid level in pneumonectomized pleural space on CXR.
- Bronchoscopy confirms diagnosis: allows the stump and any defects in it to be visualized directly, as well as permitting bronchial toilet.

Management
Management first involves preventing the patient from aspiration of pleural fluid through the BPF, and treating the infection
- Nurse the patient with the operated side lowest to prevent spillage into the airway. This is a contraindication to CPAP.
- *Immediate chest tube* after discovery of new air fluid level in the pneumonectomized pleural space. Occasionally this is all that is required to drain the space and allow the defect to close.
- Failure to close and contamination of the pleural space requires:
  - Creation of a chest wall window and primary closure of the BPF.
  - Serial debridements of the infected space with either continuous packing or wound vacuum dressing.
  - Filling of space either with space-occupying tissue (omentum, muscle) or antibiotic solution and primary closure of chest wall (*Clagett procedure*) 📖 p707.
  - Early fistulas are usually associated with technical difficulty at surgery, repeat thoracotomy and resuturing of stump is indicated.
  - Fistulae occurring >2 weeks postoperatively are usually associated with empyema: iv antibiotics should be administered.

Empyema

Key facts

• Defined as **pus in the pleural space**: often from the lung parenchyma or translocated through the chest wall, mediastinum, or abdomen.
• An empyema may grow organisms or it may be sterile (1/3 of cases), depending how long the patient has been on antibiotics.
• The aim of treatment is to drain and sterilize the space, and re-expand the lung which can done using VATS with limited decortication in early stage empyemas, but in recurrent empyema ± bronchopleural fistula (🕮 p702) may require a chest wall window for chronic debridement.

Pathology

• A **parapneumonic pleural effusion** is common. The majority resolve with antibiotic therapy. **Postpneumonic empyema** forms when bacteria infect the pleural fluid or pleural space. It is the commonest cause of an empyema.
• **Postsurgical empyema** accounts for 20% of cases of empyema and can follow surgery to the mediastinum, esophagus, and lungs, most commonly following pneumonectomy. It can also follow surgery or injury to the abdomen. Presentation is usually in the early postoperative period, but it may develop several years after surgery.
• Empyema may also follow rupture of a lung abscess or infected pleural bleb, inhaled foreign bodies or bronchopleural fistula.
• Empyema may also result form thoracic trauma, ruptured esophagus, pericarditis, abdominal processes such as cholangitis and diverticulitis with translocation of bacteria across the diaphragm, mediastinitis, chest wall or spine osteomyelitis, rupture of lung abscess or infected pleural bleb, and inhaled foreign body.

Stage I: acute exudative phase

• Typically occurs 2–5 days after a pneumonia.
• Accumulation of fluid with low cellular content and viscosity.
• Characterized by low WBC, LDH, glucose, and a normal pH.
• Can be successfully treated with antibiotics only.

Stage II: fibrinopurulent phase

• Typically occurs 5–14 days after a pneumonia.
• Turbid or purulent fluid with heavy fibrin deposits.
• Appearance of simple loculations and septations.
• May have bacterial invasions, and high numbers of polymorphonuclear leukocytes (PMNs) and lymphocytes.
• Characterized by low pH, glucose, and increased LDH.
• Antibiotics and chest tube drainage is required, ± VATS decortication.

Stage III: chronic organizing phase

• Lung trapping by collagen, visceral and parietal pleural peel with ingrowth of fibroblast and capillaries.
• Antibiotics and aggressive decortications, generally by thoracotomy.
• Bacteriology.

- Includes staphylococcus, *Haemophilus influenza*, Gram −ve bacilli, *Streptococcus pneumonia*, *Streptococcus pyogenes*, *Mycoplasma*.
- Empyema that has been present for >2 weeks has a higher risk of conversion from VATS to open for decortication.

Presentation

Patients may complain of fever, productive cough, dyspnea, chest wall pain, malaise, fatigue. Physical examination may reveal decreased ipsilateral chest wall expansion, egophony, dullness to percussion, chest wall tenderness. Complications include **empyema necessitans** (discharge of empyema through the chest wall), pulmonary fibrosis, chest wall contractures, osteomyelitis, pericarditis, subphrenic, or mediastinal abscesses.

Investigation

- CXR, PA and lateral, and/or decubitus films to determine loculation.
- Chest CT: provides anatomy, and helps planning for chest tube placement of surgery, as well as showing thickened pleural peel, and presence of calcifications in the peel which help determine if thoracotomy rather than VATS necessary.
- Thoracentesis: Gram's stain and culture, **Light's criteria** distinguishes transudative effusion from exudative:
  - Exudative if specific gravity is >1.02, protein content >2.0 g/dL, and at least one of the following: ratio of pleural fluid protein to serum >0.5, ratio of pleural fluid LDH and serum >0.6, total pleural fluid LDH >2/3 upper limit of normal, ratio of pleural fluid albumin and blood <1.

Management

Stage I
- Sensitivity-appropriate antibiotics.

Stage II
- Chest tube drainage (small or large bore).
- Thrombolytics most likely to be effective during early stage empyema, and should be reserved for patients who are poor surgical candidates.

Stage III and failure of stage II to resolve
- If pleural space drainage is ineffective, or the effusion has loculated appearance on imaging, a **VATS decortication** should be performed without delay
- If complete lung expansion is not achieved by VATS, then should convert to open thoracotomy: in processes that have been going >14 days, or in patients who have chest wall tenderness, need for conversion for open thoracotomy is higher.
- *Open decortication* (📖 p706) indicated for late stage II, stage III, and incomplete lung expansion with VATS.
- *Chest wall window* (Eloesser flap) (📖 p707) may be required if lung cannot expand and empyema chronically reaccumulates, or in the case of a BPF that cannot be closed.

Decortication

Key facts

- This is a major undertaking usually performed through a posterolateral thoracotomy attempting to completely remove what is usually densely adherent of visceral peel off the lung to allow it to completely re-expand.
- It is indicated for treatment of stage III empyemas: early stage II decortications are difficult because there is less of a plane between the lung and the peel than in later stage III empyemas.

Procedure

Set-up

- General ET anesthesia with invasive arterial monitoring, and usually a central line.
- A flexible bronchoscopy (🕮 p654) is performed via a single lumen tube, before lung isolation is obtained using a bronchial blocker or a double lumen tube.
- The patient is then positioned in the *lateral, decubitus position* (🕮 p39) with spine parallel to and close to the edge of the table, using sandbags, or rolls and tape, usually with the upper arm positioned on a rest, the lower arm flexed in front of the head.

Procedure

- The aim is complete removal of the rind, leaving the visceral pleura intact allowing complete expansion of the lung.
- Entry into the pleural space is not like a normal thoracotomy: once through the intercostal muscles the first thing encountered may be a thick, cream-coloured rind, and there may be no plane between this and the lung parenchyma.
- In order to safely get enough space to place a retractor and spread the ribs it is usually safest to start with a local pleurectomy, carefully wiping the rind off the chest wall with finger tips. This leaves raw surface area which should be cauterized.
- Once a retractor can be safely introduced the correct plane to elevate the rind off the lung parenchyma should be found: it's easiest to do this cutting carefully into the rind with a 15 or a 23 blade with the lung inflated.
- As soon as the plane is identified then counter-traction on the lung and traction on the rind, with careful blunt dissection using peanuts or multiple blades and or/a periosteal elevator, similarly usually permits most of the rind to be removed without damaging the lung parenchyma.
- The most difficult areas are the fissures (although air leaks here usually seal up postoperatively) and along the diaphragm.
- Careful hemostasis to avoid retained hemothorax and reinfection of space is mandatory.

Postoperative management

- Lung expansion is encouraged by leaving chest tubes on water seal suction.
- Chest tubes should remain until output is minimal.
- Excessive bleeding from raw surfaces is an occasional problem that may require re-exploration, whereas air leaks often resolve quickly due to the sticky nature of the pleural space.

Eloesser window

- This is used in the setting of chronic recurrent empyema, including after pneumonectomy, and it allows chronic drainage to the skin.
- It involves removal of ribs over an accessible location (ideally in a dependent posterior area to improve drainage) with preservation of muscle, soft tissue, and skin.
- 1/3 of scapula may need to be removed with a sternal saw to avoid locking of the scapula tip in the window.
- Muscle and skin is marsupialized by sewing to parietal pleura of chest wall (Figure 14.3).
- After serial debridements, when the space is sterile and any BPF has resolved, the space may be closed by filling with antibiotic solution (*Clagett procedure*) or omentum or muscle and the marsupialized tissue is released and used to close the surface of the wound.
- A stoma bag can be placed over the site.

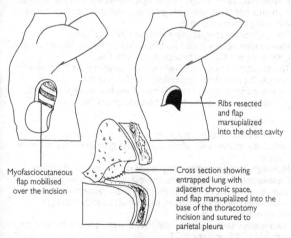

Myofasciocutaneous flap mobilised over the incision

Ribs resected and flap marsupialized into the chest cavity

Cross section showing entrapped lung with adjacent chronic space, and flap marsupialized into the base of the thoracotomy incision and sutured to parietal pleura

Fig. 14.3 Eloesser window marsupialization of chest wall tissue.

Fungal lung disease

Key points

Pathogens include histoplasmosis, coccidioidomycosis, blastomycosis, and opportunistic infections, e.g., aspergillosis, cryptococcosis.

Histoplasmosis

- Endemic in midwestern US states such as Michigan, Ohio, and Indiana.
- *Histology:* budding yeasts consistent with *Histoplasma capsulatum*.
- *Presentation:* fever, malaise, pleuritic chest pain, flu-like symptoms, but often asymptomatic. Can also lead to insidious *mediastinal fibrosis, broncholiths, traction diverticulum* of the esophagus.
- *Investigation:* sputum culture, CXR, chest CT which show solitary pulmonary nodules, calcified nodules, and lymph nodes.
- *Treatment:* if symptomatic, amphotericin B.
- Surgery for medical refractory disease, symptomatic broncholiths, traction esophageal diverticulum, or mediastinal fibrosis resulting in destruction of lung tissue.
- Surgery can have high mortality or catastrophic bleeding: consider cardiopulmonary bypass or stand by for difficult hilar disease.

Coccidioidomycosis

- Infection from inhalation of *Coccidioides immitis* spores. Also called *valley fever.* Endemic to western and southwestern USA and Mexico.
- *Histology:* demonstrates spherule containing endospores.
- *Presentation:* fever, cough, fatigue, dyspnea (valley fever), arthralgias, erythema nodosum, rarely progressive pneumonia, cavitary lesions, thin wall pulmonary cavities.
- Extrapulmonary complications includes CNS infections.
- *Investigation:* serum testing for IgM or IgG antibodies, sputum culture, CXR and chest CT, and bronchoscopy with BAL.
- *Treatment:* most infections self-limiting—amphotericin B for severe disease, fluconazole or itraconazole for 3–6 months.
- Indications for surgery include failure of medical management with persistent cavitary lesion, hemoptysis, secondary infection, or BPF.

Blastomycosis

- Caused by *Blastomyces dermatidis.* Endemic to southeastern USA, as well as the midwest. Results in suppurative granulomatous pulmonary disease.
- *Histology:* broad-based budding yeasts and neutrophil infiltration.
- *Presentation:* flu-like symptoms, myalgias, non-productive cough, acute pneumonitis, ARDS, chronic pyogranulomatous lung disease, with extrapulmonary symptoms, e.g., skin ulcers and multiorgan dissemination.
- *Investigation:* serodiagnosis unreliable, sputum cultures, bronchoscopy with BAL, CXR, and chest CT.
- *Treatment:* most infections self-limiting, amphotericin B for severe disease, fluconazole or itraconazole for 6–12 months.
- Indications for surgery include failure of medical management with persistent cavitary lesion, hemoptysis, secondary infection, or BPF.

Aspergillosis

- *Aspergillus fumigatus* is an opportunistic fungus that is found in soil and is inhaled. Especially in patients with AIDS, immunosuppression including prolonged periods of neutropenia, and chronic steroid use.
- **Presentation:** fever, cough dyspnea, hemoptysis, anorexia, malaise, may be complicated by aspergilloma, chronic necrotizing aspergillosis, invasive pulmonary aspergillosis.
- **Investigation:** sputum cultures (negative in 50% of cases), bronchoscopy with BAL, CXR, and chest CT.
- **Treatment:** IV voriconazole for invasive pulmonary aspergillosis, with amphotericin B as an alternative therapy for 6–12 weeks, with subsequent maintenance therapy, voriconazole for necrotizing aspergillosis for 6 months, amphotericin B for severe disease.
- Indications for surgery: asymptomatic aspergilloma can be left alone. Anatomic resection for aspergilloma, persistent hemoptysis, BPF, invasive disease, potential invasion of great vessels or pericardium.

Mucormycosis

- Opportunistic fungal infection caused by *Mucor*, *Rhizopus* and other zygomycetes. Found in soil. Can affect lungs in patients with AIDS, transplant patients, and other immunosuppressed patients.
- **Histology:** non-septate hyphae, right angle branching, vascular invasion.
- **Presentation:** bronchopneumonia, hemoptysis, lung infarction, chest wall invasion.
- **Investigation:** sputum cultures are not sensitive, CXR and chest CT.
- Tissue diagnosis demonstrating right angle branching non-septate hyphae is the gold standard.
- **Treatment:** amphotericin B for aggressive disease, long-term to lifetime posaconazole therapy for less aggressive disease.
- Surgery: anatomic resection of lung and adjacent tissue followed by long-term to lifetime posaconazole therapy.

Cryptococcosis

- Caused by the encapsulated yeast *Cryptococcus neoformans*. In addition to pulmonary disease, also associated with CNS disease, specifically meningitis. Commonly found in pigeon droppings.
- **Histology:** by budding yeasts.
- **Presentation:** cough, low-grade fever, fatigue, meningitis, pulmonary masses, and mediastinal lymphadenopathy.
- **Investigation:** serology for cryptococcal antigen is sensitive, CSF should always be examined, sputum cultures, bronchoscopy with BAL, CXR, and chest CT.
- **Treatment:** medical therapy is the gold standard with amphotericin B for aggressive disease including meningitis, fluconazole for less aggressive disease for 3–12 months.
- **Surgery:** mediastinoscopy to diagnosis suspicious mediastinal lymphadenopathy for diagnosis, wedge resection of suspicious lung nodules for diagnosis.

Other lung infections

Lung abscess

Etiology
- *Primary:* direct infection via aspiration, esophageal disease, necrotizing pneumonia, primary tuberculosis, or fungal infections.
- *Secondary:* bronchial obstruction, malignancy, hematogenous bacterial spread, such as endocarditis, cystic disease, collagen vascular disease such as Wegner granulomatosis.

Presentation
- Productive cough, fever, rigors, fatigue, malaise, pleuritic chest pain, dyspnea, hemoptysis.
- Absence of fever or leucocytosis may suggest non-infectious causes of abscess, such as malignancy.

Investigation and management
- *Investigation:* sputum and blood cultures, CXR and chest CT, bronchoscopy for BAL.
- Avoid FNA, as may contaminate the pleural space and result in empyema.
- Medical management is 6–8 weeks appropriate antibiotics: 90% of patients respond to targeted antibiotic therapy alone and do not require surgical intervention, and aggressive chest physiotherapy.
- 1/3 of percutaneous drainage attempts fail, and should be avoided if possible.
- *Indications for surgery:*
  - Failed medical therapy.
  - Persistent endobronchial obstruction.
  - Formation of an empyema.
  - Hemorrhage.
  - Bronchopleural fistula.
  - Inability to rule out malignancy.

Surgical options
- Anatomic lobectomy.
- Pneumonectomy (avoid where possible for benign disease).
- All bronchial stumps should be covered with viable tissue.
- Intercostal muscle, omentum, pleural flap, pericardial fat pad.
- Cavernostomy.
- Thoracoplasty is rarely required to obliterate an apical space.

Hydatid pulmonary disease
- Caused by tapeworm infestation of *Echinococcus*. Results of invasion of lung and/or rupture of hydatid cyst into the pleural space from adjacent structures (such as transdiaphragmatic from the liver).
- *Presentation:* cough, dyspnea, hemoptysis, expectoration of cyst material, acute pleural drainage can cause pain and **anaphylactic shock**.
- *Diagnosis:* serology (IgG, IgM, hemagglutination), Casoni skin test, CXR and chest CT.
- *Treatment:* albendazole is drug of choice (3–6 months).

- *Surgery:* avoid spillage. Cystectomy ± anatomic resection, may require concurrent liver resection or cystotomy and capitonnage, concurrent albendazole therapy.

Amoebiasis

- Parasitic infection with *Entamoeba histolytica*. Transmitted via feco-oral route forming **liver abscess**, which ruptures or extends into surrounding tissues, producing **pleuro-pulmonary contamination**.
- *Presentation:* right-sided chest pain, pain radiating to shoulder, cough initially unproductive becoming productive of purulent chocolate brown sputum, fever, malaise, anorexia and weight loss, dyspnea. Parasites found in sputum.
- *Investigation:* sputum culture.
- *Treatment:* metronidazole, drainage of pleural fluid.

Actinomycosis

- Gram +ve actinomyces.
- *Presentation:* chest pain, dyspnea, hemoptysis, cough, fever, weight loss, invasion of chest wall with drainage.
- *Investigation:* wound and sputum culture.
- *Treatment:* penicillin for 5 weeks, drainage of pleural fluid.

Nocardiosis

- Aerobic Gram +ve organism. *Norcardia asteroides*.
- Presentation: cough, fever, malaise.
- Investigation: culture of sputum or pleural fluid.
- Treatment: Sulfonamide therapy, drainage of pleural fluid.

Interstitial lung disease

Key points

- Role of surgery is for tissue diagnosis.
- Lung biopsy helps determine diagnosis and mode of therapy (i.e., corticosteroids or lung transplantation).
- Severely diseased or 'burned out' tissue should be avoided for biopsy as histological architecture may be distorted.
- If both sides are equally diseased, VATS biopsy is performed on the left, as right lung is better equipped to tolerate single-lung ventilation.
- Open biopsy on ventilated lung should be performed on patients with severe respiratory distress.

Pathology

- Diffuse inflammation and fibrosis of the lung parenchyma characterized by inflammatory cells, fibroblastic foci, collagen accumulation.
- The underlying aetiology include a number of conditions (Table 14.5). as well as collagen vascular disease, SLE, rheumatoid arthritis, and environmental exposure (silicosis, berylliosis), drug-induced (smoking, amiodarone, bleomycin), granulomatous disease, sarcoidosis, Wegener granulomatosis, idiopathic interstitial pneumonia, TB, lymphangiomyotosis, Langerhans cell histiocytosis.

Investigation

- Chest CT: reticular pattern, ground glass infiltrates, honeycombing
- Pulmonary function tests: restrictive lung disease pattern, reduced DLCO, TLC, FRC and RV, while FEV_1, and FVC may be normal.
- Transbronchial needle biopsy has low yield, low accuracy.

Lung biopsy

- Lung biopsy is the gold standard and provides the most accurate diagnosis. Indications for lung biopsy include no definitive diagnosis before starting steroid therapy, need to exclude neoplasm infection.
- Goals are to biopsy areas of parenchymal that both appear normal and abnormal on CT, avoiding severely diseased or 'burned out' areas of parenchyma that have severe amount of fibrosis such as lingula and middle lobe which often have the highest areas of 'burned out' disease.
- 2–3 biopsy specimens, specimen $\geq 3 \times 2 \times 1 cm^3$ in size.
- Open biopsy: in critically ill patients who would not tolerate single-lung ventilation (can be done in ICU via an anterior thoracotomy).
- VATS: procedure of choice for elective lung biopsy.
- Accuracy and outcomes equivalent to open lung biopsy, 5% 60-day mortality, 20% morbidity.
- If both sides are equally diseased, then choose left side for biopsy, as the right lung is best equipped to tolerate single-lung ventilation.

Complications of surgical lung biopsy

- Exacerbation of underlying lung disease: avoid by limiting FiO_2 level to avoid O_2 toxicity and free radical production.
- Limit barotrauma and excessive tidal volumes, and use staple line reinforcement to avoid prolonged air leak.

Table 14.5

Etiology	Presentation	CT findings	Histology	Treatment	Survival
AIP	Acute onset respiratory failure mimicking ARDS	Ground glass opacities with areas of consolidation	Proliferative phase: Hyaline membranes, diffuse alveolar injury Organizing phase: Abundant type II pneumocytes and fibroblasts	Supportive therapy with mechanical ventilation	Poor survival
COP	Subacute onset with short duration of symptoms. Associated with infectious pneumonia	Areas of consolidation, small nodules and subpleural and/or peribronchial ground glass attenuation	Patch areas of organizing pneumonia	High-dose steroids	Usually good recovery after 4–6 week course of steroids
DIP	Occurs in heavy smokers and patients with environmental or drug exposures	Lower lobe predominant ground glass attenuation and consolidation	Diffuse distribution of alveolar macrophages	High-dose steroids	Good prognosis after steroid therapy
LIP	Slow progression of dyspnea and cough	Ground glass attenuation, interstitial thickening, and pulmonary nodules	Diffuse interstitial lymphoid hyperplasia	Steroids	Good prognosis after steroid therapy, but may progress to lymphoma

(continued)

Table 14.5 (*Continued*)

Etiology	Presentation	CT findings	Histology	Treatment	Survival
NSIP	Derivative of UIP, but milder symptoms. Progressive dyspnea and cough	Reticular markings with bronchiectasis, ground glass attenuation, and volume loss	Diffuse fibrosis and inflammation	Steroids, cyclophosphamide, colchicines, azathioprine, IFN-γ1b	Median survival of 56 months
RBILD	Occurs in heavy smokers. Progressive dyspnea	Ground glass attenuation with centrilobular nodules	Centriacinar proliferation of alveolar macrophages in respiratory bronchioles	Smoking cessation, steroids	Usually reversible after smoking cessation
UIP	Progressing cough, dyspnea, and reduced vital capacity	Patch reticular fibrosis pattern and honeycombing	Fibrosis with without fibroblastic proliferation	Steroids, cyclophosphamide, colchicines, azathioprine, IFN-γ-b	Median survival of 33 months

Hemoptysis

Key facts

- Hemoptysis is expectoration of (coughing up) blood, either mild or catastrophic: minor is streaks in sputum, moderate <400mL/24h, massive >400mL/24h, exsanguinating>1L.
- In *massive hemoptysis* patients generally do not die from exsanguination, but 'drowning' of unaffected lung because of inability to secure the airway.
- Consider bronchoscopic-guided selective intubation to protect the unaffected lung, with coil embolization to stop bleeding.
- Definitive surgery often requires thoracotomy and anatomic resection.

Pathology

Broad range of causes of hemoptysis:

- Bronchiectasis.
- Infectious, e.g., TB, fungal infection, pulmonary abscess.
- Malignant, including primary and secondary tumors of the lung and airway.
- Trauma, usually penetrating airway injury.
- Iatrogenic: chemotherapeutics such as bevacizumab (Avastin®), TIF after tracheostomy, pulmonary artery rupture from PA catheter.
- Other causes include cystic fibrosis, congenital atriovenous malformations, Wegener granulomatosis, Goodpasture syndrome.

Investigation

- CBC, PT, PTT, INR, DIC panel including fibrinogen, Chem 7.
- If stable, chest CT angiogram to determine relevant anatomy and extravasation.
- Bronchoscopy either flexible or rigid can identify which lung is the source of hemoptysis, and allow for selective intubation of non-involved lung.
- Rigid bronchoscopy is advantageous as it allows for concurrent ventilation and large tools for evacuating clot.
- Bronchial artery angiogram can be diagnostic and therapeutic, permitting coil embolization may stop or temporize bleeding.

Therapy

- Correction of all coagulopathy.
- Administration of antifibrinolytics such as factor VIIa.
- Bronchial artery embolization.
- Often indicated for fungal aetiology such as aspergillosis.
- Bronchoscopic techniques for localized area of hemoptysis.
- Iced saline lavage.
- Epinephrine or phenylephrine lavage.
- Cryoprobe.
- Argon beam coagulation.
- Laser coagulation.

Indications for surgery
- Failure of medical management in medical diseases and localization of disease.
- TIF.
- Congenital abnormalities such as known pulmonary artery aneurysms or AVM.
- Failed bronchial artery embolization.

Contraindications for surgery
- Generalized source of hemoptysis—consider ECMO and treatment of underlying lung disease.
- Palliative condition.
- Metastatic end-stage malignancy.

Surgical technique
- Thoracotomy.
- Anatomic resection: lobectomy or pneumonectomy.

Congenital disorders of the lung

Key facts

- Many of the disorders of the lung can be diagnosed *in utero*.
- All should be part of the differential diagnosis for neonatal respiratory distress and cyanosis.
- Most are treated with anatomical resection.

Congenital lobar emphysema

- *Pathology:* this is over-distension of one or more lobes of the lung, leading to life-threatening compression of the unaffected lung and mediastinal shift. The left upper and right middle lobes are the most commonly affected.
- Due to dysfunctional cartilage development of involved bronchus, resulting in air trapping, associated with congenital cardiac anomalies.
- *Presentation:* usually affects newborns and infants, and is diagnosed in the first 6 months of life due to life-threatening conditions including respiratory distress and cyanosis. Less acute symptoms include dyspnea, wheezing, cough and tachypnea. Late symptoms include recurrent pneumonia, failure to thrive, and chest wall deformity.
- *Investigation:* CXR demonstrates hyperinflation of the affected lobe, with contralateral mediastinal shift. Paucity of lung markings on the ipsilateral side. Chest CT usually diagnostic.
- Surgical management consists of anatomic lobectomy.

Pulmonary sequestration

- *Pathology:* congenital mass of non-functioning lung tissue that has no communication with the tracheobronchial tree, and derives its blood supply from systemic artery system (thoracic aorta, the abdominal aorta travelling via the inferior pulmonary ligament, or the intercostal arteries), not the bronchial arterial circulation. Two types: venous drainage for *intralobar* (most common) is the pulmonary venous system, while venous drainage for *extralobar* is the systemic circulation.
- *Histology:* bronchiectasis and vascular hypertrophy.
- *Presentation:* cyanosis, respiratory distress in younger patients, in older patients may result in recurrent infections, empyema, chronic pleuritic chest pain. Extralobar sequestrations can be associated with congenital heart defects, vertebral defects, and diaphragmatic abnormalities. Extralobar has a 3:1 male to female ratio.
- *Investigation:* chest CT angiogram, interventional angiogram can identify anomalous arterial supply, and at the same time coil embolize subdiaphragmatic feeding arteries to limit risk of resection (Fig. 14.4).
- *Management:* surgical resection (VATS or open). Failure to identify feeding artery can result in retraction beneath diaphragm and catastrophic exsanguination: pre-op coil embolization of feeding artery mitigates the this risk.
- Identify and ligate feeding artery often in the inferior pulmonary ligament. Only sublobar resection needed. Ventilation of lung will identify demarcation of non-ventilated sequestration and normal lung tissue.

Congenital cystic adenomatoid malformation

- *Pathology*: hamartomatous type lesion with overgrowth of bronchioles with increased terminal respiratory structures that are connected to the tracheobronchial tree.
- Histology: cyst-like bronchioles lined with either pseudostratified columnar or cuboidal epithelium. Absence of cartilage in the cyst wall.
- Results from bronchial atresia with subsequent dysplastic lung growth beyond the atretic segment. Lesions occur on either side, most commonly in the lower lobes. They are classified into three types:
  - Type I (70%): large cystic spaces confined to one lobe.
  - Type II (20%): numerous small cysts, <2cm in size.
  - Type III (10%): multiple small cysts, <0.5cm in size, with large amount of solid adenomatoid hyperplasia or bronchial structures.
- *Presentation*: in newborns with respiratory distress, cyanosis, dyspnea, tachypnea, pneumothorax, poor feeding, pulmonary hypoplasia. Older children and adults may have milder symptoms or are asymptomatic.
- Investigation: most are diagnosed *in utero* by ultrasound. Newborn plain babygram may reveal cystic or solid mass, with contralateral mediastinal shift. Cysts may contain air fluid level.
- CT scan can distinguish from congenital diaphragmatic hernia.
- *Management*: some regress spontaneously, most require anatomic lobectomy. Type I: good prognosis. Type II and III: 50% mortality.

Bronchogenic cysts

- *Pathology*: abnormal non-communicating bronchogenic tissue that may be intrapulmonary or mediastinal. Represents 10–15% of mediastinal masses in children. In children, 65% are located in the mediastinum.
- Derived from the embryonic foregut.
- *Histology*: squamous or ciliated columnar epithelium. They may also contain hyaline cartilage, smooth muscle cells, and glands.
- Cysts occurring early in gestation tend to be centrally located, while those developing late in gestation tend to be peripheral.
- *Presentation*: respiratory distress from compression symptoms especially in newborns. Dysphagia from extrinsic compression of the esophagus, recurrent infections, fever, pain, dyspnea, anorexia. Often are asymptomatic and found incidentally.
- *Investigation*: CXR and chest CT. FNA is not necessary.
- *Management*: if surgical excision is not possible, than the cyst is opened and the lining excised and fulgurated to prevent recurrence.

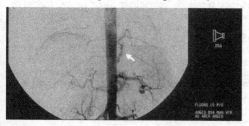

Fig. 14.4 Subdiaphragmatic feeding artery in left intralobar pulmonary sequestration.

Pulmonary tuberculosis 1

Key facts

- Airborne infection caused by *Mycobacterium tuberculosis*, more rarely *M. bovis* or *M. africanum*, transmitted as aerosol, or in the case of *M. bovis* by ingestion of contaminated milk.
- Increased incidence in patients with HIV infection. Low socioeconomical status, substance abuse, immigrants, inhabitants of nursing homes and prisons.
- Surgery is indicated for failure of medical therapy to remove destroyed lung, deal with secondary infections, e.g., *Aspergillus*, and complications such as massive hemoptysis and bronchopleural fistula.
- Although 2 billion patients worldwide are infected with TB, <15 000 cases annually are diagnosed in the USA: the numbers of operations for TB in the west are correspondingly very limited in number.

Pathology

- The characteristic lesion is **tuberculous granulomas** with **central caseation**. The primary infection is characterized by a *Ghon focus*, usually at the apex of the upper lobe.
- Later reactivation results in growth of mycobacterium within the liquefied caseum. Bronchial involvement results in expectoration of infected material. Seeding via the bloodstream also occurs.
- Following primary infection healing a **dormant phase** follows, which may last many decades. During this phase the patients are asymptomatic and the only evidence of infection is radiographical visualization of the Ghon focus and a **positive tuberculin skin test**.
- There is a 10–15% reactivation rate, usually involving the lungs.

Presentation

Presentation is extremely variable, but classically symptoms include low-grade fever, weight loss, night sweats, malaise, productive cough, hemo-ptysis, chest pain, and dyspnea. Complications include destroyed or cavitated lung, bronchostenosis with middle lobe atrophy (Lady Windermere or middle lobe syndrome), bronchopleural fistula, and secondary infection with aspergillosis.

Investigation

- For definitive diagnosis one of the described *Myobcacteria* species must be cultured, most commonly from sputum (which can be obtained by bronchoalveolar lavage, bronchial washings), but also from pus, CSF or biopsied tissue (FNA, mediastinoscopy, etc.).
- For detection of acid-fast bacilli, fluorescence microscopy is more sensitive than conventional Zieh–Nielson staining, confirmed by PCR.
- CXR may show consolidation or cavities in the upper lobes, with mediastinal and hilar lymphadenopathy and pleural effusions in active pulmonary TB. Miliary TB described as many sub-cm nodules throughout both lungs.
- CT is used to identify parenchymal destruction, caseous granulomas, Ghon foci, lymphadenopathy.

- A +ve tuberculin skin test (*Mantoux test*) of more than 5mm induration indicates TB infection, except in people previously immunized with the BCG vaccine where there is a high number of false positives. Thoracentesis for pleural effusion: pleural fluid analysis may demonstrate protein >5.0gm/dL, 50% lymphocytes, high ednosine deaminase level.

Management

Medical

- Avoid chest tubes in TB pleural effusion as high rate of superinfection and they generally resolve with appropriate antibiotic therapy.
- 2–3 months of triple therapy (isoniazid, rifampin, and pyrazinamide) followed by 4 months of dual therapy (isoniazid and rifampin).

Two months of triple therapy (isoniazid, rifampicin, and pyrazinamide) followed by 4 months of dual therapy (isoniazid and rifampicin). Drug resistance may require alternative drugs such as ethambutol or streptomycin. Multidrug resistant TB is often responsible for lesions in patients requiring surgery. All surgical patients should be on antituberculous medical therapy for 3 months preoperatively, and undergo aggressive nutrition and physiotherapy to correct their anabolic state where clinical presentation permits.

Indications for surgery

Surgery is indicated for failure of medical therapy to remove destroyed lung, deal with secondary infections, e.g., *Aspergillus*, and complications such as massive hemoptysis, bronchopleural fistula, bronchostenosis, and re-expansion of trapped lung.

Pulmonary tuberculosis 2

Surgery

The aim of surgery is complete resection of diseased lung tissue along with conversion of sputum. Should be complemented with neo- and adjuvant antituberculous multidrug therapy. Surgery may be hazardous due to previous infection/surgery. May require extrapleural lobectomy or pneumonectomy. Care is needed not to contaminate pleural space.

- General ET anesthesia, invasive arterial and central venous monitoring, bronchoscopy, and lung isolation.
- Patients is positioned in the lateral decubitus position.
- *Posterolateral thoracotomy:* 5th intercostal space incorporating bronchopleural fistulas or prior Eloesser flaps, preserving latissimus dorsi for a muscle flap to cover the bronchial stump, and preserving serratus to close the thoracotomy wound (and reduce the risk of winging of the scapula, which would compromise wound healing posteriorly).
- Omentum may also be mobilized to cover the bronchial stump.
- Rib resection is necessary in patients with hemithorax contracture.
- Dense adhesions between the parietal and visceral pleura mean that an *extrapleural dissection* is needed to mobilize the lung, taking great care to avoid the aorta on the left side, and the azygos, IVC, and esophagus on the right side, and the subclavian vessels at the apex.
- Lobectomy and pneumonectomy are performed in the standard fashion after mobilizing the lung: occasionally dense adhesions at the hilum necessitate intrapericardial division of vessels.
- The pleural cavity is irrigated with antibiotic solution, and the thoracotomy closed in layers with multiple absorbable sutures, and bronchoscopy performed to remove any secretions.

Outcomes

- Operative mortality 3–5%, sputum conversion 95%.
- Complications include empyema, late bronchopleural fistula—this is managed with *Eloesser window* (📖 p705) until the space is sterilized, and then the stump dehiscence is covered with a muscle flap, omentum or a *thoracoplasty* (where the chest wall is partially resected so that it collapses into effectively obliterating the pleural space).
- Bleeding, infection of the pleural space with TB empyema, BPF, acute lung injury.
- 95% sputum conversion.

Multidrug resistant tuberculosis (MDR-TB)

- Defined as resistance to both rifampin and isoniazid.
- Medical treatment involves addition of a fluoroquinolone such as levofloxacin and amikacin.
- Indications for surgery include refractory to medical therapy, localized disease or persistent cavity, complications such as hemoptysis.
- Outcomes: 93% disease free-outcome.

Non-tuberculosis mycobacteria (NTM)

- Defined as new and old species other than TB that affect public health, such as Mycobacterium avium, Mycobacterium bovis, and Mycobacterium africanum.
- Medical treatment includes isoniazid, rifampin, ethambutol, with addition of a macrolide and a fluoroquinolone if resistant to any of the described regimen.
- Indications for surgery include disease refractory to medical therapy, localized disease or persistent cavity, complications such as hemoptysis.

Bronchiectasis

Key facts

- Bronchiectasis is irreversible dilatation of the bronchi usually associated with inflammation.
- It is caused by the destruction of the elastic and muscular components of the bronchial wall and is either a localized or diffuse process.

Pathology

Three main types are described: *cylindrical*—often seen with TB, *varicose*, and *saccular*—usually seen after infection or obstruction.

Congenital

Congenital bronchiectasis usually results in diffuse disease (the exception being cystic fibrosis which tends to primarily affect the upper lobes). Congenital bronchiectasis may be due to a congenital immunoglobulin deficiency, cystic fibrosis, ciliary dysmotility disorders, or connective tissue disorders.

Acquired

- Bronchiectasis secondary to tuberculous infection usually affects the upper lobe and that secondary to any other bacterial or viral chest infection affects the lower lobes. More common causative organisms include adenovirus, influenza virus, HIV, *Staphylococcus aureus*, *Haemophilus influenzae*, anaerobes, *Mycobacterium tuberculosis*.
- Chronic external compression of a bronchus, due to tumor mass (carcinoid more common than malignancy) or enlarged lymph nodes.
- Gastric aspiration, pneumonia secondary to foreign body aspiration and inhalational injury, e.g., ammonia.
- Allergic bronchopulmonary aspergillosis.
- Other diseases: rheumatoid arthritis, ulcerative colitis, Sjögren syndrome.

Presentation

Recurrent productive cough. Sputum is purulent. More advanced disease may present with hemoptysis. If disease affects the upper lobes the cough may be non-productive.

Investigations

- CXR: may be normal or may show cystic lesions with air–fluid levels. Bronchial wall thickening may be evident.
- CT scan: high-resolution scans routinely used to demonstrate the dilated airways.
- *Sputum culture*: pathogens often identified. Commonly *H. influenzae*, *P. aeruginosa*, *S. pneumoniae*.

Management

The aim of therapy is to treat any infection, any underlying cause for bronchiectasis, optimize clearance of secretions, and reduce air flow limitation with bronchodilators. Physiotherapy is very important, using postural drainage techniques, chest percussion, and vibration. Aggressive antibiotic therapy for acute exacerbations prolongs periods of remission.

Surgical options

Lung resection, e.g., lobectomy (📖 pp680–689) or segmentectomy (📖 p694) is indicated in those patients with sufficient pulmonary reserve who remain symptomatic despite optimal medical therapy. Massive hemoptysis may also necessitate surgical resection of the affected lung. The aim is to preserve as much normal lung parenchyma as possible, hence surgical candidates tend to be those with limited disease. In those with insufficient pulmonary reserve embolization may be an option but is associated with rebleeding.

Emphysema

Key facts

- Pulmonary emphysema results from the destruction of air spaces, with a loss of elastic recoil of the lungs and alveolar capillary surface for gas exchange.
- 4 million Americans are currently affected by emphysema.
- The only medical therapy that has shown to impact survival is O_2 therapy: surgery is indicated for selected patients.

Pathology

Destruction of pulmonary parenchyma reduces functional lung mass, resulting in impaired gas exchange; as well as loss of elastic recoil which leads to hyperinflation (bullae), loss of the mechanical advantages seen in normal lung volumes, and compression of relatively normal areas.

Presentation

Patients present with insidious onset of dyspnea. Chronic productive cough is common. Cyanosis. May present with acute infective exacerbation, pneumothorax. Smoking history is common. Physical examination reveals characteristic barrel chest, widened intercostal spaces.

Investigation

- *CXR:* large bullae may be visible, flattened diaphragm, reduction in lung markings.
- *CT chest:* destruction of lung parenchyma, bullous disease.
- *Lung function:* increased residual capacity, decreased DLCO.

Rationale for lung volume reduction surgery

Medical management is supportive, (smoking cessation, physiotherapy, bronchodilators and steroids, home O_2) and associated with poor functional and prognostic outcomes. Rationale for surgery is that removal of hyperinflated and underperfused lung parenchyma will allow expansion of functional ventilated and perfused lung, restoring mechanical advantage by normalizing lung volume and diminishing dyspnea.

- 1957 Brantigan and Mueller[1] first described excision of hyperinflated lung parenchyma with 18% mortality.
- 1996 Cooper *et al.*[2] reported on 150 patients undergoing LVRS: 2.5% mortality, 14.4% mortality at 3 months, and 23% mortality at 12 months.

National practice

- Because of poor national results, the Health Care Finance Administration (HCFA) halted reimbursement for LVRS until a 'definitive' study published.
- The Center for Medicare and Medicaid Services (CMS, formerly HCFA) and the National Heart, Lung and Blood Institute (NHLBI) developed the National Emphysema Treatment Trial (NETT) (limited to 17 centers).

National Emphysema Treatment Trial (NETT)

Study design

- Prospective randomized clinical trial comparing LVRS with medical management of emphysema in patients with Medicare, or private insurance that would pay for therapy.

- Presence of bilateral emphysema with severe airflow obstruction, hyper-inflation on imaging, and the ability to participate in an exercise program.
- Optimal medical therapy: smoking cessation, bronchodilators, O_2 therapy, pulmonary rehab, pneumococcal and influenza vaccines.
- Surgery: LVRS via a sternotomy, VATS, or thoracotomy.
- All patients had 6–8 weeks of pulmonary rehab prerandomization.
- Patients randomized to medical therapy received pulmonary rehab for 8–9 weeks postrandomization.

Initial results

Initial results identified a high-risk group that had higher mortality after surgery compared to medical therapy and these were removed from further analysis:[3]

- Patients with FEV_1 <20% and homogenous emphysema.
- Patients with FEV_1 <20% and DLCO <20%.

Longer-term results[4,5]

- Short- and long-term survival advantage for surgery in patients with upper lobe emphysema and low exercise capacity.
- Survival advantage for medical therapy for patients with non-upper-lobe emphysema and high exercise capacity.
- Improvements in both exercise capacity and quality of life as a result of surgery in patients with upper lobe emphysema and both low or high exercise capacity.
- Improvements in quality of life only (no survival advantage) as a result of surgery for patients with upper lobe emphysema and high exercise capacity, and patients with non-upper-lobe emphysema and low baseline exercise capacity.

Impact of NETT on Medicare coverage

- Non-coverage of LVRS was extended for high-risk patients.
- Coverage for LVRS was provided for upper lobe emphysema and low or high exercise capacity for survival and palliative benefit respectively.
- Coverage for LVRS was extended for non-upper-lobe emphysema and low exercise capacity for palliative benefit.
- Types of facilities that are allowed Medicare coverage of LVRS:
  - NETT approved research centers.
  - Centers accredited by the Joint Commission on Accreditation of Healthcare Organizations (JCAHO) under the Disease Specific Certification Program for LVRS.
  - Centers approved for lung or heart and lung transplantation.

References

1. Brantigan OC, Mueller, F. Surgical treatment of pulmonary emphysema. *Am Surg* 1957; **23**(9): 789–804.
2. Cooper JD et al. Results of 150 consecutive bilateral lung volume reduction procedures in patients with severe emphysema. *J Thorac Cardiovasc Surg* 1996; **112**: 1319–30.
3. NETT Group. Patients at high risk of death after lung-volume-reduction surgery. *New Engl J Med* 2001; **345**: 1075–83.
4. NETT Group. A randomized trial comparing lung-volume-reduction surgery with medical therapy for severe emphysema. *New Engl J Med* 2003; **348**:2059–73.
5. Naunheim KS et al. Long-term follow-up of patients receiving lung-volume-reduction surgery versus medical therapy for severe emphysema by the National Emphysema Treatment Trial Research Group. *Ann Thorac Surg* 2006; **82**(2):431–43.

Lung volume reduction surgery

Key facts

- In the USA, Medicare will only reimburse lung volume reduction surgery (LVRS) for very specific patient types and defined surgeon and institution qualifications.
- The goal of surgery is to remove ventilated but poorly perfused lungs in patients with upper lobe emphysema and low exercise capacity (see Fig. 14.5).
- VATS approach is as effective as open techniques and is the preferred approach.
- Prolonged air leak is the most common postoperative complication and staple line buttressing is a necessity.

Open approach

Set-up

- General ET anesthesia with invasive arterial monitoring, and usually a central line.
- The patient is then positioned in the *supine position* (📖 p39).
- Median sternotomy, both mediastinal pleura are opened.

Lung resection

- The pulmonary ligaments are divided.
- The hyperinflated lung tissue can be punctured to allow for deflation.
- A clamp can be used to mark the area of resection, and a stapler is used to resect the lung tissue.
- The line of stapling is parallel and 3–4cm above the major fissure.
- Staple line buttress material should be used to avoid air leaks.
- Multiple commercially available staple line buttressing products.
- Care should be taken to avoid crossing fissures into the lower lobes.

VATS approach

Set-up

- General ET anesthesia with invasive arterial monitoring, and usually a central line.
- The patient is then positioned in the *lateral, decubitus position* (📖 p39) with spine parallel to and close to the edge of the table, using sandbags, or rolls and tape, usually with the upper arm positioned on a rest, the lower arm flexed in front of the head.
- Incisions are similar to VATS lobectomy (see 📖 p686).

Lung resection

- The bullous disease in the apex of the lung can be decompressed with cautery or scissors.
- Resection of tissue follows the same principles as the open technique.

Postoperative care and complications

- Patients should be extubated in the operating room.
- Epidural catheters should be liberally used or PCA.
- Aggressive pulmonary toilet is essential.

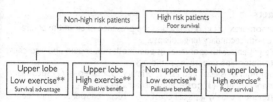

Fig. 14.5 Algorithm for surgical treatment of emphysema. ** Low and high exercise refers to exercise capacity.

- Supraventricular arrhythmias occur in 20% of patients and should be treated, though amiodarone should be avoided secondary to risk of pulmonary fibrosis.
- Bowel prophylaxis to avoid stress ulcers, and laxatives to avoid constipation secondary to narcotic use.
- 30-day hospital mortality, 3% after sternotomy and 2.1% after VATS (P=0.74).[1]

Prolonged air leak
- Most common complication is air leak.
- 54% after sternotomy and 66% after VATS.[1]
- Chest tubes should remain on water seal.
- Patients may eventually go home with Heimlich valves.

Reference
1. NETT Research Group. Safety and efficacy of median sternotomy versus video-assisted thoracic surgery for lung volume reduction surgery. *J Thorac Cardiovasc Surg* 2004; **127**:1350–60.

Pneumothorax

Key facts

- Pneumothorax (PTx) is defined as the presence of air in the pleural space with secondary lung collapse.
- Stable patients with spontaneous pneumothorax should undergo chest CT to determine underlying pathology.
- Pneumothorax is classified as: (1) primary spontaneous, (2) secondary spontaneous, and (3) post-traumatic/iatrogenic.
- Treatment is usually a pigtail chest tube: recurrent penumothoraces secondary to apical blebs may require VATS pleurodesis.

Primary spontaneous pneumothorax

Commonly seen in young, tall, male smokers. The lifetime risk of primary spontaneous PTx in smoking males is 12% vs. 0.1% in non-smoking males. More common on the right side. ≈10% of cases are bilateral. Usually caused by rupture of small subpleural blebs (collections of air <2cm). Usually found at the apex of the upper lobe or the apical segment of the lower lobe. The rest of the lung parenchyma is normal. May also be caused by rupture of bullae.

Presentation

- Dyspnea, chest pain, cough, tachypnea.
- Ipsilateral decreased chest wall movement, hyper-resonant hemithorax to percussion, absent breath sounds on auscultation, pleural rub, tachycardia. Rarely as tension pneumothorax (🔲 p823).

Investigations

- PA CXR usually diagnostic.
- CT scan gives an accurate estimate of size of pneumothorax and is useful for assessment of remaining lung parenchyma and contralateral lung. High-resolution fine slice CT will demonstrate apical blebs.

Complications

- Tension PTx (emergency chest tube, 🔲 p248).
- Pneumomediastinum.
- Haemopneumothorax.
- Recurrent PTx.

Conservative management

- Observation (unilateral, small <20% pneumothorax, no apical blebs).
- Trial of needle aspiration if minimal symptoms and moderate PTx.
- Tube thoracostomy if compromised or very large PTx.

Surgery

- Surgery is indicated in the following cases;
- *First episode:* prolonged air leak (>72h) tension PTx, hemothorax, bilateral pneumothoraces, residual collapse of lung, 100% PTx, occupational hazard, PTx secondary to giant bulla, previous contralateral pneumonectomy.
- *Recurrence of PTx:* the aim is to resect the blebs or bullae and obliterate the pleural space with adhesions either using chemical or abrasion pleurodesis or parietal pleurectomy (apical or full). It may be performed through a minithoracotomy, axillary incision, or thoracoscopically.

Recurrence rate
- <2% following surgical pleurectomy via minithoracotomy.
- 5% after VATs pleurodesis, 5–10% following chemical pleurodesis.

Secondary spontaneous pneumothorax

These patients are frequently sicker patients with primary spontaneous PTx, less likely to resolve with needle aspiration, more likely to be compromised. Formal chest tube is usually the first-line option.

Causes
- Cystic fibrosis, asthma, COPD and other bullous disease. Be wary of confusing a large bulla with a pneumothorax—inserting a chest tube could cause a tension pneumothorax. Get a CT if any doubt.
- Interstitial lung disease.
- Infections, e.g., mycobacterial, *Pneumocystis jiroveci (carinii)*, parasitic, mycotic.
- Malignancy: bronchogenic, metastatic (sarcoma and lymphoma).
- Collagen diseases, catamenial, Ehlers–Danlos syndrome, histiocytosis X, scleroderma, lymphangioleiomyomatosis, Marfan syndrome.
- Rupture of the esophagus.
- *Cystic fibrosis:* PTx found in 10% of patients. Remember these patients are possible candidates for future lung transplantation when considering management options. Full parietal pleurectomy is a contraindication to lung transplantation, but pleurodesis is not.
- *COPD:* the most common cause of secondary pneumothorax. Age usually >50 years. Patients often have very little pulmonary reserve. They may not tolerate surgical management and single-lung ventilation. Treatment options are tube thoracoscopy and chemical pleurodesis or long-term tube thoracoscopy.
- *Infection:* cavitating pulmonary lesions rupture into pleural space.
- *AIDS:* Usually secondary to *Pneumocystis jiroveci (carinii)*, and pneumonia. May be presenting feature of AIDS. Most effective treatment is surgical.
- *Catamenial:* age 20–30 years. Incidence 3–6% of women. Occurs 2–3 days following onset of menstruation. Right side more commonly affected. Usually small, presenting with dyspnea and chest pain. Pathogenesis unclear. May be a result of ectopic endometrial tissue on the diaphragm, or pleura, and possible diaphragmatic defects. Treatment is VATS resection of endometrial deposits, blebs, mechanical pleurodesis, and oral contraceptive therapy.

Primary spontaneous pneumomediastinum

- Uncommon. Males affected more frequently than females. Occurs after exertion or increased intra-abdominal pressure. Associated with cocaine, marijuana, and crack cocaine use. Caused by rupture of alveolar sacs with air tracking along peribronchial and perivascular spaces into neck.

Presentation: sudden onset chest pain, dyspnea, dysphagia, cough, subcutaneous emphysema over chest wall, Hamman's sign. CXR confirms diagnosis. *Management:* non-operative. Need for emergency surgical decompression rare.

Pleural effusion

Key facts

- Pleural effusions are abnormal collections of pleural fluid in the pleural space, which exceed the lymphatic drainage capacity.
- Pleural effusions are determined by Light's criteria to be transudative or exudative.

Exudate versus transudate

- *Exudate*: specific gravity is >1.02, protein content >2.0g/dL, and at least one of the following: ratio of pleural fluid protein to serum >0.5, ratio of pleural fluid LDH and serum >0.6, total pleural fluid LDH >2/3 upper limit of normal, ratio of pleural fluid albumin and blood <1.2.
- Other lab results that are not part of **Light's criteria**, but are suggestive of an exudative effusion are glucose <60 mg/dL, leukocyte count >10 000/mL, pH <7.20, and elevated amylase.
- *Transudates* are generally 'simple' effusions that result from capillary leak syndromes, or increases in hydrostatic or oncotic pressure. Examples of transudative effusions include congestive heart failure, cirrhosis of the liver, nephrotic syndrome, sarcoidosis, and increased pulmonary hydrostatic pressure from pulmonary emboli.
- Examples of exudates include malignant effusions, chylothorax, hemothorax, empyema, pancreatitis, esophageal leak, collagen vascular disorders, autoimmune disorders, uremia, and postmyocardial infarction syndrome.
- Transudates are caused by cirrhosis of the liver, nephrotic syndrome, glomerulonephritis, congestive heart failure, myxedema, sarcoidosis, multiple pulmonary emboli.

Clinical presentation

- Small effusions are often asymptomatic. Larger effusions cause cough, chest pain, dyspnea.
- Decreased ipsilateral chest expansion, dullness to percussion, decreased breath sounds over the effusion on auscultation, crepitations may be heard.

Investigations

- *CXR:* small effusions are demonstrated by blunting of the costodiaphragmatic angles, larger effusions produce a fluid level with a meniscus. Decubitus films can determine free-flowing fluid versus loculated fluid. Blunting of the costophrenic angle on a PA view often represents at least 400mL of fluid.
- *US scan:* useful for loculated effusions, helps to localize optimal site for chest drainage.
- *CT scan:* useful when looking at underlying lung and pleural lesions. Gold standard in identifying fluid loculations, entrapped lung, and surgical planning.
- *Pleural aspiration cytology:* may obtain diagnostic information, helpful when planning treatment. Can provide Light's criteria information as well as other analysis such as Gram's stain.

Management

- Chest tube placement, either small bore or large bore (28F). May not be completely successful in loculated effusions.
- VATS evacuation of pleural fluid ± decortication, ± pleurodesis (see 🕮 p734).
- For effusions that have been present >2 weeks or are associated with chest wall tenderness, or have a calcific peel or rind, VATS may not allow for successful lung expansion.[1]
- During VATS exploration, a pleural biopsy should be performed to evaluate for cause of effusion.
- Thoracotomy with decortication (see 🕮 p706).

Malignant pleural effusion

- Malignant pleural effusions are exudative and are the result of tumor invading pleural lymphatics and reducing the absorptive capacity of the pleural space.
- Pleural effusions as the result of lymphoma may respond to chemotherapy, but most malignant pleural effusions have a poor prognosis.
- Symptoms include insidious progressive dyspnea, with eventual mediastinal shift.
- Only 20% of thoracentesis yield diagnostic cytology.
- Malignant pleural effusions are often bloody.
- Treatment: thoracentesis should be done initially to determine if the lung expands or not. 98% of malignant effusions recur within 30 days.
- If the lung expands, then a VATS evacuation and pleurodesis can be successful.
- VATS also provides pleural tissue to confirm tumor deposits.

Complications

- Supper infections causing empyema.
- Treatment failure with recurrence of pleural effusion.
- Damage to underlying lung parenchyma, resulting in prolonged air leak.

Reference

1. Luh SP et al. Video-assisted thoracoscopic surgery in the treatment of complicated parapneumonic effusions or empyemas: outcome of 234 patients. Chest 2005; 127(4): 1427–32.

Pleurodesis

Key facts

- Pleurodesis is any procedure designed to cause the parietal and visceral pleura to adhere together, obliterating the pleural space with a view to preventing recurrent pneumothoraces or pleural effusions.
- This can be achieved by two mechanisms: abrasion pleurodesis (where the parietal pleura is abraded) or chemical pleurodesis (where talc or other agent is instilled into the pleural space).
- Pleurodesis can be performed via a chest tube, VATS, or open.

Procedure

Set-up

- General ET anesthesia.
- The patient in the *lateral, decubitus position* (📖 p39) using sandbags, or rolls and tape, usually with the upper arm positioned on a rest.
- Incisions are as for VATS lobectomy without the large working port.

Dealing with underlying pathology

- Evacuate any pleural effusion to dryness, sending samples for cytology (the more, the better), microbiology, and biochemistry. Inspect whole hemithorax, sending samples of abnormal pleural plaques for histology.
- If pleurodesis is being performed for pneumothorax, carefully inspect the lung parenchyma, particularly the apices of the upper lobe for any apical blebs, which should be stapled and send for histology. Blebs commonly appear in the apical or anterior segments of the upper lobes, the lateral segment of the middle lobe, and the superior segment of the lower lobes.
- If no blebs are found, the lung apex is resected prophylactically.

Pleurodesis

- Mechanical pleurodesis uses an electrocautery scratch pad or sterile scratch paper to abrade the parietal pleural of the chest wall to the point of visual tissue disruption and hyperemia.
- Chemical pleurodesis can be done by insufflating talc, docycline, or bleomycin.
- Talc is cheaper and probably more effective.
- 4–6g of aerosolized talc is insufflated into the pleural space, taking care to occlude all ports (so that it does not simply mostly escape) and carefully coat all areas of the lung and chest wall. Mechanical pleurodesis does not prevent additional blebs from forming and subsequent spontaneous PTx but may prevent complete lung collapse and tension pneumothorax.
- Talc pleurodesis are avoided in young patients, as the long-term side effects of talc are unclear, and talc pleurodesis leads to false-positive PET activity in the pleura, which may confound potential cancer staging in the future.
- Talc may be used in elderly patients, secondary spontaneous PTx, and patients with primary spontaneous PTx who have failed initial mechanical pleurodesis.
- The lung is inflated under thoracscopic vision after chest tubes placed.

- Chest tubes remain on continuous suction for 72h, and are removed when output is <200mL for 24h.

Stage I empyema
- Talc should be avoided where coinciding pleural space infection is suspected.
- Docycline may be useful for pleurodesis for effusions where infection cannot be ruled out.
- Instil solution of 500mg of doxicycline in 50mL of saline.
- If the lung does not expand, then a pleurodesis will not be effective, and a chronic indwelling pleural catheter should be placed.

Malignant pleural effusion
- An entrapped lung secondary to malignant pleural effusion should not be decorticated.
- There are commercially available indwelling pleural catheter kits.
- These catheters can be placed in the OR or at the bedside.
- Patients can drain their own pleural space when symptomatic.
- Often the catheters can eventually be removed if no need for drainage for 2 weeks.
- Complications include infection, discomfort, purchasing of catheter and bottle system.

Bedside (chest tube) pleurodesis
- If the patient is a poor surgical candidate, then a pleurodesis can be done at the bedside by inserting pleurodesing agent through a large-bore chest tube (24–28F).
- 4–6g of talc is suspended in 120mL saline to form a slurry, and inserted into the chest tube.
- The chest tube is clamped for 1h, and the patient undergoes position changes every 15min: supine left lateral decubitus, right lateral decubitus, and reverse Trendelenburg.
- The tube is unclamped, and the patient is placed on continuous suction for 72h. The chest tube is removed if total output is <200mL for 24h.

Outcomes
- VATS talc pleurodesis is 95% effective, bedside pleurodesis 75%.
- Pain is common secondary to inflammation of the parietal pleura.
- Often talc slurries can be mixed with 1% lidocaine to limit the pain. Patients may need a PCA. NSAIDs such as ibuprofen and ketorolac should be avoided as they may decrease inflammatory response and subsequently limit an effective pleurodesis.
- Fever caused by local inflammation, treated with acetaminophen.
- SIRS due to over-administration of talc: pulmonary insufficiency and hypotension.
- Two or more of the following: tachypnea >20 breaths/min, tachycardia >90bpm, temperature >38°C or <36°C, or WBC >12 000 or <4000.
- Limiting the amount of talc used to ≤ 6g, and not performing bilateral talc pleurodesis during the same setting.

Pleurectomy

Key facts

- Removal of the parietal pleura is another way of getting the visceral pleura to adhere completely to the chest wall, obliterating the pleural space and preventing recurrent pneumothorax.
- It is usually performed via VATS or a minithoracotomy in the axilla or posterolaterally

Pleural anatomy

- The pleura consists of mesothelial cells forming the visceral pleura which lines the outer aspects of the lung and the parietal pleura which lines the chest wall, mediastinum, pericardium, diaphragm, and other extrapulmonary organs of the chest cavity.
- The potential space between the visceral and parietal pleura contains pleural fluid, which lubricates the space, and allows for easy movement of the lung.
- The amount of pleural fluid produced is 0.01mL/kg/h or 200mL/24h.
- Pleural fluid is reabsorbed via the pulmonary lymphatics for the visceral pleura and direct lymphatic channels permeating the parietal pleura.
- Venous drainage is via the peribronchial veins.
- The parietal pleura contains afferent nerve fibers which can transmit pain signals, and is the layer that should be anesthetized during chest tube placement.

Procedure

Set-up

- General ET anesthesia with lung isolation if VATS.
- The patient is positioned in the *lateral, decubitus position* (🕮 p39) with spine parallel to and close to the edge of the table, using sandbags, or rolls and tape, usually with the upper arm positioned on a rest, the lower arm flexed in-front of the head.

Procedure

- The aim is removal of the parietal pleura from the 4th intercostal space up to the apex, as well as addressing likely causes which are usually apical blebs which should be stapled first as they are easiest to see at the beginning of the case.
- The parietal pleura is then peeled off the chest wall either starting at the minithoracotomy incision or at the port site opposite the camera in a VATS.
- Once you have a lip of pleura big enough to grab with a tonsil clamp or a Roberts, then a gentle winding action wraps the pleura around the clamp, peeling it off the chest wall.
- An apical and basal chest tube are replaced and the lung carefully checked to make sure it re-expands.

Closure

Insufflation with 10–20mL 0.25% bupivacaine helps postoperative pain, along with the usual costal block.

Chylothorax

Chylothorax

Key facts

- Chylothorax is the abnormal collection of lymphatic fluid in the pleural space, usually as a result of disruption of the thoracic duct or one of its tributaries.
- It usually occurs after inadvertent damage to the thoracic duct or its tributaries during mediastinal dissection, rapidly accumulating in chest tubes as a milky fluid once the patient resumes normal diet, or forming a pleural collection.
- Pleural fluid triglycerides >110mg/dL and pleural fluid to cholesterol level ratio <1 is diagnostic.
- It usually resolves with adequate pleural drainage and a low-triglyceride diet, but occasionally surgical repair is required.

Pathology

- The thoracic duct is a valved lymph channel that originates in the abdomen as the **cisterna chyli**, forming from vessels draining the lower limbs and vessels, entering the right thoracic cavity via the esophageal hiatus at T10–T11, travelling cephalad between the spine, descending aorta, esophagus, and azygos vein, crossing over to the left side at T4–T6. It drains into the left subclavian or jugular vein above the clavicle.
- 1.5–2.5L of chyle is produced per day, and may decrease or increase depending on the level of fat in the diet.
- Aetiology includes: trauma, iatrogenic surgical injury, malignancy, tuberculosis, mediastinitis, pancreatitis, SVC, left jugular or subclavian vein thrombosis, idiopathic, and congenital thoracic duct atresia or fistula.
- Chyle leaks have been described after almost all thoracic procedures, including left subclavian central venous line placement, but most commonly after procedures involving extensive posterior mediastinal dissection at the base of the heart, or around the esophagus.
- Spontaneous chyle leaks in adults are almost always associated with malignancy, and are secondary to obstruction of the lymphactics.

Presentation and investigation

- Diagnosis is often clinical, based on clinical suspicion and the presence of milky white fluid (pink if mixed with blood postoperatively).
- Patients who are nil by mouth may exhibit only straw-colored chyle fluid.
- Pleural fluid triglycerides >110 mg/dL and pleural fluid to cholesterol level ratio <1 is diagnostic.

Management

- Initial management is medical: nil by mouth, drainage of pleural space with chest tubes, parental nutrition, and/or medium-chain triglyceride diet.
- Octreotide (80mg, sc, 3 times daily) may reduce lymphatic flow.
- Some reported success of the percutaneous thoracic duct embolization, however this is a selective skill set that that not many interventional radiologists possess.
- Pleuroperitoneal shunts have been used for diffuse leaks, e.g., SVCO and lymphangiomatosis: they can be placed under local anesthetic.

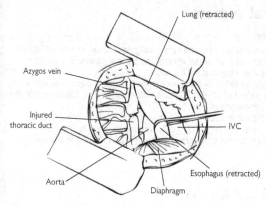

Fig. 14.6 Right thoracotomy approach to ligation of thoracic duct.

Indications for surgery
- Hypoalbuminemia, leukopenia, malnutrition secondary to chyle loss.
- 1–2L loss per day, for 1–2 weeks.

Surgical repair of thoracic duct
- Goal of surgery is thoracic duct ligation ± talc pleurodesis.
- May be done by VATS or open thoracotomy on the side of the chylothorax (or in the case of bilateral chylothorax starting on the right).
- Prior to surgery, patient is fed a high-fat diet, 6h before surgery, via a nasogastric or feeding tube, the patient is fed 80–100mL of cream per hour. This allows for marked expression of milky fluid from the disrupted thoracic duct, and facilitates identification of the injury.

Set-up
- General ET anesthesia.
- The patient in the *lateral, decubitus position* (🕮 p39) using sandbags, or rolls and tape, usually with the upper arm positioned on a rest.
- Posterloateral thoracotomy in 7th or 8th intercostal space, unless previous incision in which case reopen this.
- If a specific leak is identified this is ligated with non absorbable sutures, and the thoracic duct is also ligated as it enters the thorax through the aortic hiatus by retracting the esophagus anteriorly (Fig. 14.6).
- If the duct cannot be specifically clipped or ligated, then a mass ligation where the duct should be is performed near the diaphragmatic hiatus. This involves opening the parietal pleural overlying the descending aorta, mobilizing the distal esophagus, and mass ligating all tissue between the azygos vein, esophagus, aorta. and spine.

Results of surgery
Resolution of chyle leak after surgical ligation in 85% of patients.

Pleural tumors

Key facts

- Mesothelioma is a rare and highly malignant tumor, usually unilateral, of mesothelial cells of the visceral and parietal pleura. The median survival after diagnosis is 12 months.
- The majority (80%) of cases is caused by asbestos exposure, with a latency period of at least 20 years, incidence is rising. Often seen in the 6th to 7th decade of life.
- Other pleural masses include benign pleural plaques or asbestosis (which have no potential for deteriorating to mesothelioma); metastatic tumors to pleura, e.g., thymoma, NSCLC, and fibrous tumors.

Mesothelioma

Pathology

- Male to female ratio of 5:1.
- There is no direct link between smoking and mesothelioma.
- The majority (80%) of cases are caused by asbestos exposure, with a latency period of at least 20 years, incidence is rising due to industrial exposure in previous decades. Two types of asbestos fiber have different risk of causing mesothelioma:
  - *Serpentine fibers* are large, and have poor tissue penetration, so lower risk of causing mesothelioma.
  - *Amphibiole fibers* are small, and travel through the bronchioles to the pleural surface, associated with higher risk of mesothelioma.
- Other risk factors include radiation exposure, liquid paraffin, rubber, copper, fiberglass, nickel, aerosolized glass, industrial mineral oil, tuberculosis, pleuritis and other chronic pleural infections, hereditary, familial Mediterranean fever.
- At-risk individuals include construction workers, mechanics, pipe fitters, military personnel with contact with pre-Vietnam era ships and planes, and family members of all of these individuals who would have been exposed to their clothing.
- *Histology:* vimentin –ve and cytokeratin +ve. Three tumor types:
  - Epithelial: commonest histology and most favorable prognosis.
  - Sarcomatoid: least favorable prognosis.
  - Mixed epithelial and sarcomatoid: also with poorer prognosis than pure epithelial.
- Tumor usually unilateral, (although majority of patients have occult metastases at death—abdomen, contralateral lung). Progresses locally encasing lung, and invading chest wall, diaphragm, and mediastinum.

Presentation

May be asymptomatic. Patients usually present in their 6th or 7th decade with fatigue, chest pain, dyspnea, weight loss, cough, fever, weakness, anorexia (Horner's syndrome, hemoptysis, spontaneous pneumothorax, dysphagia). *Examination:* pleural effusions are an early finding. Diminished lung expansion on affected side. Dullness to percussion. Decreased breath sounds on auscultation. Much less commonly palpable chest wall mass, palpable supraclavicular lymph nodes.

Investigation
- CXR may demonstrate pleural thickening and any pleural effusion.
- CT scan helpful when staging tumor and monitoring response to treatment: PET CT to identify distant metastases.
- MRI useful for detection of mediastinal and brain involvement.
- Pleural biopsy to obtain histological diagnosis (tumor seeding of incision common: liaise with surgeons/oncologist to plan site).
- Pleural fluid cytology is positive in up to half of patients.

Treatment
- Primarily palliative: VATS talc pleurodesis (📖 p734) can ameliorate symptoms from malignant pleural effusion, and is often the route to obtaining definitive histological confirmation of diagnosis.
- Pleurodesis may make subsequent pleurectomy easier.
- Curative intent: multimodality therapy combining radiation and often doxorubicin-based chemotherapy with surgery (extrapleural pneumonectomy 📖 p745) is the therapeutic approach of choice.

Outcomes
Median survival from diagnosis is 12–18 months.

Fibrous pleural tumors
Pathology
- Rare tumors that tend to occur in the 6th decade of life; may be benign (80%) or malignant and have no association with asbestos exposure.
- Originate from the mesenchymal layer beneath the mesothelial layer.
- Men and women are affected equally.
- May be pedunculated or sessile.
- *Histology:* vimentin +ve and cytokeratin −ve:
  - Benign: arise from parietal or visceral pleura, though more commonly the visceral pleura. Usually small. Few mitosis with <4 per high powered field (HPF).
  - Malignant: often sessile and non-pedunculated, characterized by increased cellularity and >4 mitosis per HPF, with pleomorphism.

Presentation and investigation
Often asymptomatic, dyspnea, pleural effusion, pleuritic chest pain, hypertrophic pulmonary osteoarthropathy (clubbing), and hypoglycemia from tumor secreting insulin-like growth factors. CXR and chest CT.

Treatment
- Pedunculated lesions may require only VATS local resection.
- Sessile and large lesions may require VATS or open resection with associated lobectomy or *en bloc* resection of adjacent tissue such as the chest wall.

Outcomes
- Benign tumors with R0 resection have a <10% recurrence rate.
- Malignant tumors with R0 resection have a 14–63% recurrence rate and 30% mortality.

Staging mesothelioma

Key facts

- Staging based on thoracic surgical anatomic principles.[1]
- Staged using TNM tumor classification, but various other staging systems exist.

Stages

- Stage I: disease confined within the capsule of the parietal pleura (including the ipsilateral pleura, lung, pericardium, and diaphragm).
- Stage II: all of stage I with positive N1 and/or N2 lymph nodes.
- Stage III: local extension into the chest wall, mediastinum, heart, through the diaphragm or peritoneum, but no N3 or distal node involvement.
- Stage IV: distant metastatic disease.
- Staging based on the International Mesothelioma Interest Group [2]

Tumor stage

- T1a: tumor limited to ipsilateral parietal pleura with no involvement of the visceral pleura.
- T1b: tumor limited to ipsilateral parietal pleura with involvement of the visceral pleura.
- T2: tumor involving all of the ipsilateral pleural surfaces with at least one of the following features: Extension from visceral pleura into the underlying pulmonary parenchyma or involvement of the diaphragm.
- T3: locally advanced but resectable tumor. Tumor involving all of the ipsilateral pleural surfaces with at least one of the following features: extension into mediastinal fat, involvement of the endothoracic fascia, non-transmural involvement of the pericardium or solitary foci of tumor extending to the soft tissues of the chest wall.
- T4: locally advanced and technically unresectable tumor. Tumor involves all of the ipsilateral pleural surfaces with at least one of the following features: direct extension to mediastinal organs, contralateral pleura, spine, or peritoneum.

Nodal stage

- Nx: lymph nodes cannot be assessed.
- N0: no regional lymph node metastasis.
- N1: ipsilateral hilar or peribronchial lymph nodes.
- N2: ipsilateral mediastinal lymph nodes.
- N3: contralateral mediastinal lymph nodes, or ipsilateral or contralateral supraclavicular lymph nodes.

Metastases

- Mx: distant metastases cannot be assessed.
- M0: no distant metastases.
- M1: distant metastases.

Staging
- Stage Ia: T1aN0M0.
- Stage IB: T1bN0M0.
- Stage II: T2N0M0.
- Stage III: T3N0M0 or any T and N1 or N2.
- Stage IV: T4N0M0, or any TN3M0 or any T, any N and M1.

Staging for possible curative resection

Curative resection, which is invariably combined with multimodal therapy, carries substantial morbidity, and patients who will benefit from this strategy must not have metastatic disease, and must be able to tolerate not only pneumonectomy, but also the additional respiratory embarrassment caused by diaphragmatic resection. Routine staging (in addition to a detailed cardiopulmonary assessment) of patients being considered for extrapleural pneumonectomy includes:
- MRI brain and chest (to identify metastatic spread and local mediastinal invasion).
- CT of chest and abdomen with contrast with PET scan.
- Bronchoscopy and EGD.
- Staging laparoscopy with peritoneal lavage.
- Mediastinoscopy.

References

1. Sugarbaker DJ et al. Node status has prognostic significance in the multimodality therapy of diffuse, malignant mesothelioma. *J Clin Oncol* 1993; **11**(6):1172–8.
2. Rusch VW. A proposed new international TNM staging system for malignant pleural mesothelioma. From the International Mesothelioma Interest Group. *Chest* 1995; **108**(4):1122–8.

Treatment of mesothelioma

Key facts
- *Multimodality therapy* combining radiation and often doxorubicin-based chemotherapy with surgery is the therapeutic approach of choice: there is almost no role for surgery in isolation.
- At presentation the majority of patients are candidates only for palliation: VATS talc pleurodesis palliates malignant pleural effusion.
- *Tumor seeding* means that surgical biopsy and pleurodesis, even in palliative patients, should be planned with the involvement of the oncologist and the surgeon likely to perform pneumonectomy, as the port site should be where it can readily be excised as part of the thoracotomy incision, or irradiated without causing radiation pneumonitis.
- *Extrapleural pneumonectomy*, and occasionally *lung-sparing tumor resection* are the two options for surgery with curative intent. Choice is partially dictated by planned adjuvant therapy—if radiation is planned then pneumonectomy must be performed to avoid radiation pneumonitis.

VATS biopsy and pleurodesis for mesothelioma
- This differs from VATS biopsy and pleurodesis for other conditions, because of the high incidence of *tumor seeding* along incision and biopsy sites.
- A single-port technique is used.

Procedure
- In advanced cases where extensive pleural plaque is shown on CT but large effusion is not a component, it is often possible and desirable to obtain a biopsy of the parietal plaque without entering the pleural space to reduce the risk of air leak and infection.
  - A small skin incision (10mm in thin individuals 3–4cm in obese patients) is made based on where the CT scan indicates extensive parietal involvement, and the tissue carefully separated until the thick white rind is encountered.
  - This is biopsied taking care not to breach the pleural space, and checked by irrigating the wound with saline and ventilating the lung: the saline should not disappear, and there should be no air bubbles.
  - This is closed in layers with absorbable sutures.
- Where the primary goal is biopsy of less advanced disease or pleurodesis, a 15mm port site is created at a suitable location.
  - A 30° angled scope is introduced carefully into the pleural space.
  - A biopsy forceps is introduced using the same incision.
  - Avoid biopsying visceral lesions to minimize the risk of an air leak.
  - Take multiple biopsies from multiple sites.
  - After insufflating talc inflate the lung under direct vision, ensuring it expands as fully as possible without air leaks, and close the incision in layers carefully, with absorbable sutures.

Extrapleural pneumonectomy

Set-up

- General ET anesthesia, bronchoscopy (contralateral endobronchial mesothelioma is a contraindication to curative resection).
- Place NG tube (enables esophagus to be readily palpated).
- Reposition the patient in the *lateral, decubitus position* (📖 p39) using sandbags, or rolls and tape, and recheck lung isolation.
- Posterolateral thoracotomy in 7th or intercostal space, excising previous biopsy sites as full thickness ellipses down to muscle, trying to keep serratus intact, and excising 7th rib in subperiosteal fashion.

Extrapleural pneumonectomy

- The plane between the 8th rib and the parietal pleura is developed with a combination of cautery, scissors, and finger dissection, and the same is done with the 6th rib so that a retractor can be inserted.
- Dissection results in diffuse bleeding which can be cauterized using argon beam or spray settings on standard electrocautery.
- Structures to pay particular attention to include the azygos, esophagus, and IVC on the right, and the descending aorta on the left.
- The lung and tumor mass is bulky, usually making it difficult to complete the hilar dissection before the lung is completely mobilized.
- Once the tumor is completely separated from the bony chest wall, it is dissected off the pericardium which occasionally offers a reasonable plane. Pericardial involvement mandates resection: the pericardium is repaired using a Gore-Tex patch ensuring adequate 'give' to prevent hemodynamic compromise, and incised to prevent tamponade.
- The diaphragm is preserved is possible: if a small resection is performed the defect is closed primarily. Large defects are patched, taking care to preserve the phrenic nerve.
- The pulmonary artery and veins are divided, and the bronchus is divided flush with the carina, full mediastinal lymph node dissection is carried out, on right-sided resections the thoracic duct is ligated.
- Meticulous care is taken closing the wound.

Outcomes

- Operative mortality is 4–10% depending on patient selection.
- Mesothelioma generally carries a poor prognosis regardless of therapy; some studies have reported up to 50% survival in the most favorable of clinical characteristics, but 10-year survival is near 0%.
- Intraoperative instilled intrathoracic heated cisplatin immediately after extrapleural pneumonectomy has been described.

Diaphragmatic hernia

Key facts

- These hernias may be congenital hernia defects in the diaphragm that occur at anatomic points of weakness (Fig. 14.7). With time, these points of weakness allow the herniation of abdominal contents into the mediastinum or hemithorax.
- Acquired hernias can be sliding esophageal, or paraesophageal hernias (📖 p788), or occasionally due to trauma, presenting early or late after both penetrating and blunt trauma.
- Treatment is usually surgical, to prevent intestinal obstruction and respiratory compromise: repair must take into account blood and nerve supply of the diaphragm (Fig. 14.7) to preserve function.

Bochdalek hernia

- *Pathology:* rare hernia that occurs in 1 in 5000 births. Due to *in utero* failure of pleuro-peritoneal folds to join, resulting in a left-sided posterior defect (Fig. 14.7). 1/3 have other congenital abnormalities.
- *Presentation:* often asymptomatic. If occurs *in utero*, may develop pulmonary hypoplasia: these infants may be critically ill. In adulthood dyspnea, atypical chest pain, tachycardia, bowel obstruction.
- *Investigation:* ultrasound, CXR, and chest CT.
- *Management:* surgical therapy is recommended even if asymptomatic, although timing challenging as infants may require ECMO support.
  - Reduction of hernia contents and primary closure best accomplished via transverse incision 3cm below costal margin.
  - Identify and resect the hernia sac to prevent cyst formation.
  - Defect can be closed primarily if small or closed with mesh.
  - Viscera may need to be accommodated in prosthetic silo.
  - Mortality 12–50%.

Hernia of Morgagni

- *Pathology:* represents only 5% of the congenital defects of the diaphragm. Occurs in the space of Larrey between the xiphoid process and distal body of the sternum and the costochondral attachments of the diaphragm (Fig. 14.7) where IMA passes through diaphragm to become superior epigastric artery. More commonly occurs on the right side. Predilection towards females. Rare in children.
- *Presentation:* often asymptomatic, but can have symptoms of dyspnea, bowel obstruction, and atypical chest pain.
- *Investigation:* CXR and chest CT.
- *Management:* surgical repair. Usually via subcostal or midline laparotomy, or laparoscopy. Principles include reduction of hernia contents, resection of the hernia sac, and reinforcement of the hernia repair with mesh if of significant size.

Traumatic diaphragmatic hernias

- *Pathology:* occasional complication of penetrating or blunt trauma. Usually stomach or small intestine herniates. Predominantly left-sided.

- *Presentation:* often asymptomatic, but can have symptoms of dyspnea, bowel obstruction, and atypical chest pain. May present months or years after trauma with symptoms of intestinal obstruction.
- *Investigation:* CXR and chest CT.
- *Management:* surgical repair. Usually via posterolateral thoracotomy. . Principles include reduction of hernia contents, resection of the hernia sac, and reinforcement of the hernia repair with mesh.

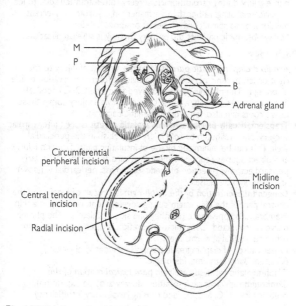

Fig. 14.7 Top image shows location of most common diaphragmatic hernias M (Foramen of Morgagni), B (Bochdalek), P (paraesophageal). Bottom image shows the relationship of phrenic nerve branches to the most commonly used diaphragmatic incisions.

Diaphragmatic paralysis

Key facts

- Congenital (*eventration*) or acquired, where the hemidiaphragm does not contract appropriately.
- This results in paradoxical motion of the diaphragm with respiration, reducing RV, TLC, and VC, and causing respiratory insufficiency.
- Acquired diaphragmatic paralysis is most commonly due to phrenic nerve injury during cardiothoracic surgery (often transient due to ice in pericardial sling, rather than permanent injury from inadvertent division), or to spinal cord injuries at or above C4–5.
- For symptomatic patients the primary therapy is surgical plication.

Pathology

- *Acquired diaphragmatic paralysis* is often a result of injury to the right or left phrenic nerves, which provide efferent innervation to the diaphragm. The phrenic nerve is derived from the C3–C5 cervical nerve roots. As a result, a spinal cord or cervical injury above those nerve roots can also cause diaphragmatic paralysis.
- Transient, usually unilateral, diaphragmatic paresis is seen after cardiac surgery, and attributed to *cold injury* from slush in the pericardial well. This can be minimized by use of insulating pads. Traction injuries, and direct injuries (during thymectomy, cardiac surgery particularly pericardiectomy, resection of mediastinal mass, pericardial window) are less common causes.
- *Congenital eventration of the diaphragm* is a result of a defect in the central part of the diaphragm during development, resulting in a thin membranous appearance of either one side or bilateral. The phrenic nerve is unaffected. Congenital eventration is often associated with other congenital abnormalities.
- Other causes of diaphragmatic paralysis includes viral illness (Guillain–Barré), trauma, idiopathic.
- Diaphragmatic paralysis results in **paradoxical motion of the diaphragm** (upwards on inspiration, downwards on expiration), reducing RV, TLC, and VC, and causing respiratory insufficiency.

Presentation and investigation

- Dyspnea, orthopnea, air hunger. Failure to wean mechanical ventilation.
- CXR shows ipsilateral elevation of the hemidiaphragm in unilateral paralysis, bilateral paresis may be less obvious.
- Fluoroscopy (**sniff test**): documents paradoxical motion of the diaphragm as the patient sniffs quickly, or breathes in, the unaffected diaphragm displaces caudally, while the ipsilateral diaphragm displaces cephalad paradoxically, causing the reduction of ipsilateral lung capacity, and movement of the mediastinum to the contralateral side.
- US: similar principle as the fluoroscopic sniff test, documenting paradoxical motion of the ipsilateral diaphragm with inspiration.
- Pulmonary function tests: spirometry is obtained to have a baseline values, and document improvement post surgical therapy. Spirometry values themselves are not diagnostic.

Management

- Primary therapy is surgery.
- For patients with phrenic nerve injury, surgical therapy of choice is **diaphragm plication.**
- For patients with high cervical lesions (i.e., quadriplegics with lesions above C3, and intact phrenic nerve) **diaphragmatic pacing** may enable patients to wean off of mechanical ventilation.

Indications for surgery

- Presence of symptoms.
- Documented paradoxical motion of the diaphragm.
- No improvement after 6 months.
- In postsurgical or idiopathic etiology, the phrenic nerve may be paretic and not completely disrupted, and may recover with time.

Diaphragmatic plication

- The aim of plication is to immobilize the hemidiaphragm, preventing it from moving in a paradoxical manner.
- Can be performed via posterolateral thoracotomy (6th intercostal space), VATS, or laparoscopically.
- Using a running U stitch (0 Ethibond) and felt pledgets to limit injury to the diaphragmatic muscle, several rows are placed, and when tied, the diaphragm shortens (plicates; Fig. 14.8).
- Care must be taken to grasp and elevated the diaphragm with Allis clamps, to avoid suturing bowel on the other side of the diaphragm (generally not an issue on the right given the presence of the liver).

Diaphragmatic pacing

- Performed in patients with spinal cord injuries, to help wean mechanical ventilation. Pacing electrodes can be placed in the intact phrenic nerve in the neck, chest via VATS or directly into the diaphragm laparoscopically.
- A pacing transmitter controls respiratory rate and duration of inspiration.

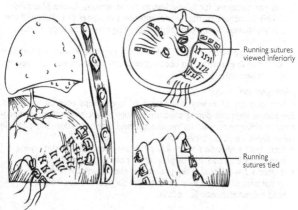

Running sutures viewed inferiorly

Running sutures tied

Fig. 14.8 Diaphragmatic plication.

Tracheomalacia and stenosis

Key facts

- *Tracheomalacia* is characterized by progressive weakening of the walls of the trachea, leading to dynamic (>90%) collapse of the airway with expiration.
- *Tracheal stenosis* is narrowing due congenital or acquired disorders, commonly pressure injury from ET intubation or previous tracheostomy.

Tracheomalacia

Pathology

- May be due to a congenital structural abnormality in the tracheal wall. Associated with esophageal atresia, tracheoesophageal fistula, and double aortic arch. It may occur in isolation.
- Acquired tracheomalacia may occur as a result of trauma, intubation injury, COPD, extrinsic compression of the trachea (e.g., thyroid goiters) and mediastinal tumors.

Presentation

Symptoms are due to respiratory airways obstruction. Barking cough and recurrent pneumonia are common in children. Most severe cases are characterized by cyanosis, apnea, bradycardia and, if untreated, cardiac arrest. This particularly occurs at 2–3 months of age, during or shortly after feeding. In adults some cases of tracheomalacia are not diagnosed until there is failure of extubation following a surgical procedure: most commonly after resection of massive goiters or mediastinal masses.

Investigations

- CXR: shows a narrowing of the trachea on a lateral view.
- Bronchoscopy: confirms diagnosis. The patient must be self-ventilating and not paralyzed for full evaluation of the airways. *Awake fiberoptic flexible bronchoscopy* may reveal anterior and posterior collapse of the tracheal lumen during expiration. Coughing may cause total airway obstruction.
- Dynamic expiratory chest CT also is very sensitive. Pulmonary function tests may demonstrate an obstructive pattern, but are not very specific for tracheomalacia.

Management

Minor degrees of airway collapse in all age groups may be observed. Symptoms improve during childhood. More severe respiratory compromise in children and adults require tracheal stent insertion and possible subsequent surgical intervention.

- *Stent trial*: a silicone Y stent (◻ p753) may be placed to determine if symptoms improve. Mucus plugs are a potential complication.
- If after a 2-week trial, if the patient has marked improvement in symptoms, then they may benefit from surgical therapy from a *tracheobronchoplasty* (◻ p755).

Tracheal stenosis

Pathology

- Congenital: caused by absence of part of membranous portion of tracheal segment. Manifests as multiple, complete, and stenotic tracheal rings. Often associated with other abnormalities of the tracheobronchial tree. Children usually present within the first few months of life with stridor or recurrent pneumonias. Less severe cases may present with exertional stridor.
- Intubation injuries:
  - Prolonged ET intubation with elevated (>20mmHg) cuff pressures (usually circumferential full-thickness lesion).
  - Prior tracheostomy (usually anterior triangular shaped full thickness defect from erosion around the tracheostomy site due to constant movement of the patient relative to the ventilator tubing).
  - If tracheostomy too high, subglottic injury results.
- Chronic inflammatory conditions, e.g., Wegner's granulomatosis.
- Chronic infection such as tuberculosis.

Presentation and investigation

- Symptoms usually appear up to 6 weeks following extubation.
- Clinically significant lesions present as upper airways obstruction, with exertional dyspnea, progressing to wheeze, and finally stridor (which may herald imminent *complete airway obstruction*). At this point the residual airway lumen may be <1cm, and has the potential to be rapidly and completely obstructed by mucus, aspirate, or inflammation, including attempts to intubate.
- Spiral CT scanning with 3D reconstruction (tracheal tomogram) is the investigation of choice, MRI.
- Bronchoscopy is essential in all patients:
  - Flexible awake to evaluate vocal cord function: *do not attempt to pass lesion*—this may result in loss of the residual airway due to inflammation, secretion, or bleeding.
  - Equipment for emergency dilatation and tracheostomy should be available.

Medical management

Observation may be indicated in the very young, especially those with long segment stenosis. Results may be improved if surgery is delayed until the patient is larger.

Surgery

There are several surgical options including:

- Dilation: balloon, Savary guidewire dilation, Jackson dilation via a rigid bronchoscope—this is most use in the setting of inflammation in the region where tracheal resection is planned, and buys time for this to settle before definitive surgery.
- Rigid bronchoscopy for dilation or core-out of granulation tissue.
- Tracheoplasty (🕮 p755) for congenital tracheal stenosis.
- Tracheal resection and reconstruction of the stenotic segment (🕮 p755).

Tracheal tumors

Key facts
Tracheal tumors are rare.

Primary tumors
Incidence rare, <2 per million persons per year. In children most are benign (90%), in adults most are malignant (>90%), mainly squamous cell carcinoma and adenoid cystic carcinoma.

Benign primary tumors
- Epithelial origin: trapilomas (viral etiology HPV6 & 11) increased risk of malignant change in patients HPV11 +ve. Carcinoid tumor: neuroendocrine tumor. Hypervascular.
- Mesenchymal origin: chondroma (most frequent, usually found in the upper trachea), Schwannoma, fibroma, lipoma, neurilemmoma hemangioma, leiomyoma, myoblastoma, polyps.

Malignant primary tumors

Adenoid cystic carcinoma
Male to female ratio 1:1. All age groups. Not related to smoking. Slowly progressive tumors. Spread occurs both circumferentially and longitudinally. Metastatic spread most commonly to lungs, also occasionally to brain, bone, and liver.

Squamous cell carcinoma
Male to female ratio 3:1. Age range 6th and 7th decades. Strongly associated with cigarette smoking. Hemoptysis common. Lymph node metastases at time of diagnosis common.

Rare, malignant primary tracheal tumors
- Spindle cell carcinoma.
- Adenocarcinoma.
- Small-cell carcinoma.
- Chondrosarcoma.
- Leiomyosarcoma.
- Carcinosarcoma.
- Melanoma.
- Synovial cell sarcoma.
- Mucoepidermoid carcinoma.

Presentation and investigation
Clinically significant lesions present as upper airways obstruction, with exertional dyspnea, progressing to wheeze, and finally stridor (which may herald imminent **complete airway obstruction**). At this point the residual airway lumen may be <1cm, and has the potential to be rapidly and completely obstructed by mucus, aspirate, or inflammation, including attempts to intubate. Evaluation includes bronchoscopy ± rigid bronchoscopy, endoscopic biopsy to confirm malignant or benign, neck and chest CT with 3D reconstruction of the trachea, and PET/CT if malignant for staging.

Management

- For malignant tracheal tumors, there is no data to support neoadjuvant chemoradiation.
- Endoscopic techniques such as laser, argon plasma coagulation, cryotherapy, endoluminal stenting can be considered in patients who are poor operative candidates and/or palliative intent.
- Tracheal resection and reconstruction.
- Adjuvant radiation may be considered after resection of aggressive tumors or R1 resections.

Tracheobronchial stents

Indications

Used for both benign and malignant strictures, usually unsuitable for surgical resection, either due to anatomical position or general condition of patient. Most common tracheal strictures are a result of prolonged mechanical ventilation or long-term presence of tracheostomy. Also indicated in the palliation of malignant obstruction either secondary to intraluminal tumor or extrinsic compressions.

Types of stents

Airway stents should be easy to place and replace. They are placed under bronchoscopic visualization. They should not interfere with normal respiration and should have adequate intraluminal diameter to allow clearance of secretions.

- *T-tubes:* made of silicone rubber. Generally very well tolerated. May be left *in situ* for many years. T-tubes are placed through an existing stoma, or a stoma created in the centre of a tracheal stenosis.
- *T-Y tube:* similar to T-tube but longer with Y-shaped extension for placement in to left and right main bronchi.
- *Y-stents:* ideal for patients with distal tracheal, carinal, or proximal main bronchial strictures. Various lengths available.
- *Bronchial stents:* made of silicone. Flanged on both ends to prevent dislodgement.
- *Self-expanding stents:* made from stainless steel or nitinol (nickel + titanium). Uncovered stents are useful when crossing the origin of lobar bronchi as aeration of that lobe is uninterrupted. A covered version of these stents prevents intraluminal growth of either granulation tissue or tumor. Particularly useful in palliation of malignant disease. Also, often covered stents can be temporary.

Complications

- Obstruction secondary to mucous plugging, granulation tissue, tumor, displacement, or anatomical obstruction.
- Erosion into adjacent structures.

Tracheal reconstruction

Contraindications to surgery

- Metastatic disease.
- Long segment (>5cm) of involved trachea, where an anastomosis cannot be accomplished despite releases. Usually in an adult, up to 50% of the trachea can be resected with successful reconstruction.
- Invasion of tumor into adjacent structures other than the esophagus.

Reconstruction of the upper half of the trachea

Set-up

- The patient is positioned with the neck extended. General anesthesia is obtained. A rigid bronchoscopy may need to be performed to dilate and establish an airway. The chest is prepped to allow for a partial sternotomy if needed.
- A collar incision is performed, and skin flaps are made extending to the sternocleidomastoid muscles laterally, cricoid cartilage superiorly and the sternal notch inferiorly.
- The thyroid and anterior trachea is exposed.
- The isthmus of the thyroid is divided and dissected off of the trachea. The pretracheal plane is bluntly dissected. There should be minimal use of cautery, or alternatively a bipolar cautery can be used to avoid injury to the recurrent laryngeal nerves.
- An intraoperative bronchoscopy is performed to identify the location of the stenosis or tumor, and externally a needle is placed to mark the area of the lesion. Traction sutures are placed on either side of the marked area.

Tracheal resection and reconstruction

- The affected area of trachea is resected, and the patient is ventilated using a sterile armored ET tube and cross-table ventilation.
- The traction sutures are used to bring the trachea together, and the head is flexed to relieve tension.
- The trachea is re-anastomosed or reconstructed using 3/0 Vicryl sutures as corner stitches, a 4/0 running PDS for the membranous wall, and interrupted figure-of-eight 3/0 Vicryl sutures for the anterior cartilaginous wall.

Closure

- The wound is closed in layers, no drain is needed.
- A guardian or 'Grillo' 0 silk stitch is placed suturing the chin to the anterior chest wall, not as strength but to remind the patient not extend their neck.

Reconstruction of the lower half of the trachea

- Lower tracheal lesions are best approached via a right posterior lateral thoracotomy through the 4th intercostal space.
- The general surgical techniques and principles are the same for surgical tracheal resection and reconstruction.

Tracheobronchoplasty

Tracheobronchoplasty reconstitutes the normal morphology D shape of the trachea in *tracheomalacia*, and prevents collapse of the membranous wall against the cartilaginous rings.

Set-up
- General ET anesthesia, lung isolation, lateral decubitus.
- Right posterolateral thoracotomy.
- Dissection of the posterior wall.

Reconstruction
- The distal trachea, main bronchi and bronchus intermedius are measured and a Y-shaped polypropylene mesh with 0.5cm lateral overlap fashioned to size.
- Using 4/0 polypropylene interrupted, partial thickness, mattressed sutures, the membranous wall is plicated to the mesh, restoring the anatomic D shape of each ring.

Outcomes
- Perioperative mortality around 5%, with morbidity including respiratory infection (11%) and cardiac arrhythmia (8%).
- Results in significant improvement of quality of life as defined by the St. George Respiratory Questionnaire, Karnofsky performance status, and 6-minute walk test.

Releases

Generally in the adult, 4–5cm of the trachea can be resected and a reconstruction can be performed without tension. A release can be performed to provide an additional 1–2cm of mobility, e.g., *thyrohyoid (Dedo)* or *suprahyoid (Montgomery)* release for upper half reconstructions, and a *hilar release* for lower half reconstructions. The suprahyoid release is favored as it results in less risk to the superior laryngeal nerve.

Suprahyoid release
- Transverse incision is made over the hyoid bone, and the insertions of mylohyoid, geniohyoid, and genioglossus tendons are divided.
- The attachments of the digastric muscles are divided.
- The greater cornu of the hyoid bone are divided. Drain placed.

Hilar release
On the side of the thoracotomy, the pericardium surrounding the pulmonary hilum is incised, and the pulmonary ligament is divided.

Postoperative care and outcomes
- Ideally patients should be extubated at the end of the procedure. There should be aggressive pulmonary toilet. The patient is nil by mouth for 24–48h. A fiberoptic bronchoscopy is performed at the end of the operative procedure and prior to discharge.
- Postoperative complications include pneumonia, arrhythmia, and anastomotic breakdown, especially in patients obese and diabetic patients. Anastomotic complications can be managed with an appliance or stent.
- 1% mortality and 9% anastomotic complications in expert centers.

Foreign body inhalation

Presentation

- Infants and toddlers mainly.
- Male to female ratio 2:1.
- Children usually inhale vegetable matter or nuts whereas adults commonly inhale bones.
- Immediately following inhalation there may be violent bouts of coughing, choking, and gagging with possible complete airway obstruction.
- This is usually followed by an asymptomatic interval, where there is an absence of signs and symptoms as the foreign body becomes lodged.

Upper airway foreign bodies

Usually bone or eggshell. They become lodged between the vocal cords and usually cause complete obstruction.

Tracheal foreign bodies

Usually causes a partial obstruction. There may be an audible slap and palpatory thud.

Bronchial foreign bodies

Signs change rapidly until foreign body lodges within a bronchus. There is wheezing, coughing, and decreased ipsilateral air entry.

Complications

- Obstruction with infection distal to the foreign body.
- Cough, hemoptysis, and fever.
- Atelectasis, lung abscess, pneumonia.
- Bronchial granulation tissue, fistula formation.

Investigation

The majority of foreign bodies are radiolucent. Early radiography will demonstrate air trapping with mediastinal shift to the unaffected side. Radioopaque objects will be seen on chest radiographs. Radiographs taken a week or more after the event may demonstrate atelectasis distal to a foreign body.

Treatment

Usually not a surgical emergency. Endoscopic removal usually performed within 24h of presentation. Flexible instruments should not be used as they are unable to adequately control the airways. A rigid bronchoscope and retrieving forceps are the instruments of choice. If the foreign body is spherical a balloon may be passed deflated beyond the foreign body. It is then inflated and the balloon is withdrawn. This dislodges the object and allows easier extraction.

Postoperative course

Usually uneventful. Any evidence perioperatively of infection should be treated with antibiotics and physiotherapy. Patients are usually admitted for observation overnight.

Esophagus

Epidemiology and clinical features

Key facts

- The commonest malignant esophageal tumors (Box 15.1) worldwide are *squamous cell carcinoma* and *adenocarcinoma*: adenocarcinoma is commonest in the USA where the incidence of squamous cell is falling.
- Most patients present with dysphagia to solids, and eventually liquids.
- 50% of patients have metastatic disease at the time of diagnosis.

Epidemiology and risk factors

- The commonest esophageal cancer in the West is adenocarcinoma. In the USA the incidence of adenocarcinoma is rising faster than the incidence of melanoma, prostate, breast, lung, and colorectal cancer.
- The incidence of squamous cell carcinoma is decreasing.
- In the USA, in 2010 there were an estimated 16 640 new cases of esophageal cancer, with 14 500 deaths (National Cancer Institute, 2010).

Squamous cell carcinoma

Most commonly occurs in the upper 2/3 of the esophagus.

- Smoking and alcohol consumption: synergistic (↑risk 44×).
- Nitrosamines: associated with pickled vegetables and cured meats.
- Diets deficient in vitamins A, C, and riboflavin.
- Previous SCCs of the head and neck.
- Previous external beam therapy.
- Chronic stasis injury:
  - Achalasia.
  - Esophageal webs.
  - Esophageal diverticulum.
- Chronic irritation: caustic burn injury, chronic ingestion of hot foods.
- Celiac disease.
- Tylosis.

Box 15.1 Etiology of esophageal tumors

- Common primary tumors (accounting for >95% of USA cases):
  - Adenocarcinoma.
  - Squamous cell carcinoma.
- Unusual primary tumors:
  - Adenoid cystic carcinoma.
  - Mucoepidermoid carcinoma.
  - Verrucous carcinoma.
  - Small-cell carcinoma.
  - Melanoma.
  - Lymphoma (1–2% of USA cases).
  - Mesenchymal tumors.
- Secondary tumors:
  - Breast.
  - Lung.
  - Stomach.

Adenocarcinoma

Most commonly found in the lower 2/3 of the esophagus.

- Barrett's metaplasia (see 📖 p780):
  - Due to chronic acid exposure (gastroesophageal reflux disease (GERD), 📖 p778).
  - Transformation of usual non-keratinizing stratified squamous epithelium to intestinal columnar epithelium with goblet cells.
  - Estimated annual incidence of malignant transformation 1–2%.
- Male gender:
  - 7× more likely to develop adenocarcinoma than SCC.
  - 3:1 male to female ratio.

Clinical features

- Most patients present with *dysphagia*, initially to solids, then progressing to liquids.
- With cervical lesions, patients often can point directly at point of obstruction, whereas with distal 2/3 lesions, patients have only a vague sense of the point of obstruction.
  - Odynophagia (pain on swallowing).
  - Weight loss.
  - Bleeding, anemia.
  - Aspiration, regurgitation, cough.

Diagnosis

- This is covered in more detail on 📖 pp760–763.
- Patients with dysphagia should undergo a barium esophagram to identify a stricture, and assess its site, length, and severity.
- Abnormalities on esophagram are evaluated with esophagogastroduodenoscopy (EGD). Brushings for cytology, and biopsy of suspicious lesions should be performed.
- Contrast CT of chest and upper abdomen allows accurate assessment of spread, and mediastinal lymph nodes but is less sensitive at assessing invasion into adjacent structures: PET is a useful adjunct to assess spread.

Imaging for diagnosis and staging

Key facts

- Accurate staging of esophageal cancer includes: (1) endoscopy, (2) chest and abdominal CT, (3) PET, and (4) EUS.
- EUS and CT together offer a 79% accuracy for T staging and 82% accuracy for N staging.

Chest and abdominal CT scan

Chest and abdominal contrast CT helps define locoregional spread, invasion of local structures, distant metastasis, and key anatomic structures.

Endoscopic ultrasound

- This is the gold standard for defining T stage: it allows detailed assessment of esophageal wall and surrounding structures.
- Also allows fine needle aspiration (FNA) of suspicious lymph nodes.
- EUS identifies five sonographic layers (Fig. 15.1):
  - Layers 1–2: mucosa.
  - Layer 3: submucosa.
  - Layer 4: muscularis propia.
  - Layer 5: adventitia.
- EUS has several limitations: it is poor at assessing tracheobronchial invasion, may be unable to pass through very tight stenoses, and cannot detect distant metastases.

PET scan

PET is most useful as a combination PET/CT fusion where it has a 78% sensitivity for identifying nodal disease and distant metastasis.

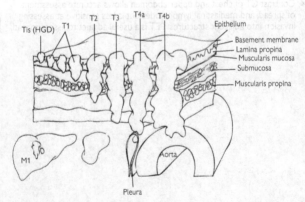

Fig.15.1 Layers of the esophageal wall, as they correspond to the five layers seen in an EUS image.

Staging esophageal cancer

Key facts

See Tables 15.1–15.3 for stage grouping of different cancers.

- Stage 0, I, and IIA cancers are treated with esophagectomy, with postoperative chemoradiotherapy for postsurgical stage IIB and III cancers.
- Localized stage IIB and III are treated with trimodality therapy (📖 p772).

Table 15.1 Stage grouping for esophageal cancer

Primary tumor (T)	
T0:	No evidence of primary tumor
Tis:	Tumor in situ or high-grade dysplasia (HGD)
T1:	Tumor invades lamina propria or submucosa
T2:	Tumor invades muscularis propria
T3:	Tumor invades adventitia
T4a:	Tumor invades resectable structures (e.g., pleura, pericardium, diaphragm)
T4b:	Tumor invades unresectable structures (e.g., aorta, vertebral body, trachea)
Clinical regional lymph nodes (cN)*	
N0:	No regional lymph node metastasis
N1:	Regional lymph node metastasis
Pathologic regional lymph nodes (pN)*	
N0:	No regional lymph node metastasis
N1:	1–2 positive regional lymph nodes
N2:	3–6 positive regional lymph nodes
N3:	≥7 positive regional lymph nodes
Distant metastasis (M)	
M0:	No distant metastasis
M1:	Distant metastasis
Histologic grade (G)	
Gx:	Grade cannot be assessed
G1:	Well differentiated
G2:	Moderately differentiated
G3:	Poorly differentiated
G4:	Undifferentiated

* Defined as periesophageal lymph nodes extending from cervical to celiac nodes.

Adapted from Rice TW et al. Cancer of the esophagus and esophagogastric junction: data-driven staging for the seventh edition of the American Joint Committee on Cancer/ International Union Against Cancer Cancer Staging Manuals. *Cancer* 2010; **116**(16):3763–73.

Table 15.2 Stage groupings for adenocarcinoma

Stage	T	N	M	G
0	Tis (HGD)	0	0	1
IA	1	0	0	1–2
IB	1	0	0	3
	2	0	0	1–2
IIA	2	0	0	3
IIB	3	0	0	Any
	1–2	1	0	Any
	1–2	2	0	Any
IIIA	1–2	2	0	Any
	3	1	0	Any
	4a	0	0	Any
IIIB	3	2	0	Any
IIIC	4a	1–2	0	Any
	4b	Any	0	Any
	Any	3	0	Any
IV	Any	Any	1	Any

Adapted from Rice TW et al. Cancer of the esophagus and esophagogastric junction: data-driven staging for the seventh edition of the American Joint Committee on Cancer/International Union Against Cancer Cancer Staging Manuals. *Cancer* 2010; **116**(16):3763–73.

Table 15.3 Stage groupings for squamous cell carcinoma

Stage	T	N	M	G	Location
0	Tis (HGD)	0	0	1	Any
IA	1	0	0	1	Any
IB	1	0	0	2–3	Any
	2–3			1	
IIA	2–3	0	0	1	Upper[a], middle[b]
	2–3	0	0	2–3	Lower[c]
IIB	2–3	0	0	2–3	Upper[a], middle[b]
	1–2	1	0	Any	Any
IIIA	1–2	2	0	Any	Any
	3	1	0	Any	Any
	4a	0	0	Any	Any
IIIB	3	2	0	Any	Any
IIIC	4a	1–2	0	Any	Any
	4b	Any	0	Any	Any
	Any	3	0	Any	Any
IV	Any	Any	1	Any	Any

[a]Upper thoracic esophagus, bordered superiorly by the thoracic inlet and inferiorly by the azygos vein. Distance from incisors is 20cm to <25cm; [b]Middle thoracic esophagus bordered superiorly by the azygos vein and inferiorly by the inferior pulmonary veins. Distance from incisors is 25cm to <30cm; [c]Lower thoracic esophagus is bordered superiorly by the inferior pulmonary veins and inferiorly by the stomach. It includes EGJ. Distance from incisors is 30–45cm. Stages 0–IIB are amenable to surgical resection.

Esophagectomy: overview

Key facts

- Numerous approaches to esophagectomy, most of which can be divided into esophagectomy *with thoracotomy* and esophagectomy *without thoracotomy* (Table 15.4).
- There is no survival difference between esophagectomy with thoracotomy and esophagectomy without thoracotomy.[1]
- The stomach is the most common conduit. Conduits include:
  - Stomach: right gastric and right gastric epiploic artery pedicles.
  - Left colon: ascending branch of left colic artery pedicle.
  - Right colon: middle colic artery pedicle.
  - Jejunal free graft: microsurgery implantation of mesenteric arcade.
  - Myocutaneous tube flaps: radial forearm, pectoralis major, TRAM.
- Route of enteric reconstruction is most commonly the posterior mediastinum. If the posterior mediastinum is obliterated, then the conduit can be passed substernally, subcutaneous (anterior to the sternum), or via the right or left pleural space.
- Distal adenocarcinomas are divided by *Siewert classification* (Fig. 15.2).
  - *Siewert I:* tumors confined to the distal esophagus, just above the gastroesophageal junction (GEJ), spread to mediastinal and celiac nodes: esophagectomy only required, with negative gastric margins.
  - *Siewert II:* tumors with epicenter in the GEJ, which may invade the proximal gastric cardia: generally esophagectomy only is required, with negative gastric margins. Spread is to abdominal lymph nodes.
  - *Siewert III:* tumors with epicenter within the cardia, and extensive gastric involvement: best treated with total gastrectomy, with possible esophagectomy. Spread is to abdominal lymph nodes.

Choice of esophagectomy (Table 15.4)

- *Transhiatal:* portion of esophagus which needs to be blindly mobilized (distal trachea to subcarinal region) should be extrinsically normal as it cannot be directly visualized. Previous thoracotomy, especially if mediastinal pleura opened, mid to upper esophageal transmural cancers, inflammation (e.g., from caustic ingestion injury) are contraindications.

Table 15.4 Esophagectomy

Esophagectomy without thoracotomy	Transhiatal esophagectomy (THE)
Esophagectomy with thoracotomy	1. Ivor Lewis esophagectomy (transthoracic esophagectomy, TTE) 2. McKeown esophagectomy (3-hole) 3. Esophagectomy with three field lymphadenectomy 4. Left thoracoabdominal esophagectomy
Esophagectomy with complete laparoscopic and thorascopic mobilization	Minimally invasive esophagectomy

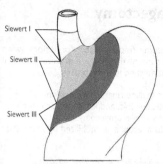

Fig. 15.2 Siewert classification of distal esophageal tumors.

- *Transthoracic:* allows mediastinal lymphadenectomy, and accurate resection of tumors in distal tracheal to subcarinal region.
- A VATS approach is limited to patients without N1 or M1 disease.
- Three-field dissection has significant physiologic burden: patients with FEV_1 <1.5L, significant cardiac disease, age >75 years are probably not candidates.

General principles

Esophagectomy should be preceded by esophagoscopy by the operating surgeon to confirm tumor location, extent of tumor and Barrett's mucosa, pyloric narrowing, and duodenal ulceration. Avoiding incomplete tumor resection, anastomotic leaks, and much of the other major morbidity associated with this operation depends on strict adherence to basic general surgical principles:

- This is a major operation conducted in patients who may be elderly, malnourished and immunocompromised, and who often have cardiovascular risk factors:
  - Nutritional support, e.g., NG feeds may be needed preoperatively.
  - Pulmonary physiotherapy including smoking cessation and ambulation may help reduce the high risk of respiratory complications.
  - Normalization of hematocrit and immunological status in patients undergoing preoperative chemotherapy.
  - Careful evaluation of cardiovascular status.
- Gentle handling of tissues.
- Meticulous hemostasis and avoidance of dead space.
- Adequate conduit length to create a tension-free anastomosis.
- Adequate arterial supply.
- Adequate venous drainage (do not dissect out more distal esophagus more than necessary to mobilize it).
- Gastric decompression, including pyloroplasty or pyloromyotomy in patients where gastric tube reconstruction is chosen, and placement of an NG tube to reduce risk of vomiting.

Reference

1. Chang AC et al. Outcomes after transhiatal and transthoracic esophagectomy for cancer. *Ann Thorac Surg* 2008; **85**:424–9.

Transhiatal esophagectomy

Key facts

Esophagectomy without thoracotomy (most suitable for lesions when esophagus from distal trachea to subcarinal region is extrinsically normal as this is blindly mobilized). It is performed in three phases:

- *Abdominal phase* (Fig. 15.3, top left):
  - Performed through an upper midline laparotomy incision.
  - Divide short gastric, left gastroepiploic, and left gastric arteries.
  - Kocher maneuver followed by a pyloromyotomy.
  - Esophageal hiatus, and the distal esophagus mobilized by sharp and blunt dissection.
- *Cervical phase:*
  - Standard left neck incision anterior to sternocleidomastoid.
  - Middle thyroid vein and inferior thyroid artery are divided.
  - The superior esophagus is mobilized down to the carina.
- *Mediastinal phase* (Fig.15.3, bottom left):
  - Mobilize posterior mediastinum—sharp and blunt dissection.
  - The cervical esophagus is divided and the proximal stomach is divided with a 4–5cm margin from the tumor.
  - Gastric conduit delivered via posterior mediastinum to neck.
  - A feeding jejunostomy is placed and the abdomen closed.
  - A cervico-esophagogastric anastomosis is performed end-to-side either stapled or hand sewn, after a NG tube is positioned.

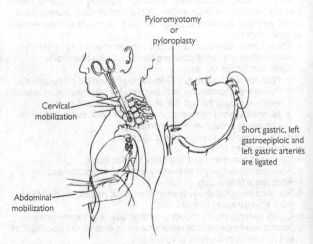

Pyloromyotomy
or
pyloroplasty

Cervical
mobilization

Short gastric, left
gastroepiploic and
left gastric arteries
are ligated

Abdominal
mobilization

Fig. 15.3 Transhiatal esophagectomy.

Set-up

- Single lumen ET tube, NG tube, arterial line, Foley catheter.
- CVP line optional.
- Supine with left arm tucked, right arm extended on arm board.
- Roll under neck improves cervical exposure.
- Prep neck, chest, and abdomen to groin as continuous field.

Operative procedure

Gastric mobilization

- Upper midline laparotomy, extending over xiphoid to lower sternum.
- Retractor with bladder blade to lift xiphoid, malleable blade on right to retract left hepatic lobe exposing esophageal hiatus and EGJ.
- Gastric mobilization preserving left gastroepiploic arcade.
- Left gastric vessels exposed and ligated individually with 3/0 silk (or staple/Harmonic scalpel) via lesser sac or anteriorly via divided gastrohepatic ligament.
- Kocher maneuver to straighten duodenum (peritoneum incised to right of duodenum which is reflected to left to expose structures behind).
- Pyloromyotomy (15 blade or electrocautery on low longitudinal incision muscularis down to mucosa), cover with omental patch.

Esophageal mobilization

- Performed from below through esophageal hiatus.
- Widen hiatus anteriorly after ligating crossing phrenic vein, or by dividing left crus (more risk breaching left pleural space).
- Blunt mobilization of esophagus into upper mediastinal space (NG tube helps stay on esophagus).

Cervical phase

- Modified left collar incision.
- Anterior border sternomastoid is retracted laterally, prevertebral space accessed medial to carotid sheath.
- Distal cervical esophagus encircled, bimanual mobilization to complete intrathoracic dissection.
- Laryngeal nerve injury a risk.

Creation gastric tube and cervical anastomosis

- Based on greater curvature stomach, 4–5cm diameter using serial firings of 7.5cm GIA stapler, oversew staple line to prevent fistula/leaks.
- Deliver esophagus and gastric cardia from chest—either pull esophagus through neck, or divide distal cervical esophagus and deliver tumor through abdomen.
- Attaching a 32F chest tube to stomach tip helps prevent twisting.
- Hand-sewn anastomosis (4/0 silk two-layer, inverting).
- Direct NG tube across anastomosis under direct vision before completing.
- Replace anastomosis in midline, prevertebral space.

Closure

- Irrigate and close cervical incision in layers.
- Place adjuvant jejunostomy, abdominal incision closed in layers.
- Abdominal and cervical drains.

Esophagectomy with thoracotomy

Key facts

- Four main types of esophagectomy involve thoracotomy (or thoracoscopic approaches), improving exposure of the thoracic esophagus, with anastomoses in either the thorax or the neck.
- *Transthoracic esophagectomy (Ivor Lewis)* allows mediastinal lymphadenectomy, and accurate resection of tumors in the distal tracheal to subcarinal region (Fig. 15.4).
- A *three-hole (McKeown)* approach combines the excellent exposure of the Ivor Lewis with the advantages of a cervical anastomosis, as well as the option of performing lymph node dissection in three fields (Fig. 15.4).
- *Three-field dissection* has significant physiologic burden: patients with FEV_1 <1.5L, significant cardiac disease, age >75 years are probably not candidates.
- A *left thoracoabdominal approach* employs a single incision in patients with tumors at the gastroesophageal junction (Fig. 15.4).

Ivor Lewis (transthoracic) esophagectomy

Rationale

- Esophagectomy with right thoracotomy named after Welsh surgeon, Mr Ivor Lewis, designed to provide excellent exposure of the intrathoracic mid to upper thoracic esophagus.
- It also allows the surgeon to perform a regional lymph node dissection under direct vision.
- The main drawbacks compared to a transhiatal esophagectomy are the additional morbidity of a thoracotomy incision, and an intrathoracic anastomosis (leaks from a cervical anastomosis are easier to treat and less likely to result in respiratory and systemic complications).

Technique

- Performed through two incisions in two phases.
- *Abdominal phase:*
  - Performed through an *upper midline laparotomy* incision.
  - Steps similar to transhiatal esophagectomy.
  - Abdomen is closed after mobilization of the stomach conduit.
- *Thoracic phase:*
  - Performed through a *right posterolateral thoracotomy* after repositioning the patient in the right lateral position.
  - The esophagus is mobilized and the azygos vein is divided.
  - The thoracic duct is mass ligated prophylactically near the hiatus.
  - The stomach conduit is brought into the chest. The esophagus is divided at the level of the azygos vein, and the proximal stomach is divided as mentioned on 📖 p767). The thoracic esophagogastric anastomosis (TEGA) is performed either end-to-side stapled or hand sewn, or stapled end-to-end, after a NG tube is positioned.

McKeown or three-hole esophagectomy

- Three incisions; modified left collar cervical incision, upper midline laparotomy, and right posterolateral thoracotomy.
- This combines the advantages of exposure of an Ivor Lewis esophagectomy, with the advantages of a cervical anastomosis.
- No part of the dissection is performed blindly.
- The abdominal and thoracic phases are performed similarly to Ivor Lewis esophagectomy, although the thoracic phase is performed first.
- A cervico-esophagogastric anastomosis is performed in a similar way to the transhiatal esophagectomy.

Left thoracoabdominal approach

- This employs a single incision extending from the left 5th or 6th intercostal space in the anterior axillary line, across the costal margin to the abdomen.
- It provides best exposure of the lower 1/3 of the esophagus, so is used in patients with tumors at the gastroesophageal junction.
- The disadvantages are that the amount of proximal esophagus that can be visualized and therefore mobilized is limited (the aortic arch is in the way), and division of the costal margin contributes to post-thoracotomy pain and respiratory dysfunction.

Minimally invasive esophagectomy

Many different approaches, including robotic, but common approach is similar to Ivor Lewis, with a thoracic esophagogastric anastomosis, however, the abdominal and thoracic phases are performed laparoscopically and thorascopically respectively.

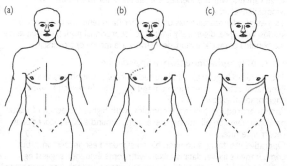

Fig. 15.4 Esophagectomy approaches. (a) Ivor Lewis. (b) McKeown or three-hole. (c) Left thoracoabdominal.

Lymphadenectomy

Key facts

- The optimal extent of lymph node dissection in esophageal cancer is controversial.
- The esophagus has an extensive lymphatic drainage, which is divided into three zones (fields): abdominal, intrathoracic, and cervical.
- Lymph node resection strategies at the time of esophagectomy range from standard regional and one-field lymphadenectomy, to radical approaches involving two- or three-field lymphadenectomy.

Anatomy of lymphatic drainage

- The esophagus has a dense network of mucosal and submucosal lymphatics: hence tumors as early as stage II have access to draining lymphatics and therefore regional spread.
- Tumors of the cervical and middle esophagus generally drain to upper mediastinal lymph nodes.
- The middle and lower 1/3 of the esophagus drains to lymph nodes along the lesser curvature of the stomach, celiac axis nodes, cardiac and upper and lower paraesophageal nodes.
- Celiac axis and lesser curvature nodes are involved in 60% of tumors of the lower 1/3 of the esophagus: celiac nodal involvement represents distant spread and precludes surgical cure.
- The *Siewart classification* of distal esophageal tumors (☐ p765) differentiates between type I lesions which tend to drain to mediastinal and celiac lymph nodes, as opposed to the more distal type II and III lesions which drain to celiac, splenic, and para-aortic nodes.
- Squamous cell cancers are characterized by extensive local and regional involvement with skip metastases even in relatively early stage cancers, which underlies the rationale for more extensive lymphadenectomy.
- Early-stage adenocarcinomas on the other hand tend not to have skip lesions, with spread generally limited to locoregional nodes; consequently the benefits of radical lymphadenectomy are more controversial.

Results of lymphadenectomy approaches

- There are no large-scale randomized studies to support radical lymphadenectomy over more limited lymph node resection with chemoradiotherapy.
- Radical procedures are more complex, with higher incidence of major postoperative complications: there is still around a 20% locoregional recurrence rate.
- Operative mortality is comparable to standard esophagectomy, but comparative survival data is mixed with some evidence suggesting enhanced survival with en bloc esophagectomy in early and later stage cancers, compared to standard transhiatal technique, but other studies finding no difference.
- Variation in surgical technique, and discrepancies in preoperative staging, and intraoperative lymph node sampling and resection may account for some of these differences.

Chemotherapy and radiotherapy

Key facts

- Treatment options include primary surgery, neoadjuvant chemoradiation followed by surgery, postoperative adjuvant chemoradiotherapy, definitive or primary chemoradiation, palliative chemotherapy ± radiotherapy.
- Neoadjuvant chemoradiotherapy followed by surgery probably offers best survival in patients with locally advanced resectable tumor: cure rate is <50% due to a combination of inadequate pathologic response and distant metastases:
  - Stage 0, I, and IIa should be offered primary surgery.
  - Stage IIB and III tumors should be offered trimodality therapy.
  - Stage IV tumors are treated with primary chemoradiotherapy.
- Nutritional status should be optimized before treatment, possibly requiring either NG or jejunal tube feeds.
- PEG should be avoided, if possible, if the stomach is planned as a conduit. PEG may injure the right gastroepiploic artery which is a necessary vascular pedicle for a gastric conduit.

Definitions

- *Neoadjuvant therapy* is treatment (chemotherapy and/or radiotherapy) given *before* surgery. Also called *induction* or *preoperative therapy*.
- *Adjuvant therapy* is treatment (chemotherapy and/or radiotherapy) given *after* surgery.
- *Chemoradiotherapy* is chemotherapy and radiotherapy given simultaneously.
- *Primary therapy* is therapy given as the first line of treatment with intent to cure (as opposed to palliative therapy).
- *Trimodality therapy* comprises neoadjuvant therapy, surgery, and then adjuvant therapy.
- *Clinical stage* is the tumor stage determined by multiple imaging including laparoscopic assessment, but without pathologic examination of the resected tumor.
- *Pathologic stage* is the tumor stage determined by inspection of the resected specimen.

Treatment options

Neoadjuvant chemoradiation

- Rationale for neoadjuvant chemoradiation:
  - Chemotherapy and radiation offer synergistic effect on the locoregional level.
  - Chemotherapy treats *micrometastatic* disease.
  - Chemotherapy is better delivered to primary tumor when the blood supply is intact.
  - Downstaging by chemoradiation may increase resectability.
- Two major studies demonstrate survival advantage for neoadjuvant chemoradiation followed by surgery compared to surgery alone for stage IIB-III esophageal cancer.
  - Urba et al.[1] Regimen included 5-FU/cisplatin/vinblastine/concurrent 45Gy. Significant decrease in local recurrence and trend in survival at 3 years.

- • Walsh et al.[2] 5-FU/cisplatin/concurrent 40Gy. Significant increase in survival at 3 years.
- Two major meta-analyses demonstrate advantage for neoadjuvant chemoradiation followed by surgery compared to surgery alone for stage IIB–III esophageal cancer.
  - • Urschel et al.[3] showed improved 3-year survival, reduced locoregional tumor recurrence, higher rate of complete (R0) resection, overall complete pathologic response rate of 21%.
  - • Gebski V et al.[4] showed improved 2-year survival, survival benefit for both adenocarcinoma and SCC. There was no survival benefit for sequential chemoradiotherapy for SCC.
- Common neoadjuvant regimen: cisplatin or carboplatin and 5-FU or taxol with concurrent 45Gy or 50.8Gy external beam radiation, 3–8 weeks of rest, followed by surgery.

Adjuvant therapy

Patients with R1 or R2 resection or residual postoperative N1 disease should be considered for adjuvant chemotherapy ± radiation, though there is no conclusive data that supports this regimen.

Primary chemoradiation

- Should be considered in patients who from a cardiopulmonary or anatomic standpoint are poor surgical candidates, or who refuse surgery, and for stage IV tumors.
- Two studies suggest role for definitive chemoradiation in patients who are otherwise surgical candidates.
  - • Stahl M et al.[5] randomized 172 patients with locally advanced (T3,4, N0–1, M0) SCC of the esophagus who received induction (5-FU/etoposide/cisplatin) chemotherapy followed by chemoradiotherapy (40Gy to surgery, or continued chemoradiotherapy (65Gy)). No 2-year survival difference. 31% to 24% survival advantage for surgery, not statistically significant. Survival curves widened after 3 years.
  - • Bedenne et al.[6] randomized 259 patients with locally advanced (T3, N0–1, M0) cancer (88% SCC) of the esophagus. Received induction (5-FU/cisplatin) chemotherapy followed by concomitant radiotherapy (46Gy) conventional or split course. Patients with tumor response were then randomized to surgery or continued chemoradiotherapy. No difference in 2-year survival. Patients undergoing surgery had lower local recurrence (34% vs. 43%) and less need for additional palliation (24% vs. 43%).

References

1. Urba et al. Randomized trial of preoperative chemoradiation versus surgery alone in patients with locoregional esophageal carcinoma. *J Clin Oncol* 2001; **19**(2):305–13.
2. Walsh et al. A comparison of multimodal therapy and surgery for esophageal adenocarcinoma. *New Engl J Med* 1996; **335**(7):462–7.
3. Urschel JD et al. A meta-analysis of randomized controlled trials that compared neoadjuvant chemoradiation and surgery to surgery alone for resectable esophageal cancer. *Am J Surg* 2003; **185**:538–43.
4. Gebski V et al. Survival benefits from neoadjuvant chemoradiotherapy or chemotherapy in esophageal carcinoma: a meta-analysis. *Lancet Oncol* 2007; **8**:226–34.
5. Stahl M et al. Chemoradiation with and without surgery in patients with locally advanced squamous cell carcinoma of the esophagus. *J Clin Oncol* 2005; **23**(10):2310–17.
6. Bedenne L et al. Chemoradiation followed by surgery compared with chemoradiation alone in squamous cancer of the esophagus: FFCD 9102. *J Clin Oncol* 2007; **25**(10):1160–8.

Postoperative care

Key facts

- 40–50% of esophagectomy patients have some sort of postoperative complication (📖 pp776–777).
- Postoperative pathways and protocols can be helpful.

Immediate perioperative and postoperative care

- Intraoperative pressors should be avoided, and adequate intravascular volume should be maintained.
- Transfusion of blood products in the setting of cancer may increase the incidence of recurrence. Transfusion may be considered if the hemoglobin level drops below 8g/dL.

Pulmonary toilet

- Aggressive pulmonary toilet and early ambulation to prevent pneumonia.
- Patients should ambulate 4x/day.
- Head of bed at 45° to reduce aspiration risk.

Nutrition

- An intrathoracic anastomosis should be examined with a thin barium esophagram before instituting an oral diet (day 4–5). Oral diet can be instituted in a stepwise fashion for cervical anastomosis.
- Diet should start with sips of liquids, to clear liquids, full liquids, and finally soft, ground diet.
- Tube feedings via the jejunostomy tube can be initiated beginning postoperative day 3 and advanced to goal within 48–72h. Rate of tube feeds may need to be adjusted or held if development of an ileus.

Deep venous thrombosis prophylaxis

- Prophylaxis dose of LMWH is used (e.g., 5000U heparin sc bid or tid) until the patient is discharged from the hospital.
- In addition, sequential compression devices are worn while the patient is in bed or sitting in a chair.
- Early ambulation also assists in DVT prevention.

Gastrointestinal prophylaxis

- Although outside of a vagal-sparing esophagectomy, the vagi are removed and acid production by the conduit is diminished; however, IV and then PO PPI are used to prevent gastric secretions of the conduit.
- The NG tube is generally removed postoperative day 3–7.
- IV antiemetics are used if necessary, though incidence of nausea after esophagectomy is no higher than other general surgeries.

Palliation
- Attempts at palliation are generally directed to alleviating or minimizing dysphagia.
- Photodynamic therapy (PDT):
  - The patient is injected with a 2mg/kg photosensitizer such as sodium porfimer (Photofrin®)
  - After 48h the tumor is exposed to 300–400J/cm of 630nm light.
  - <5% perforation rate.
  - Skin injury from light exposure is common.
- Brachytherapy:
  - Catheter-based administration of iridium-192.
  - Risk of fistula formation.
- Esophageal stents:
  - Endoscopy-directed plastic or self-expanding metal stents (SEMS).
  - Plastic stents are easily removed, but frequently migrate.
  - Nickel/titanium (nitinol) stents are common. Covered stents (silicone or polyurethane) are beneficial in temporarily sealing trachealesophageal fistulas. 95% effective in alleviating dysphagia.

Complications and outcomes

Perioperative

Pneumothorax

During the gastric mobilization and distal mediastinal dissection, both mediastinal pleural spaces are inspected to determine pleural disruption. Chest tubes are placed if identified. Prior to extubation in the operating room, an intraoperative CXR is obtained to determine pneumothorax of pleural effusion, and a chest tube is placed if necessary.

Hemorrhage

Although arterial branches from the aorta to the thoracic esophagus are avulsed during THO, significant bleeding is rarely an issue as such vessels usually undergo spasm. If the azygos vein is disrupted during dissection during a THO, simple packing usually stops bleeding, as the azygos vein is part of a low-pressure system.

Tracheal injury

Tracheal injury during esophagectomy should be repaired once identified. Usually the injury involves the membranous wall of the trachea, and is identified by release of air from the wound. If this occurs during the cervical dissection, a partial sternal split can be performed to provide exposure for repair, or the patient should be positioned for a right thoracotomy if the injury is more distal on the trachea.

Postoperative

Recurrent laryngeal nerve injury

• Rare complication after THE.
• Hoarseness occurs in 5% of patients, permanent chordal paralysis in <1%.
• Injury to the recurrent laryngeal nerve can be avoided by keeping dissection close to the surface of the esophagus, avoiding the tracheo-esophageal groove, and not using metal to retract the trachea medially.

Supraventricular tachyarrhythmias

• AF occurs in up to 30% of thoracic surgical patients.
• AF prophylaxis can be utilized, including magnesium and β-blockade (see 📖 pp262–263).

Chylothorax

• Rare complication. Higher after THE (1%).
• Chylothorax should be dealt with immediately with diet modification, and possible surgical intervention.
• During esophagectomy with thoracotomy, the thoracic duct can be ligated prophylactically.

Pleural effusions

• Pleural effusions should be drained with small- or regular-bore chest tubes.
• Late development of a pleural effusion with an ipsilateral intrathoracic anastomosis should raise suspicions of an anastomotic leak.

Anastomotic leaks

- *Cervical esophagogastric anastomosis* (4–12%) have higher incidence of anastomotic leaks than intrathoracic anastomosis.
- Once an anastomotic leak develops, 50% of those anastomoses go on to develop strictures.
- *Cervical leaks* should undergo early dilation.
- 90% of cervical esophagogastric anastomosis leaks occur within first 10 postoperative days.
- Risk factors for developing CEGA leaks include higher number of preoperative comorbidities, advanced pathologic stage, postoperative arrhythmia, increased number of prior esophagogastric surgeries, and active smoking history.
- Previous chemoradiation does not seem to be a risk factor for anastomotic leak.
- CEGA leaks often present as foul discharge from the wound, low-grade temps, wound erythema, leukocytosis, halitosis.
- Cervical leaks are treated by bedside opening of the wound and twice daily packing. The patient finds a position where they can drink and eventually eat without leaking. The fistula usually heals within 2 weeks. Early dilation stretches an edematous anastomosis and promotes antegrade movement of swallowed food.
- *Intrathoracic leaks* present as fever, tachycardia, tachypnea, new ipsilateral pleural effusion, and can be treated by adequate drainage with chest tube(s) and an endoscopic-placed covered stent across the anastomosis.

Outcomes

- Esophagectomy with and without thoracotomy have similar perioperative and long-term outcomes.
- Univariate analysis demonstrates that THE has reduced overall complications (P = 0.01) including pulmonary and GI complications. However, after controlling for confounding factors, multivariate analysis, THE and TTE have similar overall complication rates, though TTE has slightly higher gastrointestinal and systemic complications.[1]
- In regards to cancer specific survival, studies demonstrate that the number of lymph nodes obtained as well as the number of surgical fields dissected, may improve overall cancer specific survival. However, adjusted for patient characteristics (hazard ratio (HR) 0.91) and patient and provider characteristics (HR 0.95) THE and TTE have no difference in oncologic survival.[2]
- Cancer specific survival after neoadjuvant chemoradiotherapy followed by surgery is largely dependent on the pathologic stage of the tumor. Complete pathologic (yp) response demonstrates a 2- and 5-year survival of 80% and 58% respectively. A yp stage of I–IV combined yields a 2- and 5-year survival of 45% and 22% respectively.[3]

References

1. Connors RC et al. Comparing outcomes after transthoracic and transhiatal esophagectomy: a 5-year prospective cohort of 17,395 patients. J Am Coll Surg 2007; 205:735–40.
2. Chang AC et al. Outcomes after transhiatal and transthoracic esophagectomy for cancer. Ann Thorac Surg 2008; 85:424–9.
3. Orringer MB et al. Two thousand transhiatal esophagectomies: changing trends, lessons learned. Ann Surg 2007; 246:363–72.

Gastroesophageal reflux disease

Key facts

- GERD is the reflux of acid or bile from the stomach into the esophagus caused by dysfunction of the lower esophageal sphincter (LES); or changes in the type or volume of refluxate, the mucosal barrier, or esophageal clearance.
- GERD can result in substernal chest pain, but the primary rationale for treating it remains the risk of Barrett's esophagus (📖 p780) and potential for malignant transformation.
- If antacids, and dietary modification fails, laparoscopic Nissen fundoplication and wrap is the procedure of choice.

Pathology

- The normal 'anti-reflux barrier' is made up of the intrinsic pressure of the LES, its intraabdominal location, the crural diaphragm, the acute angle of His between the esophagus and stomach.
- The normal LES has a resting amplitude of 12–20mmHg and length of 3–5cm. A dysfunctional LES has sphincter pressure <6mmHg and/or overall sphincter length <2cm. Causes of LES dysfunction include:
  - Cephalad displacement of LOS, e.g., sliding hiatal hernia.
  - Obesity and increased intra-abdominal pressure.
  - Foods and drugs, including nicotine, nitrates, benzodiazepines, mint, caffeine, chocolate, tomato-based products, spiced foods, alcohol.
- Changes in refluxate (increased acid and pepsin, or bile salts), reduced esophageal clearance (type II hiatus hernia), pregnancy, previous gastric surgery, scleroderma, and diabetes can contribute to GERD.

Presentation and investigation

- May be asymptomatic. Atypical substernal chest pain (heartburn), belching, halitosis, cough, wheeze, dysphagia, reflux esophagitis, stricture.
- Barium esophagram can identify a sliding hiatal hernia, after reflux of contrast material and presence of strictures.
- Endoscopy (📖 p658) determines the presence of esophagitis, and biopsy abnormal mucosa, and identifying malignancy or Barrett's metaplasia.
- Manometry is used to determine the location of the LES or high-pressure zone (HPZ) and document abnormal LES tone.

24h pH monitoring

- The patient holds H2 receptor blockers or proton pump inhibitors (PPIs) for 48–72h prior to the exam.
- The pH probe is placed 5cm above the HPZ. Six components are recorded to determine a composite DeMeester score:
  - Total percentage of time pH <4.
  - Percent upright and supine time pH <4.
  - Number of total reflux episodes.
  - Number of reflux episodes that are ≥5min in duration.
  - Longest reflux episode duration in minutes.
- Abnormal esophageal acid exposure is diagnosed if composite DeMeester score >14.7, or the percent total time pH <4 is >4%.

Management

Medical management includes diet modification (eliminating precipitants listed on 📖 p776), antacids, i.e. H_2 receptor blockers, e.g. cimetidine 150mg twice daily, or proton pump inhibitors (PPI), e.g. omeprazole 20mg daily.

Indications for surgery

Diagnosis of GERD as defined by barium esophagram, manometry and 24h pH monitoring, and:

- Failed medical management, but responsive to PPI therapy.
- Presence of esophagitis.
- Barrett's metaplasia.
- Recurrent aspiration.

Laparoscopic Nissen fundoplication

- 360° wrap.
- Should be avoided in patients with a concurrent motility disorder as complete wrap may cause dysphagia.
- Nissen fundoplication can be done open or laparoscopically. Unless a multiple redo fundoplication, most cases can be done laparoscopically.
- Five ports may be used, with one port used for specifically for liver retraction.
- The gastrohepatic ligament (pars lucida) is divided, as well as the phrenoesophageal ligament exposing the esophageal hiatus, and the right and left crus.
- The short gastric arteries are divided.
- Opening the hiatus, the distal mediastinum is dissected. To avoid tension and a slipped wrap, at least 2.5cm of esophagus must be within the abdomen without tension, otherwise an esophageal lengthening procedure (Collis gastroplasty) is necessary.
- The crural is closed to the approximation of the esophagus with a 56F Maloney dilator.
- Cural closure can be reinforced with biodegradable reinforcement (xeno- or allograft patches).
- Synthetic mesh should not be used to avoid extrinsic stricturing and perforation.
- The fundus of the wrap is slid posteriorly and around the esophagus to form a 360° wrap, and secured with interrupted sutures.

Postoperative care

- The patient is started on clear liquids and advanced to soft solids.
- Carbonated beverages and thick foods like bread and steak are avoided.
- Complications include:
  - Esophageal perforation and other perforated viscus, splenic injury, liver injury or injury during initiating pneumoperitoneum.
  - Slipped Nissen, or herniation of the wrap into the mediastinum may occur if the abdominal esophagus is under tension.
- Can be repaired laparoscopically if found early.

Barrett's metaplasia

Key facts

- Barrett's metaplasia describes the situation where *the squamocolumnar junction is cephalad to the gastroesophageal junction* (GEJ). Initially described by Australian thoracic surgeon Norman 'Patsy' Barrett in 1950.
- It is an adaptive response to esophageal mucosal injury from gastric acid or bile reflux. It is found in 6–12% of patients with GERD.
- Its clinical relevance is the increased risk of malignant transformation (around 1% of patients per year with Barrett's metaplasia progress to adenocarcinoma of the esophagus).

Pathology

- Presence of columnar mucosa (intestinal metaplasia) with goblet cells, with progressive disorganization of cells and glands, above the GEJ:
  - No dysplasia.
  - Low-grade dysplasia (LGD)
  - High-grade dysplasia (HGD).
  - Adenocarcinoma.
- 5–10% of patients per year will progress to dysplasia.
- 15–25% of patients have concurrent LGD.
- 5–10% of patients have concurrent HGD.
- Risk for adenocarcinoma is increased 30–125-fold.
- 0.5–1% per year will progress to adenocarcinoma.
- Occult cancer is found in 25–73% of esophagectomy specimen for HGD.
- Primary Barrett's results from esophageal mucosal injury from gastric acid or bile reflux. Other causes include salivary nitrates, tobacco, oral flora, obesity, increased insulin-like growth factors, bacterial colonization, *Helicobacter pylori* eradication, hypergastrinemia, and chronic use of proton pump inhibitors.

Management

Surveillance

- Barrett's metaplasia without dysplasia: endoscopy every 2–3 years with four-quadrant biopsies at 2cm intervals.
- LGD: endoscopy and four-quadrant biopsies at 2cm intervals ever 6 months for 1 year, then annually if still LGD.
- HGD: confirm diagnosis with repeat endoscopy and two separate pathologists. If confirmed then procedural intervention:
  - Flat and unifocal HGD may be treated with endoscopic techniques
  - Multifocal HGD, HGD with dysplasia-associated lesions or masses (DALM) and long segments of dysplasia are best treated by esophagectomy.

Endoscopic therapy

- PDT: injection of photosensitizing agent followed by treatment with 630nm laser causes oxygen-radical dependent tissue necrosis. Complications include 30% esophageal stricture, 10% sunburn odynophagia. Key limitations:

- Depth of penetration limited to submucosa.
- Invasive cancers are inadequately treated.
- *Radiofrequency ablation*: ablates tumor to the level of the muscularis mucosae. Does not provide intact histology architecture and therefore provides no information on deep or lateral margins.
- *Endoscopic mucosal resection*: injection of air or saline in submucosa beneath lesion, and then endoscopic snaring, or suctioning. Provides large specimen with intact histology architecture to assess deep and lateral margins.

Surgery

Esophagectomy is indicated for HGD (📖 pp764–765).

Esophageal strictures and webs

Key facts

- Esophageal rings and webs are the most common structural abnormalities in the esophagus (found in around 10% esophagrams).
- Strictures should be biopsied to rule out malignancy (📖 p658).
- Esophageal webs and most strictures respond well to dilatation and rarely need surgery.

Benign esophageal strictures

Etiology
See Table 15.5.

Pathology
Abnormal narrowing of the esophageal wall. Most commonly as a result of chronic inflammation leading to fibrosis. Peptic strictures represent 75% of benign esophageal stricture.

Presentation and diagnosis
- Symptoms may include dysphagia to solids and then liquids, odynophagia, hemoptysis, impaction of food.
- *Barium esophagram* can identify stricture location. Important to evaluate esophagram at multiple images, in order to distinguish a stricture from a transient peristaltic indentation.
- *Endoscopy* is important for visual characterization and biopsy. Never push a food impaction forward, as there may be a stricture behind the impaction, and esophageal perforation may result.

Management
- *Blind dilation* using *Maloney dilators* can be performed for cervical anastomotic strictures after esophagectomy.
- *Endoscopic dilation* with either wire-guided Savary dilators or pneumatic balloon dilation.
- Refractory symptomatic strictures may require *esophagectomy* (see 📖 p764).

Esophageal rings and webs

Pathology
- Thought to be congenital, or due to inflammation, postcricoid webs associated with Plummer–Vinson syndrome.
- The terms rings and webs are often used interchangeably. An esophageal ring is a concentric smooth, thin (3–5mm) extension of normal esophageal tissue including the three anatomic layers (mucosa, submucosa, and muscle) found anywhere along the esophagus, but usually distal. Three types:
  - A ring: uncommon. Several cm proximal to squamocolumnar junction (SQJ). Not a fixed structure, may not appear in esophagrams.
  - B (Schatzki) ring: most common, composed of mucosa and submucosa only, usually located at the SQJ marking proximal margin of a hiatal hernia (📖 p788).
  - C ring: rare finding, caused by indentation of diaphragmatic crura.
  - Webs: thin, eccentric, extension of esophagus mucosa and submucosa occurring anywhere along esophagus but usually postcricoid.

Presentation

- Most asymptomatic. Almost all patients with lumen <13mm have dysphagia, worse for solids than liquids (in contrast with motility disorders). Location of ring or web often determines location of sensation of dysphagia, or discomfort.
- Weight loss and anemia suggest underlying malignancy.

Investigation

- Barium swallow demonstrates intraluminal obstruction, competency of the LES and presence of GOR, and is more sensitive than OGD.
- OGD is useful for biopsy if malignancy is suspected.

Management

- If symptoms not managed by conservative measures such as modifying diet, esophageal dilatation can be carried out using Maloney or Savary dilators, with a high success rate and minimal recurrence.
- Surgery is rarely indicated.

Table 15.5 Etiology of benign esophageal strictures

Congenital

Webs:
  Perforate
  Imperforate

Acquired
Peptic

Webs:
  Plummer–Vinson syndrome
  Schatzki's ring

Autoimmune:
  SLE
  Scleroderma
  Polyarteritis nodosa
  Dermatomyositis

Caustic injury
Chronic foreign body reaction
Crohn's disease

Infectious:
  Tuberculosis
  Syphilis

Radiation effect
Postoperative anastomotic
Drug-induced
Idiopathic

Esophageal diverticula

Key facts

- These are blind pouches lined by epithelium arising from the esophagus: although they are usually acquired as a result of motility disorders (e.g., *Zenkers*), they may occasionally be congenital, or due to local inflammatory disease and compression.
- They may be asymptomatic, or present with dysphagia, odynophagia, regurgitation, and aspiration.
- Diverticula are excised open or endoscopically: there is no role for medical management.

Pathology

- Esophageal diverticula are classified as pulsion or traction diverticulae:
  - *Pulsion (or pseudo) diverticulae* consist of only mucosal layers herniating through a weak point as a result of increased transmural pressure gradient, and include Zenker's and epiphrenic diverticula.
  - *Traction (or true) diverticula* consist of all three muscle layers, and are caused by inflammation or fibrosis in adjacent lymph nodes.

Zenker's diverticulum

Pathology

- This is a propulsion diverticulum involving only the mucosa layer.
- It protrudes posteriorly from *Killian's triangle*, an area of anatomic weakness bounded by the inferior constrictors and cricopharyngeus muscle or upper esophageal sphincter (UES)
- Underlying mechanism is non-coordinated deglutition with premature contraction and incomplete relaxation of UES.
- The neck lies above cricopharynx lading to spontaneous emptying and regurgitation into mouth, and aspiration, and compression of pharynx.

Presentation and diagnosis

May be asymptomatic. Presents in 5th–8th decades with dysphagia, *regurgitation of fresh food*, aspiration, halitosis, hoarseness, weight loss, asthma.

- Barium esophagram is gold standard.
- Endoscopy.

Management

- There is no medical therapy: all patients are candidates for surgery.
- Diverticulectomy and myotomy are best formed electively while diverticulum is still small.
- Myotomy alone can be performed for small (<2cm) diverticulum.
- *Open approach*: the cervical esophagus is reached via a left neck incision, anterior to sternocleidomastoid, and anterior to the carotid towards the cervical spine. A long myotomy is performed from the inferior constrictors superiorly, dividing the cricopharyngeus muscle, extending inferiorly dividing both muscle layers of the esophagus towards the clavicle. The diverticulum is divided with a stapler.
- *Endoscopic approach*: intraoperative trans-oral stapling of the esophageal wall and diverticulum. A Collard–Weerda diverticuloscope

is placed simultaneously in the diverticulum and the esophagus and a stapler is used to simultaneously divide the anterior wall of the diverticulum, cricopharyngeus.

- 4% conversion rate, 4% reoperation rate. 1.5% mortality, recurrent laryngeal nerve palsy in 2%, fistula in 2%.

Epiphrenic diverticulum

Pathology

Rare pulsion-type diverticula, only involving the mucosa and submucosa, found in the distal 10cm of the esophagus, found predominantly in elderly people, and associated with achalasia and GERD.

Presentation and investigation

- Symptoms variable: dysphagia, odynophagia, regurgitation, aspiration.
- Barium esophagram is the gold standard for diagnosis.
- Chest CT aids in characterization of anatomy.

Surgery

Performed via a left thoracotomy, even if diverticulum extends into the right chest. This is a motility disorder, therefore a long myotomy is performed, extending onto the wall of the stomach. The diverticulum is divided with a stapler. To prevent reflux, a modified Belsey antireflux procedure is performed. Surgical outcomes 2.8% mortality and 5.7% leak rate.[1] Key is to perform a myotomy which limits risk of leak after diverticulum resection.

Other acquired diverticula

Traction diverticula

- These are mid-esophageal diverticula that involve all layers of the esophagus wall, and are not related to disorder in motility.
- They occur as a result of chronic traction or pulling from chronic mediastinal inflammation and fibrosis, e.g., histoplasmosis, TB.
- Symptoms are rare because their location and size, but may include dysphagia, odynophagia (due to stricture/compression), and bleeding.

Management

- Local excision or stapled resection of the diverticulum and adjacent inflammatory mass, best approached via a right thoracotomy.
- Extensive myotomy is not required.

Congenital diverticula

- These rare diverticula are true diverticula containing esophageal mucosa, submucosa, and muscular walls: embryology is uncertain.
- They usually present in late infancy with progressive dysphagia, recurrent respiratory infections, or in the case of high diverticula regurgitation, cough with feeding, excess salivation, and even cyanosis.
- They are diagnosed with a contrast esophagram and endoscopy.
- Surgical excision is via a single-stage transverse diverticulectomy.

Reference

1. Varghese TK *et al.* Surgical treatment of epiphrenic diverticula: a 30-year experience. *Ann Thorac Surg* 2007; **84**(6):1801–9.

Motility disorders

Key facts

Esophageal motility disorders include problems of hypomotility (e.g., achalasia) and hypermotility (diffuse esophageal spasm, nutcracker esophagus and hypertensive LES).

Physiology of swallowing

- Esophageal function is coordinated by sympathetic innervation (from the *cervical and thoracic chains and celiac plexus*), parasympathetic innervation from the *vagus which forms Auerbach's plexus* around the circular muscular layer) and *Meissner's submucosal plexus*.
- Peristalsis is coordinated under central control through the vagus nerve by Meissner's and Auerbach's plexus:
  - Primary peristalsis is a normal propulsive wave in response to the stimulus of voluntary deglutition.
  - Secondary peristalsis is a normal wave without voluntary deglutition.
  - Tertiary waves—abnormal low-amplitude simultaneous contractions.
- For effective swallow peristalsis is coordinated with contraction and relaxation of the *upper (UES) and lower (LES) esophageal sphincters*.
  - The UES is composed of cricopharyngeus and inferior pharyngeal constrictors at C5–C6, remains contracted between swallows due to stimulation by *CN IX and XI*, with resting tone up to 100mmHg. Swallowing involves *inhibition* of IX and XI, UES opens then closes.
  - The LES is specialized arrangement of esophageal muscle 3–4cm above GEJ, has a high-pressure zone with resting tone 15–25mmHg. Influenced by neural, hormonal and drugs: relaxes during swallow and closes with passage of food bolus through LES.

Achalasia

Pathology

- Achalasia is a rare (1:100 000) disorder characterized by *loss of peristalsis* in the distal esophagus and *failure of the LES to relax*. Some patients have abnormal vigorous tertiary peristalsis:
  - *Primary achalasia* is an idiopathic degenerative nerve process associated with loss of ganglion cells in the myenteric plexus, and reduction of vagal fibres in the esophageal wall with loss of control at the postganglionic, non-adrenergic and non-cholinergic inhibitory nerves.
  - *Secondary achalasia* is due to parasites, e.g., Chagas disease, malignancy, diabetes, infiltrative, e.g., amyloid, sarcoid, post-vagotomy.
- There is increased risk of SCC of the esophagus secondary to chronic stasis.

Presentation and investigation

Progressive dysphagia, regurgitation of undigested food, weight loss, halitosis, chronic aspiration.

- Barium esophagram shows tertiary contractions, bird's beak image at LES.
- Manometry shows normal LES pressure, but failure to relax, no progressive peristalsis, and tertiary contractions.

Medical management
- Oral nitrates and calcium channel blockers.
- Balloon dilation. 1–7% perforation rate. Most patients report symptomatic relief. Half of these will require a second dilatation within 5 years.
- Injection of bothlinum toxin (Botox) into the LES (inhibits Ach release from nerve endings). 85% of patients have symptomatic relief after Botox therapy lasting 3–12 months. 50% recurrence after 6 months.

Surgical options
- **Myotomy antireflux procedure** (wrap): main controversies are the extent of the myotomy, need for a wrap, thorascopic versus laparoscopic approach, and management of patients who fail surgery.
- Laparoscopic or robotic **Heller myotomy** with 180° wrap:
  - Port set-up is similar to laparoscopic Nissen fundoplication (📖 p779).
  - After mediastinal dissection anterior myotomy is performed through longitudinal and circular layers of esophagus, extending from inferior pulmonary vein to 2–3cm onto anterior stomach.
  - To prevent reflux a 180° wrap is performed.
- Dor anterior wrap Toupet posterior wrap.
- **Esophagectomy** (📖 p764) is reserved for end-stage achalasia, sigmoid or megaesophagus, multiple reflux strictures, two or more prior myotomies.

Nutcracker esophagus
- **Pathology:** normal peristalsis, but in the distal esophagus contraction amplitudes are up to 180mmHg, and duration >6s.
- **Presentation:** extreme atypical chest pain. Emotional triggers.
- **Investigation:** manometry shows high-amplitude contractions with contraction durations >6s, normal LES.
- **Management:** primarily medical, nitrates and calcium channel blockers.

Diffuse esophageal spasm
- **Pathology:** degenerative changes in vagus, muscle hypertrophy. Simultaneous contractions in esophagus leading to 'corkscrew' or 'rosary bead' appearance, and epiphrenic diverticulum.
- **Presentation:** substernal atypical pain that is similar to angina, anxiety, high association with psychiatric disorders.
- **Investigation:** manometry shows normal or hypertensive LES, normal relaxation of LES; simultaneous, high-amplitude esophageal contractions. Barium esophagram shows simultaneous esophageal contractions.
- **Treatment:** nitrates and calcium channel blockers, anxiolytics.
- **Surgery:** reserved only for failed medial management: long myotomy via left thoracotomy, myotomy extending from aortic arch onto the LES, with incomplete wrap such as Belsey fundoplication to limit reflux after dividing LES. Good results in only 2/3 of patients.

Scleroderma
- Atrophy of smooth muscle components, fibrous infiltration, and incompetence of LES is found in 80% of patients with scleroderma.
- Manometry shows an incompetent LES and lack of peristalsis.
- Antireflux procedures are not very successful, and may exacerbate dysphagia: occasionally esophagectomy is required.

Hernias and ruptures

Key facts

- Herniation of the body and/or fundus of the stomach through the diaphragmatic esophageal hiatus into the mediastinum, anterior or lateral to the esophagus is considered a paraesophageal hiatal hernia.
- Found in a mostly elderly population.

Pathology

- Hiatus hernia is divided into four types:
  - Type I (sliding hiatal hernia) occurs with migration of the *GEJ above the diaphragmatic hiatus* so reflux is predominant symptom.
  - Type II (rolling or paraesophageal) due to upward migration of the gastric fundus into the posterior mediastinum; however, the *GEJ remains below diaphragm* in normal position within the abdomen.
  - Type III (combination) massive or giant paraesophageal hernia where the majority of the stomach, including the fundus and GEJ have herniated into the mediastinum.
  - Type IV (complex) massive hernia where the stomach and other abdominal organs, such as the spleen, colon, small bowel have herniated into the mediastinum.
- Complications are *functional* (GERD, Barrett's, esophagitis, strictures, aspiration) and *mechanical* (obstruction, volvulus, and impaired pulmonary function in the case of massive hernias).

Presentation

- Often are asymptomatic.
- Dysphagia, odynophagia, hematemesis, vomiting, anemia, dysphagia, regurgitation, postprandial fullness.
- If a patient complaints of chest or epigastric pain, a NG tube should be placed immediately to decompress the stomach and avoid strangulation.

Investigation

- Barium esophagram defines anatomy, level of obstruction, position of stomach, and emptying of esophagus and stomach.
- EGD helps exclude other pathology, and permits biopsy to assess esophagitis and strictures.
- Esophageal function may be further assessed with manometry and pH.
- Chest CT provides information on contents and size of hernia sac.

Management

- Type I hernias may not require repair: GERD may be managed medically (🔲 p778) with antireflux surgery (🔲 p787) if medical management fails.
- Type II–IV hernias require surgical repair.

Surgery

- Can be done laparoscopically or through a left thoracotomy.
- The hernia sac and its contents is reduced (via laparoscopic, laparotomy or left thoracotomy approach).
- The sac is excised and the esophageal hiatus narrowed posteriorly with or without mesh reinforcement, to reduce recurrence (permanent mesh is avoided to prevent chronic constriction or perforation).

- If there is any tension when the GEJ is returned into the abdomen, then an esophageal lengthening procedure should be performed, e.g., Collis gastroplasty with Nissen fundoplication (📖 p787).
- A gastropexy may be performed to fix the stomach in the abdomen.
- The mortality of surgery is around 2–5%, higher in emergency repair, and the risk of recurrence around 10–20%.

Esophageal ruptures

General principles are covered on 📖 p790. Specific types include:

Boerhaave syndrome

- Boerhaave syndrome classically presents as sudden onset severe chest pain radiating to back, abdomen left shoulder, worse on swallowing, and starting after repeated and prolonged vomiting.
- In 1723 Hermann Boerhaave detailed a postmortem on Baron Jan Gerrit von Wassenaer, who suffered postemetic esophageal rupture after self-inducing emeses after a heavy meal—he found a transverse tear of the distal esophagus.
- Vomiting is the most common cause, and is thought to be secondary to simultaneous closing of the upper and lower esophageal sphincters, with resultant increase of intraluminal pressure.
- 90% of injuries occur in the lower 1/3 of the esophagus on the left side.
- Unlike originally described, commonly a longitudinal tear (3–10cm).
- Usually in men age 35–55, often occurs in alcoholics.
- Repair of esophageal rupture is described on 📖 p790.

Esophageal foreign body and food impaction

- Foreign body impaction is common in children and psychiatric patients. Children commonly ingest coins. Elderly people may accidentally ingest their dentures. Represents 12% of esophageal perforations.
- Common area of impaction is the broncho-aortic constriction point.
- Meat impaction is dissolved by having the patient swallow 5mL of 20% papain (meat tenderizer) in 10% of alcohol every 5min for 1h.
- Flexible endoscopy or rigid esophagoscopy is often adequate.
- Do not push the impacted object forward, as there may be a distal obstructing lesion, especially if the impacted object is in the distal 1/3 of the esophagus. Pushing against a fixed obstruction may perforate.
- Esophagotomy may be required if the foreign body cannot be removed endoscopically: objects in the distal 1/3 of the esophagus should be approached via a left posterolateral thoracotomy, objects in the proximal 2/3 of the esophagus should be approached via a right posterolateral thoracotomy.

Esophageal mucosal dissection

- Mucosal injury after ingestion of sharp food, e.g., bone or shell, resulting in dissection along the submucosa, causing exquisite odynophagia.
- Thin barium esophagram demonstrates migration of contrast within the wall of the esophagus, but no extravasation.
- Therapy is supportive therapy with pain control. Self-limiting.

Esophageal perforation

Key facts

- Esophageal perforation is a full-thickness injury to the cervical, thoracic, or abdominal esophagus, resulting in extravasation of luminal contents into the neck, mediastinum, pleural space, or abdominal cavity.
- Overall mortality associated with esophageal perforation is 18%.
- Mortality is determined by cause, location, and treatment delay:
  - Spontaneous esophageal perforation carries a 36% mortality; iatrogenic 19% mortality; traumatic 7% mortality.
  - Cervical perforations carry a 6% mortality; thoracic perforation a 27% mortality; abdominal perforations a 21% mortality.
  - Diagnosis <24h, mortality 14%; >24h, mortality 27%.

Pathology

- Instrumental (60–75%), e.g., endoscopy, dilation, balloon and bouginage, intubation errors, laser therapy.
- Non-instrumental: barogenic trauma (15%), postemetic *Boerhaave syndrome* (📖 p789) (excess vomiting results in rupture of esophagus).
- Penetrating trauma (9%), operative trauma (2%), caustic injury (📖 p792).
- Swallowed foreign bodies or meat impaction (12%), malignancy (1%).

Presentation

- Symptoms depend on location, common points of perforation occur at three naturally occurring areas of esophageal narrowing (📖 p659):
  - Cervical constriction point: cricopharyngeus muscles and Killian's triangle (14–16cm from the incisors).
  - Mid-esophageal constriction point: bronchoaortic constriction (22–24cm from the incisors).
  - Distal esophageal constriction point: esophagogastric junction (40–45cm from the incisors).
- Cervical perforation: low severity, with contamination limited by neck, but may extend down anterior to the prevertebral fascia ('danger space') into the mediastinum. May present with neck pain, dysphagia, dysphonia, subcutaneous emphysema.
- Thoracic perforation: may rapidly contaminate the mediastinum and the pleural space, resulting in chemical irritation, inflammation, marked fluid shifts, and sepsis. May present with chest pain, tachycardia, fever, leukocytosis, hypotension.
- Abdominal perforation: extravasation of luminal contents into the abdomen. May present with abdominal pain, and a clinical examination demonstrating epigastric tenderness and peritoneal signs.

Investigation

- CXR shows pneumomediastinum and subcutaneous emphysema.
- All stable patients should undergo a thin barium esophagram: water-soluble contrast has poorer sensitivity and poses a risk of pneumonitis if aspirated. If patients are going to the OR for other reasons, and an

esophageal injury is suspected, then a flexible endoscopy should be performed—it may not always identify the lesion.
- Concurrent tracheal injury repairs should be separated from esophageal repairs with viable tissue, such as strap muscle, intercostal muscle, pericardial fat, pleural patch, or omentum.

Operative management

Cervical perforation

- A cervical esophageal perforation is approached via a standard left neck incision, anterior to the sternocleidomastoid muscles, and the carotid–jugular bundle. The omohyoid muscle is divided, and the incision is carried down to the esophagus and anterior spine.
- If a cervical perforation cannot be primarily repaired, leaving the neck open to allow for drainage is adequate, and the injury should heal with packing in 2 weeks.
- The mucosa injury is always more extensive than the muscular injury.
- The muscularis propria (longitudinal and circular) layers are divided with cautery, exposing the entire mucosal defect; devitalized tissue is debrided. The mucosal defect is closed using running 4/0 PDS. The muscular layer is closed with running or interrupted 4/0 PDS and the neck wound is closed in layers over a drain (1/4 inch Penrose).

Intrathoracic perforation

- All intrathoracic injuries in the absence of intrinsic disease, e.g., malignancy should undergo primary repair regardless of time from diagnosis.
- In achalasia (📖 p786), a myotomy should also be performed, whereas in the setting of malignancy, an esophagectomy is necessary.
- Distal 1/3 lesions are reached via a left posterolateral thoracotomy. Middle and upper 1/3 lesions are reached via a right thoracotomy.
- The esophagus is mobilized.
- The mucosal injury is always more extensive than the muscular injury.
- The longitudinal and circular muscle layers are divided with cautery, revealing the entire extent of the mucosal injury. A 48–52F Maloney bougie is passed to prevent narrowing of the esophagus by the repair.
- The submucosal edges are grasped with Allis clamps; the defect is closed with a stapler and reinforced with an intercostal muscle flap.

Esophageal stents

- With small perforations, or patients who are poor surgical candidates, there have been numerous reports documenting success with endoscopically placed temporary covered esophageal stents.
- In the setting of intrathoracic perforation, the pleural space still needs drainage either with tube thoracostomy or by VATS.

Outcomes

- Complications after primary repair of esophageal perforation include leak, empyema, soft tissue infections, recurrent laryngeal nerve injury.
- Overall mortality <10%.

Caustic esophageal injuries

Key facts

- There are 5000 caustic ingestion injuries per year in the USA.
- Occurs in young children and adults attempting suicide.
- Offending agents include acids, alkalis, and household materials such as detergents and bleach.
- Acids and alkali cause reflex pyloric and cricopharyngeal spasm resulting in pooling in the gastric antrum. Contractions in the esophagus and stomach distribute the corrosive agents. As a result can have full tissue destruction of the distal esophagus and the stomach.

Pathology

Strong alkali

- Includes household drain cleaners.
- Alkali causes liquefaction necrosis with deep tissue penetration.

Strong acids

- May relatively spare the esophagus and cause severe gastric injury.
- The depth of tissue injury is often less than that of alkali.

Presentation and investigation

- Thin barium esophagram is helpful in identifying areas of perforation.
- Chest CT.
- Flexible endoscopy is critical in determining extent of mucosal destruction. Mucosal injuries are described similar to burns:
  - *First-degree:* mucosal hyperaemia and oedema.
  - *Second-degree:* mucosal ulceration with blisters and exudates with pseudomembrane formation.
  - *Third-degree:* deep ulcerations with charring and eschar formation, with massive edema and luminal obliteration.

Management

Initial management

- Airway control, fluid resuscitation and broad-spectrum antibiotics.
- No role for prophylactic corticosteroids.

First-degree injury

- Expectant management with observation for 24–48h.

Second-degree injury

- Careful observation for perforation.
- These patients will often need long-term surveillance as stricture formation is common.
- Dilations should not be performed until 6–8 weeks after initial injury.
- Patients with strictures intractable to dilation may require esophagectomy with gastric reconstruction if available, or colon conduit.

Third-degree injury

- Complete necrosis and/or perforation of the esophagus requires esophagectomy with delayed reconstruction.

- A THE is often made easier due to edema in the mediastinum.
- The esophageal hiatus is closed.
- A feeding jejunostomy is placed, and if the stomach is viable, then a draining gastrostomy is performed.
- A diverting end esophagostomy (spit fistula) is performed.
- The residual esophagus is brought out via a standard left neck incision, and tunnelled along the chest and exteriorized as an ostomy just below the clavicle via interrupted 4/0 Vicryl. This allows for a flat surface on which to place an ostomy bag (Fig. 15.5).
- The end esophagostomy should be dilated with a finger every day to prevent stricture formation.

Esophageal discontinuity

- If during attempt at primary repair of the esophagus, the patient is too unstable to move forward, or the tissues are too compromised by sepsis, the area in question can just be stapled closed and adequately drained.
- The patient can be brought back when stable for an end oesophagostomy or 'spit fistula' (Fig. 15.5), and placement of an enteral feeding tube, for long-term nutrition.
- Eventually completion esophagectomy with gastric or colon conduit reconstruction can be performed.

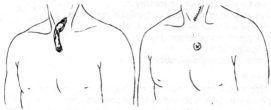

Fig. 15.5 Formation of a 'spit' fistula.

Benign tumors and cysts

Key facts
- Benign esophageal tumors are rare lesions which can appear anywhere within the wall of the esophagus. Most common etiology is leiomyoma, lipomas, and hemangiomas (Table 15.6).
- Esophageal cysts are rare; they may be congenital or acquired.
- Symptoms depend upon tumor location: dysphagia, odynophagia, aspiration, hematemesis, regurgitation of lesion into mouth or airway if pedunculated, atypical chest pain.
- Chest CT and MRI are useful for delineation of anatomy, endoscopy and EUS provides biopsy and histology, and location within wall of esophagus.
- Treatment if required for symptom control is surgical extirpation via myotomy; need for esophagectomy is rare.

Esophageal duplication cysts

Pathology
- These rare congenital cysts result from a developmental failure of the posterior division of the primitive foregut.
- Intramural and enclosed within the esophageal wall, lined with squamous epithelium, though may contain gastric epithelium.
- Frequently found on the right inferior aspect of the esophagus, and do not have continuity with the esophagus.
- May be associated with other congenital abnormalities:
  - Vertebral defects and spinal cord defects.
  - Congenital tracheoesophageal fistula.
  - Esophageal atresia.
  - Other GI visceral duplications.

Presentation
- In children they may obstruct the esophageal lumen or cause respiratory symptoms secondary to compression effect.
- Adults are often asymptomatic. Symptoms include dysphagia, dyspnea, atypical chest pain. Perforation, bleeding, and malignant degeneration is rare.

Diagnosis
- Chest CT and MRI are useful for delineation of anatomy and fluid or viscous contents.
- Biopsy should be avoided.
- Endoscopy and EUS rules out intraluminal pathology, and confirms intramural location.

Treatment
- Surgical extirpation via a myotomy.

Other congenital cysts

Bronchogenic esophageal cysts
These congenital intramural cysts are found in the distal 1/3 of the esophagus, and contain cartilage.

Esophageal gastric cysts
- These intramural cysts are lined with gastric mucosa.
- May present with a peptic ulcer.

Inclusion cysts
Intramural. Contain respiratory or squamous epithelium.

Acquired cysts
- Retention cysts.
- May be single or multiple.
- Found in the upper 1/3 of the esophagus.

Leiomyoma
- Most common benign tumor of the esophagus.
- Usually found in the middle and lower 1/3 of the esophagus.
- Intramural location.
- 2:1 male to female ratio, rare in children.
- Usually single intraluminal polyp found in the cervical esophagus.

Lipoma
- Commonly presents as an intraluminal polyp, in the upper esophagus.
- Can grow to large size and may present as a mass in the throat which disappears upon swallowing.

Haemangioma
- Submucosal lesion.
- Usually asymptomatic. Symptoms include atypical chest pain, dysphagia, and hematemesis.

Table 15.6 Location of benign tumors and cysts within the esophageal wall

Lesion	Location
Squamous papilloma	Mucosa
Fibrovascular polyp	
Retention cyst	
Lipoma	Submucosa
Fibroma	
Neurofibroma	
Granular cell tumor	
Hemangioma	
Salivary gland type tumor	
Leiomyoma	Muscularis
Duplication cyst	
Adventitia	
Foregut cyst	

Mediastinum and chest wall

Mediastinal masses

Key facts
- Most mediastinal masses in children and young adults are malignant.
- Anterior mediastinal masses should be removed, unless lymphoma is likely, which is better treated with adjuvant therapy.
- *Thymoma* should be resected (🕮 p800). VATS approach is reasonable unless large thymoma or thymic carcinoma which require sternotomy.

Mediastinal compartments
Mediastinal compartments are depicted on 🕮 p41.
- *Anterior superior:* borders are the thoracic inlet superiorly, sternum anteriorly, pleura laterally, and anterior pericardium posteriorly. Contents include the thymus, lymphatics, and great vessels.
- *Middle:* borders are the anterior and posterior pericardium, and pleura laterally. Contents include the heart, phrenic nerves, tracheal carina and bronchi, and lymphatics.
- *Posterior:* borders are posterior pericardium anteriorly, spine posteriorly, and pleura laterally. Contents include esophagus, vagi, sympathetic chain, thoracic duct, descending aorta, azygos, and hemiazygos.

Pathology
- *Etiology:* neurogenic (20%), thymomas (20%), primary cysts (20%), lymphomas (13%), germ cell tumors (10%).
- *Location:* anterosuperior (54%), posterior (26%), middle (20%).
- *Malignancy:* 25–50% are malignant. Mediastinal malignancy has highest incidence between the first and fourth decades of life. Malignant neurogenic tumors and non-Hodgkin's lymphoma are the most common mediastinal tumors in children.

Presentation and investigation
1/3 of patients are asymptomatic. Symptoms include chest pain, cough, fever, mechanical compression, and invasion of vital structures. Paraneoplastic syndromes (🕮 p670) may be present.
- *CXR:* provides relative location, incidental discovery.
- *Chest CT:* defines anatomy and distal spread, bony involvement.
- *MRI:* able to determine spinal involvement and vascular invasion.
- *Echo:* evaluation of cardiac tumors and cysts.
- *Fine needle aspiration or core biopsy:* able to make diagnosis of malignancy in 80–90% of cases. FNA is not reliable for the diagnosis of lymphoma, as additional tissue is needed for adequate flow cytometry.
- *Mediastinoscopy or anterior mediastinotomy* (Chamberlain procedure) (🕮 p662). Mediastinoscopy is helpful for paratracheal lymphadenopathy (middle compartment) but cannot reach an anterior mediastinal mass. Chamberlain procedure for large anterior mediastinal masses.

Middle mediastinal masses
- *Pathology:* lymphoma, paratracheal lymph nodes (LNs), bronchogenic cysts.

- *Lymphoma* is best diagnosed by mediastinoscopy.
- Although diagnosis by EBUS has been described, often an FNA does not provide enough tissue for diagnosis.
- Hodgkin's lymphoma may be difficult to diagnosis as lymph tissue can be markedly inflamed with ill-defined histology.
- *Bronchogenic cysts* account for 5% of mediastinal masses and the most common mediastinal cyst, usually located in the subcarinal area. The majority are asymptomatic, but can cause atypical pain, and symptoms related to compression. May become infected if it communicated with the tracheobronchial tree. If symptomatic, then surgical resection by thoracotomy or VATS.
- *Thoracic duct cysts*. Very rare. Can present with symptoms of tracheal or esophageal compression. Surgical resection if symptomatic.

Posterior mediastinal masses

- *Pathology:* esophageal duplication cysts (see benign disease of the esophagus), neurogenic tumors.
- *Neurogenic tumors* make up to 25% of mediastinal masses in adults and 40% in children (most common mediastinal tumor in children). 85% are autonomic ganglia and may produce catecholamines. Occur in the right and left paravertebral sulci, usually in the upper chest, and may involve spinal, intercostal, phrenic, vagus, and sympathetic chain.
- Symptoms include atypical pain, cough, and symptoms of extrinsic compression including dyspnea, dysphagia, and symptoms of neurogenic involvement such as Horner's syndrome, spinal cord compression, also fever and malaise.
- Chest CT and MRI delineate anatomy. MRI especially useful for determining spinal involvement. FNA biopsy.
- Thoracotomy or VATS resection. *Dumbbell tumors* or tumors that invade neuroforamina require surgical assistance from orthopedic or neurosurgery, as laminectomy may be required for a R0 resection. Disease-specific adjuvant chemotherapy and/or radiotherapy if malignant.

Thymoma

Key facts

Abnormal persistent growth of the thymus gland instead of the usual involution and atrophy seen in adulthood.

Pathology

- Thymus develops embryonically from the third pharyngeal pouch.
- Lies posterior to the sternal manubrium and anterior to the great
  vessels, receives its blood supply from the IMAs.
- Venous drainage is to the innominate vein and internal thoracic veins.
- Lymphatic drainage is to the lower cervical, internal mammary,
  anterior mediastinal, and hilar lymph node lymphatic basins.
- *Thymoma* is characterized by thymic epithelial cells with variable
  lymphocytes, subdivided by fibrous bands.
- *Thymic carcinoma* lacks features of normal thymus, characterized by
  cellular atypia, and increased proliferation of cells.

Presentation

- Usually incidental finding, or paraneoplastic syndromes including:
  - *Endocrine disorders,* e.g., Addison's disease, hyperthyroidism,
    hyperparathyroidism, panhypopituitarism.
  - *Hematologic disorders,* e.g., red cell aplasia,
    hypogammaglobulinemia, T cell deficiency syndrome, pancytopenia,
    erythrocytosis, amegakaryocytic thrombocytopenia.
  - *Neuromuscular syndromes,* e.g., *myasthenia gravis* (MG),
    Eaton–Lambert syndrome, myotonic dystrophy, and myositis.
- 30% of patients with thymoma have MG, 10–20% of patient with
  MG have thymoma. Thymic carcinoma with MG is rare.
- 5% of patients with thymoma have RBC aplasia and 50% of patients
  with RBC aplasia have thymoma.
- 2% of patients with thymoma have hypogammaglobulinemia.
- Hypogammaglobulinemia and RBC aplasia indicate poor prognosis.

Classification and staging

Classification includes Muller–Hermelink and World Health Organization
(WHO) systems (Table 16.1) and Masaoka clinical stage:

- Stage I: macroscopically completely encapsulated with no invasion.
- Stage II: microscopic capsular invasion or macroscopic invasion into
  surrounding fatty tissue or mediastinal pleura.
- Stage III: macroscopic invasion into surrounding organs such as the
  pericardium, great vessels, and pleura.
- Stage IVa: pleural or pericardial dissemination.
- Stage IVb: haematogenous or lymphogenous spread.

Surgery

Main principles include wide resection of entire thymus from phrenic
nerve to phrenic nerve, en bloc resection of invaded structure, and marking residual disease with clips for irradiation if unresectable. Preoperative
plasmapheresis for thymectomy for MG.

Sternotomy approach
- Upper sternotomy (📖 p467) rather than VATS is approach of choice for larger thymomas or suspicion of thymic carcinoma.
- Open bilateral pleural spaces, divide vein extending from the innominate vein, identify phrenic nerves bilaterally.
- Exenteration of anteromediastinal tissue from phrenic to phrenic nerve, including the pericardial fat, with skeletonization of the innominate vein, and removal intact of all four poles of the thymus.

Transcervical thymectomy
Useful for smaller thymomas, via collar incision in the neck. Surgeon stands at the head of the patient, and a 'thymus retractor' is used to distract sternum anteriorly and expose contents of anterior mediastinum.

VATS thymectomy
- Useful for smaller thymomas, performed from one side, or bilaterally.
- CO_2 insufflation to push the lung aside. May be difficult to identify the contralateral phrenic nerve—bilateral approach limits phrenic injury.
- The patient is placed in the supine position with arms extended, and a shoulder roll along the spine, to allow shoulders to drop posteriorly.
- The pericardial fat pad and thymus is mobilized inferiorly and meticulously moving cephalad and both pleural spaces are opened.
- After freeing the inferior poles, and identifying the contralateral phrenic nerve, the superior poles are mobilized and the thymic vein is divided with a Harmonic scalpel. The specimen is removed in a bag.

Chemotherapy and radiation
- Adjuvant radiation for R1 resection, Stage IIa or higher.
- Adjuvant chemotherapy is platinum based and indicated for R1 resection of thymic carcinoma, R2 resections of thymoma, unresectable disease, or stage III or higher.

Outcomes
- Thymectomy for MG often takes up 1 year to see improvement.
- At 5 years, 30–50% patients will experience some improvement and 25–30% of patients will have complete resolution of symptoms.
- Thymectomy for thymoma, 5-year survival for Masaoka stage— Stage I: 94–100%, Stage II: 86–95%, stage III: 56–69%, stage IV: 11–50.

Table 16.1 Thymoma classification

Muller–Hermelink	WHO
Thymoma	Thymoma
Medullary type	Type A
Mixed type	Type AB
Predominantly cortical	Type B1
Cortical type	Type B2
Well-differentiated carcinoma	Type B3
Thymic carcinoma	Type C (thymic carcinoma)

Anterior mediastinal masses

Key facts

* Masses in the anterior mediastinum are more likely to be malignant (60%) than middle (30%) or posterior (<20%) mediastinal masses.
* Common causes are thymomas (📖 p800), lymphomas (📖 p799) and germ cell tumors, as well as cysts, e.g., pericardial and bronchogenic (📖 p802) which account for around 20% of anterior mediastinal masses.
* Thyroid goiters may have retrosternal extension.
* Thymomas (📖 p800) are the commonest cause of anterior mediastinal masses, although they are rarely seen in children. These should be removed via VATS or sternotomy.

Thymic cysts

* Uncommon in adults. Often found incidentally. May occur in association with syphilis (DuBois abscess) or MG.
* Treatment: thymectomy.

Germ cell tumors

* Same as germ cell tumors in gonads, but are primary and not metastatic. Represent 15–25% of all anterior mediastinal masses.
* More common in young adults and children. 60% are malignant.
* Majority of benign tumors are teratomas.
* Malignant tumors (Table 16.2) include non-seminomas (60%) (embryonal cell, choriocarcinoma, yolk-sac tumors, teratocarcinoma), and seminomas (40%).

Lymphangioma (cystic hygroma)

* Multiloculated cystic mass of lymphatics. Often extends from a cervical or axillary origin. Usually involves the anterior mediastinum.

Table 16.2 Germ cell tumors

α-fetoprotein and β-HCG	Seminomas	Non-seminomas
	Unusual	90%
Associated pathology	None	Chromosomal defects
Metastasis	Unusual	Frequent
Radiosensitive	Very	No
Therapy	Radiation	Platinum-based neoadjuvant chemotherapy; resection if residual disease
Remission	> 80%	Complete response in 55%
		Partial response 35%
Outcomes	5-year survival 50–80%	5-year survival 50–60%

- Chest CT.
- Surgical resection if symptomatic. May be difficult to achieve a R0 resection, especially if it extends into vital structures.

Pericardial cysts

- Most commonly occurs at the right pericardiophrenic angle. Often are found incidentally, but may have symptoms of atypical chest pain. Has no malignant potential.
- Chest CT.
- Surgical resection if symptomatic. VATS resection is the procedure of choice. Care must be taken to avoid injury to the phrenic nerve.

Parathyroid adenoma

- Ectopic anteromediastinal location of a parathyroid adenoma, often found with in a residual thymus gland or area as a result of common embryogenesis from the third branchial cleft.
- Symptoms of primary hyperparathyroidism.
- Sestamibi scan locates tumor in the anterior mediastinum.
- Chest CT confirms location.
- Surgery is VATS resection.
- Preoperative and intraoperative PTH levels are measured to confirm removal.
- The patient can also be injected with sestamibi 1h before surgery, and the lesion can be confirmed after resection with a gamma probe and counter.

Sclerosing fibrosis of the mediastinum

- *Pathology*: it is a chronic granulomatous proliferative inflammatory process involving the anterior and middle mediastinum. The process can encase mediastinal structures leading to compression-type abnormalities.
- Causes include histoplasmosis, aspergillosis, *Cryptococcus*, TB, nocardiosis, actinomycosis, autoimmune diseases, sarcoidosis.
- More common in females, higher incidence in the midwest USA.
- *Presentation:* symptoms include fever, cough, dyspnea, recurrent pneumonias, fistulas of luminal origins, SVC syndrome, cardiac tamponade, cor pulmonale.
- *Investigation:* chest CT identifies loss of normal tissue plains, calcified lymph nodes and invasion of adjacent structures.
- *Management:* surgical biopsy of lymph nodes for tissue diagnosis.
- Treatment of underlying disease process, including antifungals.
- Alleviation of sequelae, such as repair of SVC syndrome, resection of fibrosed dysfunction tissue, such as pulmonary resection. As tissue planes are lost, may be difficult to identify and control vascular structures. Consider cardiopulmonary bypass for difficult resections.

Thoracic sympathectomy

Key facts

- Interruption of the upper thoracic sympathetic chain (between T2 and T4) usually via bilateral VATS approach: the precise level of interruption remains controversial.
- Indicated for primary hyperhidrosis of the face, and upper extremities and axilla.
- Medical treatment includes topical aluminium chloride, systemic or topical anticholinergic agents, iontophoresis, or localized botulinum toxin injections. Surgery is reserved for failed medical management.
- Secondary hyperhidrosis, i.e., hyperthyroidism or other systemic entities, should be ruled out before surgical therapy.

Hyperhidrosis

- Most patients report excessive (pools of water rather than just dampness) plantar and palmar sweating since childhood, which has significant impact on work and social life. Commonly associated with axillary hyperhidrosis.
- Incidence around 1–2% depending on definition, and familial history in around 2/3 of patients. It affects females slightly more than males.
- Secondary hyperhidrosis.
- Preganglionic sympathetic fibers responsible for palmar sweating arise from T3–T6, ascending via T2 to reach the hand via the brachial plexus. The sympathetic chain is located just under the rib heads: T2 ganglion is between the heads of the 2nd and 3rd ribs.

Procedure

- Principles of the procedure involve transection of the appropriate level of sympathetic chain that corresponds to the anatomic location of the patient's symptoms, which can be achieved in several ways:
  - *Sympathectomy* is removal or ablation of a sympathetic ganglion, as well as transection of the sympathetic chain above and below.
  - *Sympathicotomy* is transection of the sympathetic chain.
  - *Clipping* refers to application of clips at a particular level, or above and below a specific ganglion.
- The level of division may be based on clinical findings, although multiple trials with conflicting results have been published:
  - For facial sweating the sympathetic chain is isolated by dividing the chain overlying the 2nd and 3rd ribs.
  - For palmar sweating, the chain overlying 2nd, 3rd and 4th ribs is divided.
  - For axillary sweating, the ramus overlying 3rd, 4th, and 5th ribs is divided.
  - Isolated axillary hyperhidrosis is treated by transection of the chain between the 3rd and the 4th rib.
- Care must be taken to avoid injury to the T1 or stellate ganglia, which may lead to Horner's syndrome.

Set-up
- The patient is placed in the semi-Fowler's position (sitting up at about 30–45° to allow the lungs to fall away from the apex), with the arms extended at 90°.
- Two 5mm trocars are placed in the 2nd and 4th intercostal space in the anterior axillary line.
- CO_2 insufflation can be used to further displace the lung (10mmHg).

Sympathectomy
- The sympathetic chain is divided over the appropriate rib with hook cautery (Fig. 16.1). Great care is taken to correctly identify the 2nd rib:
  - It is usually the most proximal rib that can be seen in the thorax.
  - It is the only rib crossed lateral to the sympathetic chain by a small arterial branch of the subclavian that forms the 2nd intercostal artery.
- Both sides are done during the same operative setting.
- The accessory nerve of Kuntz is divided, cauterizing the parietal pleura running along the rib lateral from the rib head.

Outcomes
- Improvement or resolution of symptoms occurs in >90% of patients.
- Compensatory symptoms occur in up to 40% of patients.
- Compensatory sweating includes Frey syndrome or gustatory sweating, sweating of the back, chest, or feet.
- Treatment of compensatory symptoms is generally supportive.
- Asians may have a risk of compensatory sweating of up to 90%.
- Horner's syndrome (ptosis, miosis, anhidrosis) occurs in <1%.
- Resting and peak heart rate decreases by 5–10% as a result of division of sympathetic cardiac nerve supply: this is the rationale for use of sympathectomy in refractory tachyarrhythmias.

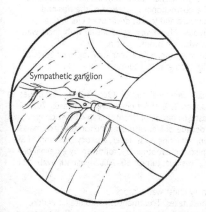

Sympathetic ganglion

Fig. 16.1 Sympathectomy. The cut is ideally made on the surface of the rib, not between them.

Primary chest wall tumors

Key facts

Primary chest wall tumors comprise 5% of all thoracic neoplasms, and approximately 26% of all chest wall tumors, with 50% being malignant.

Primary bone tumors

- *Pathology*: 85% occur in the ribs and 15% in the sternum, 90% are malignant. Most common benign tumors are chondroma, fibrous dysplasia, osteochondroma (see Table 16.3).
- Most common malignant tumors are chondrosarcoma, Ewing sarcoma, osteosarcoma, benign primary bone tumors.

Chondroma

- 15% of benign rib tumors, occurs in the second and third decades of life, found in the costochondral junction, difficult to distinguish from chondrosarcoma, histology demonstrates lobules of hyaline cartilage.
- Managed as a malignant lesion (see Chest wall resection, 📖 p808).

Fibrous dysplasia

- Fibrous replacement of the medullary cavity of the rib, slow growing, and generally asymptomatic. Occurs equally in males and females.
- Characteristic radiographic appearance is an expansile lesion with cortical thinning and a ground-glass center.

Osteochondroma

Occurs at the metaphyseal area of the rib, bony stalk with cartilaginous cap, occurs in children. Has ability to transform into a malignancy.

Malignant bone tumors

Chondrosarcoma

- Represents 1/3 of primary malignant bone tumors, and is the most common. Occurs at the costochondral junction of the ribs and sternum. Occurs in the third and fourth decades of life, with a predilection towards males. May have a relationship with chest wall trauma. Grows slowly, with symptoms of pain.
- Treatment is complete resection, 65% 5-year survival, predictors of survival are R0 resection and grade of tumor.

Ewing sarcoma

- 15% of malignant primary chest wall tumor. Occurs in the flat bones and midshaft of long bones, 25% of patients have metastases. 70% of patients develop metastases during up-front therapy. Most commonly occurs in the second decade of life, with predilection towards males.
- Symptoms include pain, enlarging mass, fever, leukocytosis, and ↑ESR.
- Treatment involves upfront chemotherapy, followed by external beam radiation or resection if residual tumor. 60–70% 5-year survival.

Osteosarcoma

- 10% of malignant primary chest wall tumors.
- 1/3 of patients have metastases. Treatment is complete resection.
- Associated with previous radiotherapy, chemotherapy, Paget disease.

- Painful rapidly enlarging mass with elevated alkaline phosphatase. Often in patients age 10–25 and >40 years. 15% 5-year survival.

Plasmacytoma
- Located in the ribs. Occurs in sixth decade of life, commoner in males.
- Treatment is radiotherapy, followed by surgical excision if radioresistant, and chemotherapy for disease progression. 60% 5-year survival.

Primary soft-tissue tumors
- Common benign tumors include connective tissue tumors, e.g., fibroma, lipomas, hemangiomas. Malignant degeneration is rare.
- Treatment is local excision.

Desmoid tissues
- Though technically benign, behaves in an aggressive 'malignant' manner. Originate in the muscle and fascia, and grows along tissue planes and surrounds local structures. histology demonstrates fibroblasts and fibrocytes. Associated with Gardner syndrome.
- Treatment is wide complete resection. High recurrence rate.

Sarcoma
- 50% of all primary malignant chest wall tumors, majority of secondary or metastatic chest wall tumors. 2:1 male to female ratio. Most common in adults, though rhabdomyosarcoma occurs more commonly in children. Most common sarcomas are fibrosarcoma, liposarcoma, rhabdomyosarcoma. Prognostic factors include tumor grade, presence of metastases, and symptoms of pain.
- Treatment is wide complete resection, 82% 5-year survival with low grade tumors compared to 39% with high grade.
- Adjuvant chemotherapy 9 radiation should be considered.

Table 16.3 Primary tumors of the chest wall

	Bone and cartilage	Soft tissue
Benign	Aneurysmal bone cyst	Fibroma
	Chondroblastoma	Haemangioma
	Chondroma	Lipoma
	Giant cell tumor	Lymphangioma
	Eosinophilic granuloma	Neurofibroma
	Fibrous dysplasia	
	Osteoblastoma	
	Osteochondroma	
Malignant	Condrosarcoma	Desmoid
	Ewing's sarcoma	Leiomyosarcoma
	Lymphoma	Liposarcoma
	Osteosarcoma	Lymphangiosarcoma
	Solitary plasmacytoma	Malignant fibrous histiocytoma

Secondary chest wall tumors

Key facts
These include tumors of direct invasion such as breast and lung and meta-static tumors.

Directly invasive secondary chest wall tumors

Breast cancer
- Treatment is resection *if* locoregional disease is controlled, *and* the chest wall is the only site of recurrence *and* R0 resection is achievable.
- 34–58% 5-year survival.

Lung cancer
- Chest wall invasion is considered a T3 tumor. Occurs in 2–8% of patients with NSCLC. Treatment is en bloc resection with 2cm margins.
- 25–10% 5 year survival.

Metastatic secondary tumors of the chest wall
- *Pathology:* sarcomas and carcinoma are most common: 20% of all chest wall tumors. Resection *if* locoregional disease is controlled, *and* chest wall is the only metastatic site, *and* R0 resection achievable.
- *Presentation:* generally asymptomatic, pain as the lesion becomes larger; painful masses are generally malignant. Bone and cartilage tumors have pain as a common symptom. Systemic symptoms include fever, leukocystosis, eosinophilia, elevated ESR.
- CT: imaging of choice, provides anatomy and delineates associated thoracic pathology. MRI not always necessary. Helpful in determining tissue planes.
- Tissue diagnosis: fine needle or core biopsy. 790% diagnostic. Excisional biopsy for tumors <5cm.
- Reoperation with wide en bloc resection if malignant.
- Incisional biopsy for tumors ≥5cm.

Chest wall resection
- Margins should include one rib above and below the lesion.
- 2cm margins for benign or metastatic lesions.
- 4cm margins for primary malignant lesions such sarcoma.
- En bloc resection of adherent structures.
- Frozen section intraoperative histology of soft tissue and bone marrow to confirm R0 resection.

Chest wall reconstruction
- Defects that are <5cm and/or are covered by the scapula generally do not need reconstruction.
- Reconstruction of large defects avoids paradoxical movement of chest wall with respiration, protects vital organs and improves cosmetics.

Reconstruction options
- Prosthetic materials:
  - Meshes, e.g., Gore-Tex, Marlex, Prolene, PTFE, Vicryl.

- Concrete, e.g., methyl methacrylate, a plastic monomer that is used often in orthopedics. Hardens after drying into cement-like substance. Applied wet between layers of mesh to assist in suturing, and then allowed to dry and harden.

Muscle flaps

- *Latissimus dorsi*: arterial pedicles are the thoracodorsal and lumbar/intercostal arteries. Can cover large areas of the anterior or posterior chest wall. May not be usable if divided during a posterolateral thoracotomy.
- *Pectoralis major*: arterial pedicles are the thoracoacromial artery internal mammary artery perforators and the perforators from the lateral thoracic artery. Excellent for lateral and anterior chest wall defects. Often used as a myocutaneous flap.
- *Rectus abdominus*: pedicles include the superior epigastric artery superiorly and the inferior epigastric artery inferiorly. Useful for sternal defects. Also can be used as a myocutaneous flap.
- *Serratus anterior*: pedicle is derived from the subscapular artery at the origin of the thoracodorsal artery. Primarily used or intrathoracic applications as it has a limited arc of rotation. Often spared during previous posterolateral thoracotomy.

Omentum

- Durable 'wonder' flap that can be used to cover many defects: with skilled mobilization, it can reach the top of the skull.
- The pedicle is either the right (for right-sided defects) or left (for left-sided defects) gastroepiploic artery. Prior to dividing either artery a vascular clamp should be placed on the proposed pedicle to insure that it is adequate to supply all arcades of the omentum.

Chest wall deformities

Pectus exavatum ('funnel chest')

Pathology

- Anterior thoracic wall deformity with depression of the sternum and lower costal cartilages. Frequently asymmetrical with the right side more depressed than the left. The manubrium and first two costal cartilages are usually normal.
- 1 in 300–400 live births, 5:1 male to female ratio. 90% noted with the first year of life. Family history in 37% of patients.
- Posterior traction of sternum due to diaphragm abnormalities or excessive pressure in utero. Abnormal production of connective tissue.

Presentation

- Often asymptomatic, presenting for cosmetic reasons. Dyspnea and easy fatigability. Transient atrial arrhythmias manifesting as palpitations.
- Cardiovascular changes: up to 28% drop in CO and 31% drop in SV.
- Pulmonary function changes: decreases in VC, TLC, and MVV.

Indications for surgery

- Cosmetic reasons causing emotional distress, symptoms, high degree of deformity (severity index >3.2). Severe sternal depression.
- Repair after age 8.
- *Modified Ravitch procedure* (see Fig. 16.2): submammary incision. Subperiosteal excision of the affected costal cartilages with elevation of the sternum via a sternal wedge osteotomy. Insertion of a pectus bar to maintain position of the elevated sternum.
- *Nuss procedure* (see Fig. 16.2): a Nuss bar is placed thoracoscopically with no costal cartilage excision. The bar is rotated, causing elevation of the sternum.
- Complications include wound infection, pain, pneumothorax, migration of the Nuss bar, recurrence and avulsion of pectus muscles.

Pectus carinatum ('pigeon breast')

Pathology

- Anterior chest wall deformity with protrusion of the mid to lower sternum, with lateral depression of the ribs.
- 4:1 male to female ratio. 22% of patients have concurrent scoliosis and 20% congenital heart disease. 25% family history chest wall disorders.

Presentation

Often symptomatic. Dyspnea, with diminished respiratory excursion of the chest. Easy fatiguability and atypical chest pain. Psychological distress from poor cosmetics.

Options for reconstruction

Submammary incision with subpericondral resection of deformed costal cartilages, sternal wedge osteotomy for posterior displacement of the sternum, removal of the xiphoid process.

Complications

Wound infection, recurrence, and pneumothorax.

Poland's syndrome

Pathology

- Congenital absence of the pectoralis muscles. Varying degrees of breast, hand, and anterior chest wall bony defects.
- 1 in 30 000 live births. Unknown etiology.

Surgical options

- Small deformities limited to the absence of the medial part of the pectoralis muscles may not require major reconstruction.
- Extensive deformities require major reconstruction with sternal wedge osteotomy, rib grafts taken from the contralateral side, resection of depressed costal cartilages, insertion of polypropylene mesh, latissimus dorsi flap for soft tissue coverage, and breast augmentation in females.

Other chest wall deformities

- Cleft sternum.
- Thoracic ectopia cordis.
- Rib dysplasia.
- Asphyxiating thoracic dystrophy (Jeune syndrome).
- Spondylothoracic dysplasia (Jarcho–Levin syndrome).

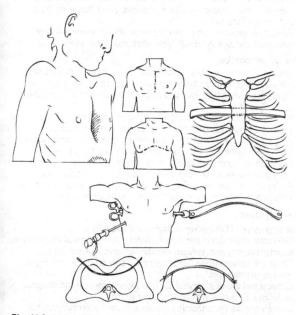

Fig. 16.2 Options for pectus excavatum. Top: modified Ravitch procedure. Bottom: Nuss procedure.

Thoracic outlet syndrome

Key facts

Compression of the brachial plexus and subclavian vessels at the apical opening of the thorax (thoracic outlet).

Pathology

Congenital narrowing of the thoracic outlet may be caused by:
- Congenital lesions: cervical rib, first thoracic rib, abnormal anterior scalene muscle, biphid clavicle, enlarged transverse process of the C7 vertebrae, anomalous course of the transverse cervical artery, adventitious fibrous bands.
- Trauma causing narrowing of the thoracic outlet, e.g., clavicular fracture, head of humerus dislocation, crush injury, cervical spondylosis, cervical scar tissue, severe atherosclerosis.

Presentation

- **Neurologic symptoms** are the most common: pain paresthesias of the ulnar brachial plexus C8 and T1 distribution, motor weakness of the hands, atypical anterior chest wall pain, headaches.
- **Arterial compression** symptoms are the next common: poikilothermia, Raynaud's phenomenon in 7.5% of patients, effort fatigue of the arm and hand, diffuse pain.
- **Venous compression** symptoms are rarer: effort thrombosis of the subclavian and axillary vein (Paget–Schroetter syndrome).

Physical examination

There are a number of physical tests that make diagnosis of TOS likely:
- *Adson (Scalene) test*: occludes the radial pulse and/or symptoms are reproduced when the head is turned to the ipsilateral side and the patient breathes in.
- *Halsted test*: occludes the radial pulse and/or symptoms are reproduced when the shoulders are displaced caudally (military position).
- *Wright test*: occludes radial pulse and/or symptoms are reproduced when the ipsilateral arm is abducted cranially and the elbow is extended, and arm is elevated for 1min. Symptoms may occur sooner if digital pressure is placed in the ipsilateral supraclavicular fossa.
- *Roo's test*: occludes the radial pulse and/or symptoms are reproduced with 3min of rapid opening and closing of the ipsilateral hand.

Investigations

The diagnosis of TOS is often a diagnosis of exclusion:
- Differential diagnosis includes carpal tunnel syndrome, cervical disc prolapse, superior sulcus tumors, collagen vascular disorders, Raynaud disease.
- Chest and cervical plane films may reveal cervical rib or prolonged transverse processes.
- Cervical and thoracic cervical CT may identify cervical and thoracic pathology. Commonly, imaging is unremarkable.
- Sensory and nerve conduction studies are often unremarkable, but may be helpful in ruling out other causes.

Management
- Physical therapy is the first-line treatment.
- Surgery is reserved for patients who fail physical therapy and involves (1) resection of the first rib, (2) vascular and brachial plexus decompression, (3) division of costoclavicular ligament, (4) resection of the anterior and middle scalene muscles, and (5) sympathectomy C8 through T3.

Transaxillary approach
- This is preferred for symptoms of nerve compression: as it allows the first rib and soft tissues to be completely resected.
- The patient is placed in the lateral decubitus position.
- Transaxillary incision just below the hairline between the pectoralis major and latissimus dorsi.
- The assistant should elevate the upper arm towards the ceiling to open up the axilla.
- The insertion of the anterior scalene muscle is divided where it is attached to the first rib.
- A middle wedge of the first rib is resected with bone cutters.
- Anterior rib is resected to the costocartilage of the sternum and the posterior rib is resected to the transverse process.
- A T1–T3 sympathectomy is optional.

Supraclavicular approach
- This is used for reoperations (the posterior approach shown in Fig. 16.3) is an alternative for reoperations.
- A supraclavicular cervical incision is made parallel to the clavicle.
- The scalene fat pad is removed to identify the phrenic nerve running anterior to the anterior scalene muscle.
- The anterior scalene is divided revealing the subclavian artery.
- The brachial plexus is retracted to reveal the first rib.
- The first rib is removed.

Complications
- 10% recurrence rate.
- Resection of the wrong rib (second rib), pain, injury to vessels or nerves.

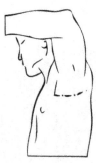

Fig. 16.3 Transaxillary approach to first rib resection.

Chest trauma

Traumatic aortic dissection is described on 📖 p452.

Principles of trauma management

Key facts

- Cardiothoracic surgeons are usually called to see trauma patients after initial evaluation and management has been carried out, but it is important to be aware of the general principles of trauma management.
- Initial approach consists of a focused *primary survey* aimed at detecting and treating immediately life-threatening conditions, followed by a more detailed secondary survey.
- Emergency department anterior thoracotomy (📖 p818) is reserved for loss of a pulse in the emergency department or en route. Survival depends on mechanism of injury (poor with blunt trauma and gunshots, better with stabbing).
- Chest trauma can be divided into blunt and penetrating: the majority of blunt chest trauma does not require operative intervention.
- Chest trauma is the third most common cause of trauma-related mortality behind head and spinal cord respectively.

Primary survey

This is aimed at identifying immediately life threatening injuries (see Box 17.1), and it consists of:

- A: Airway maintenance and cervical spine care.
- B: Breathing and ventilation.
- C: Circulation and control of hemorrhage.
- D: Disability and neurological state.
- E: Exposure.

Airway and maintenance of cervical spine

- Establish an airway: using basic life support maneuvers, simple Venturi mask, suction, nasopharyngeal tubes, oropharyngeal airways, endotracheal intubation, or rarely emergency cricothyroidotomy (📖 p248).
- The *cervical spine is immobilized, and all patient movements performed with in-line traction,* if the nature of the injury includes a significant impact or fall, until it is possible to exclude instability with a complete AP and lateral C-spine radiograph or CT.

Breathing and ventilation

Check ventilation by looking at chest expansion, auscultating for breath sounds, and monitoring O_2 saturations and blood gases where appropriate.

Box 17.1 Immediately life-threatening injuries

- Tension pneumothorax.
- Massive hemothorax.
- Open pneumothorax.
- Cardiac tamponade.
- Flail chest.

Causes of inadequate ventilation, all of which need immediate treatment are:
- Upper airway obstruction.
- Malplacement ET tube if used.
- Pneumothorax.
- Hemothorax.
- Massive lung contusion.
- Flail segment.

Circulation and control of hemorrhage

Signs of hypovolemic shock include confusion, pallor, tachycardia, tachypnea, oliguria. If peripheral access is difficult place a large lumen catheter into the femoral vein, or perform saphenous vein cut-down. Fluid resuscitation is aimed at expanding the intravascular space and may initially be titrated against pulse, BP, and later against urine output and central venous pressure. Causes of circulatory collapse include:
- Cardiac arrest.
- Hypovolemia: obvious bleeding site, or occult, e.g., fracture of femur or pelvis, intra-abdominal bleed, hemothorax.
- Cardiac tamponade.
- Cardiac contusion.
- Aortic transection.

Disability and neurological state

Crucial in the evaluation of head and spinal injury, this is of less importance to the cardiothoracic surgeon than:

Exposure

Examine the patient front *and* back, swiftly but carefully for any evidence of penetrating or blunt trauma. Penetrating wounds below the fourth intercostal space may well have crossed the diaphragm, raising the specter of abdominal injury.

Secondary survey

This is a more detailed and complete clinical examination aimed at elucidating some form of basic history, and identifying and managing the following potentially life-threatening injuries:
- Rib fractures and flail chest.
- Pulmonary contusion.
- Simple pneumothorax.
- Blunt aortic injury.
- Blunt myocardial injury.

Investigations

First-line investigations performed once the primary survey and management is established include:
- CXR (C-spine and pelvis as indicated).
- TTE if pericardial effusion suspected.
- CT if there is any suspicion about injury to major thoracic structures, and the patient is hemodynamically stable.
- Aortography if aortic injury is suspected.

Emergency thoracotomy

Key facts

- Emergency thoracotomy is used to provide access to the chest for evaluation of the heart and descending aorta, and temporize catastrophic blood loss by cross-clamping the descending aorta, or alleviating cardiac tamponade.
- A *clamshell* provides rapid and excellent access to most areas of the chest except subclavian vessels, and does not require sternal saw: it carries significant morbidity in survivors but it is the incision of choice in the emergency room where the exact location of the problem may be unclear and rib retractors not immediately available.
- Indications include **loss of cardiac output during transport or in the emergency department.**
- Knowledge of the causative agent, all entry and exit points is crucial in planning investigation and management of thoracic trauma.

Emergency thoracotomy in the emergency room

Where at all possible, every effort should be made to get the patient to an operating room where equipment, sterility, and personnel are readily available, approach can be more precisely tailored to the injury, and the patient resuscitated in a more controlled environment. If the patient has lost cardiac output clearly this is not possible.

Indications

- Cardiac arrest or imminent cardiac arrest after penetrating trauma.
- Limited role in cardiac arrest in setting of blunt trauma.

Incision

The approach is dictated by available expertise (do what you are able to do), and equipment (there may not be a sternal saw, or rib retractors), as much as by the nature of the injury. The options are:

- *Median sternotomy*: fast if a sternal saw and power source are available, excellent exposure to heart, both pleural cavities, hilums, but dependent on availability of sternal saw and suitable power source.
- *Anterior thoracotomy*: very fast, can be performed using just a scalpel, can be extended to improve what is very limited access to the pericardium and ipsilateral pleura. Difficult to carry out internal cardiac massage through this incision. Impossible to carry out definitive procedure if rib retractor not available.
- Bilateral extended anterior thoracotomy or *clamshell*: Fast, needs heavy scissors to divide sternum in addition to scalpel, excellent access to mediastinum and both pleurae. May have significant bleeding from IMAs bilaterally. Significant morbidity from wound in survivors.
- *Subxiphoid approach*: fast, but limited access to pericardium only.

Findings

Cardiac tamponade is the commonest finding, secondary to:

- RV lacerations more commonly than LV lacerations.
- Occasionally injury to coronary vessels, or great vessels.
- VSD is the commonest intracardiac injury.

- Occasionally there is no cardiac injury—the heart is empty from massive hemorrhage elsewhere: in this case internal cardiac massage is more effective than external chest compressions at getting resuscitation drugs to circulate while volume is replaced.

Emergency room clamshell

- Do not stop to place lines, or anesthetize or intubate the patient. Most of this can be done concurrently while you are opening chest, and once the patient has lost cardiac output time is critical.
- At a minimum you need gloves, a scalpel, a scissors and suction. Four clamps, a rib retractor, forceps and sutures are helpful.
- Stay calm, and communicate clearly with the person responsible for managing the airway, and the lead nurse who should be able to bring an emergency thoracotomy set and set up sterile suction with a Yankauer tip: there is usually an excited crowd of people trying to help perform a procedure most of them have never seen.
- Pour betadine on the patient's chest, put on sterile gloves (and gown if available), place drape over abdomen if available.
- Take scalpel and make incision following right to left inframammary crease across the midline, take it down to ribs and with care to intercostal muscles, protecting lung with forceps handle.
- Spend a minute to identify and clamp the proximal and distal ends of both internal mammary arteries: these retract and then bleed a lot once the patient gets a cardiac output.
- Divide the sternum with a heavy scissors or bone cutter.
- Place a retractor in if available, open the pericardium widely and carefully with a scissors.

Procedure

- Ventricular lacerations are repaired with pledgets of Teflon on 3/0 Prolene sutures, taking full thickness bites with great care to avoid iatrogenic trauma to the coronary arteries, particularly over the LV.
- Atrial and vessel lacerations are simply oversewn.
- Bleeding from the lung hilum is often best packed, especially if this is due to a deceleration injury.

Emergency thoracotomy in the operating room

- This is the optimal place to perform emergency surgery: if clinical condition permits the patient should be transferred immediately it becomes clear that thoracotomy is indicated.
- Do not delay transfer to insert additional monitoring lines.
- If you are dealing with an emergency from the invasive cardiology lab (e.g., tamponade after PCI, or catheter ablation) plan for a **sternotomy** and do not be persuaded to try a minimally invasive approach: these patients are sick, need rapid access, and may require a definitive procedure difficult via thoracotomy (repair of SVC, CABG, VAD, ECMO).
- Communicate clearly with the anesthesiologist so that they know your planned incision, timing, and findings.
- Generally, operating in a cardiac catheterization lab is even worse than trying to operate in the emergency room.

Blunt trauma

Key facts

- Emergency thoracotomy rarely indicated for management of blunt trauma: injuries may be diffuse and invariably unsuited to definitive repair or even temporizing in the emergency room.
- Diffuse bleeding is often best managed by aggressive transfusion and correction of all coagulopathy, including use of factor VII ([📖 p146).
- Diaphragmatic injuries are described on [📖 p746 and p823.

Pulmonary contusions

- Generally caused by blunt trauma: characterized by alveolar and capillary hemorrhage of lung tissue resulting in parenchymal bruising, increased capillary permeability.
- May initially be asymptomatic, but often associated with hypoxia and significant ventilation/perfusion mismatch. ARDS ([📖 p167).
- CXR demonstrates infiltrates, chest CT demonstrates areas of consolidation consistent with contusion.
- Therapy is primarily supportive. O_2, analgesia, physiotherapy. ET intubation and ventilation may become necessary. It is important to limit fluids, as the increased capillary permeability can lead to worsening and propagation of the contusion.

Tracheobronchial injury

- Tracheobronchial injuries can occur after both blunt and penetrating trauma. Blunt trauma or 'dashboard injury' is due to unrestrained motor vehicle passengers and sudden hyperextension of neck.
- The most common site of penetrating tracheal injuries is the cervical trachea, while the most common site of blunt tracheobronchial injuries is the right main stem bronchus, within 2.5cm of the carina, possibly due to an anatomic fixation point.
- Uncommon, approximately 0.5% of trauma cases, but may be life threatening and frequently associated with other major injuries.

Presentation

- Bronchial injuries may be asymptomatic, and have a delayed presentation months later with pneumothorax or bronchial stenosis.
- Dyspnea, respiratory distress, hoarseness, dysphonia. Surgical subcutaneous emphysema common. Pneumothorax in approximately half of cases and hemoptysis in a quarter.

Investigation

CXR often diagnostic. It may show disruption of the trachea or bronchial air column. Kumpe sign. CT useful in assessing the rest of the thorax. Flexible bronchoscopy diagnostic.

Management

- First step is airway control. Double lumen ET tubes should be avoided because their bulk and rigidity may exacerbate an injury. A single lumen tube should be placed beyond a tracheal injury, and lung isolation achieved by an Arndt bronchial blocker ([📖 p647).

- For tracheal injuries where intubation is impossible secondary to the injury, a tracheostomy or cricothyroidotomy should be performed. Rarely, the patient can be intubated through the cervical injury.
- Small injuries may be managed conservatively, especially if the airway is intubated past the lesion.
- Proximal 2/3 of the trachea is accessed via a cervical collar incision.
- The distal half of the trachea, carina, proximal left main stem bronchus and entire right main stem bronchus can be accessed via a right posterolateral thoracotomy, the distal left main stem bronchus is accessed via a left posterolateral thoracotomy.
- Small lacerations can be repaired primarily with absorbable suture such as 4/0 Vicryl or 4/0 PDS.
- Larger bronchial injuries should be debrided and primary bronchial anastomosis similar to bronchoplastic sleeve anastomoses (📖 p688).
- Carinal injuries should be repaired, rather than resected.
- To relieve tension of the repair, different release techniques (📖 p755) can be used: (1) division of the pulmonary ligament, (2) suprahyoid laryngeal release may provide 1–2 cm of mobilization, (3) hilar release by dividing the pericardium around the inferior hilum.
- Associated organ injuries, e.g., esophageal wounds should be repaired.
- Viable tissue should be used to reinforce the repair and prevent fistulization, such as intercostal muscle, pleura patch, pericardial fat pad.
- A guardian chin stitch is used for tracheal and carinal repairs to prevent inadvertent tension (📖 p754).

Complications
- Anastomotic dehiscence (5%), or stricture.
- Fistulization (esophageal, arterial).
- Vocal cord paralysis.
- Over 75% of patients with tracheobronchial injuries secondary to blunt trauma die before arrival at the emergency department.

Chest wall, diaphragm, and pleura

Rib fracture:

Common. 4th–9th ribs most commonly fractured. Associated with underlying lung pleural, bronchial, and cardiac injuries. Lower rib fractures associated with renal, hepatic and splenic injuries. Fracture of the 1st rib (or sternum or scapula) indicates major trauma.

Management: adequate analgesia. May require regional nerve blocks. Epidural very effective anesthesia with minimal complications.

Flail segment:

- Flail chest is the fracture of three or more ribs in a row, with two or more fractures in each rib. The resulting chest wall 'island' exhibits paradoxical motion with respiration.
- Problems with flail chest often arise from potential for underlying pulmonary contusion: symptoms include dyspnea, hemoptysis, pain, respiratory splinting, respiratory distress.
- Usually obvious on clinical exam: can confirm with CXR and chest CT.
- Therapy is supportive. Mechanical ventilation if the patient is in distress, pain control with narcotics, PCA, rib blocks, or epidural analgesia.
- Care must be taken to limit fluids, as underlying pulmonary contusion is at risk for capillary leak.
- No clear data on the efficacy of early fixation. However, external plate fixation can be used to help wean off of mechanical ventilation.
- The flail segment will often fibrose with time, eliminating paradoxical movement with respiration.

Sternal fractures

- Sternal fractures are a marker of significant blunt trauma: associated with cardiac or great vessel injuries 18–62% of the time.
- Most common area of injury is the angle of Louis or the manubrial body junction.
- Symptoms include pain, dyspnea. Late presentations include chronic non-union with a sternal click, and late mediastinal abscess formation.
- Clinical diagnosis on examination, may be confirmed by CT chest—main value is CT angiography to look for vascular injuries.
- Most fractures require only supportive therapy, with pain control and aggressive pulmonary toilet.
- Unstable fractures may require debridement; with stabilization with external plates, or sternal wires. Abscesses require aggressive debridement, followed by closure with muscle or omental pedicled flap.

Clavicular fracture

- The majority, 80%, occur in the middle area of the clavicle, 15% laterally, and <5% medially. Lateral injuries occur from impact to the shoulder, and middle and medial injuries from blunt trauma to the chest.
- They present with well-localized pain, and CXR is diagnostic.
- Most fractures can be treated conservatively, with a sling and analgesia.
- Complex and/or open fractures may require debridement and fixation.

Diaphragmatic injury

- Blunt trauma, with acute intra-abdominal pressure can lead to laceration and disruption of the diaphragm.
- More common on the left side, as the liver serves as a barrier.
- Often asymptomatic. Symptoms include dyspnea, abdominal pain, atypical chest pain, dysphagia, bowel obstruction. May present late.
- Diagnosis can be difficult: CXR may demonstrate gastric bubble above the diaphragm. Chest CT with IV and oral contrast helpful.
- Diagnostic laparoscopy.
- Treatment is primary repair of the diaphragm. This can be done laparoscopically or thorascopically, or via a laparotomy or thoracotomy (📖 p747).

Pulmonary lacerations

Most common following penetrating chest trauma. Associated with hemothorax, pneumothorax, or hemopneumothorax. Extensive pulmonary lacerations seen following high-speed motor vehicle accidents. Often centrally located disrupting large vessels and major bronchi.

Management: peripheral lacerations may be oversewn or excised. They may heal following chest tube insertion. More extensive and central lacerations require surgical repair more urgently. Control of the hilum is required prior to any repair. Bronchial and vascular injuries are repaired. Laceration is usually left open with chest tube drainage.

Traumatic pneumothorax

Cause: direct lung injury from rib fracture or rapid deceleration. May be secondary to a rapid rise in intrathoracic pressure against a closed glottis causing rupture of the distal alveoli.

Presentation: dyspnea and chest pain. Examination reveals hyper-resonance to percussion and diminished or absent breath sounds on auscultation. A *tension pneumothorax* is life threatening and in addition may present with subcutaneous emphysema, mediastinal shift, acute respiratory distress, hemodynamic instability. Immediate chest decompression is performed by placing a wide-bore needle into the pleural cavity in the 2nd intercostal space in the midclavicular line.

Definitive management: chest tube insertion in the 4th or 5th intercostal space in the midaxillary line directing the chest tube anteriorly and superiorly. Thoracotomy rarely indicated.

Hemothorax

Causes: chest wall injury, lung parenchymal laceration, bronchial artery injury, intercostal vessel injury, major thoracic vascular injury. Chest radiograph diagnostic.

Treatment: tube thoracostomy (📖 p248) inserting a wide-bore, at least a 36F, tube in the 5th or 6th intercostal space in the midaxillary line directing the tube posteriorly. Bleeding ceases in 80–90% of cases.

Indications for surgery: immediate blood loss of >1L or bleeding continues in excess of 100mL/h for 4h or more. Blunt trauma to esophagus and thoracic duct rare.

Final thoughts

- Loupes: expensive but vital. Your program may buy them for you. Start with 2.5× extended field and practice suturing with them on at home. If you can buy a lightweight headlight that clips on to them as well, do it. If you wear contacts, keep a spare pair in your loupes case.
- Kit: Littman classic or cardiology stethoscope (engrave your name on it – they all look identical), this book, pen, cash, pager/phone.
- Food: ICU nurse station usually has the best list of numbers for food.
- Top five tips:
  - Treat every patient like you'd want to be treated.
  - Always have a plan B.
  - Treasure good mentors, hard work, luck, and common sense.
  - Things usually seem better after a good night's sleep.
  - But sleep is no substitute for experience.
- Top five books recommended for residency: This one for carrying around, and:
  - *Manual of Perioperative Care in Cardiac Surgery*, 5th edn., 2011. Robert M. Bojar MD. Blackwell Publishing. The gold standard for cardiac ICU care.
  - *Sabiston and Spencer. Surgery of the Chest*, 8th edn., 2009. Frank Selke, Pedro del Nido, and Scott Swanson. Two-volume good general cardiac, thoracic, and congenital surgery early reference book.
  - *Kaiser's Mastery of Cardiothoracic Surgery*, 2nd edn., 2006. Larry Kaiser, Irving Kron, and Thomas Spray. Lippincott Williams & Wilkins. Cardiac Surgery. Strong on operative technique with great editorial comments.
  - *Cardiac Surgery: Safeguards and Pitfalls in Operative Technique*, 4th edn., 2007. Siavosh Kohnsari and Colleen Flint Sintek. Lippincott Willliams & Wilkins. Best general cardiac surgical atlas there is, sadly does not cover general thoracic surgery.
- Top five online resources:
  - http://www.tsda.org. The best collection of education material online
  - http://www.ctsnet.org. Free access to text books, videos, editorials, jobs
  - http://www.myamericanheart.org. Full text of ACC/AHA guidelines
  - http://www.ncbi.nlm.gov. Pubmed search engine
  - http://www.hsforum.com. Lively online discussion group of CT surgeons.
- Top five courses for exams
  - The Utah Core Curriculum Review Course, http://www.corereview.org
  - The Birmingham Review Course, http://www.birminghamreviewcourse.co.uk
  - Applied Basic Science for Cardiothoracic Surgical Trainees, http://www.rcseng.ac.uk
  - European school for cardiothoracic surgery, http://http://school.eacts.org
  - SESATS self assessment, http://www.sesats.org

Index

Concentrations, rates and starting doses for drug infusions

Drug	mg in 250mls	Dilution (mcg/ml)	Range (mcg/kg/min)	Patient wt (kg)		
				50	70	100
Epinephrine	4	16	0.03–0.2	9.5	13	19
Dopamine	250	1000	3.0–10.0	9.0	12.6	18
Dobutamine	250	1000	3.0–10.0	9.0	12.6	18
Dopexamine	250	1000	3.0–10.0	9.0	12.6	18
Norepinephrine	4	16	0.03–1.0	9.5	13	19
Milrinone	40	160	0.3–0.75	9.0	13	18
NTG	200	800	5–50mcg/min	4.0	5.0	8.0
SNP	50	200	0.1–3.0	8	11	16
Labetalol	250	1000	1–4mg/min	2.0	2.0	2.0
Vasopressin	2.5 units	0.01unit/ml	2.4–8 units/hr	1.0	1.0	1.0

The numbers in the table under patient weight heading show the drug infusion rate in ml/hr required to achieve the stated starting dose.

Pediatric advanced life support
Drugs

Adenosine	0.1–0.2mg/kg
Atropine sulphate	0.02mg/kg
Calcium chloride 10%	20mg/kg (0.2ml/kg)
Dobutamine	2–20µg/kg/min
Dopamine	2–20µg/kg/min
Epinephrine for asystole 1st dose	iv/io 0.01mg/kg (0.1ml/kg of 1:10,000)
Epinephrine subsequent doses	iv/io 0.1mg/kg (1ml/kg of 1:10,000)
Epinephrine infusion	0.1–1.0µg/kg/min
Lidocaine	1mg/kg
Lidocaine infusion	20–50µg/kg/min
Naloxone if <5 years/20kg	0.1mg/kg
Naloxone if >5 years/20kg	2.0mg
Prostaglandin E1	0.05–0.1µg/kg/min
Sodium bicarbonate	1mEq/kg/dose

Defibrillation and synchronized cardioversion

First shock for VF/pulseless VT	2J/kg
Subsequent shocks	4J/kg
Synchronized cardioversion	0.5–1.0J/kg

Conversions

1kPa = 7.3mmHg = 10cmH$_2$O

Reference ranges

Arterial blood gases

PaO$_2$	>10.5kPa	75mmHg
Pa CO$_2$	4.7–6.0kPa	35–54mmHg
Ph	7.35–7.45	
H$^+$	35–45mmol/l	
Base Excess	−2–+2mmol/l	
HCO$_3^-$	4.7–5.7kPa	24–30mmol/l
SaO$_2$	>95%	

Cardiac function

CO = cardiac output	4.5 0l/min
SV = stroke volume	60–100mls
BSA = body surface area	2–2.2m^2
CI = cardiac index	2.0–4.0l/min/m^2
SVI = stroke volume index	33–47ml/beat/m^2
MAP = mean arterial pressure	70–100mmHg
DP = diastolic pressure	60–80mmHg
SP = systolic pressure	110–150mmHg
SVR = systemic vascular resistance	800–1200dyne-sec/cm^5
CVP = central venous pressure	6–12mmHg
SVRI = systemic vascular resistance index	400–600dyne-sec/cm^5/m^2
PVR = pulmonary vascular resistance	50–250dyne-sec/cm^5
PAP = pulmonary artery pressure	20–30mmHg
PAWP = plmonay artery wedge pressure	8–14mmHg
PVRI = pulmonary vascular resistance index	20–125dyne-sec/cm^5/m^2

Echocardiography

Left ventricle end systolic dimension	25–41mm
Left ventricle end diastolic dimension	35–56mm
Left ventricle shortening fraction	30–40%
Left ventricle ejection fraction	50–85%
Left ventricle mass	60–124g/m^2
Septum systolic thickness	9–18mm
Septum diastolic thickness	7–21mm
Aortic root diameter	20–37mm
Left atrial diameter	19–40mm
Aortic peak velocity	0.9–1.8m/s
Mitral peak velocity	0.6–1.4m/s
Aortic valve area	2–3.0cm^2
Mitral valve area	>2.2cm^2

Pulmonary function tests (marked variation with age, height, and sex)

FVC = Forced vital capacity	3.5–5L
FEV$_1$ = Forced expiratory volume in 1 second	>2.0L
FEV$_1$ / FVC	70–80%
PEFR = Peak expiratory flow rate	450–600l/min
D$_L$CO = Diffusing lung capacity for carbon monoxide	>30%